Imaging of Central Nervous System Tumors

First Edition

Editor

Soonmee Cha, MD

Diagnostic Radiology Residency Program Director, University of California, San Francisco, California, CA
Vice Chair of Education, University of California, San Francisco, California, CA
Professor in Residence of Radiology and Neurological Surgery, University of California, San Francisco, CA

Wolters Kluwer

Philadelphia • Baltimore • New York • London
Buenos Aires • Hong Kong • Sydney • Tokyo

Acquisitions Editor: Nicole Dernoski
Development Editor: Eric McDermott
Editorial Coordinator: Remington Fernando
Marketing Manager: Kirsten Watrud
Production Project Manager: Bridgett Dougherty
Design Coordinator: Stephen Druding
Manufacturing Coordinator: Beth Welsh
Prepress Vendor: Lumina Datamatics

9 8 7 6 5 4 3 2 1

Printed in Mexico

Library of Congress Cataloging-in-Publication Data

ISBN-13: 978-1-9751-0374-3

Cataloging in Publication data available on request from publisher.

shop.lww.com

Imaging of Central Nervous System Tumors

First Edition

This book is dedicated to Heeshik, Chonghon, Oakae, Peter, Spencer, Shinae, and Sarang. Without their love and support, I will not be living today.

To all my radiology residents, past and present, to whom I owe the path to finding my calling.

Preface

I remember the day when I first saw a magnetic resonance imaging (MRI) of a patient with glioblastoma multiforme more than two decades ago. I vividly recall the stunning rim of irregular and ominous pattern of enhancement, a large dark area of central necrosis, angry looking edema and mass effect, and unmistakable destruction of the neighboring brain. From that day forward, I never lost my focus, fear, and fascination with tumors of the central nervous system (CNS), especially their variable appearance on imaging and wondering how a histologic type of tumor can look so very different on imaging.

The concept of this book was inspired by the World Health Organization Classification (WHO) of Tumors of the CNS published in 2016 where over 120 different subtypes of CNS tumors were classified, some using the novel combined histological and molecular classification, and histological grading across and within tumor entities were clarified and newly defined. Departing away from the century-long practice of tumor classification based on histogenesis and histology, the 2016 WHO Classification of CNS Tumors ushered in the new molecular genetic era of tumor classification and established the integrated pathologic diagnosis that are more objective and more precisely define each tumor entity.

This book is written for students, trainees, practicing healthcare professionals, and scientists who wish to learn more about imaging appearance of tumors of the CNS. The text is presented in a concise summary format starting with the definition of tumor and with emphasis on illustrating various imaging features of each individual CNS tumor. As much as possible, most of the CNS tumor entities in the 2016 WHO Classification of CNS Tumors are included and variable imaging appearances of the same histopathologic tumor are illustrated. The readers of this book will find it easy to navigate the text and images and become familiar with classic and unusual imaging characteristics of CNS tumors. I hope the readers will share some of my deep passion for decades-long commitment to more precisely describe the imaging characterization of CNS tumors and in so doing to positively impact the lives of those harboring the tumor.

Soonmee Cha, MD

Contents

Introduction

Advances in molecular pathology have enhanced our understanding of the molecular underpinnings of primary central nervous system (CNS) tumors and started to reshape the practice of diagnosis, classification, and therapy in neuropathology, neuro-oncology, and neuroradiology. Neuropathologic diagnostic emphasis has shifted from purely based on microscopic histology to one that combines morphologic and molecular genetic features of tumor including gene mutations, chromosomal copy number alterations, and gene rearrangements to yield integrated diagnosis. Rapid developments in next-generation sequencing techniques, multimodal molecular analysis, large-scale genomic and epigenomic analyses, and DNA methylation methods promise to fundamentally transform the pathologic CNS tumor diagnostics to a whole another level of precision and complexity. Keeping pace with the advances and discoveries in molecular signatures of CNS tumors, various targeted therapies in neuro-oncologic field to slow or block the growth of tumors by specifically targeting these molecular pathways are rapidly entering and redefining the designs of clinical trials.

The fast-evolving molecular landscapes of CNS tumors forged a new paradigm of neuroradiology where radiogenomics and surrogate imaging markers of molecular pathology are emerging to noninvasively and serially capture the biologic and clinical behaviors and assess treatment response of CNS tumors. The ground-breaking 2016 World Health Organization (WHO) Classification of Tumors of the CNS ushered in the new era of integrating morphology and molecular genetics for diagnosis and classification.

This book provides a concise summary of existing, modified, or newly recognized type, subtype, diagnostic criteria, or family of CNS tumors based on the WHO Classification with emphasis on the neuroimaging characterization.

1

Imaging Modalities for Central Nervous System Tumors

Overview

In the current state of the rapidly developing molecular genetic era of brain tumor diagnosis and classification, the imaging and clinical management of patients with brain tumor are advancing and evolving concurrently, relying heavily on physiologic imaging in addition to high-resolution structural imaging. Imaging remains a powerful noninvasive tool, especially magnetic resonance (MR) imaging, to positively impact the management of patients with brain tumor. While MR imaging remains the most essential imaging method for evaluation of brain tumors, computed tomography (CT) plays an essential role in the emergency setting to detect potential life-threatening complications of brain tumors such as hemorrhage, hydrocephalus, or herniation. In addition to structural imaging, physiology-based MR imaging, such as diffusion-weighted imaging (DWI), perfusion-weighted imaging (PWI), proton spectroscopy, functional imaging, as well as hybrid imaging, such as Positron Emission Tomography-Computed Tomography and Positron Emission Tomography-Magnetic Resonance, provide insights into biologic and physiologic alteration in brain tumors.

Imaging Modality	Indication	Strengths	Limitations
Computed Tomography	Acute hemorrhage, hydrocephalus, herniation, mass effect	Detection of acute blood, calcium, air, and metal	Ionizing radiation Suboptimal parenchymal evaluation Limited image contrast options
Catheter Angiogram	Tumor vascularity Preoperative embolization	Assessment of true vascularity	Direct arterial puncture Ionizing radiation Procedure-related complication
MRI-structural	Tumor location, size, number, associated changes	High-resolution 3D-multiplanar reformation	Structural information only
MRI-physiologic	Tumor cellularity, white matter integrity, vascularity, metabolism	Noninvasive physiologic information	Surrogate, not true biologic, markers of physiology
Hybrid Imaging (PET–CT, PET–MR)	Tumor metabolism	Specific to targeted metabolite	Ionizing radiation, low spatial resolution, uptake by normal tissue

Computed Tomography

Computed tomography (CT) combines diagnostic X-ray imaging and sophisticated computers to produce multiple images of body, including the brain, in a few minutes using relatively small amounts of ionizing radiation. In patients with brain tumor, head CT is often done as the first imaging study during acute presentation with intracranial symptoms. Unenhanced head CT is an excellent imaging study to exclude acute intracranial hemorrhage, hydrocephalus, mass effect, or herniation of brain. Latest modern CT scanners can provide a complete volume of scan data and generate a complete three-dimensional (3D) volume of data, which in turn allows the creation of multiplanar reconstruction with thick or thin slices using different algorithms. Reconstructed images can highlight abnormalities involving the three main tissue components of the brain—parenchyma, extra-axial space, and bone—to emphasize various tissue

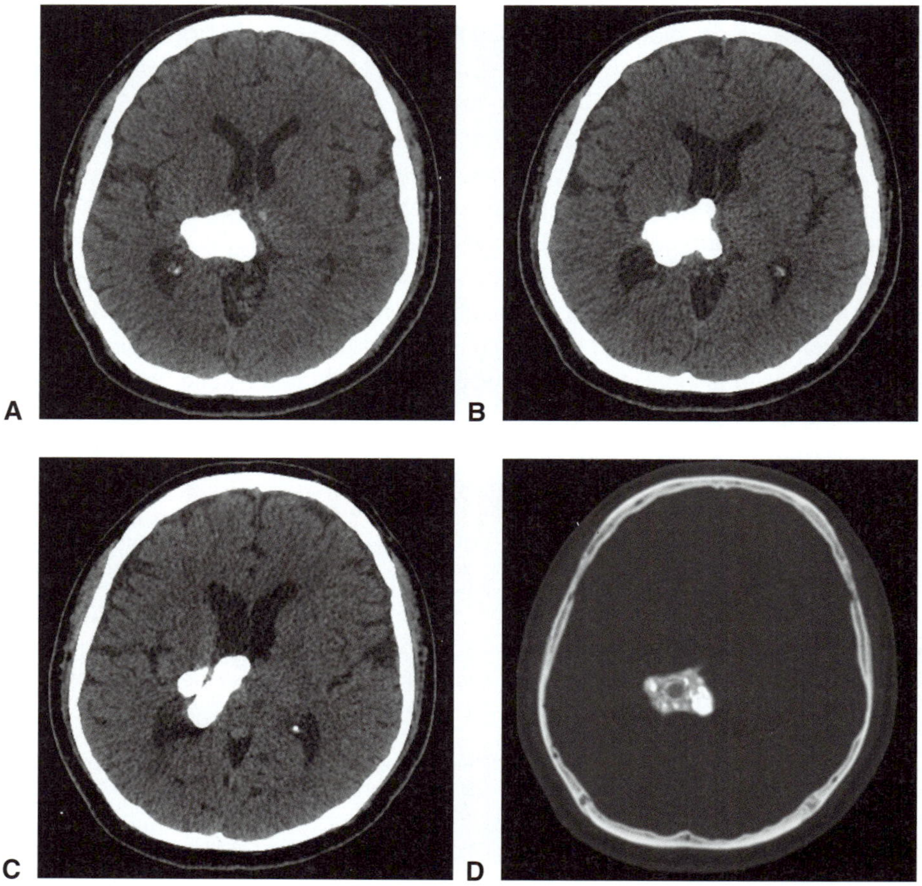

Figure 1.1. CT vs. MRI in detecting calcified central neurocytoma. A–C. Axial CT unenhanced, brain window: Heavily calcified lateral intraventricular mass. **D–F.** Axial CT unenhanced, bone window: Internal architecture of the heavily calcified component is better seen.

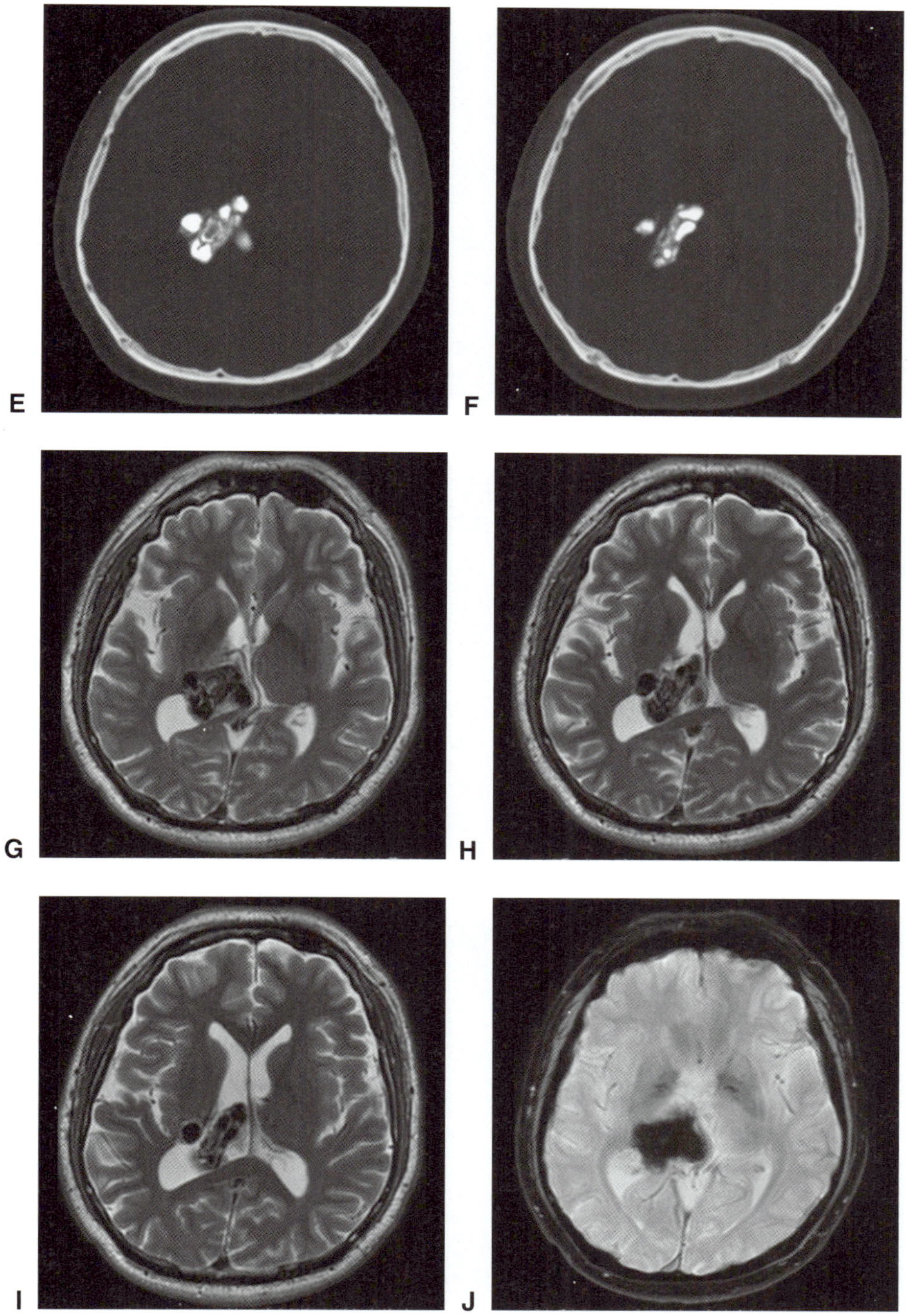

Figure 1.1. ***(continued)*** **G–I.** Axial T2: Heterogeneously hypointense mass. **J–L.** Axial SWI: Marked susceptibility due to calcium.

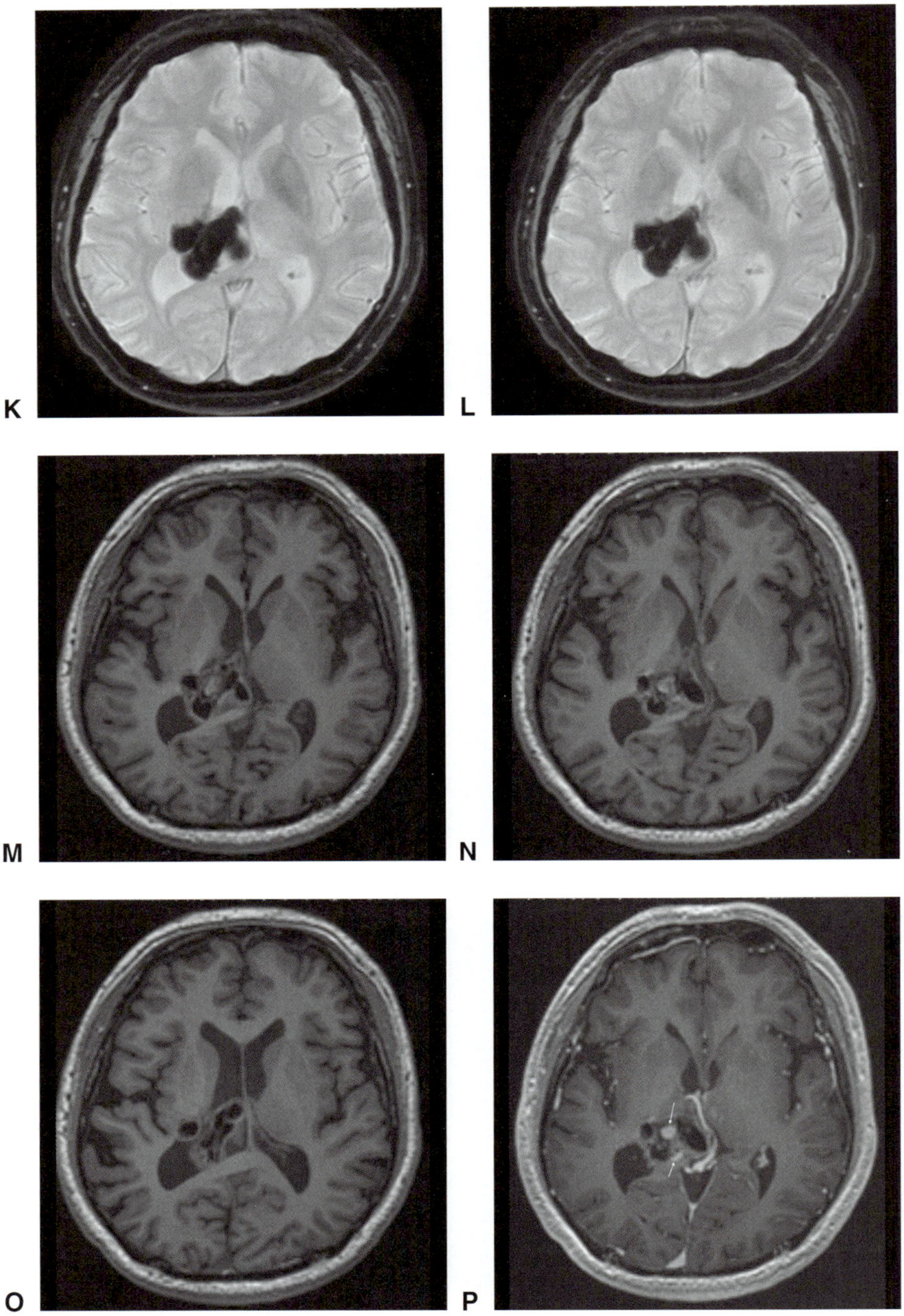

Figure 1.1. ***(continued)*** **M–O.** Axial T1-precontrast: Heterogeneously hypointense mass. **P–R.** Axial T1-postcontrast: Minimally enhancing, heterogeneously hypointense mass with small areas of enhancement (white arrows).

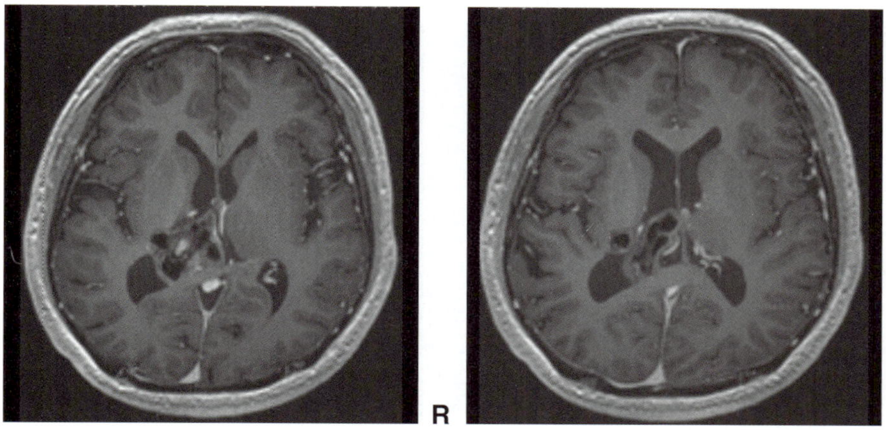

Q R

Figure 1.1. ***(continued)***

characteristics. Dynamic contrast-enhanced CT angiogram studies can provide high-resolution images of the intracranial arteries and veins that match up to the details provided by catheter angiographic studies but without the invasive catheterization of vessels.

One of the major limitations of CT is limited soft-tissue resolution of brain parenchyma. Brain tumors can be infiltrative, especially diffuse gliomas, and may not be easily detectable on CT. In fact, brain tumors that are isodense to the brain parenchyma may not be detectable at all on CT.

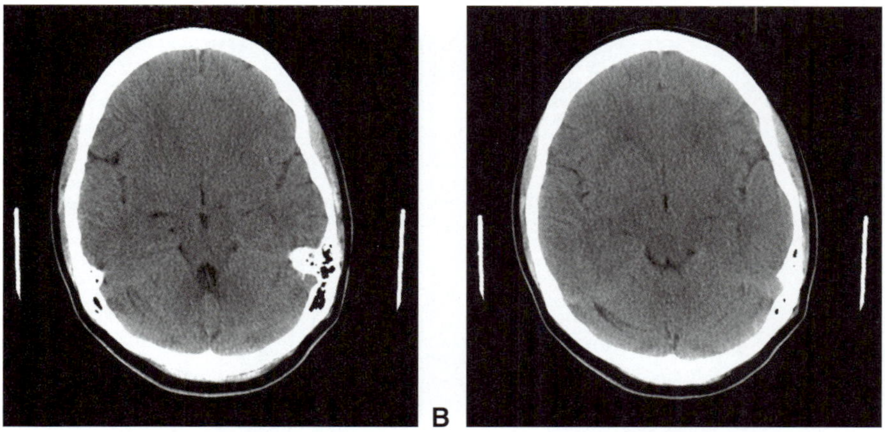

A B

Figure 1.2. Pitfall of CT in detecting isodense mass, meningioma. A–C. Axial CT, unenhanced: Midline anterior cranial fossa meningioma is hardly detectable.

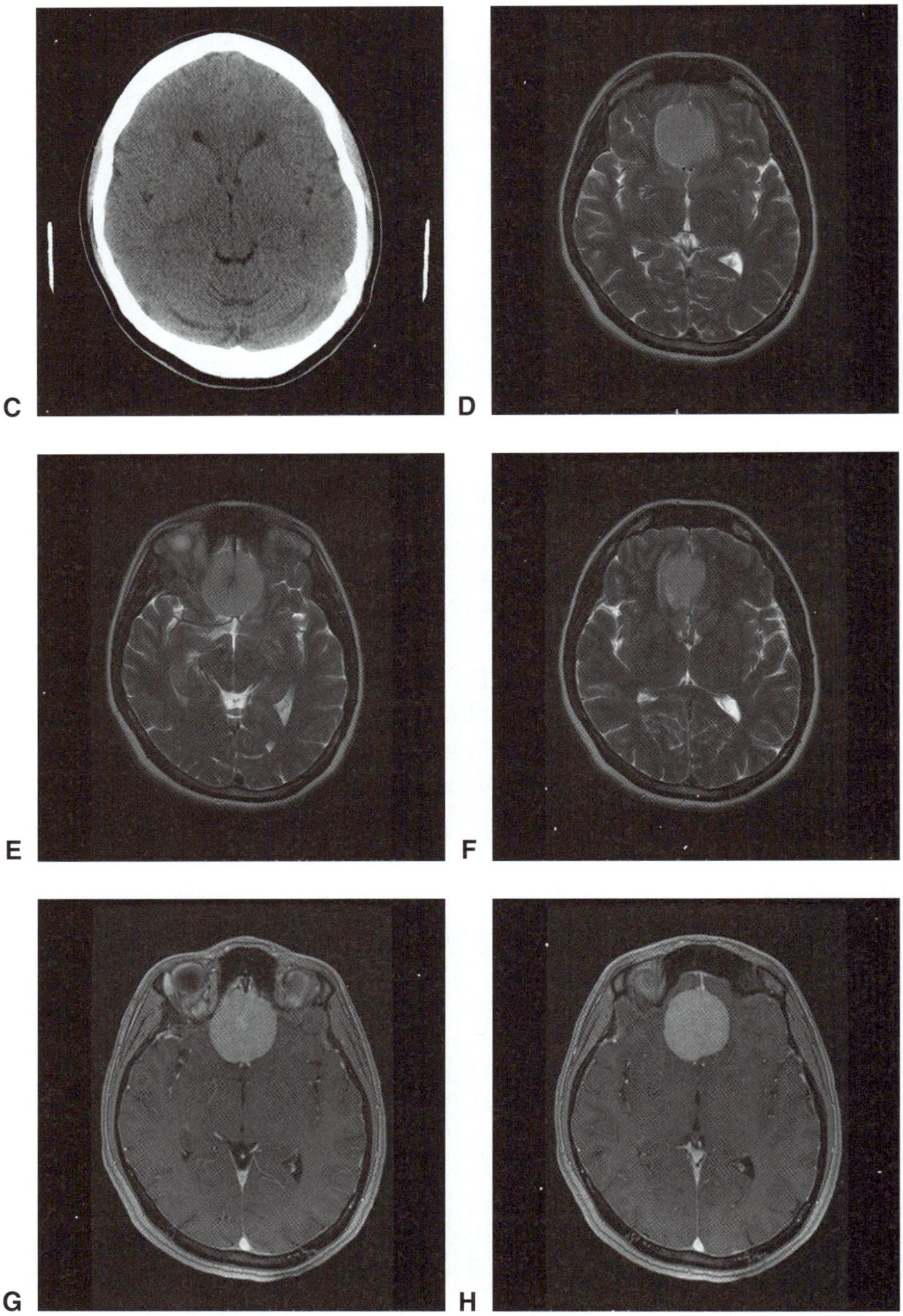

Figure 1.2. ***(continued)*** **D–E.** Axial T2: Homogeneously hypointense meningioma is clearly visible. **G–I.** Axial T1-postcontrast: Homogeneous and avid enhancement within meningioma.

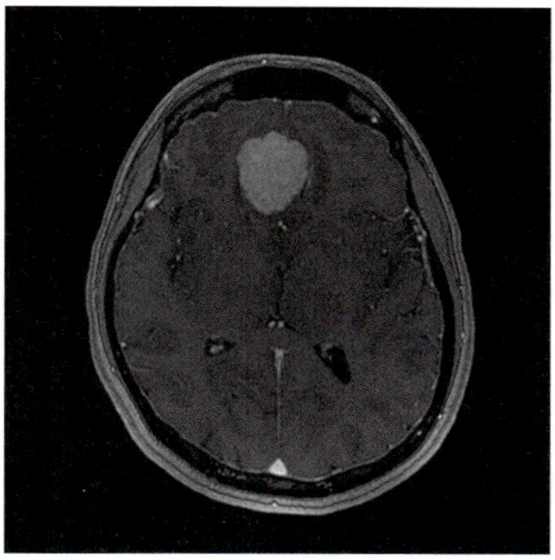

I

Figure 1.2. ***(continued)***

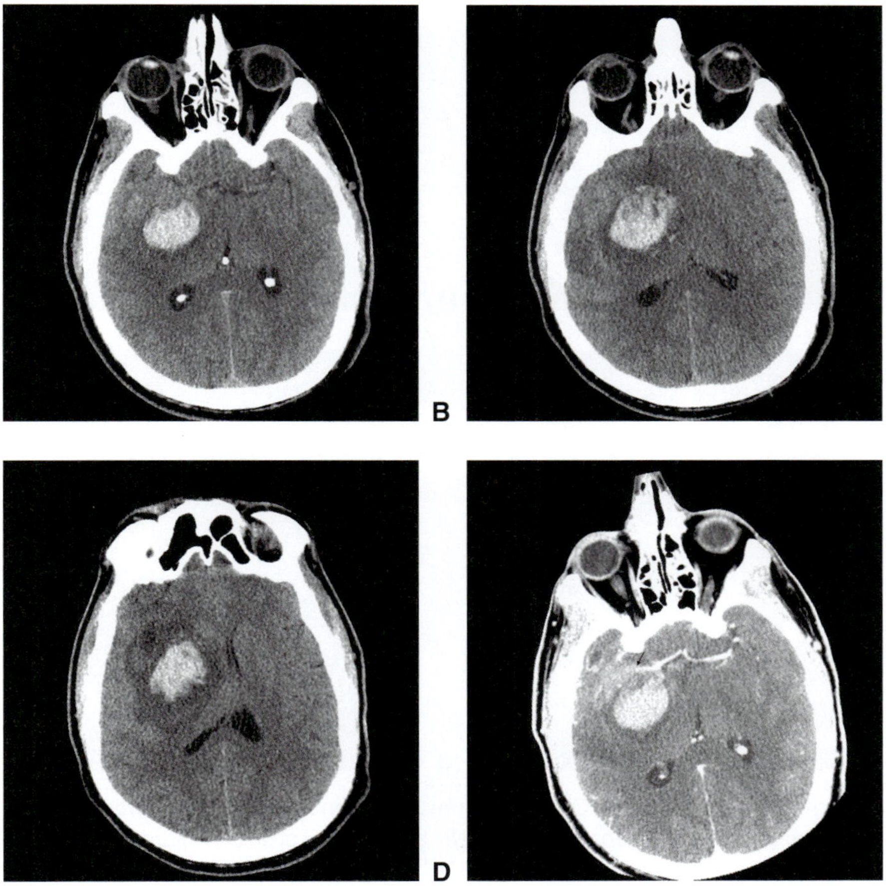

A B C D

Figure 1.3. CT and MRI of hemorrhagic glioblastoma. A–C. Axial CT, unenhanced: Hemorrhagic right basal ganglia mass. **D–F.** Axial CT, enhanced: Discontinuity of right middle cerebral artery (black arrow) along the anterior margin of the mass.

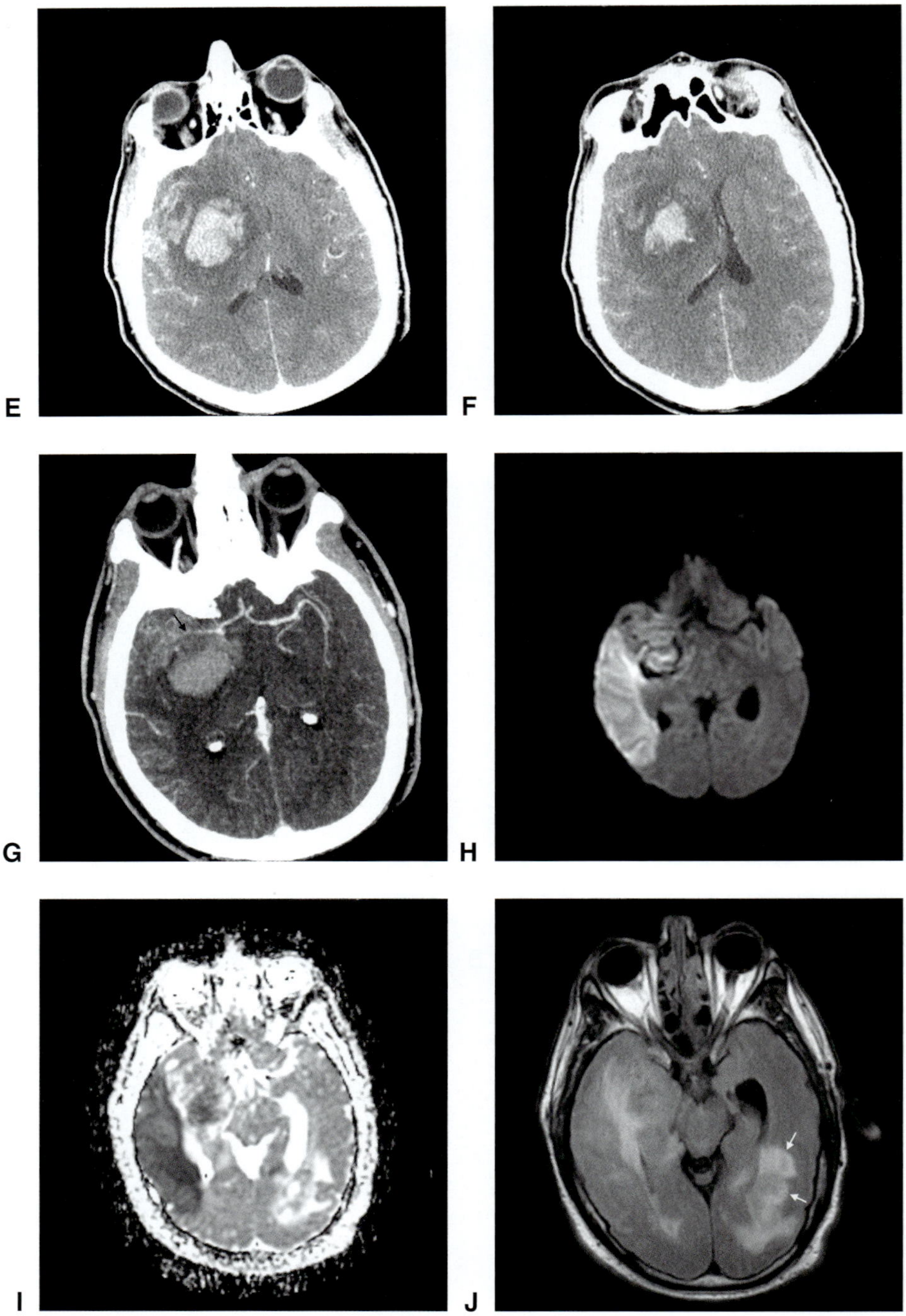

Figure 1.3. ***(continued)*** **G.** CT angiogram: Occlusion of right middle cerebral artery (black arrow) is confirmed. **H.** Axial DWI: Large area of acute infarct in the right middle cerebral artery territory. **I.** Axial ADC: Large area of acute infarct in the right middle cerebral artery territory. **J–L.** Axial FLAIR: Right basal ganglia mass is better delineated (black arrows), and the additional non-enhancing glioma (white arrows) in the left occipital lobe is more clearly seen.

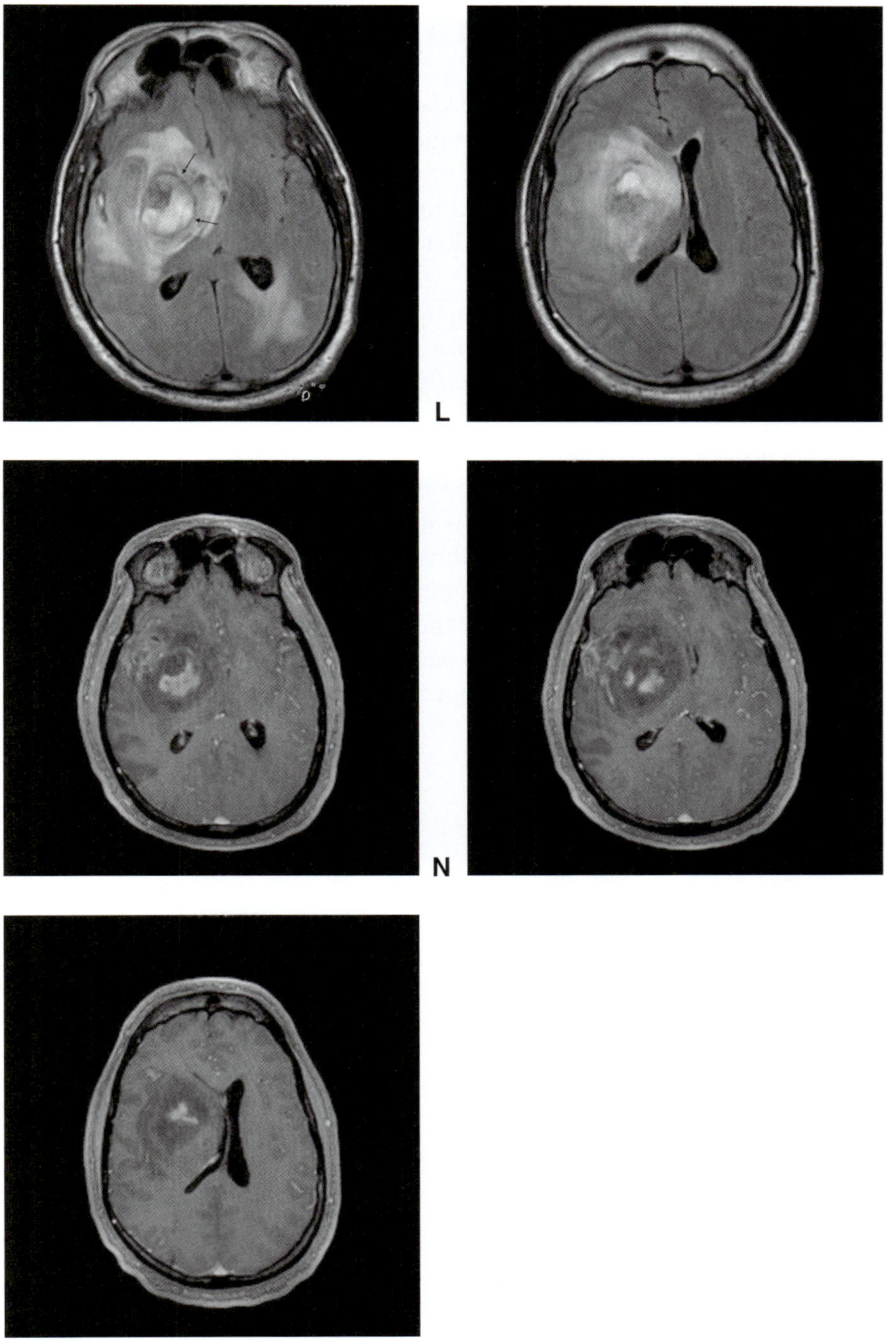

K L M N O

Figure 1.3. ***(continued)*** **M–O.** Axial T1 postcontrast: Heterogeneously enhancing right basal ganglia mass.

Cerebral Angiography

Cerebral angiography, also called cerebral angiogram, is a minimally invasive procedure that can provide a detailed, real-time imaging of blood flow, arterial supply, venous drainage, and other hemodynamics within a vascular brain tumor such as meningioma. Although safe, cerebral angiography can be associated with less than 1% incidence of neurological deficits and other non-neurological complications.

In brain tumors, cerebral angiography is not used as the primary diagnostic tool to characterize tumor location, size, or type. It is primarily used to assess tumor vascularity and to consider preoperative embolization to reduce tumor blood supply. Depending on the types of feeding vessels, the tumor's artery blood supply can be safely and precisely reduced or closed down using endovascular embolization technique prior to surgery to facilitate surgical removal of the tumor and to reduce intraoperative blood loss and operative times. Meningiomas are the most common brain tumors to undergo cerebral angiography, followed by embolization. One of the most commonly used embolic agents is polyvinyl alcohol particles, which expand in an aqueous solution due to their sponge-like quality. Other embolic agents include porous cellulose beads, hydroxyapatite, gelfoam, *N*-butyl cyanoacrylate, and platinum microcoils.

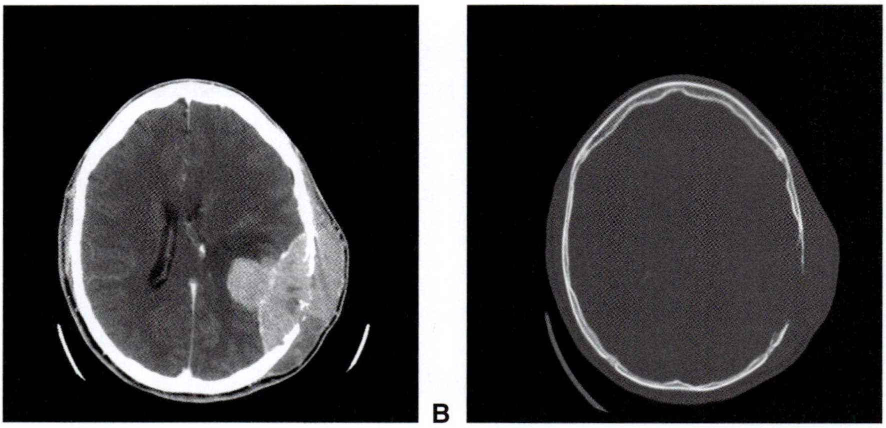

A B

Figure 1.4. Digital subtraction angiogram (DSA) of CNS lymphoma. A. Axial CT, enhanced: Large destructive left parietal skull mass with intracranial dural, intraparenchymal, and extracranial extension. **B.** Axial CT, bone window: Osseous lytic destruction of the involved skull.

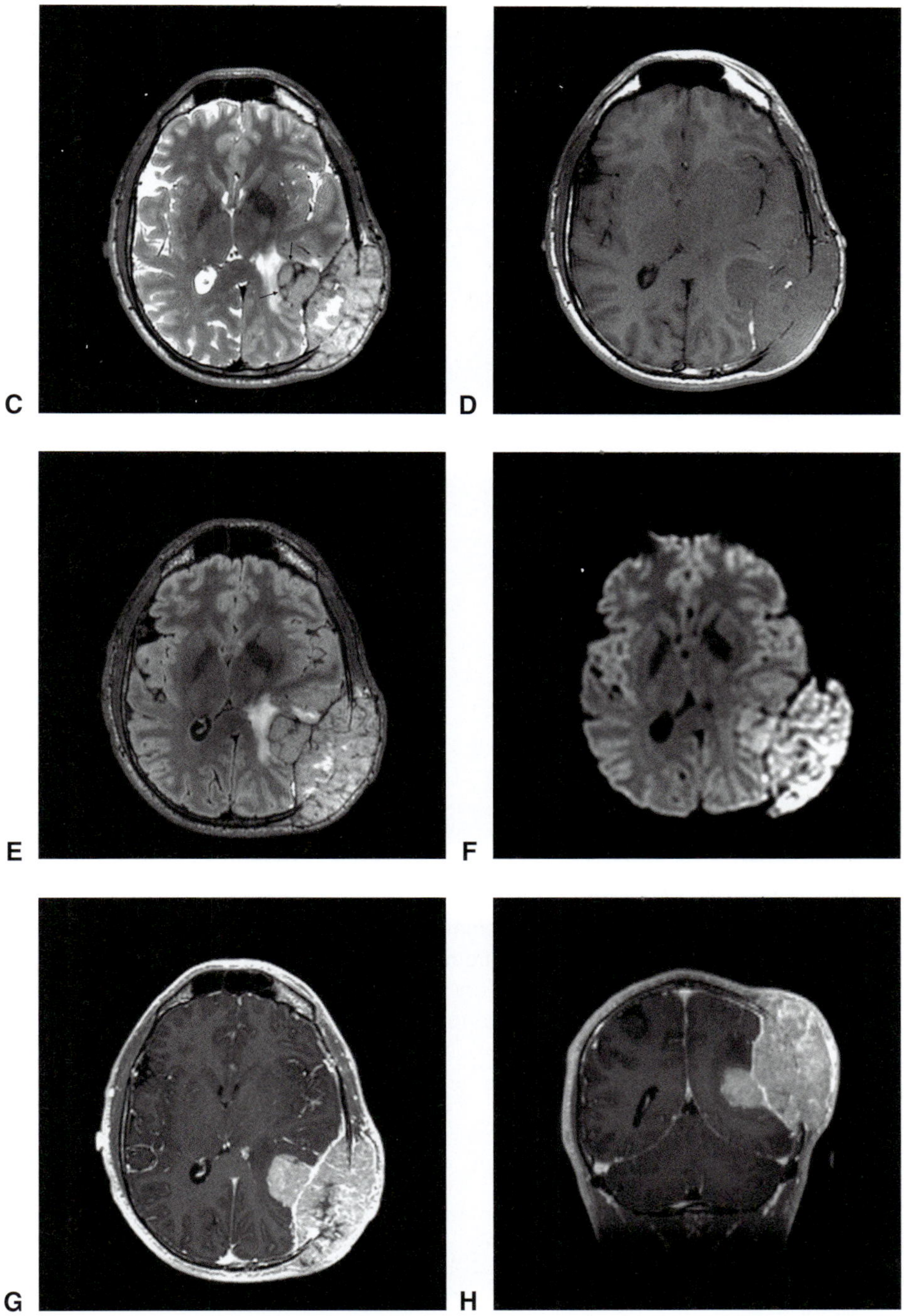

Figure 1.4. ***(continued)*** **C.** Axial T2: Heterogeneous mixed intensity mass with intraparenchymal invasion (black arrows). **D.** Axial T1-precontrast: Mostly isointense mass. **E.** Axial FLAIR: Heterogeneously isointense mass. **F.** Axial DWI: Heterogeneously reduced diffusion within the mass. **G.** Axial T1-postcontrast: Heterogeneous but avid enhancement within the mass. **H.** Coronal T1-postcontrast: Heterogeneous but avid enhancement within the mass.

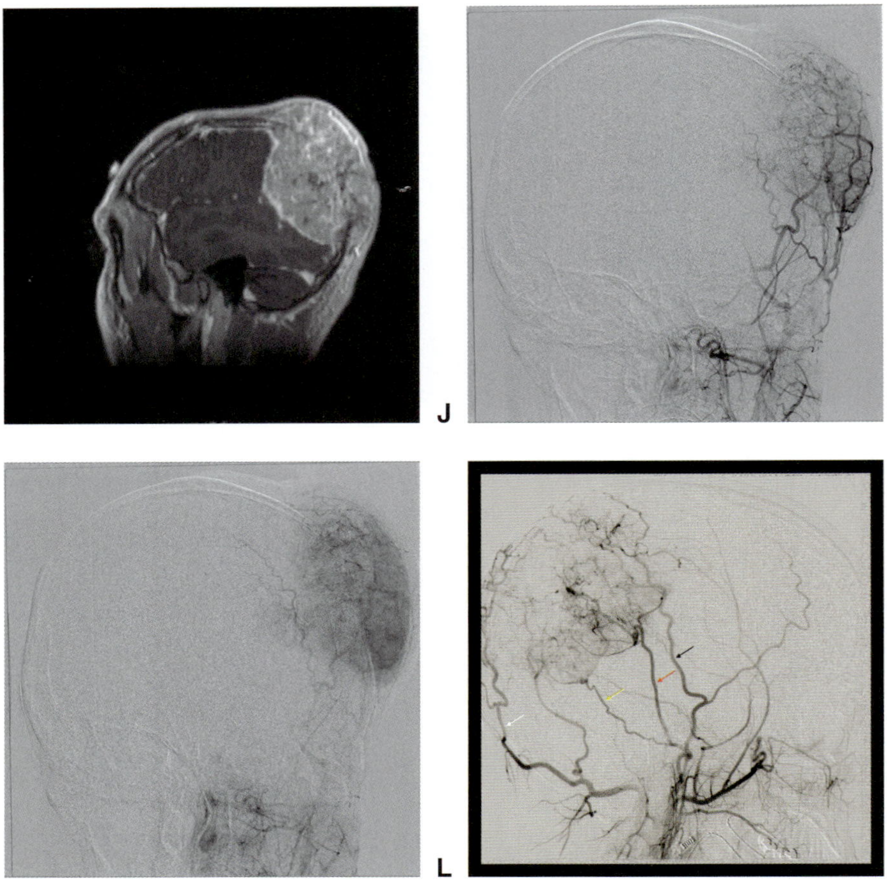

I J K L

Figure 1.4. ***(continued)*** **I.** Sagittal T1-postcontrast: Heterogeneous but avid enhancement within the mass. **J–L.** DSA, left common carotid artery injection: Hypervascular mass with dominant arterial supply from the external carotid artery, particularly branches of the left middle meningeal artery (black arrow), superficial temporal artery (red arrow), deep temporal artery (yellow arrow), and occipital artery (white arrow).

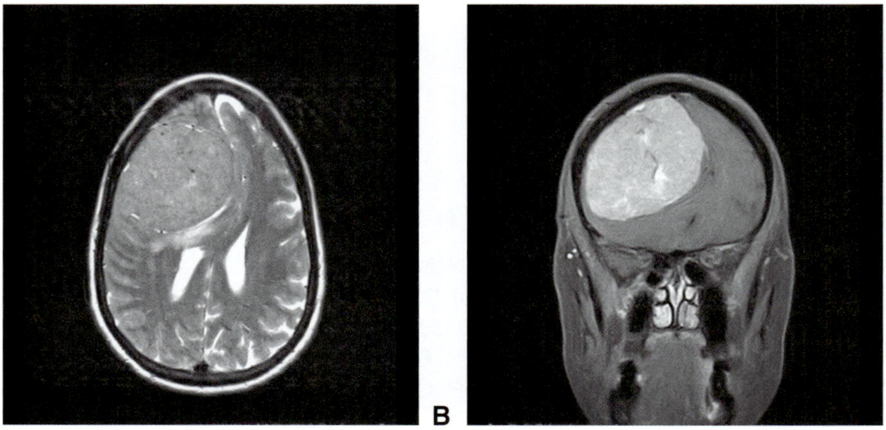

A B

Figure 1.5. DSA of meningioma, pre- and post-embolization. A. Axial T2: Heterogeneously isointense dural based right frontal mass. **B.** Coronal T1-postcontrast: Avid tumor enhancement.

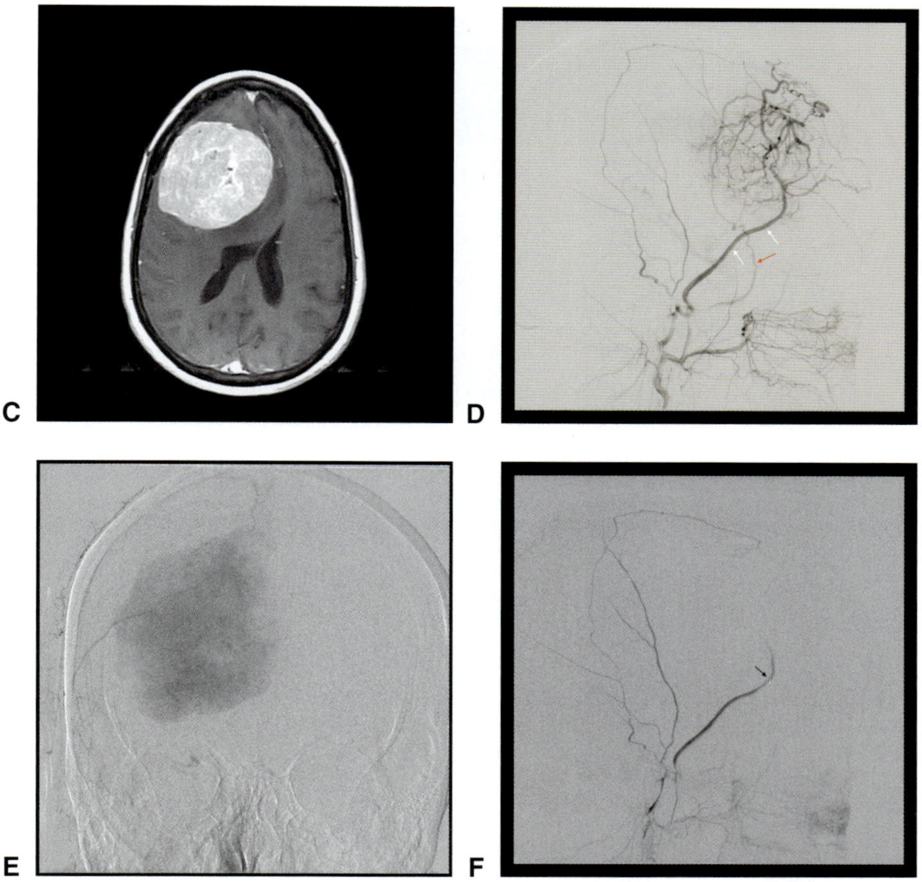

Figure 1.5. ***(continued)*** **C.** Axial T1-postcontrast: Avid tumor enhancement. **D.** DSA, right external carotid artery injection (arterial phase): Hypervascular right frontal mass with primary arterial supply from the anterior division of right middle meningeal artery (white arrows), and right superficial temporal artery (red arrow). **E.** DSA, right external carotid artery injection (delayed venous phase): Hypervascular right frontal tumor with persistent intratumoral contrast staining. **F.** DSA, right external carotid artery injection (arterial phase, post-embolization): Markedly diminished flow following embolization of the right middle meningeal artery anterior division and right superficial temporal artery using Polyvinyl Alcohol (PVA) particles (355–500 μm) and proximal coil occlusion (black arrow).

Magnetic Resonance Imaging

Magnetic Resonance Imaging (MRI) is the most commonly used imaging modality to diagnose and characterize tumors of the central nervous system (CNS). Use of intravenous gadolinium-based contrast agent is essential for detecting and evaluating brain and spinal tumors. MRI is superior to CT in soft tissue resolution, 3D data acquisition, multiplanar capability, quantitative ability, and lack of ionizing radiation. MRI provides an accurate determination of brain tumor location, extent, hemorrhage, cyst, necrosis, mass effect, edema, and any additional lesions. The typical MRI protocol for brain tumor patients

TABLE 1.1 Standard Brain Tumor MR Imaging Protocol

	TR (msec)	TE (msec)	DFOV (mm)	Slice thickness (mm)	NEX	Other
DWI	10,280	57.1	230	2	4	B = 1000; echo planar
T1-precontrast	7.68	2.95	256	1	1	3D gradient echo
SWI	43	24.58	256	2.4	0.6975	3D
FLAIR	5,952	116	256	1.2	1	TI = 1,732
ASL	4,931	10.53	240	4	3	PLD = 2,025 msec
T2-postcontrast	8389	94	256	3	1	Spin echo
T1-SPGR postcontrast	7.68	2.95	256	1	1	3D
Coronal spin echo T1-postcontrast	683.3	19	256	4	2	Spin echo

3D, three dimensional; ASL, arterial spin labeling; b, diffusion sensitivity parameter (sec/mm^2); DFOV, field of view; DWI, diffusion-weighted imaging; FLAIR, fluid-attenuated inversion recovery; NEX, number of excitations; PLD, post-labeling delay; SPGR, spoiled gradient recalled; SWI, susceptibility-weighted imaging; TE, echo time; TI-Inversion time; TR, repetition time.

includes pre- and postcontrast T1-weighted images, T2-weighted and fluid-attenuated inversion recovery (FLAIR) images, diffusion-weighted images, and susceptibility-weighted images. Perfusion-weighted imaging (PWI) such as dynamic contrast-enhanced (DCE) susceptibility-weighted imaging or arterial spin labeling imaging can be used to indirectly assess tumor vascularity. The standard brain tumor imaging protocol is listed in Table 1.1.

Although highly sensitive to pathologic alterations of normal brain, structural MRI features can be nonspecific, where both neoplastic and nonneoplastic lesions may appear similar and pose a diagnostic challenge. To complement anatomic information depicted on structural MRI, physiologic MR Imaging is widely used to image alteration in micro-architectural integrity and cellularity [diffusion-weighted imaging (DWI)], cerebral hemodynamics, and vascularity (PWI), not only the anatomical/structural but also physiologic information in normal and diseased state and to derive quantitative data. Physiologic MR imaging includes DWI, PWI, functional MR imaging, and proton MR spectroscopy.

Diffusion-Weighted Imaging

DWI is an MR imaging sequence that captures the signal contrast based on the differences in random Brownian motion and is used to evaluate alteration in proton motion within the extracellular space and micro-architectural integrity in the brain. The extent to which the image is weighted by diffusion is controlled by the b-value, diffusion sensitivity parameter, in the unit of seconds per square millimeters. Apparent diffusion coefficient (ADC) is a quantitative variable derived from DWI in units of square millimeters per second and allows generation of a map that captures difference in diffusion characteristics in different tissues of the brain. Fractional anisotropy (FA), a scalar value between zero and one that describes the degree of anisotropy of a diffusion process, can also be measured. A value of 0 means that diffusion is isotropic (unrestricted or equally restricted) in all directions, and a value of 1 means that diffusion is anisotropic (different diffusion coefficients along different directions). In normal brain, the structure with the highest FA value is the splenium of corpus callosum ranging from 0.78 to 0.8.

Diffusion Tensor Imaging

DTI is an advanced DWI method used for characterizing microstructural changes to estimate the location, direction, orientation, and anisotropy of white matter tracts of the brain. A diffusion tensor comprised of 3-by-3 matrix describes differences in diffusion anisotropy on a pixel-by-pixel basis and generates a 3D reconstruction of fiber tractography of major white matter tracts. White matter tracts of the brain are highly anisotropic because of the parallel orientation of its nerve fiber tracts. Fiber tractography, a 3D modeling technique to visually represent nerve tracts, can be derived from data collected by DTI and offers visualization of the white matter fiber architecture of neural networks such as motor, sensory, language, visual, and auditory pathways.

Perfusion-Weighted Imaging

PWI is an MR imaging sequence that depicts cerebrovascular and hemodynamic status in normal and diseased state in the brain and provides hemodynamic parameters such as cerebral blood volume, cerebral blood flow, and transit time. There are three different types of PWI: two using gadolinium contrast-enhanced techniques—(1) dynamic susceptibility-weighted contrast-enhanced (DSC) and (2) dynamic contrast-enhanced—and one using arterial blood as contrast agent—(3) arterial spin labeling imaging. In brain tumors, PWI can provide information about the tumor vascular density or volume, tumor blood flow, and capillary leakiness. Relative cerebral blood volume (rCBV) derived from DSC PWI has been shown to correlate with tumor-induced angiogenesis, higher grade of tumor, and more aggressive tumor growth. Endothelial permeability parameter, ktrans, derived from DCE, has been shown to correlate with capillary leakiness, more enhancement on standard postcontrast imaging, and higher grade of tumor. Relative cerebral blood flow (rCBF) derived from ASL has been shown to correlate with higher grade of tumor and recurrent tumor following radiation therapy.

Functional MR Imaging

Functional MRI (fMRI) measures brain activity by detecting changes associated with blood flow and maps out regional, time-varying changes in deoxyhemoglobin concentration related to task-induced or spontaneous modulation of neural metabolism.

Increased neural activity detected by fMRI is related to two primary physiologic measures—cerebral blood low and changes in oxygenation concentration, or blood oxygenation level dependent (BOLD) metabolism. Two acquisition paradigms are used to acquire fMRI data—task-activated and spontaneous. The task-related activation fMRI experiment utilizes motor, visual, auditory, language, or other stimuli to alternately induce different neural states, and activation maps are obtained by comparing the signals recorded during the different states. fMRI can be used to guide surgical resection of brain tumors located near eloquent areas such as the motor cortex or Broca's speech area so as not to injure these important functional areas of the brain.

Proton MR Spectroscopy

In vivo proton MR spectroscopy (^{1}H MRS) focuses on carbon-bound protons in the 1 to 5 ppm range of the chemical shift scale and can depict several metabolites that are present at high-enough concentrations within the micromoles per gram range (Table 1.2). Noninvasive detection and quantification of brain metabolites in normal and disease states can be assessed by ^{1}H MRS. Major types of brain biochemicals or metabolites that can be studied and detected by ^{1}H MRS include, but not limited to, choline-containing compounds (which are used to make cell membranes), creatine (a chemical involved in energy metabolism), gamma-aminobutyric acid (neurotransmitter), myoinositol, N-acetylaspartate, and lactate (a marker of hypoxia or necrosis).

TABLE 1.2 ^{1}H MRS Metabolites and Corresponding Peak Values and Biologic Correlates

Metabolite	Parts per million	Properties
Lipid (Lip)	0.9–1.4	Product of cellular membrane destruction & necrosis
Lactate (Lac)	1.33	Product of anaerobic respiration
Alanine (Ala)	1.48	Role in tricarboxylic acid cycle
N-Acetylaspartate (NAA)	2.02	Axonal viability & neuronal integrity
Glx Complex	2.25	Excitatory neurotransmission
Creatine (Cr)	3.02	Cellular energetic & respiration marker
Choline (Cho)	3.22	Cellular proliferation marker
Myoinositol (mIn)	3.56	Glial cell proliferation marker

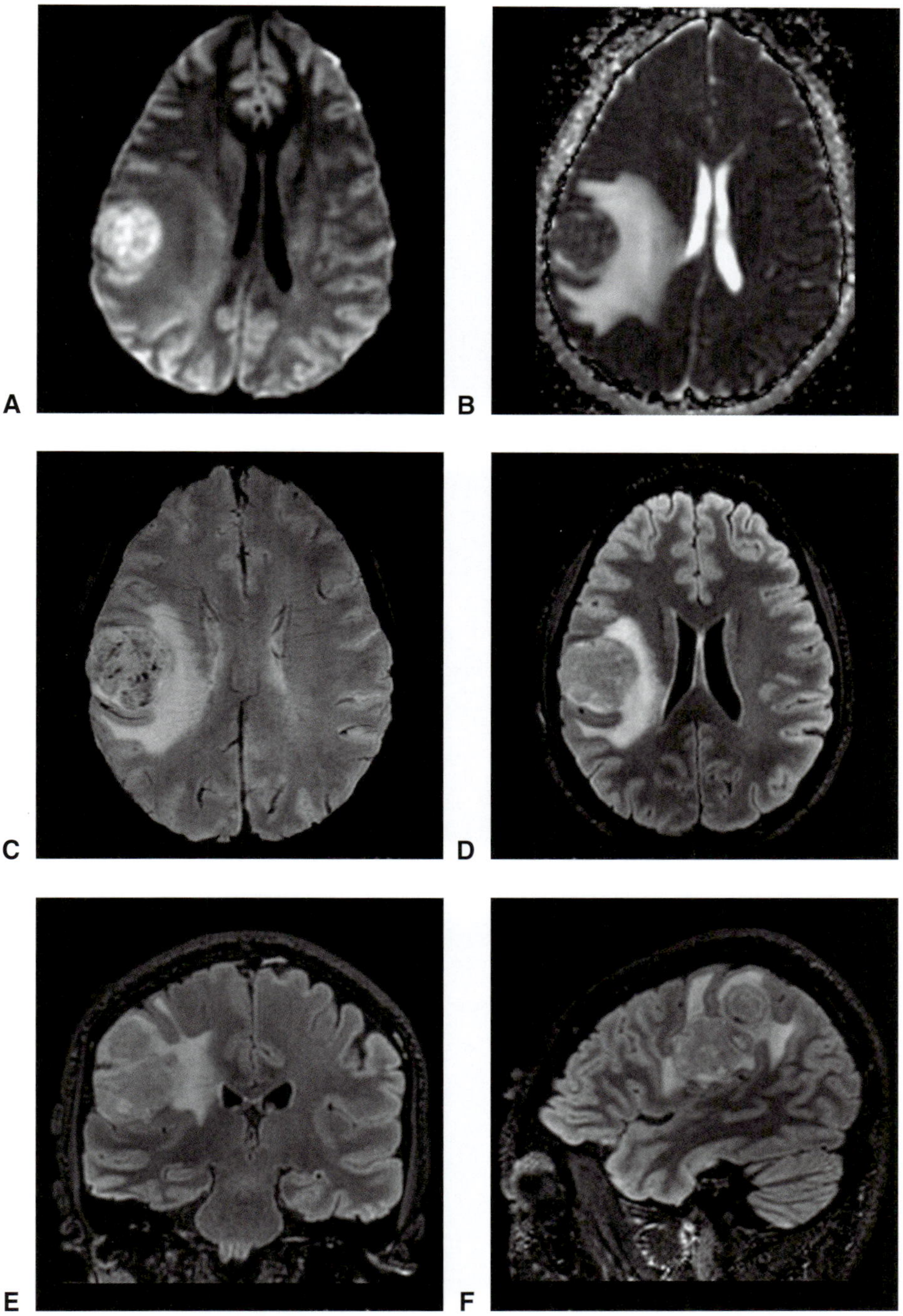

Figure 1.6. Structural MR Imaging of a glioblastoma. A. Axial DWI: Heterogeneously reduced diffusion within right parietal mass. **B.** Axial ADC: Heterogeneously reduced diffusion within right parietal mass. **C.** Axial SWI: Numerous punctate blood products within the mass. **D.** Axial FLAIR: Heterogeneously isointense mass with moderate surrounding edema. **E.** Coronal FLAIR: Heterogeneously isointense mass with moderate surrounding edema. **F.** Sagittal FLAIR: Heterogeneously isointense mass with moderate surrounding edema.

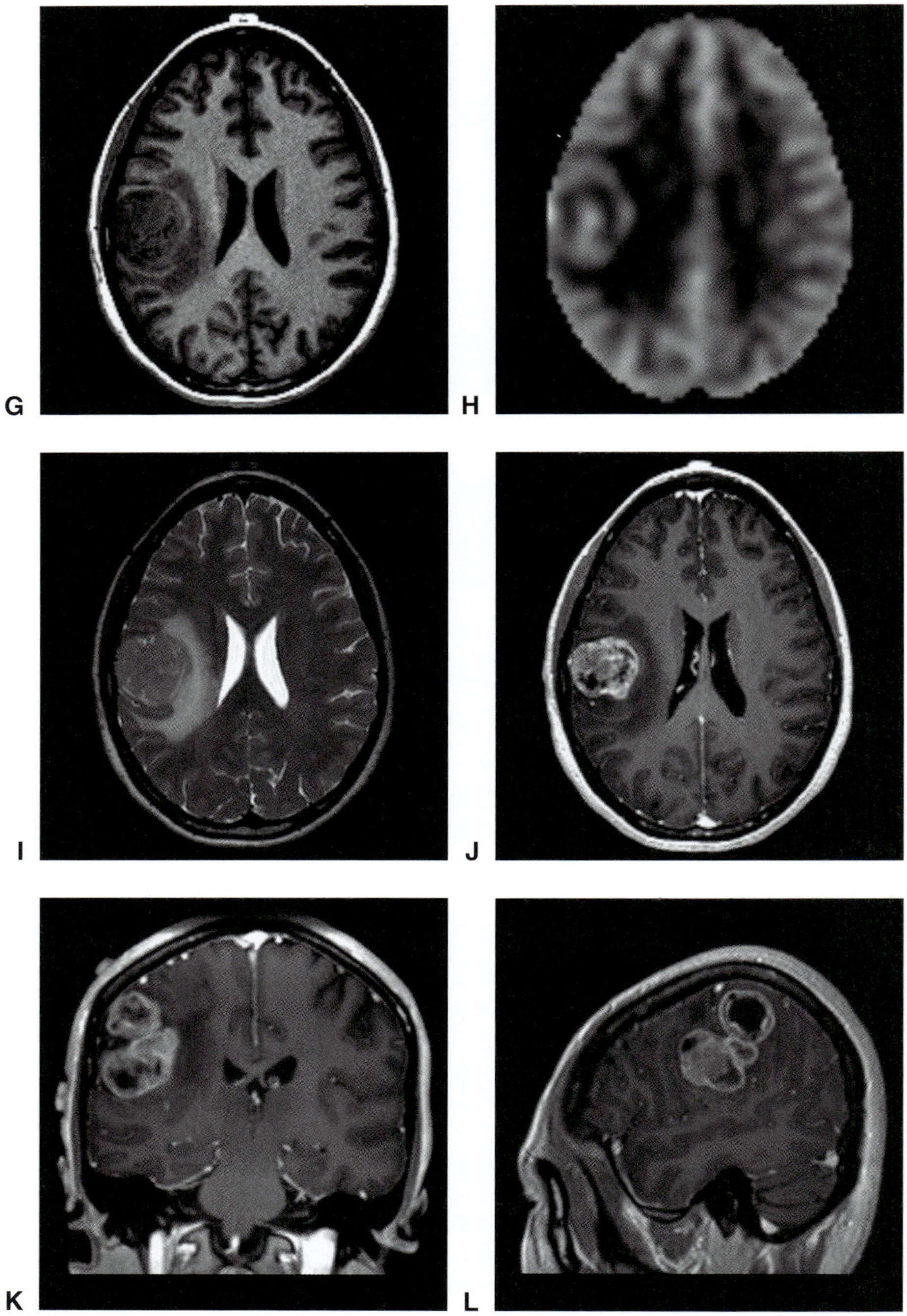

Figure 1.6. *(continued)* **G.** Axial T1-precontrast: Heterogeneously hypointense mass. **H.** Axial ASL: Rim and central areas of hyperperfusion within the mass. **I.** Axial T2: Heterogeneously hypointense mass. **J.** Axial T1-postcontrast: Heterogeneous but avid enhancement with areas of central necrosis. **K.** Coronal T1-postcontrast: Heterogeneous but avid enhancement with areas of central necrosis. **L.** Sagittal T1-postcontrast: Heterogeneous but avid enhancement with areas of central necrosis.

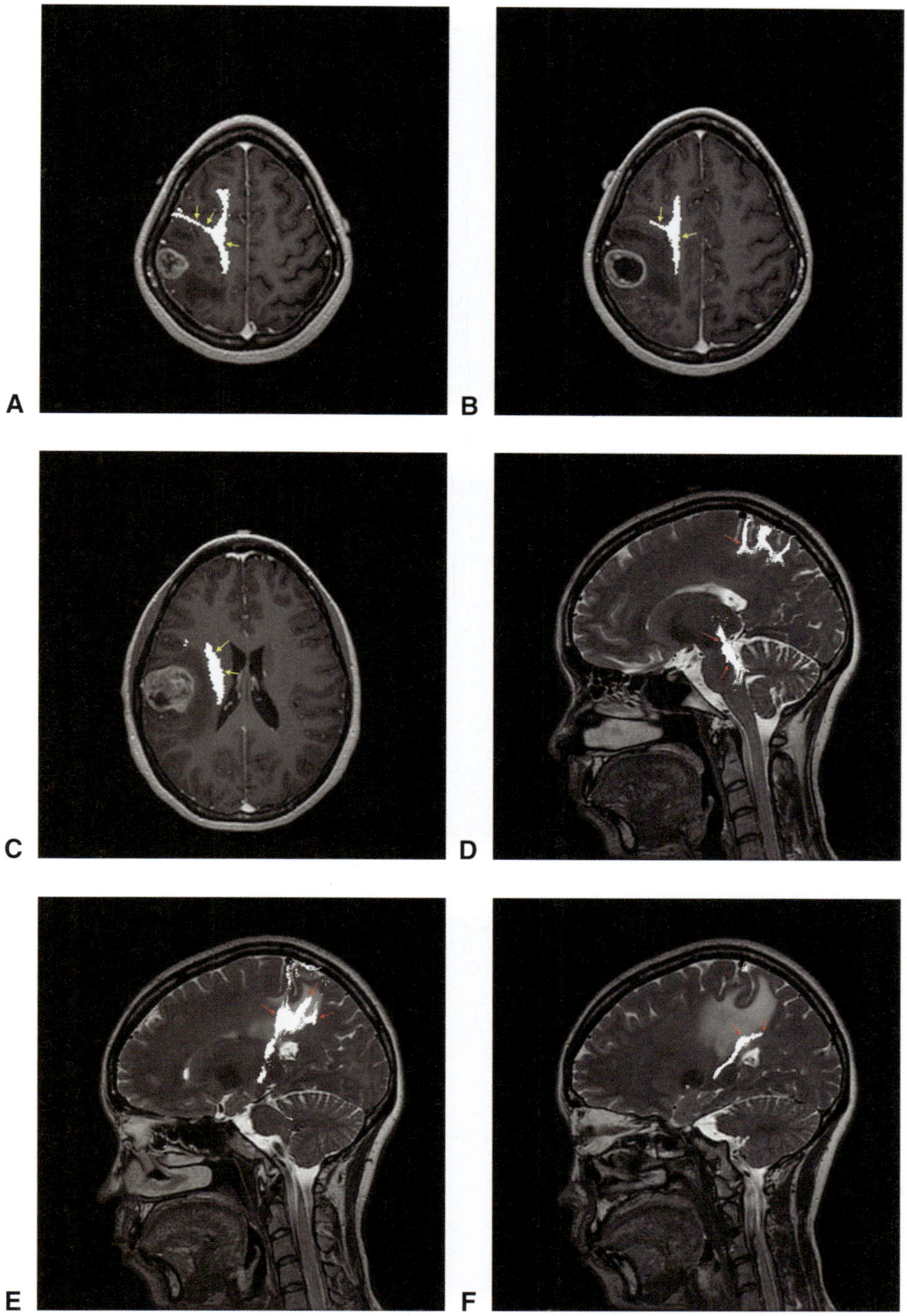

Figure 1.7. Diffusion Tensor Imaging, Tractography. **A–C.** Motor pathway: Right parietal sensory cortex glioblastoma situated posterior and superficial to the corticospinal tract (yellow arrows). **D–F.** Sensory pathway: Right parietal sensory cortex glioblastoma situated within the descending sensory tract (red arrows).

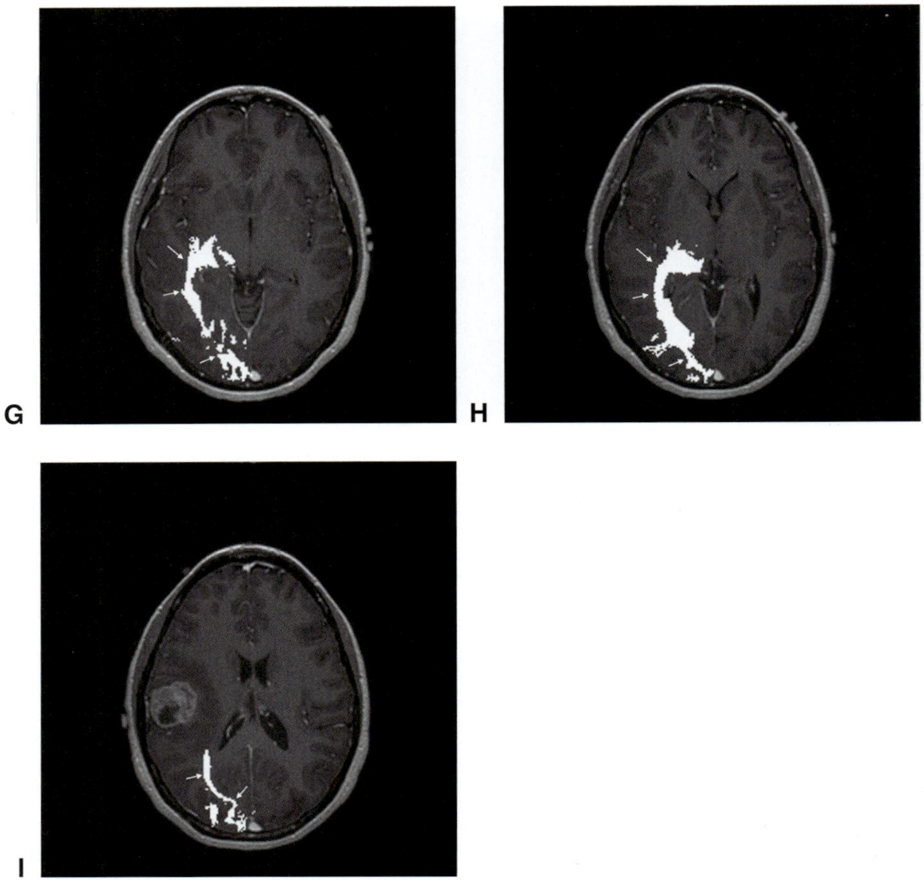

Figure 1.7. ***(continued)*** **G–I.** Visual pathway: Right parietal sensory cortex glioblastoma situated remote from the visual pathway (black yellows).

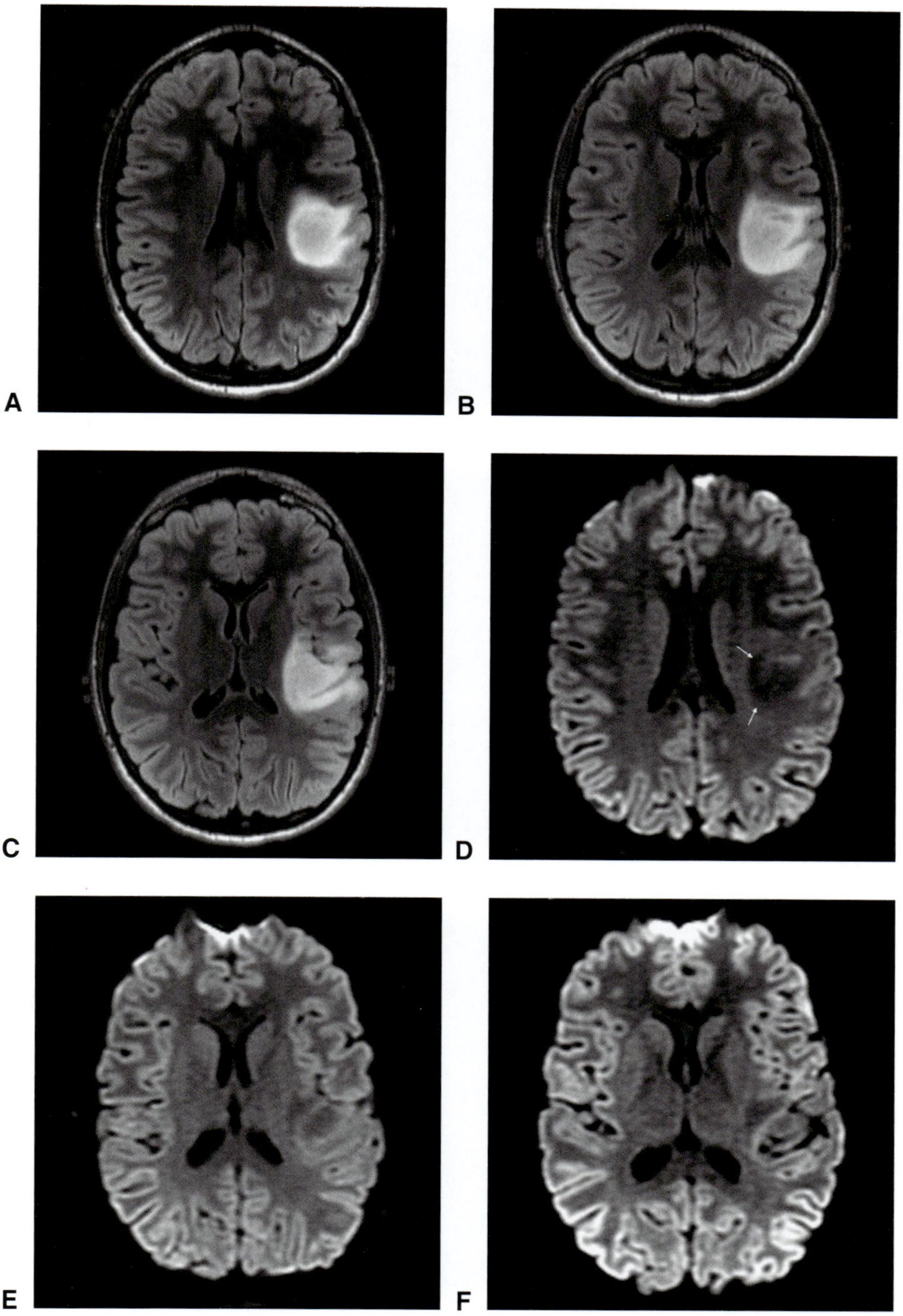

Figure 1.8. **Imaging of left frontal diffuse glioma near corticospinal tract. A–C.** Axial FLAIR: Hyperintense expansile left posterior frontal diffuse glioma. **D–F.** Axial DWI: Hypointense mass with its medial border encroaching upon the descending corticospinal tract (white arrows).

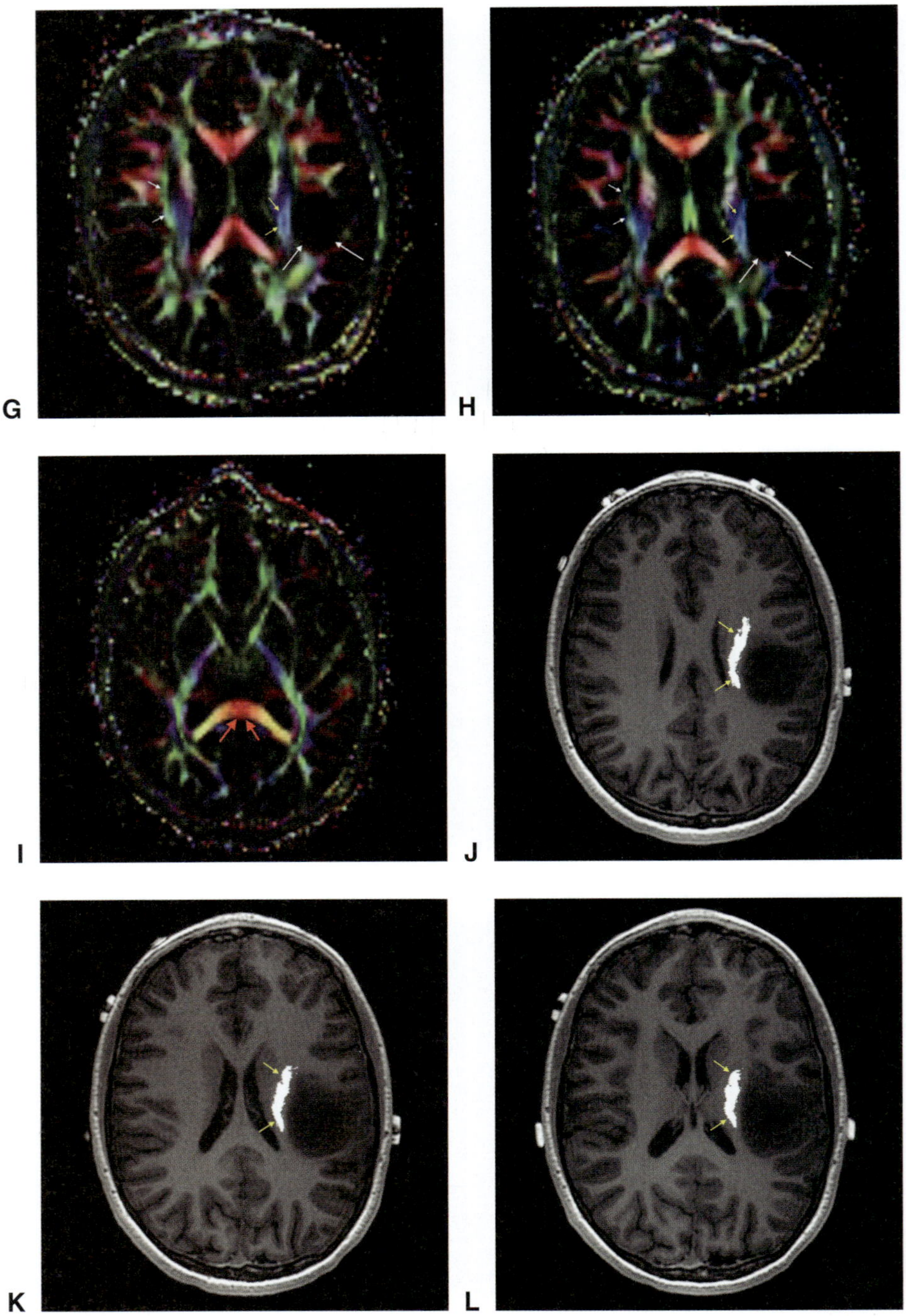

Figure 1.8. ***(continued)*** **G–I.** Axial Fractional Anisotropy map: Expansile mass seen as a marked hypointense mass (long white arrows) displacing the descending corticospinal tract (yellow arrows). Normal external capsular white matter tracts seen on the right side (small white arrows) are not seen on the left side. **J–L.** Axial T1-precontrast fused with descending corticospinal tract DTI: Motor fiber tractography confirms the descending left corticospinal tract (yellow arrows) is displaced medially but not invaded by the expansile mass.

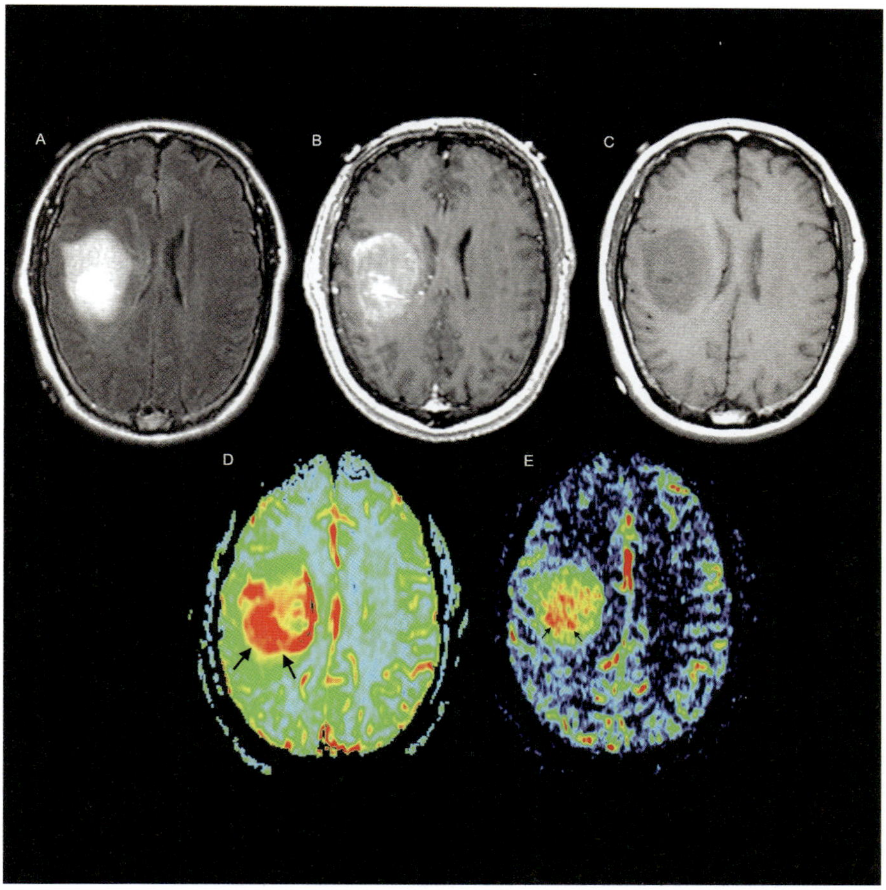

Figure 1.9. **Imaging of perfusion MRI of glioblastoma. A.** Axial FLAIR: Hyperintense right frontal mass. **B.** Axial T1-postcontrast: Heterogeneous enhancement within the mass. **C.** Axial T1-precontrast: Mostly hypointense mass. **D.** Axial DSC rCBV map: Marked elevated intratumoral blood volume mostly in the posterior aspect of the mass (large black arrows). **E.** Axial DCE ktrans map: Marked leaky intratumoral vessels are located within the center of the mass (small black arrows).

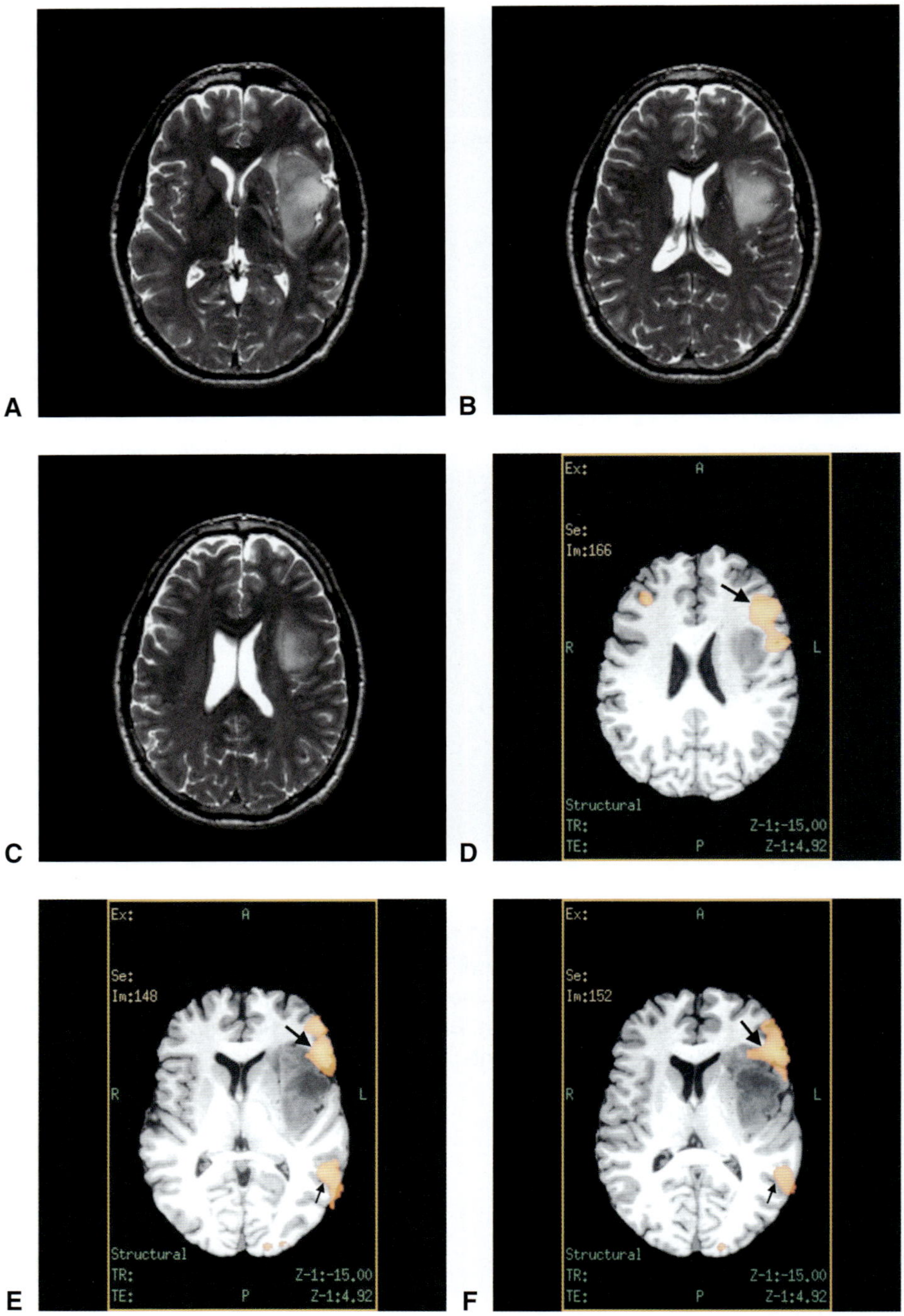

Figure 1.10. Imaging of fMRI in diffuse glioma. A–C. Axial T2: Heterogeneous mixed intensity mass centered in the left insula. **D–F.** fMRI of speech: Activation of speech area, Broca's area, anteriorly (large arrow) and angular gyrus (medium arrow) posteriorly, both of which are separate and distinct from the left insular diffuse glioma.

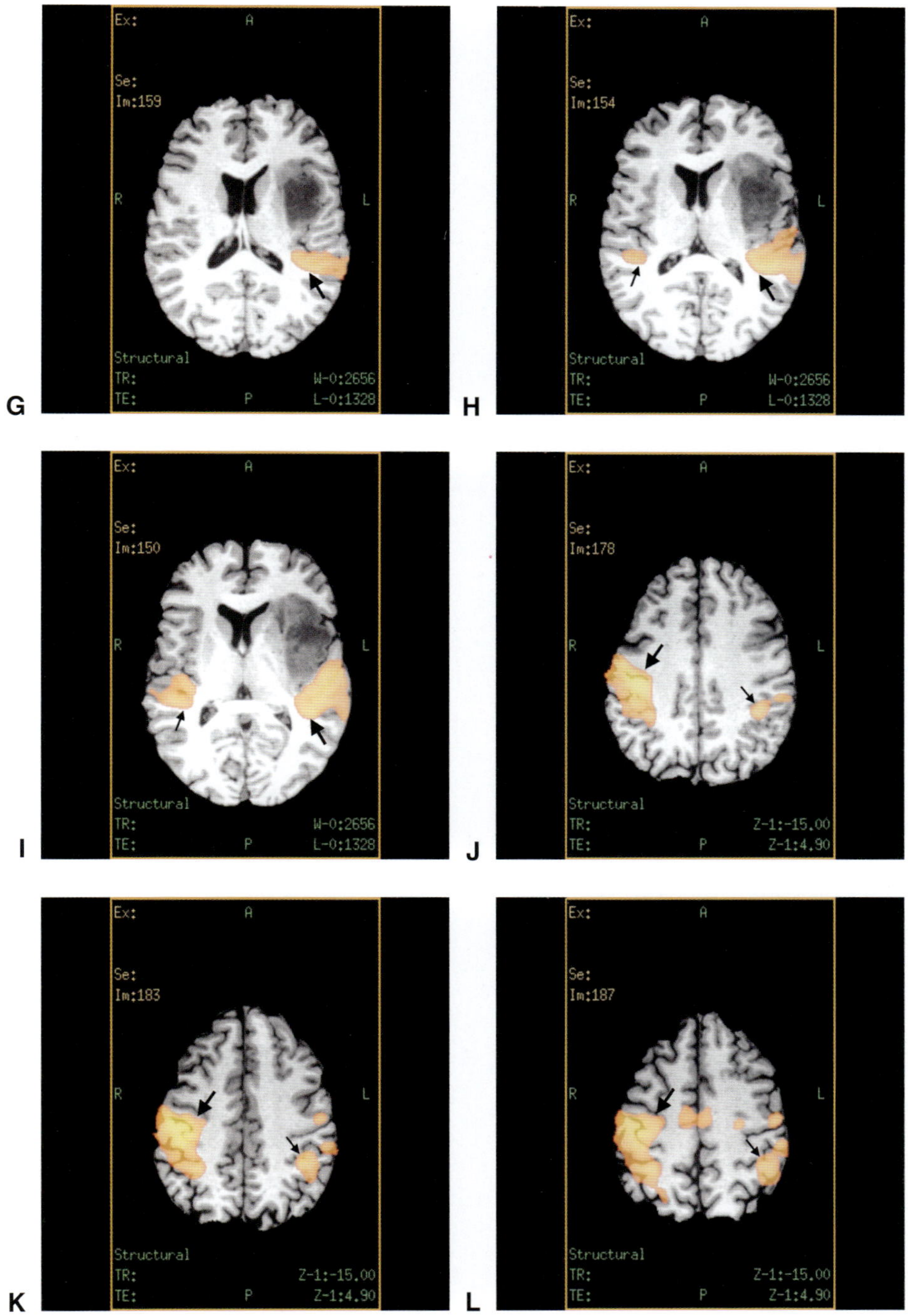

Figure 1.10. ***(continued)*** **G–I.** fMRI of primary auditory cortex: Activation of transverse temporal gyrus of Heschl, left greater than right, located posterior and uninvolved by the insular diffuse glioma. **J–L.** fMRI of motor cortex: Left hand motor task activation shows dominant right motor cortex activity (large arrow) and minor left sensory cortex (medium arrow) activity.

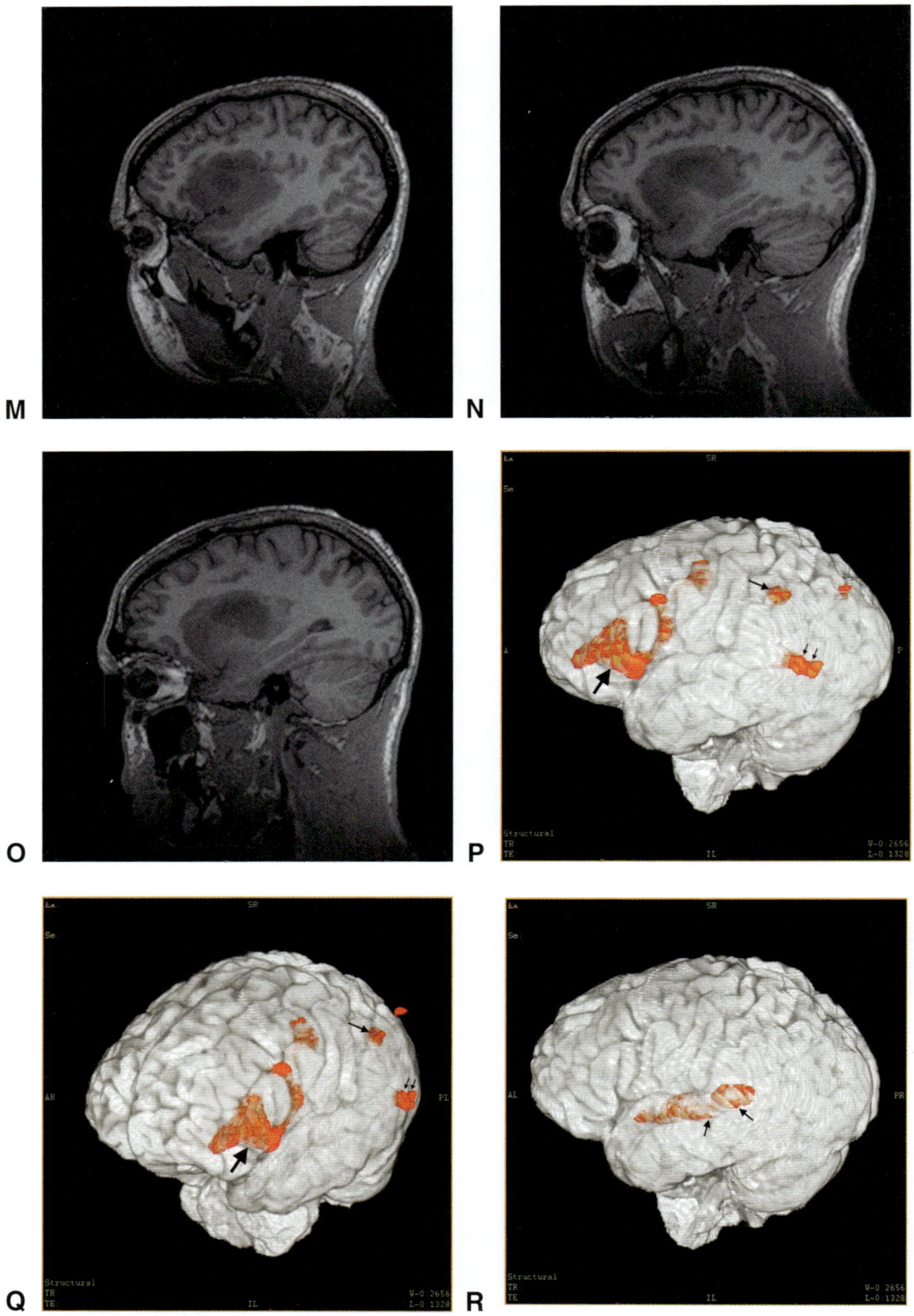

Figure 1.10. ***(continued)*** **M–O.** Sagittal T1, precontrast: Expansile hypointense left insular mass. **P, Q.** fMRI three-dimensional map of speech function: Broca's speech area (large arrow), angular gyrus (medium arrow), and Wernicke's area (small arrows). **R.** fMRI three-dimensional map of primary auditory cortex: Activation of transverse temporal gyrus of Heschl (black arrows) within the superior temporal gyrus.

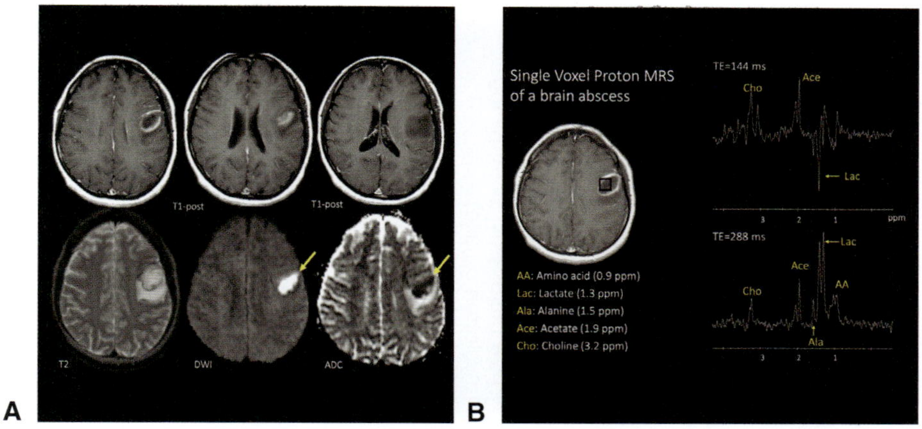

Figure 1.11. Proton MR Spectroscopy, Brain Abscess. A. Structural MRI: Rim enhancing left frontal mass with reduced diffusion on DWI and ADC (yellow arrows). **B.** Single voxel proton MR spectroscopy: Prominent lactate peak at 1.3 ppm and presence of amino acid, alanine, and acetate peaks.

Hybrid Imaging: Positron Emission Tomography and Magnetic Resonance

Hybrid imaging is an imaging technology that combines positron emission tomography (PET) and magnetic resonance (MR) imaging, allowing for superior co-registration between metabolic information from PET and higher soft-tissue contrast and resolution from MR and hence delivering precise metabolic and anatomic co-localization. The quality and specificity of radiotracers hold the future of PET–MR hybrid imaging, where more specific, reliable, and sensitive compounds will contribute to improvement on diagnosis, tumor biology, therapy response, and assessment of prognosis.

PET–MR remains a challenge for the current socioeconomic environment, where high-cost technology is questioned, particularly with unproven clinical impact and outcomes. The high costs of the hybrid system and its doubtful financial viability require cautious optimism of its potential, careful selection of clinical indication, and critical analysis of outcomes research (Table 1.3).

TABLE 1.3 Positron Emission Tomography Radiotracer for Central Nervous System Tumors

PET Radiotracer	Physiopathology	Main Strength	Main Limitation
^{18}F-Fluorodeoxyglucose (FDG)	Carbohydrate metabolism	Widely available	Lack of specificity High false positive and false negative
^{18}F-Fluoroethyl-l-tyrosine (FET)	Amino acid transport	Dynamic acquisition	Variability of uptake kinetics due to dependence of PET protocol
^{18}F-Fluoro-L-phenylalanine (FDOPA)	Amino acid transport	Early acquisition Infiltrative tumor detection	Challenges in standardization of acquisition and interpretation parameters
^{11}C-methionine	Amino acid transport	High sensitivity and specificity Suitable for tumor response evaluation	Low half-life of ^{11}C (requiring cyclotron on site)
^{18}F-Fluorothymidine (FLT)	Deoxyribonucleic Acid synthesis	High specificity Correlate to Ki-67 index (proliferation marker)	Low tumor uptake
^{18}F-Fluoromisonidazole (FMISO)	Hypoxia	Hypoxic tumor detection	High background activity
^{11}C-Choline ^{18}F-Fcholine	Cell membrane metabolism	Suitable for tumor outcome evaluation	Low half-life of ^{11}C (requiring cyclotron on site)
^{68}Ga-Prostate Specific Membrane Antigen (PMSA) ^{18}F-Prostate Specific Membrane Antigen (PSMA)	Neoangiogenesis	Suitable for detection of meningioma	High false positive

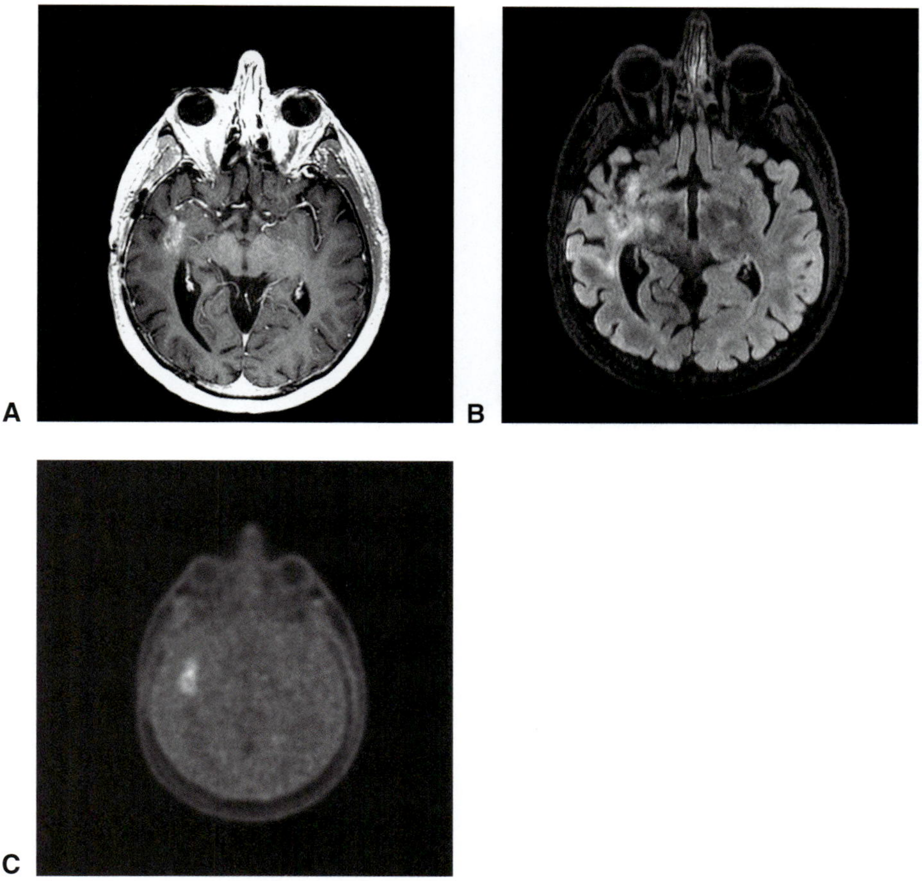

Figure 1.12. ¹⁸F-Fluoromisonidazole (MISO) PET–MR, Recurrent Glioblastoma. **A.** Axial T1-postcontrast: Mildly enhancing right temporal lesion at the site of previously resected and treated glioblastoma. **B.** Axial FLAIR: Ill-defined hyperintense lesion. **C.** FMISO PET–MR: Focal uptake in the right temporal lesion, path-proven recurrent glioblastoma.

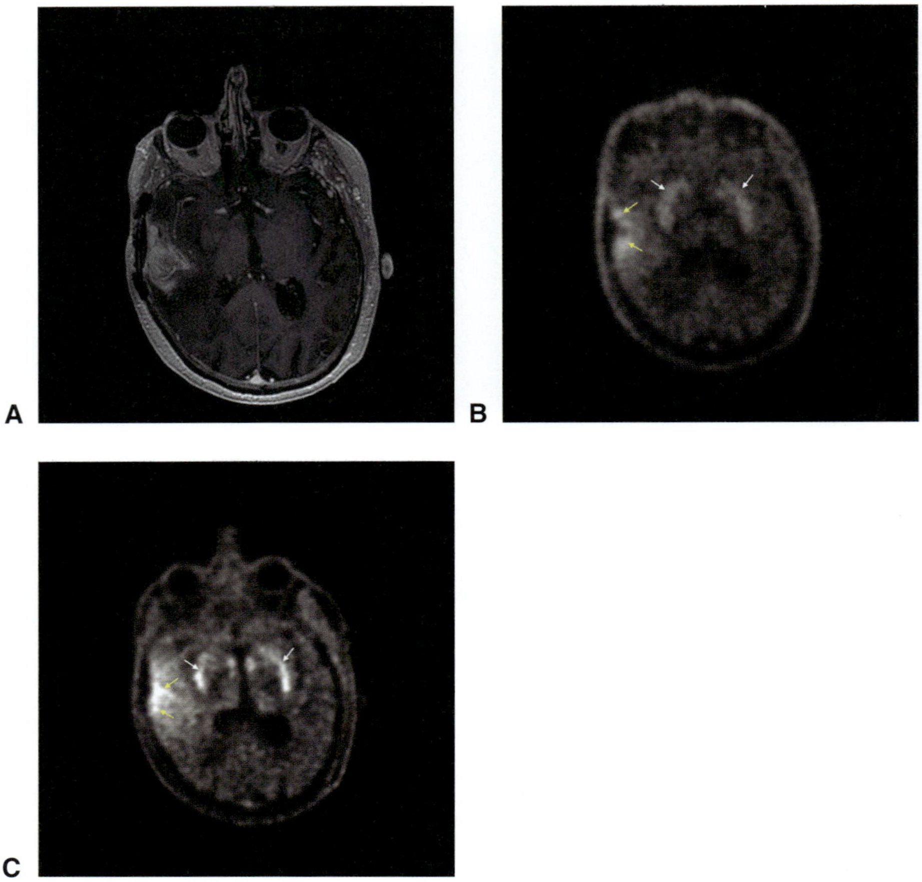

Figure 1.13. **[18]F-Fluoro-L-phenylalanine (DOPA) PET–MR, Recurrent Glioblastoma.** **A.** Axial T1-postcontrast: Avidly enhancing right temporal lesion at the site of previously resected and treated glioblastoma. **B, C.** FDOPA PET–MR: Focal uptake in the right temporal lesion (yellow arrows), path-proven recurrent glioblastoma. Notice the physiologic FDOPA uptake in bilateral basal ganglia (white arrows).

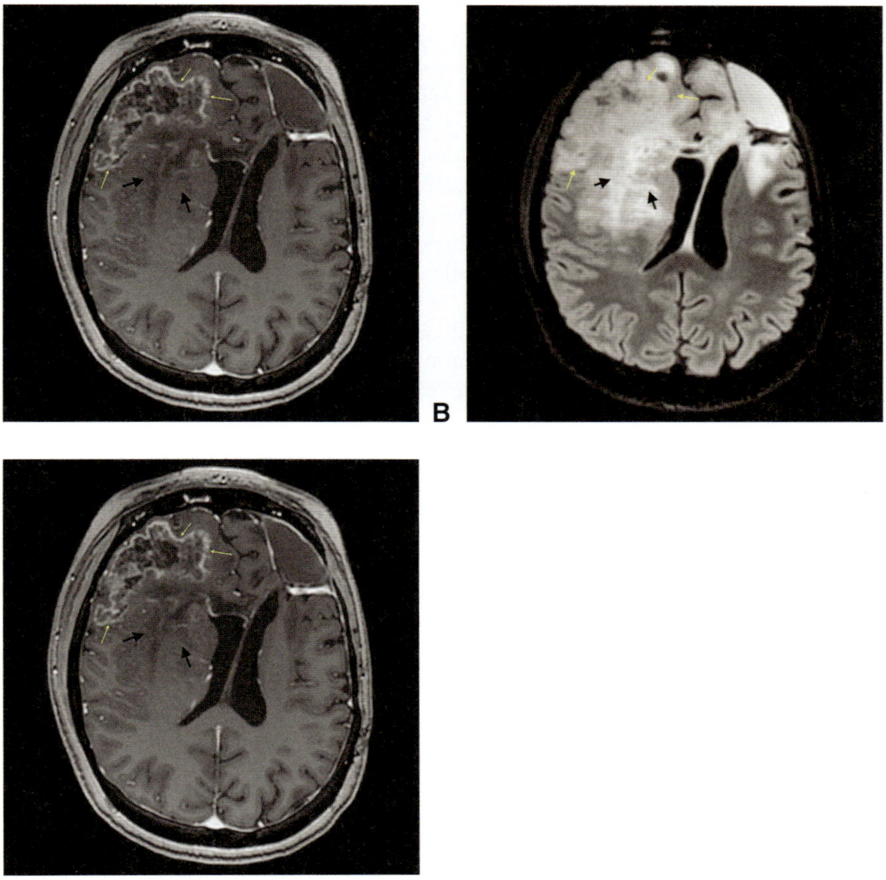
A B C

Figure 1.14. FET-PET–MR, Recurrent Glioblastoma. A. Axial T1-postcontrast: Peripheral irregular enhancing area in the right inferior frontal lobe (yellow arrows) and deeper area of nonenhancing mass-like lesion (black arrows). **B.** Axial FLAIR: Both peripheral and deeper components are heterogeneously hyperintense. **C.** FET-PET–MR fused: Marked uptake of FET within the deeper area of nonenhancing mass-like lesion (black arrows) and minimal uptake in the peripheral irregular enhancing area (yellow arrows).

Bibliography

Barajas Jr RF, Hess CP, Phillips JJ, et al. Super-resolution track density imaging of glioblastoma: histopathologic correlation. *AJNR An J Neuroradiol.* 2013;34:1319–1325.

Cha S. Perfusion MR imaging of brain tumors. *Top Magn Reson Imaging.* 2004;15:279–289.

Fink JR, Muzi M, Peck M, Krohn KA. Multimodality brain tumor imaging: MR imaging, PET, and PET/MR imaging. *J Nucl Med.* 2015;56:1554–1561.

Gharzeddine K, Hatzoglou V, Holodny AI, Young RJ. MR perfusion and MR spectroscopy of brain neoplasms. *Radiol Clin North Am.* 2019;57:1177–1188.

Glover GH. Overview of functional magnetic resonance imaging. *Neurosurg Clin N Am.* 2011:22:133–139.

Hagmann P, Jonasson L, Maeder P, Thiran J-P, Wedeen VJ, Meuli R. Understanding diffusion MR imaging techniques: from scalar diffusion-weighted imaging to diffusion tensor imaging and beyond. *Radiographics.* 2006;26:S205–223.

Hirohata M, Abe T, Fujimura N, Takeuchi Y, Shigemori M. Preoperative embolization of brain tumor with pial artery or dural branch of internal carotid artery as feeding artery. *Interv Neuroradiol.* 2006;12:246–251.

Kim EY, Park HJ, Kim DH, Lee SK, Kim J. Measuring fractional anisotropy of the corpus callosum using diffusion tensor imaging: mid-sagittal versus axial imaging planes. *Korean J Radiol.* 2008;9:391–395.

Potgieser AR, Wagemakers M, van Hulzen ALJ, et al. The role of diffusion tensor imaging in brain tumor surgery: a review of the literature. *Clin Neurol Neurosurg.* 2014;124:51–58.

Villanueva-Meyer JE, Mabray MC, Cha S. Current clinical brain tumor imaging. *Neurosurgery.* 2017;81:397–415.

2

Meningiomas

Overview

Meningiomas are the most common primary brain tumors in adults and comprise a group of mostly benign, slow-growing solid neoplasms that likely originated from meningothelial or arachnoid cells of the arachnoid layer that cover the brain and spinal cord. Meningiomas are dural based in location and can occur anywhere in the central nervous system (CNS). At least 15 different subtypes of meningiomas based on histology have been defined, some with unique molecular genetic features. Malignant meningioma, a rare variant, can metastasize outside of CNS, especially to the lung or liver.

	Age range (Yr) (mean)	Female: Male	Cell of origin	WHO Grade	Molecular/ genetic markers	Prognosis
Typical (Nine subtypes)	45–85 (65)	3:1	Meningo-thelial or arachnoid cap cells of arachnoid layer	I	Monosomy 22	Favorable; low risk of recurrence
Atypical (Three subtypes)	35–44	1:2		II	*NF2*	Less favorable; moderate risk of recurrence
Malignant (Three subtypes)	35–44	1:2		III	*NF2*	Poor; high risk of recurrence

Typical Meningiomas (WHO Grade I)

Definition: Mostly benign, slow-growing solid tumors arising from the arachnoid membranous layer of the meninges, which surrounds the brain and spinal cord.

Epidemiology: Most common primary brain tumor in adults, accounting for 36% of all brain tumors but comprise less than 3% of pediatric brain tumors. The vast majority occur as a solitary tumor (>90%) but can be multiple in the setting of prior radiation exposure or underlying syndrome such as neurofibromatosis type 2. Up to 70% of all meningiomas are benign, WHO grade I tumors, with grade II and grade III tumors accounting for 20%–25% and 1%–6%, respectively. Grades II and III tumors occur more frequently in men. Median age at diagnosis is 65 years, with higher incidence in women than in men with approximate ratio of 2.2:1. The incidence of meningioma is even higher in premenopausal women aged 35–44 years, where the ratio of women to men is 3.15:1. 2016 WHO central nervous system (CNS) Classification defines 15 different variants of meningioma based on histologic features:

Regardless of histologic features, meningiomas can be classified into at least 15 subtypes based on the anatomic location of tumor:

- Cavernous sinus, suprasellar/tuberculum sellae, cerebellopontine angle, cerebral convexity, intraorbital, intraventricular, olfactory groove, parasagittal, falcine, tentorium, petrous ridge/face, posterior fossa, sphenoid, foramen magnum and spinal.

Affected age group: Although meningioma is the most common primary brain tumor in adults, it occurs very rarely in children with predilection for clear cell and rhabdoid subtypes.

Molecular and genetic profile: There are at least 15 different histologic subtypes of meningiomas (Table 2.1). Several molecular and genetic abnormalities have been detected (Table 2.1), with characteristic differences between WHO grade I and WHO grade II/III tumors: monosomy 22, deletion of 1p, losses of chromosomes 6q, 9p, 10, 14q, and 18q, NF2 gene → truncated and presumably nonfunctional merlin protein (a.k.a. schwannomin).

Cerebrospinal Fluid (CSF) markers: None

Clinical features and standard therapy: Symptoms of meningioma depend mainly on size, location, and growth rate of tumor. Meningiomas are usually slow growing, benign, and clinically indolent. For grade I meningiomas, gross total resection of tumor leads to cure although recurrence can be seen in rare cases. For grade II and III meningiomas, gross total resection does not necessarily ensure cure because they can recur both at the site of original tumor or at a distant site.

TABLE 2.1 Histologic Subtypes of Meningiomas

	WHO Grade	Histologic hallmark	Molecular alteration	Anatomic location	Imaging hallmark
Meningothelial	I	Medium-sized epithelioid tumor cells, abundant eosinophilic cytoplasm; Epithelioid, largely uniform cells with oval nuclei forming lobules demarcated by collagenous septa	Monosomy 22	Parasagittal	Most common subtype; classic imaging features-homogeneously enhancing dural based mass with isointense T1 and T2 signal
Fibrous or fibroblastic	I	Spindle cells with intercellular collagen	NF2 EMA	Convexity	Dark on T2
Transitional	I	Meningothelial, fibrous and transitional patterns; whorls and psammoma bodies; Lobular and fascicular foci of cells with conspicuous tight whorls and psammoma bodies	NF2	Parasagittal	Partially calcified
Psammomatous	I	Psammoma bodies, calcified masses; Confluent psammoma bodies replacing tumor cells and forming irregular calcified masses and bone	–	Thoracic spine	Heavily calcified mass
Angiomatous	I	Numerous blood vessels in greater proportion than tumor mass	Aneuploid, polysomies chromo-somes 5,13,20	Convexity	Marked tumor hypervascularity; prominent peritumoral edema

TABLE 2.1 **(continued)**

	WHO Grade	Histologic hallmark	Molecular alteration	Anatomic location	Imaging hallmark
Microcystic	I	Spider-like cells with long thin processes; Cells with thin, elongated processes encompassing microcysts and creating a cobweb-like background	–	Convexity	Hyperintense on T2 & hypointense on T1; prominent peritumoral edema; micro- and macro-cystic changes
Secretory	I	Pseudo-psammoma bodies with acid-Schiff-positive eosinophilic secretions and immunoreactivity for carcinoembryonic antigen and cytokeratin	KLF4 K409Q, TRAF7 mutations	Skull base	Prominent peritumoral edema
Lymphoplasma-cyte-rich	I	Dense infiltrates of lympho-cytes & plasma cells; Chronic inflammatory infiltrates	–	Convexity, skull base, parasagittal, spine	Markedly reduced on diffusion due to high cellularity
Metaplastic	I	Focal or widespread mesen-chymal components- carti-laginous/chondroid, osseous, lipomatous, xanthomatous, myxoid patterns	–	Convexity	Scattered areas if calcium and fat within the tumor
Chordoid	II	Physaliferous-like cells resembling chordoma; Cords or trabeculae of eosinophilic, vacuolated cells set in an abundant mucoid matrix	–	–	High on T2

TABLE 2.1 *(continued)*

	WHO Grade	Histologic hallmark	Molecular alteration	Anatomic location	Imaging hallmark
Clear cell	II	Polygonal cells with clear cytoplasm; prominent interstitial & perivascular hyalinization; pattern-less or sheeting architecture, glycogen-rich cytoplasm and prominent perivascular and interstitial collagen	Switch/Sucrose non-fermentable (SWI/SNF) Related, Matrix Associated, Actin Dependent Regulator of Chromatin, Subfamily E, Member 1 mutations	Spine, posterior fossa	High on T2 with exuberant cystic architecture
Atypical	II	Meningothelial cells invading into brain parenchyma; Increased mitotic activity, brain invasion with increased cellularity, small cells with a high nuclear-to-cytoplasmic ratio, prominent nucleoli, sheeting and foci of necrosis	Loss: 1p, 6q, 10, 14q, 18q Gain: 1q, 9q, 12q, 15q, 17q, 20q	–	Irregular border with neighboring brain
Papillary	III	Epithelioid tumor cells in a papillary or pseudopapillary pattern	–	Intraventricular, tuberculum sellae	Lobular contour; lack of dural tail
Rhabdoid	III	Rhabdoid cells with eccentric vesicular nuclei & prominent eosinophilic paranuclear inclusions	SMARCB1 retained	–	Reduced on diffusion; marked peritumoral edema; irregular border with neighboring brain
Anaplastic (malignant)	III	Cellular anaplasia and excessive mitoses	LOSS: 22q, 1p, 6q, 10, 14q, 18q, 9p; NF2 & TERT mutations	–	Reduced on diffusion; irregular border with neighboring brain; metastases to lung or liver

To minimize local recurrence, adjuvant radiation therapy is often used, especially when there is any residual tumor, but it does not prevent distant recurrence.

Imaging

Meningiomas are circumscribed, dural-based masses that have similar density or signal to brain parenchyma on CT or MRI, respectively, and enhance avidly following the administration of intravenous contrast, both iodine-based and gadolinium-based intravenous contrast agents. Meningiomas often show "dural tail" enhancement, which is contiguous with the primary mass but extends farther into the adjacent dura. Most meningiomas are solid masses, but some can contain prominent cystic components. The imaging appearance of meningiomas can vary widely depending on the histologic subtypes and presence and degree of intratumoral calcium. Prominent intratumoral hemorrhage is rare in meningioma. Meningiomas can be cellular and show homogeneous reduced diffusion on diffusion-weighted imaging, and some are hypervascular, showing markedly increased vascularity on perfusion MRI.

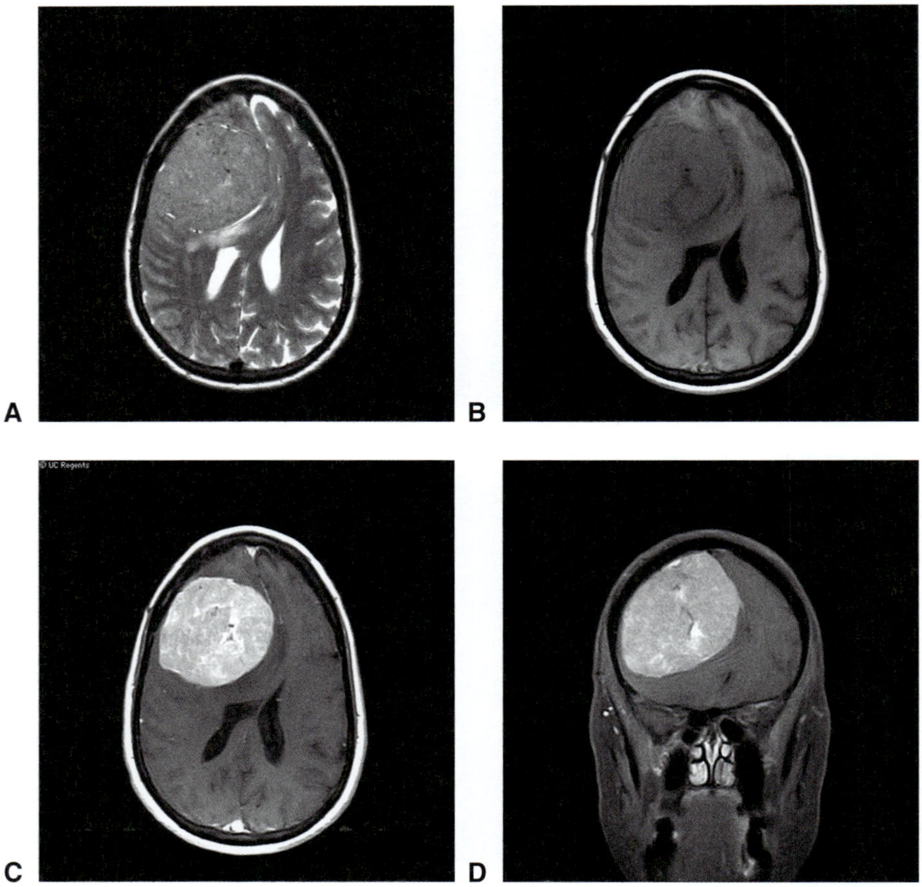

Figure 2.1. Imaging of meningothelial meningioma. A. Axial T2: hypointense mass. **B.** Axial T1-precontrast: hypointense mass. **C.** Axial T1-postcontrast: avid and homogeneous enhancement. **D.** Coronal T1-postcontrast: avid and homogeneous enhancement.

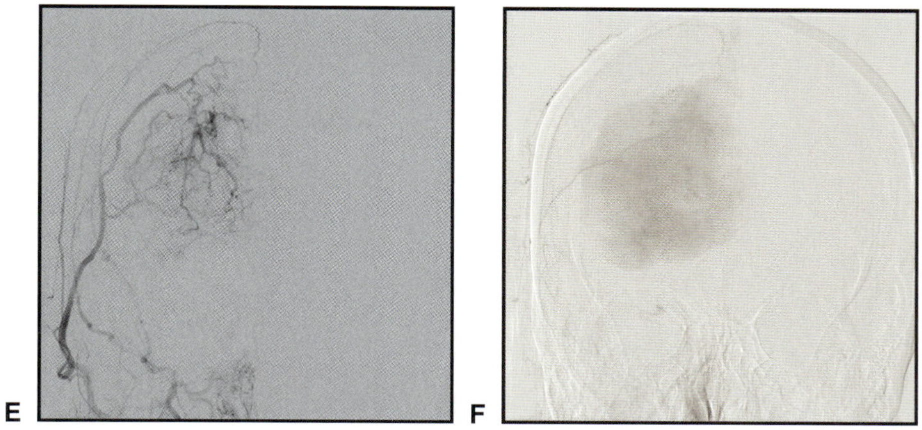

Figure 2.1. ***(continued)*** **E.** Digital Subtraction Angiography (DSA): Early arterial phase shows early tumor blush. **F.** DSA: Late venous phase shows persistent tumor blush.

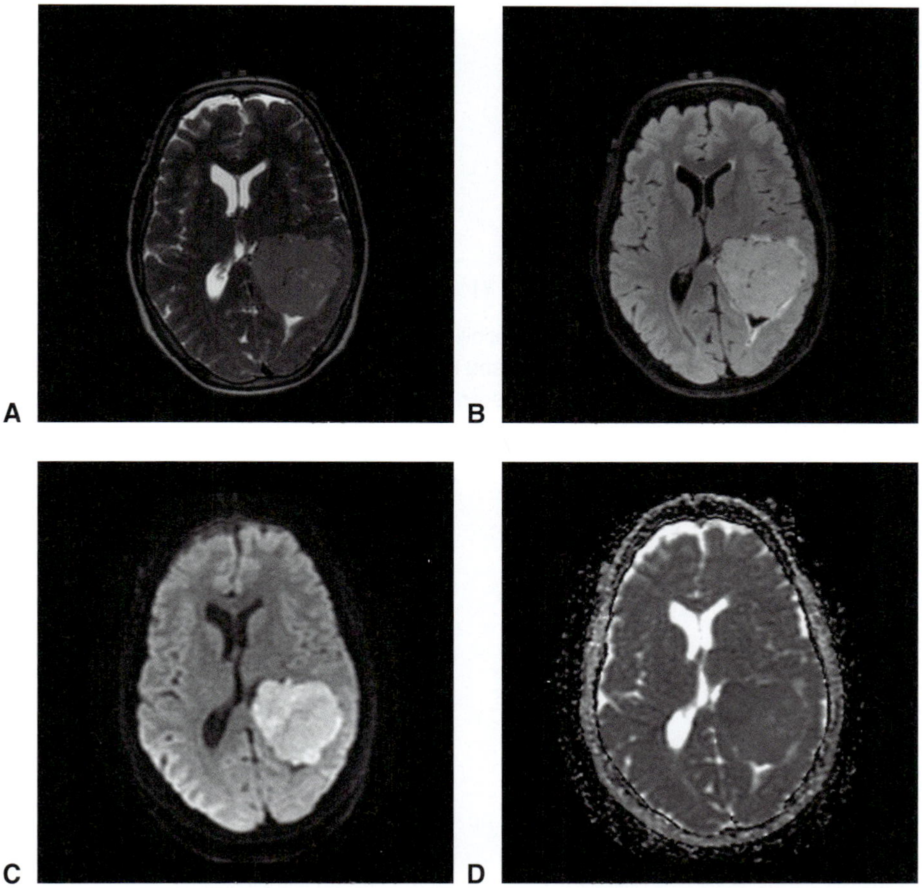

Figure 2.2. **Imaging of intraventricular fibrous meningioma. A.** Axial T2: Homogeneously hypointense. **B.** Axial Fluid Associated Inversion Recovery (FLAIR): Homogeneously hyperintense. **C.** Axial Diffusion-Weighted Imaging: Homogeneously reduced. **D.** Axial Apparent Diffusion Coefficient (ADC): Homogeneously reduced.

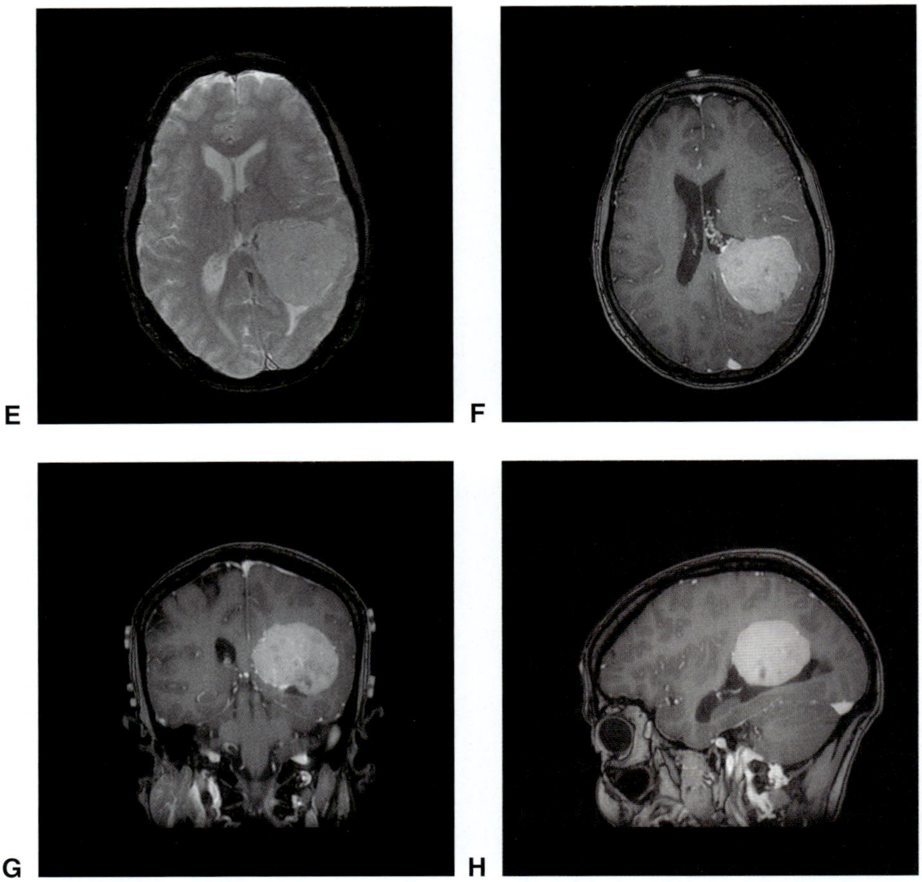

Figure 2.2. ***(continued)*** **E.** Axial Susceptibility-Weighted Imaging: No blood products or calcium. **F.** Axial T1 postcontrast: Avid and homogeneous enhancement. **G.** Coronal T1 postcontrast: Avid and homogeneous enhancement. **H.** Sagittal T1 postcontrast: Avid and homogeneous enhancement.

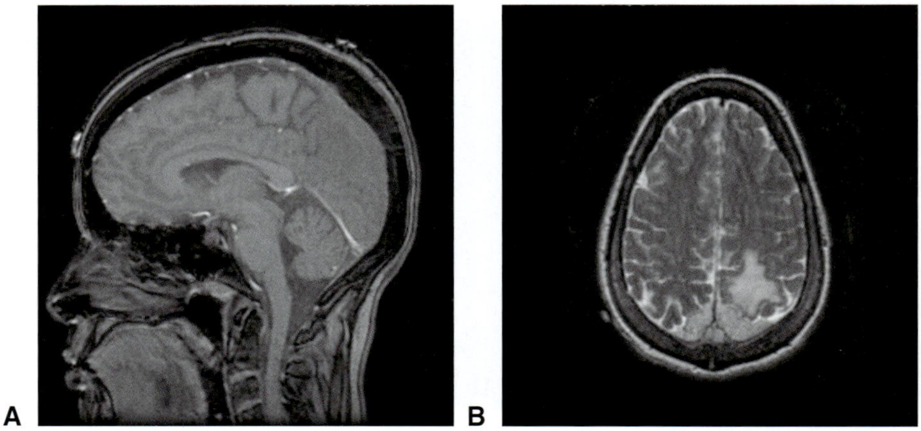

Figure 2.3. **Imaging of parasagittal transitional meningioma. A.** Sagittal T1 precontrast: Isointense to surrounding brain. **B.** Axial T2: Mildly hyperintense.

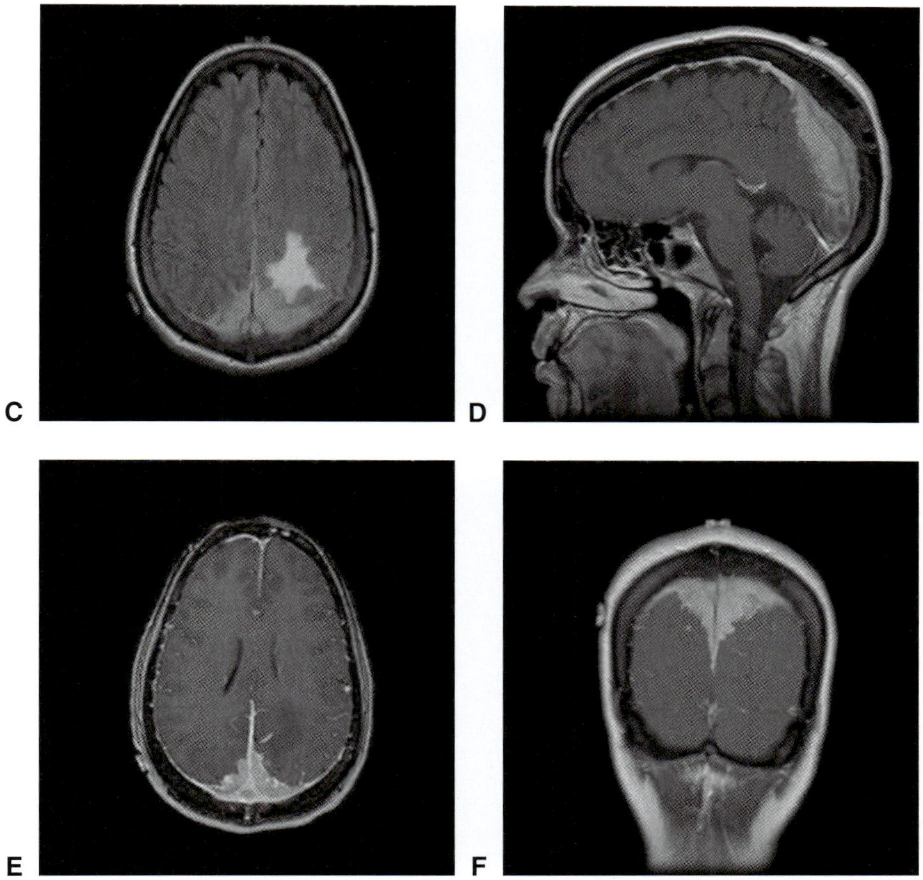

Figure 2.3. ***(continued)*** **C.** Axial FLAIR: Mildly hyperintense. **D.** Sagittal T1 postcontrast: Avid enhancement with tumor within the superior sagittal sinus. **E.** Axial T1 postcontrast: Avid enhancement with tumor within the superior sagittal sinus. **F.** Coronal T1 postcontrast: Avid enhancement with tumor within the superior sagittal sinus.

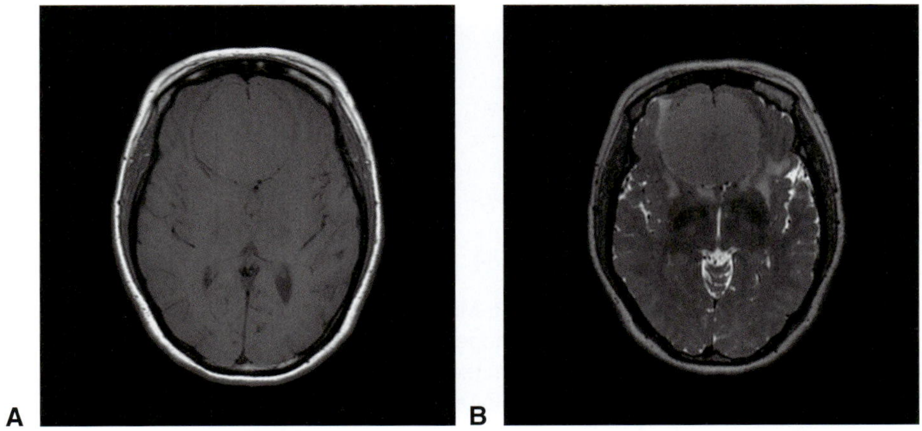

Figure 2.4. Imaging of psammomatous meningioma involving the planum sphenoidale and tuberculum sellae. A. Axial T1 precontrast: Isointense to surrounding brain. **B.** Axial T2: Homogeneously hypointense.

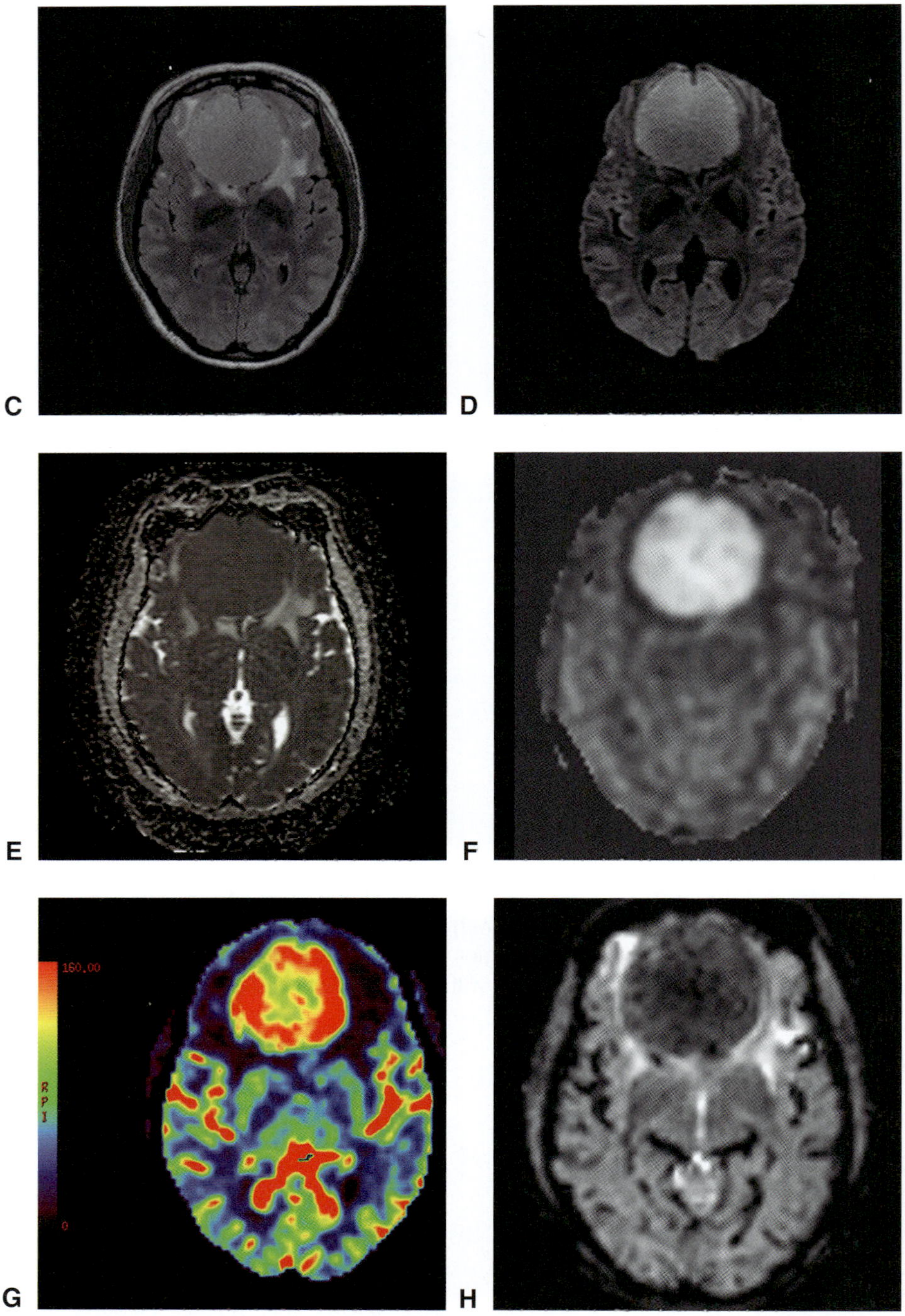

Figure 2.4. ***(continued)*** **C.** Axial FLAIR: Mildly hyperintense. **D.** Axial DWI: Homogeneously reduced. **E.** Axial ADC: Homogeneously reduced. **F.** Axial Arterial Spin Labeling (ASL) (gray-scale CBF map): Markedly hypervascular with increased blood flow. **G.** Axial Arterial Spin Labeling (color scale CBF map): Markedly hypervascular with increased blood flow, especially around the outer margin of tumor. **H.** Axial Dynamic Susceptibility-Weighted Contrast (DSC) (gray-scale CBV map): Markedly hypervascular with increased blood volume.

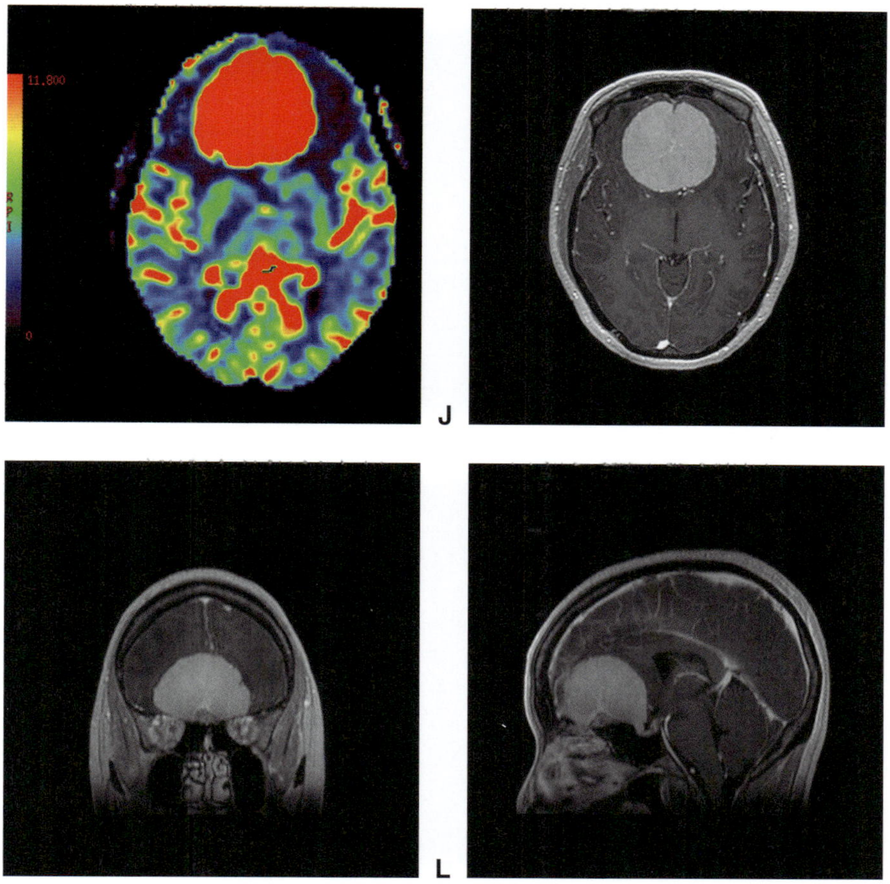

Figure 2.4. ***(continued)*** **I.** Axial DSC (color scale CBV map): Markedly hypervascular with increased blood volume. **J.** Axial T1 postcontrast: Avid and homogeneous enhancement. **K.** Coronal T1 postcontrast: Avid and homogeneous enhancement. **L.** Sagittal T1 postcontrast: Avid and homogeneous enhancement.

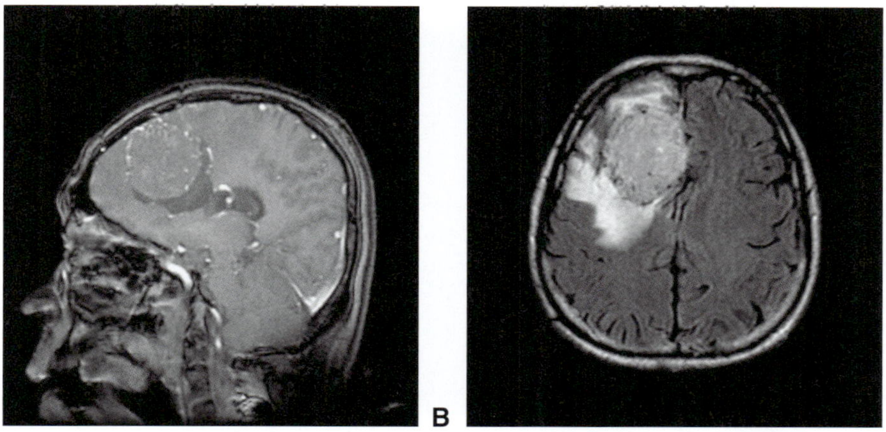

Figure 2.5. Imaging of angiomatous meningioma. A. Sagittal T1-precontrast: Isointense to surrounding brain with prominent cystic cap along inferior margin. **B.** Axial FLAIR: Mildly hyperintense with prominent vessels in and around the tumor and marked peritumoral edema.

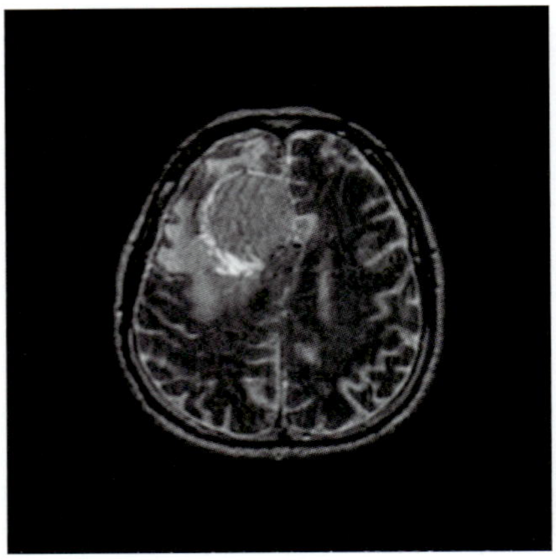
C

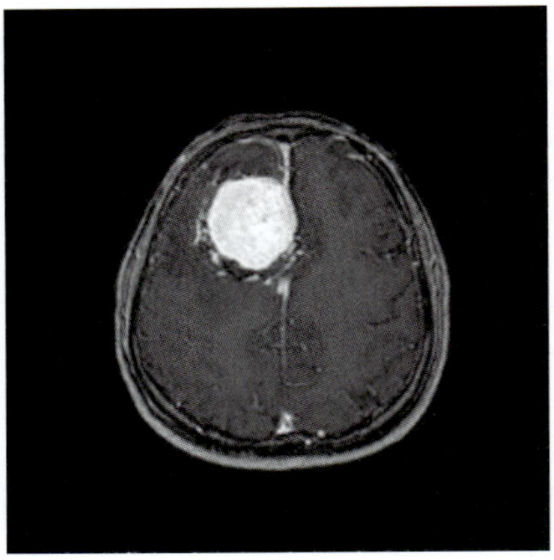
D

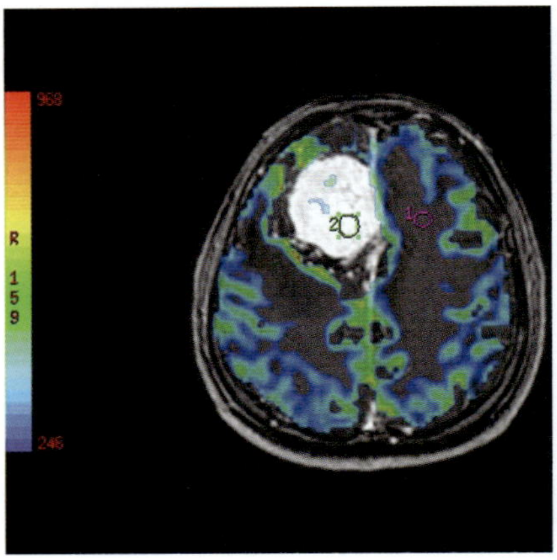

E

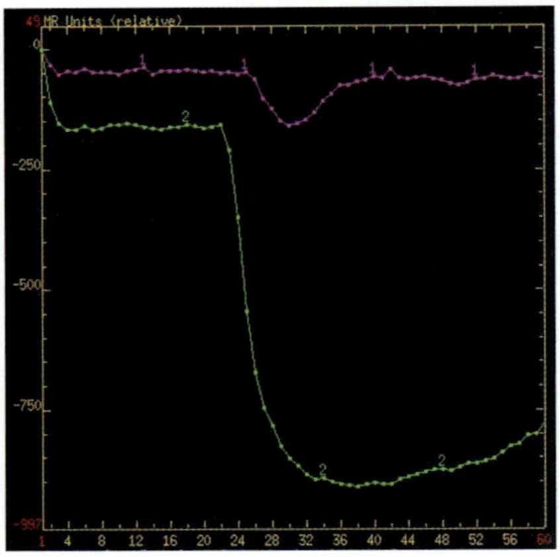

F

Figure 2.5. ***(continued)*** **C.** Axial T2: Hypointense with prominent cystic cap along the lateral and posterior margin. **D.** Axial T1 postcontrast: Avid and homogeneous enhancement with prominent peritumoral vessels. **E.** Axial T1 postcontrast and DSC fused: Region of interests in normal brain (1) and in tumor (2). **F.** Time curve from DSC: Marked tumor hypervascularity with leaky permeability compared to normal brain.

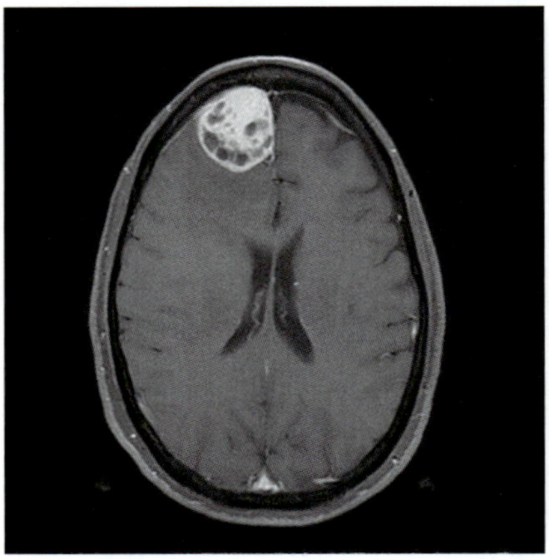
A

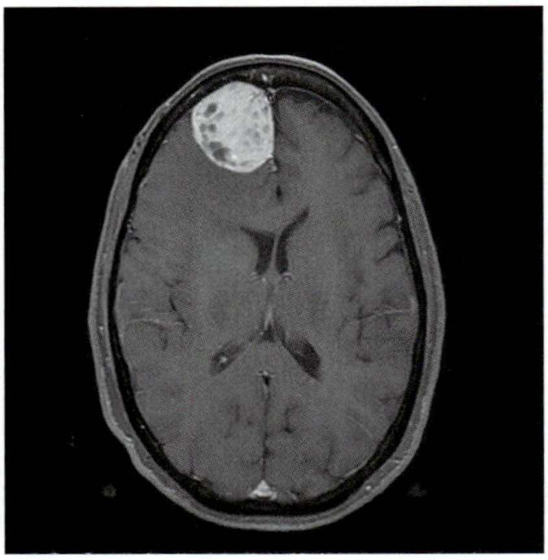
B

Figure 2.6. Imaging of microcystic meningioma. A. Axial T1 postcontrast: Avid enhancement except in areas of cysts. **B.** Axial T1 postcontrast: Avid enhancement except in areas of cysts.

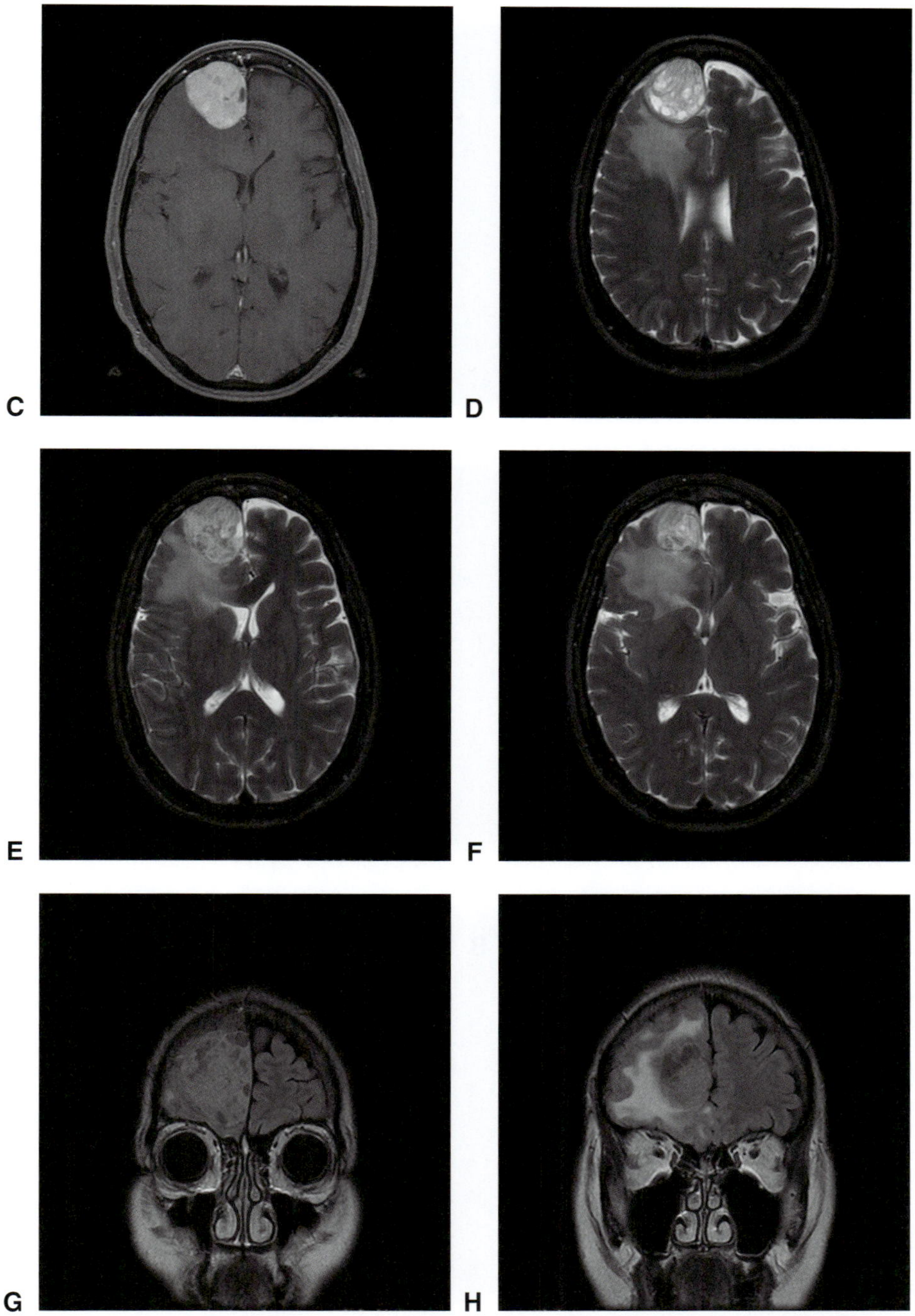

Figure 2.6. ***(continued)*** **C.** Axial T1 postcontrast: Avid enhancement except in areas of cysts. **D.** Axial T2: Heterogeneously hyperintense. **E.** Axial T2: Heterogeneously hyperintense. **F.** Axial T2: Heterogeneously hyperintense. **G.** Coronal FLAIR: Mildly hyperintense with prominent cysts. **H.** Coronal FLAIR: Macrocystic areas within the tumor.

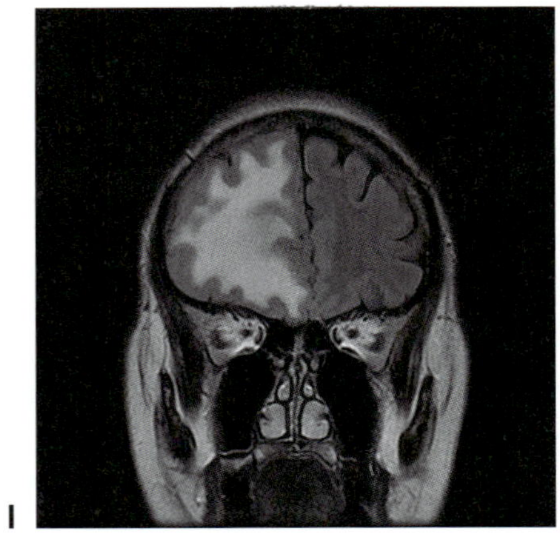

Figure 2.6. ***(continued)*** **I.** Coronal FLAIR: Marked peritumoral edema.

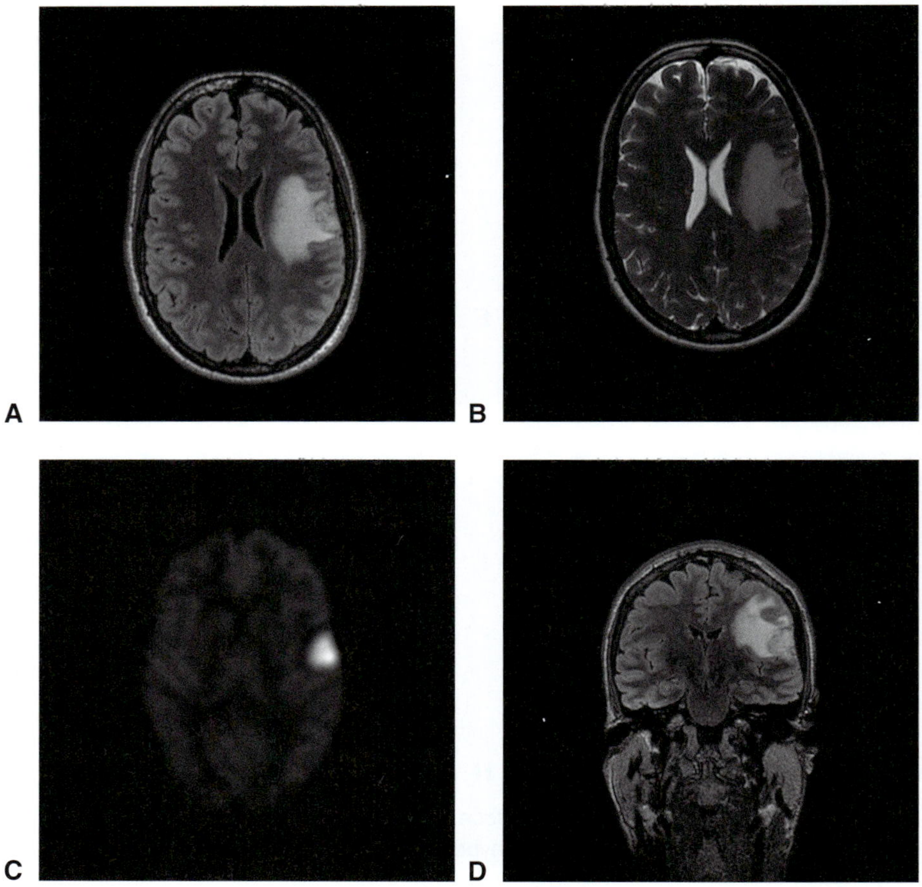

Figure 2.7. Imaging of secretory meningioma. A. Axial FLAIR: Heterogeneously hyperintense mass with prominent peritumoral edema. **B.** Axial T2: Heterogeneously hypointense mass with prominent peritumoral edema. **C.** Axial ASL: Markedly increase tumor blood flow. **D.** Coronal FLAIR: Heterogeneously hyperintense mass with prominent peritumoral edema.

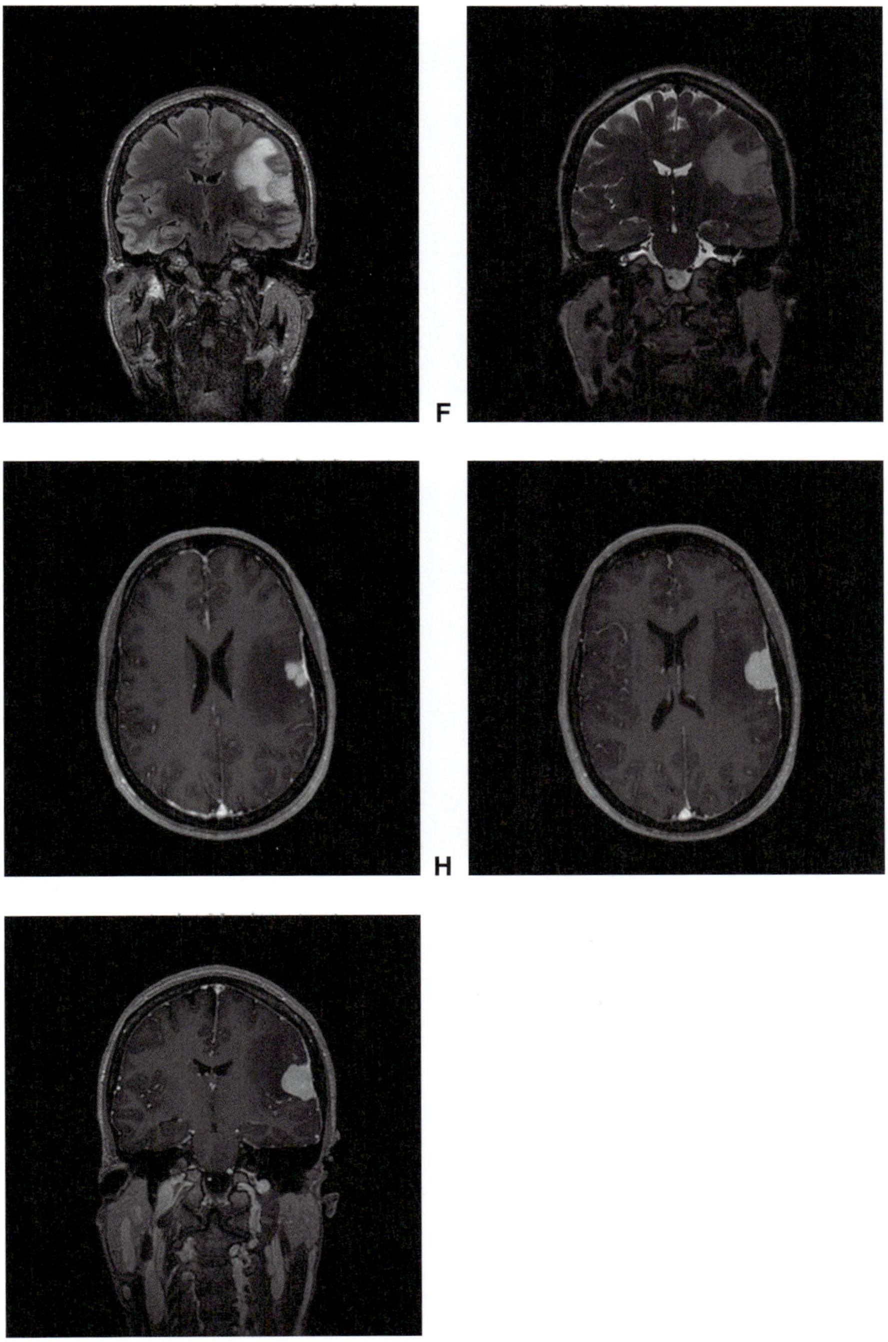

Figure 2.7. ***(continued)*** **E.** Coronal FLAIR: Heterogeneously hyperintense mass with prominent peritumoral edema. **F.** Coronal T2: Heterogeneously hypointense mass with prominent peritumoral edema. **G.** Axial T1 postcontrast: Avid enhancement with prominent dural tail. **H.** Axial T1 postcontrast: Avid enhancement with prominent dural tail. **I.** Coronal T1 postcontrast: Avid enhancement with prominent dural tail.

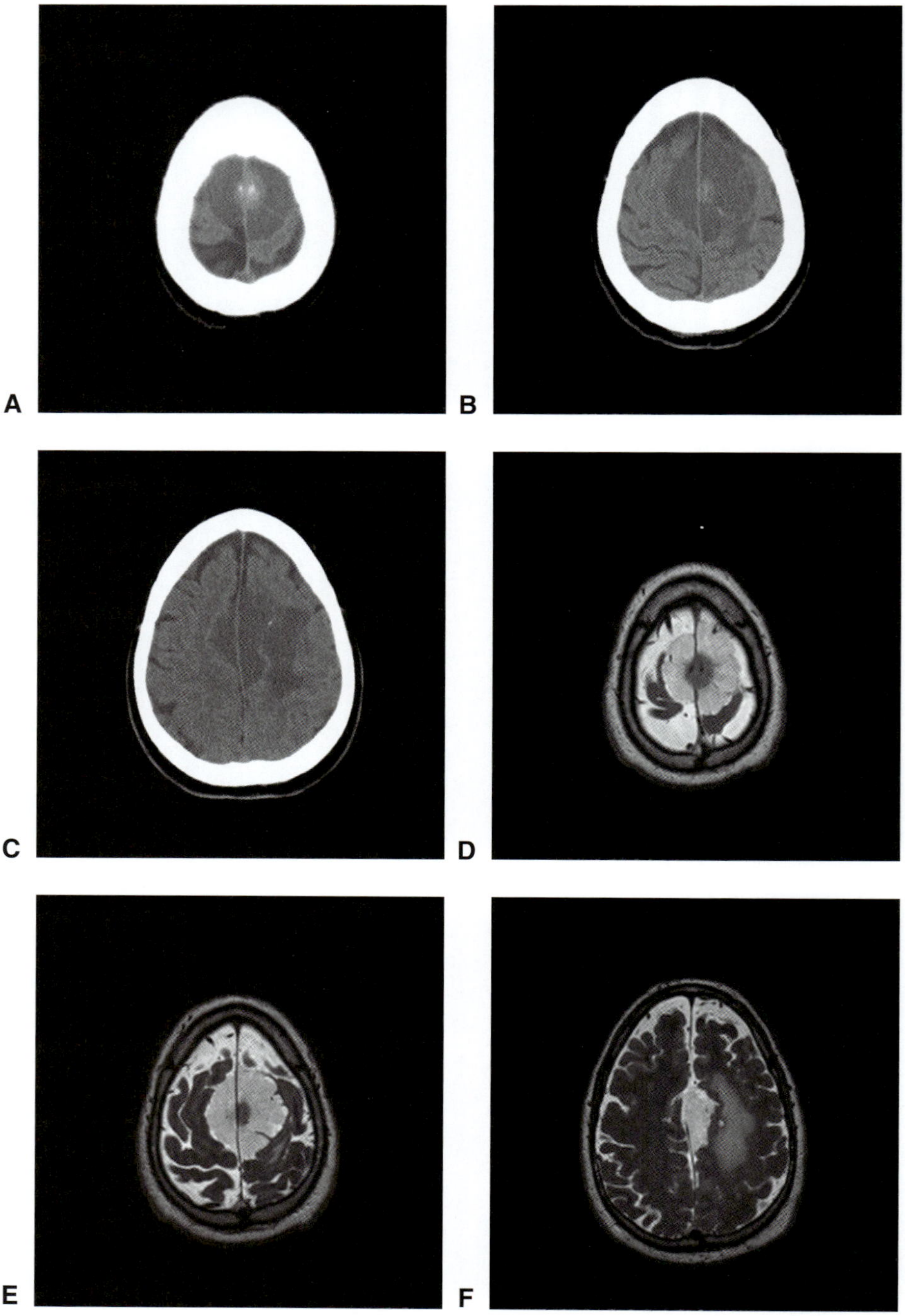

Figure 2.8. **Imaging of lymphoplasmacyte-rich meningioma. A–C.** Axial CT unenhanced: Low-density bi-falcine mass with central calcium. **D–F.** Axial T2: Hyperintense bi-falcine mass with central hypointense component.

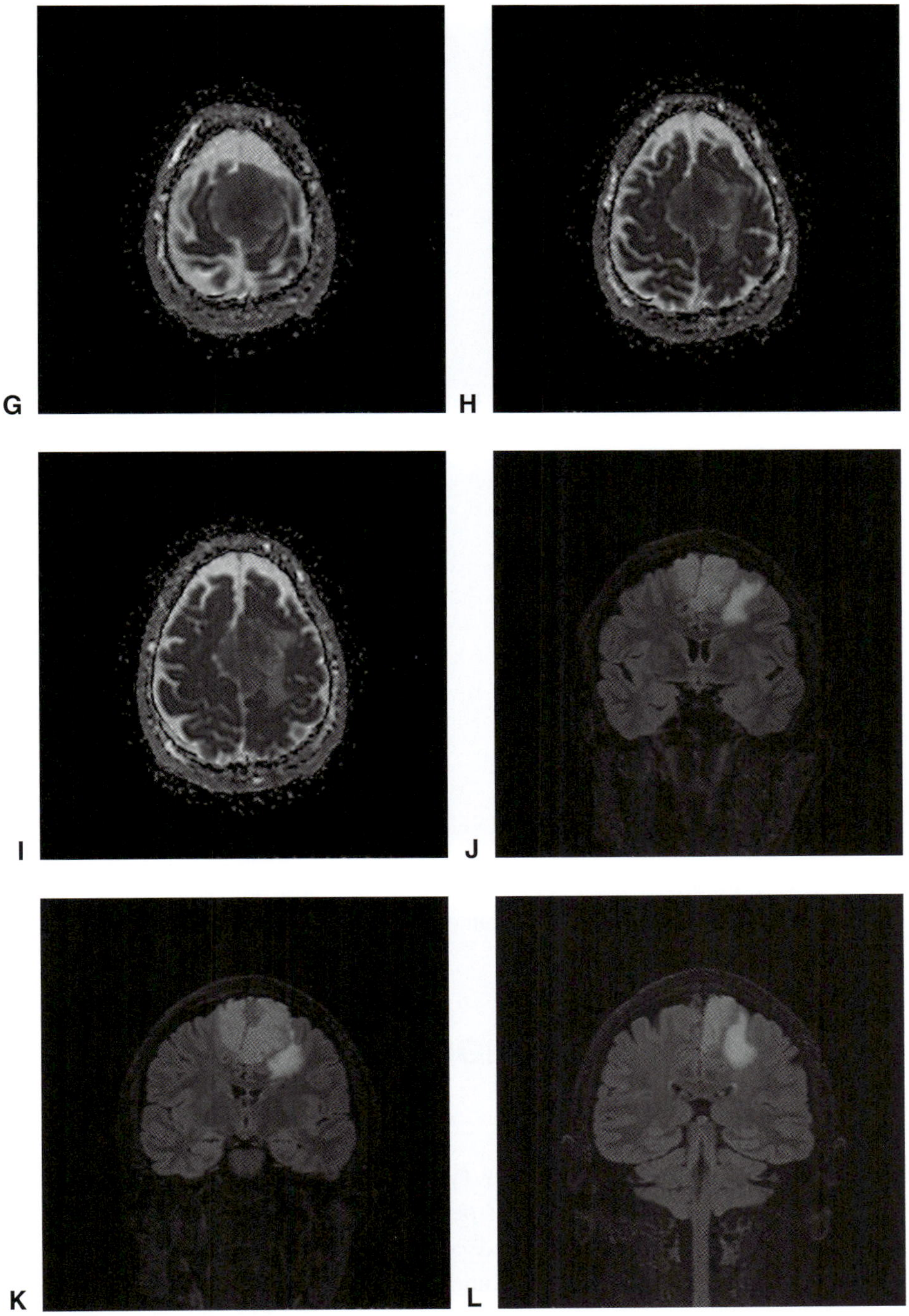

Figure 2.8. ***(continued)*** **G–I.** Axial ADC: Homogeneously reduced diffusion within the bi-falcine mass. **J–L.** Coronal FLAIR: Hyperintense mass.

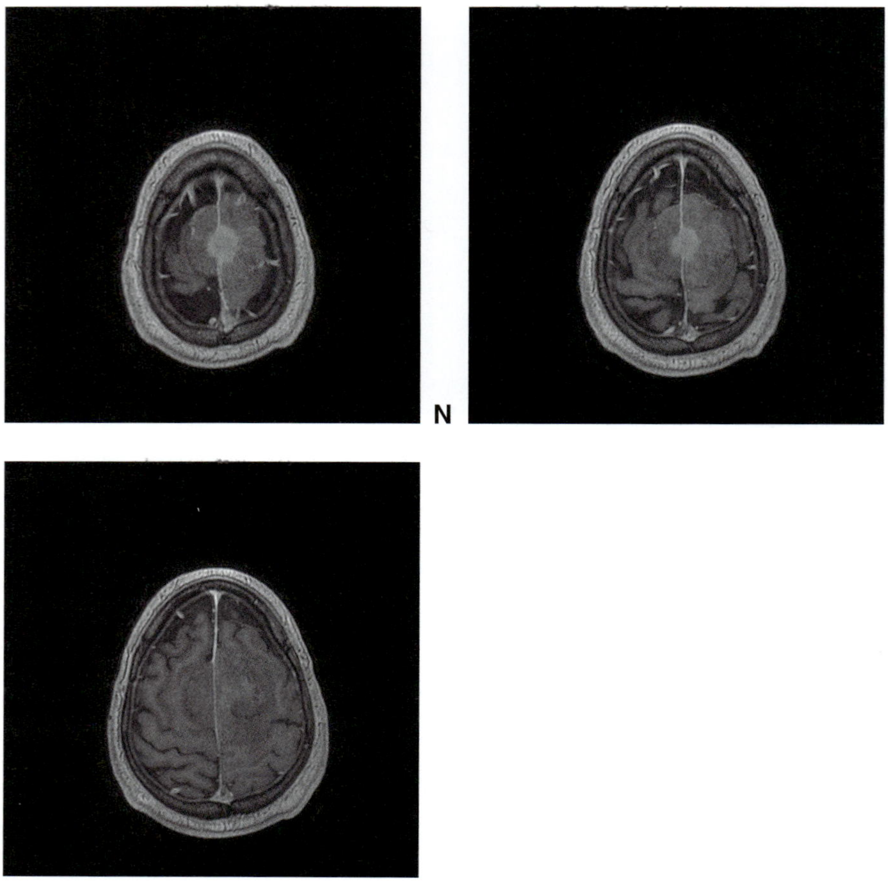

M N O

Figure 2.8. ***(continued)*** **M–O.** Axial T1 postcontrast: Avid enhancement of the central component with minimal enhancement within the bi-falcine component.

Atypical Meningiomas (WHO Grade II)

Definition: An intermediate grade (WHO Grade II) meningioma with increased mitotic activity (>4 mitoses per 10 high-powered fields), histologic evidence of brain invasion, increased cellularity, cells with a high nuclear-to-cytoplasmic ratio, and foci of spontaneous necrosis.

Epidemiology: Atypical meningiomas are rarer than the typical meningioma but tend to occur at higher rates in males. Incidence of atypical meningiomas varies significantly by race, occurring higher in African Americans.

Affected age group: Tends to affect the younger age group (third to fourth decades) compared to Atypical and malignant meningiomas have a slight male predominance.

Molecular and genetic profile: Losses of chromosomes 6q, 9p, 10, 14q, and 18q are more frequent in atypical meningiomas.

CSF markers: None.

Clinical features and standard therapy: Surgical resection is the primary treatment, and there is no effective chemotherapy or targeted agents. There is a higher recurrence rate for subtotally resected atypical meningioma.

Imaging

Overall imaging features of atypical meningiomas are similar to typical meningiomas but with higher propensity for brain invasion. Subtle brain invasion along the pial surface may not be evident on imaging, and the presence of vasogenic edema in the brain parenchyma next to meningioma does not necessarily represent brain invasion.

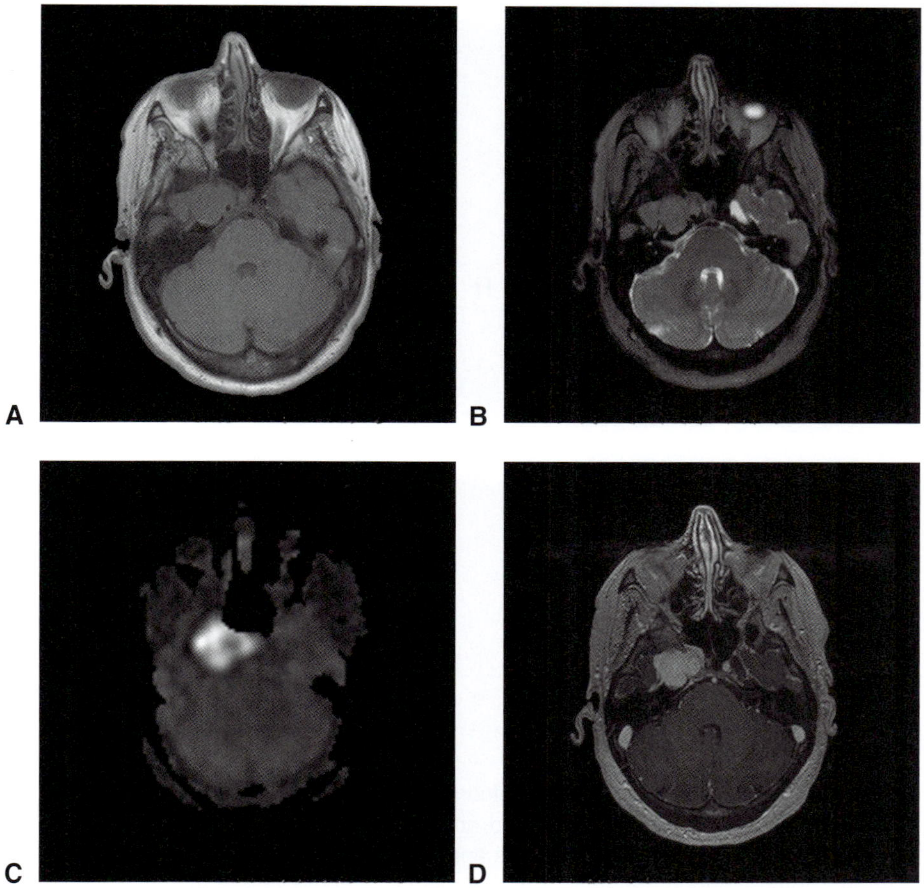

Figure 2.9. Imaging of chordoid meningioma of the cavernous sinus. A. Axial T1 precontrast: Isointense mass encasing and mildly narrowing right cavernous internal carotid artery. **B.** Axial T2: Isointense mass encasing and mildly narrowing right cavernous internal carotid artery. **C.** Axial ASL: Markedly increased tumor blood flow. **D.** Axial T1 postcontrast: Avid and homogeneous enhancement.

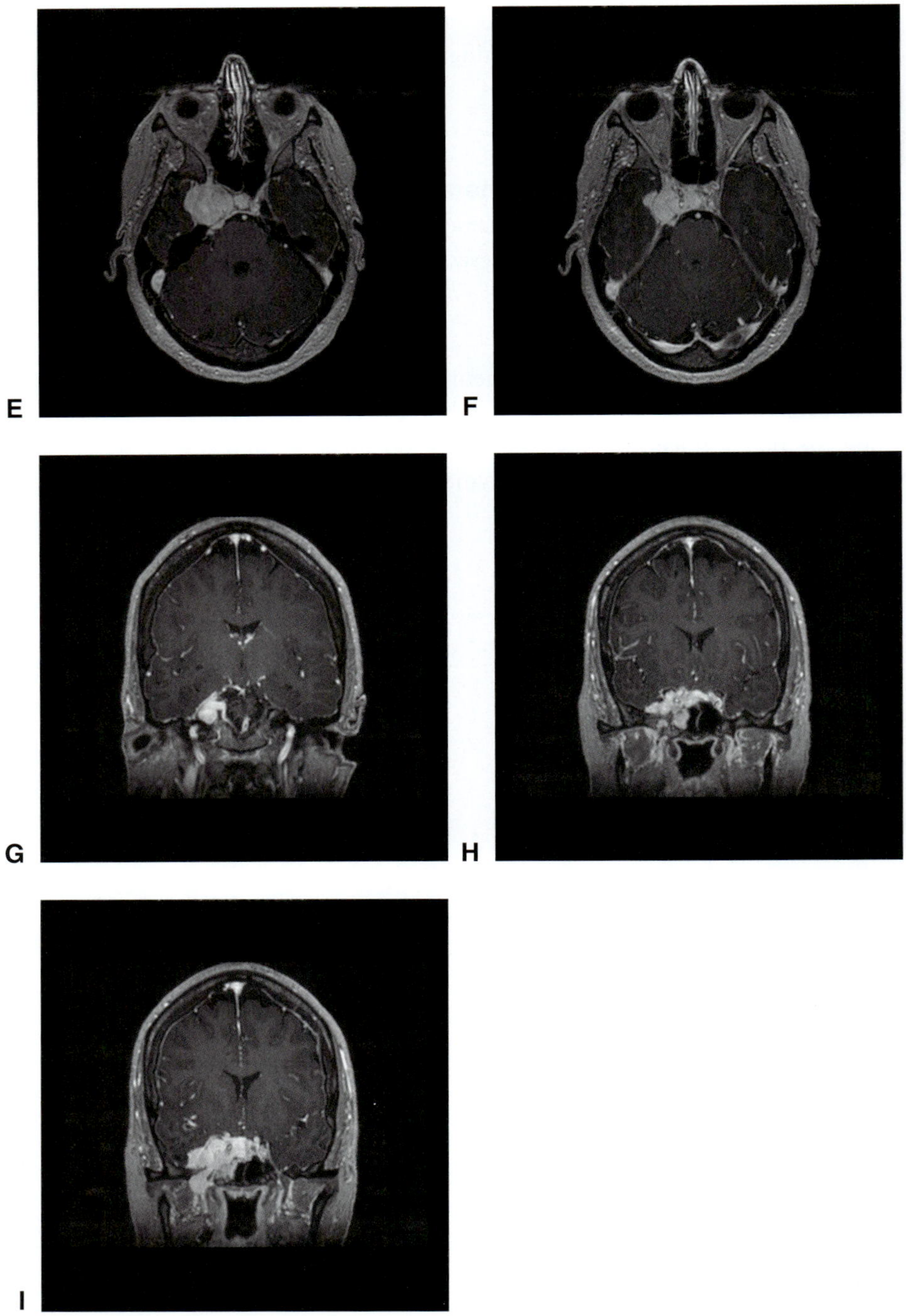

Figure 2.9. ***(continued)*** **E.** Axial T1 postcontrast: Avid and homogeneous enhancement. **F.** Axial T1 postcontrast: Avid and homogeneous enhancement. **G.** Coronal T1 postcontrast: Avid and homogeneous enhancement. **H.** Coronal T1 postcontrast: Avid and homogeneous enhancement. **I.** Coronal T1 postcontrast: Avid and homogeneous enhancement.

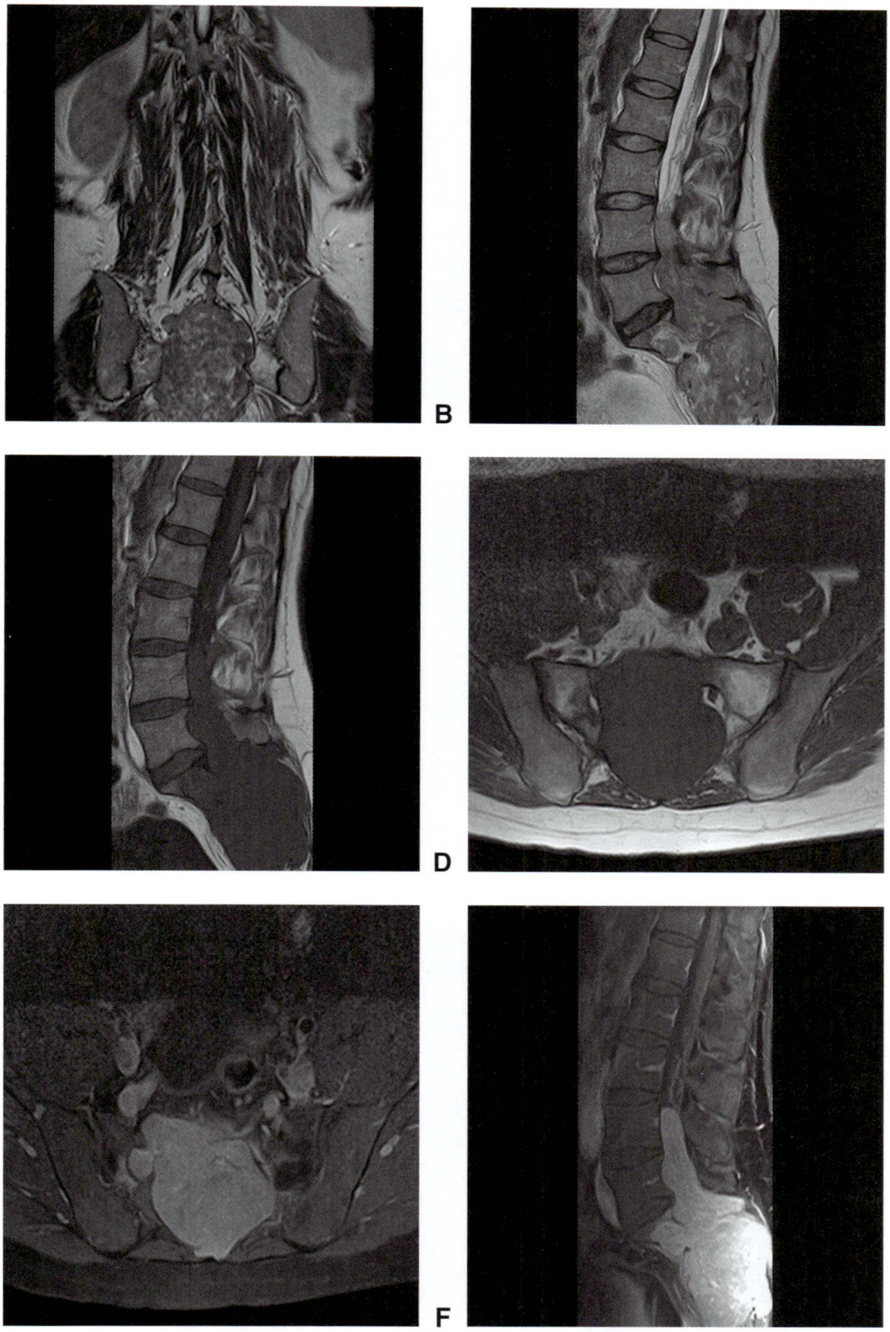

A B C D E F

Figure 2.10. Imaging of clear cell meningioma. A. Coronal T2: Heterogeneously hypointense mass centered in the sacrum. **B.** Sagittal T2: Heterogeneously hypointense mass centered in the sacrum and filling the distal lumbar and sacral thecal sac. **C.** Sagittal T1: Homogeneously hypointense mass. **D.** Axial T1 precontrast: Homogeneously hypointense and expansile mass replacing the sacrum. **E.** Axial T1 postcontrast: Avid and homogeneous enhancement. **F.** Sagittal T1 postcontrast: Avid and homogeneous enhancement.

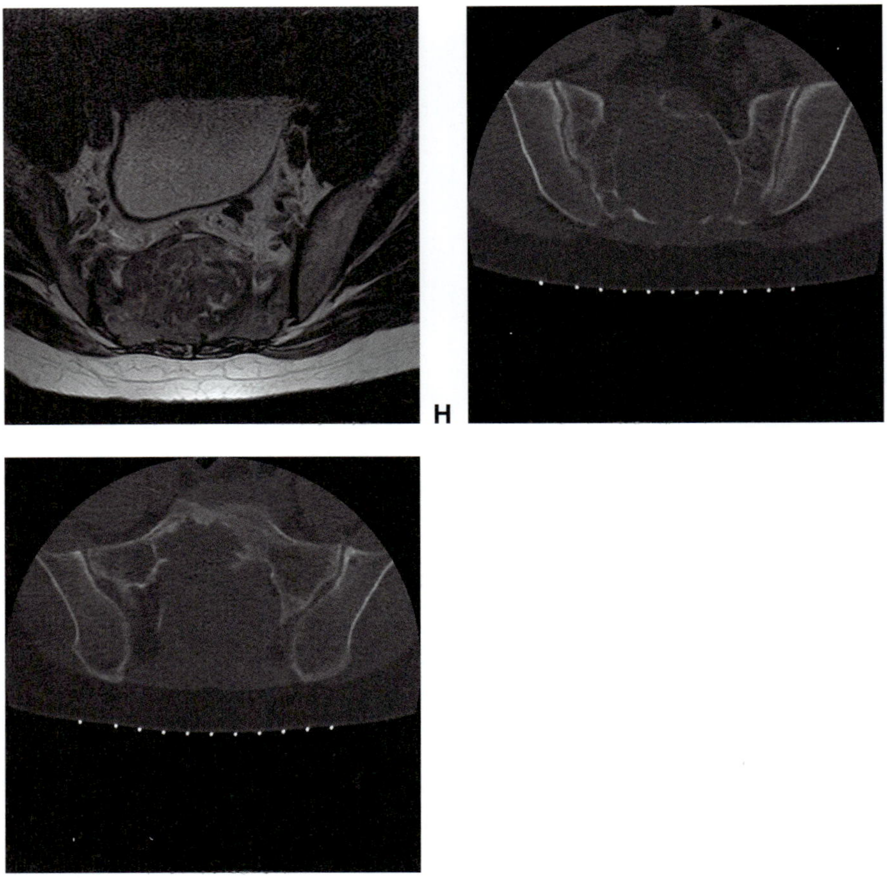

G H I

Figure 2.10. ***(continued)*** **G.** Axial T2: Heterogeneously hypointense mass. **H.** Axial CT bone window: Expansile mass with smooth bony erosion and cortical breakthrough. **I.** Axial CT bone window: Expansile mass with smooth bony erosion and cortical breakthrough.

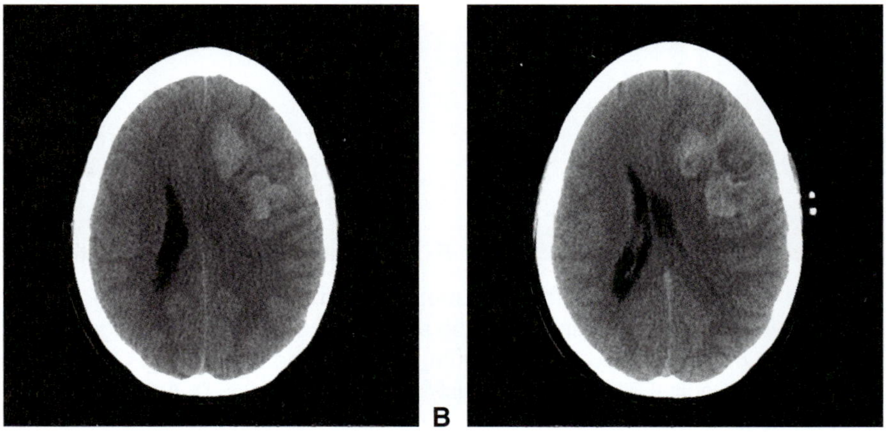

A B

Figure 2.11. Imaging of atypical meningioma. A. Axial CT unenhanced: Heterogeneously hyperdense mass. **B.** Axial CT unenhanced: Heterogeneously hyperdense mass.

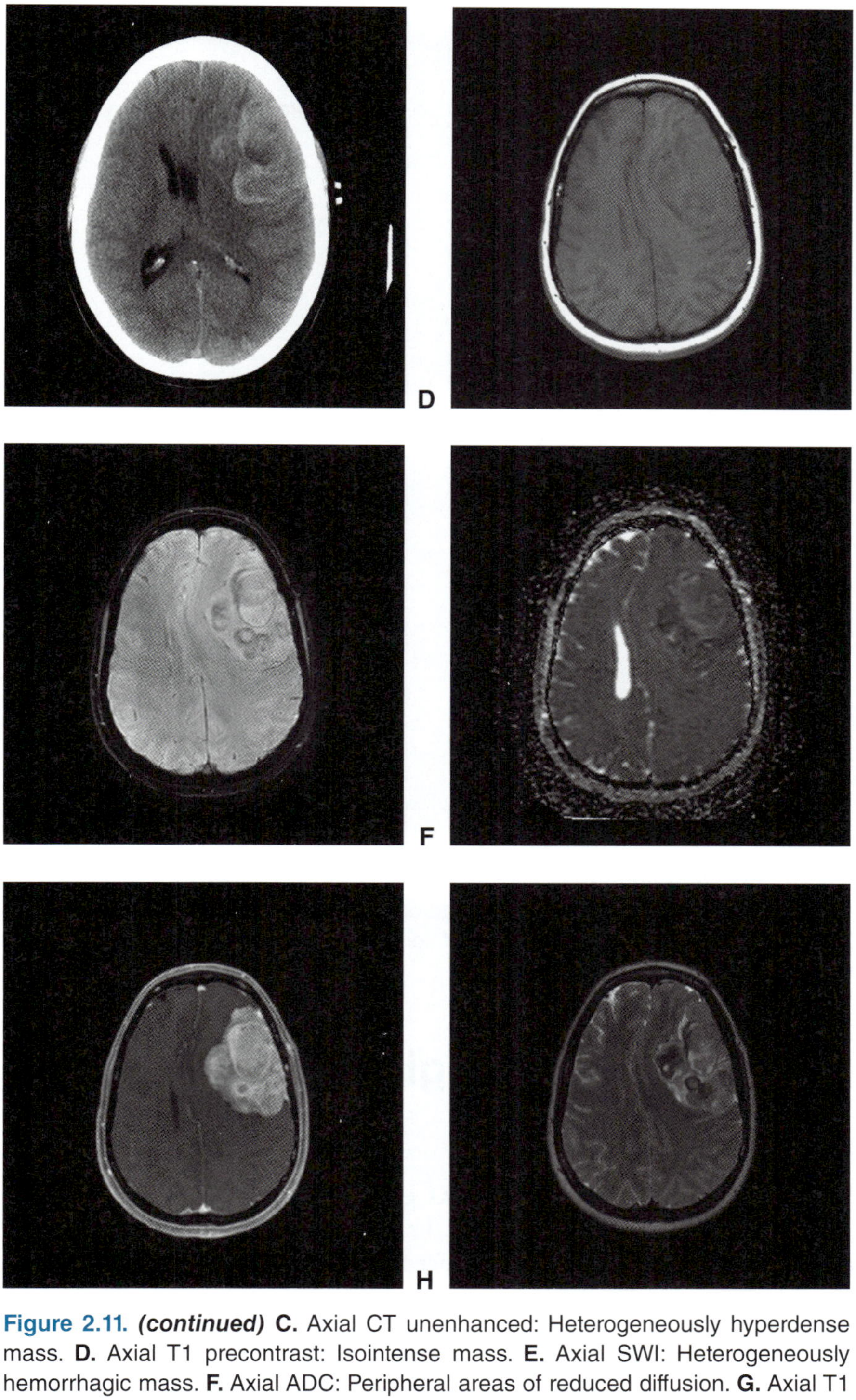

C D E F G H

Figure 2.11. ***(continued)*** **C.** Axial CT unenhanced: Heterogeneously hyperdense mass. **D.** Axial T1 precontrast: Isointense mass. **E.** Axial SWI: Heterogeneously hemorrhagic mass. **F.** Axial ADC: Peripheral areas of reduced diffusion. **G.** Axial T1 postcontrast: Avid but heterogeneous enhancement. **H.** Axial T2: Heterogeneously hypointense areas of loculation.

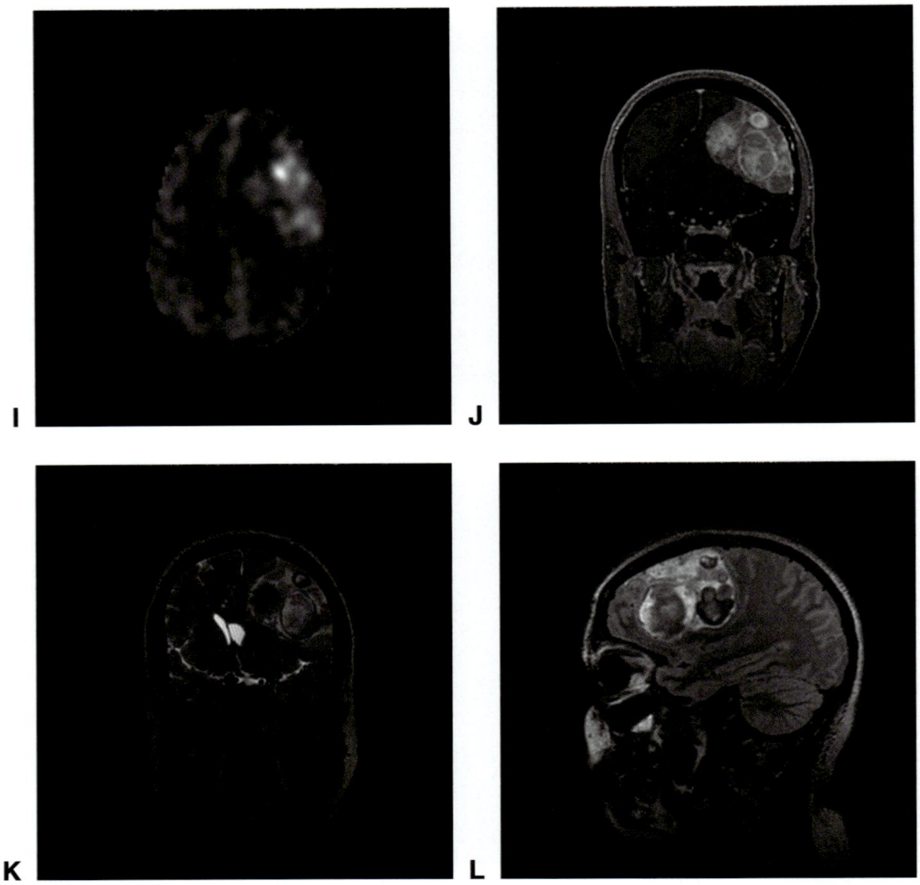

Figure 2.11. ***(continued)*** **I.** Axial ASL: Markedly increased tumor blood flow. **J.** Coronal T1 postcontrast: Avid but heterogeneous enhancement. **K.** Coronal T2: Heterogeneously hypointense areas of loculation. **L.** Sagittal FLAIR: Heterogeneously hypointense areas of loculation.

Malignant Meningiomas (WHO Grade III)

Definition: Highly aggressive, WHO grade III meningioma comprised of cellular anaplasia, geographic necrosis, brain invasion, and/or excessive mitotic activity defined as at least 20 mitoses per 10 high-power field.

Epidemiology: Malignant meningiomas are much rarer than the typical meningioma but tend to occur at higher rates in males.

Affected age group: Tends to affect younger age group (third to fourth decades) than typical meningioma, and men are more common than women unlikely typical meningioma.

Molecular and genetic profile:

- 22q, 1p, 6q, 10, 14q, 18q, and/or 9p deletions
- NF2 and Telomerase Reserve Transcriptase (TERT) promoter region mutations

CSF markers: None.

Clinical features and standard therapy: Surgical resection is the primary treatment, and there is no effective chemotherapy or targeted agents. There is a higher recurrence rate for subtotally resected malignant meningioma. Although uncommon, distant metastasis of malignancy outside of CNS, most commonly to liver and lung, has been reported.

Imaging

Overall imaging features of malignant meningiomas show aggressive features such as frank brain invasion and hemorrhage.

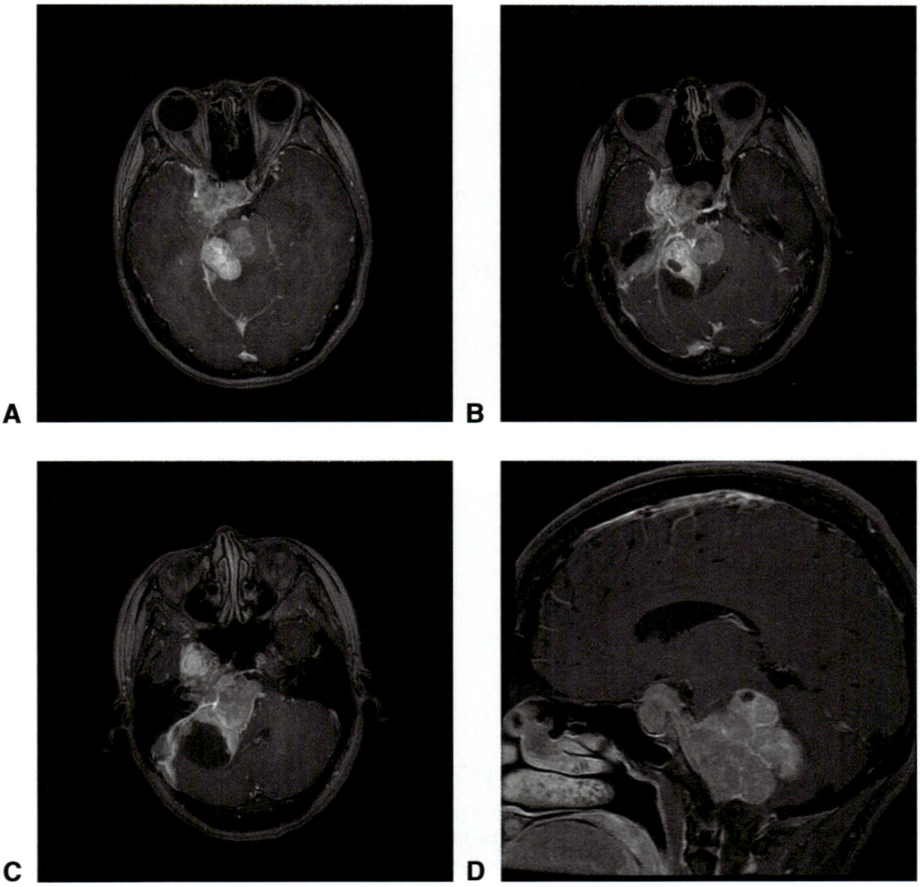

A B C D

Figure 2.12. Imaging of rhabdoid meningioma. A–C. Axial T1 postcontrast: Multicompartmental avidly enhancing masses with irregular border with neighboring brain suggestive of invasion and prominent cystic component.

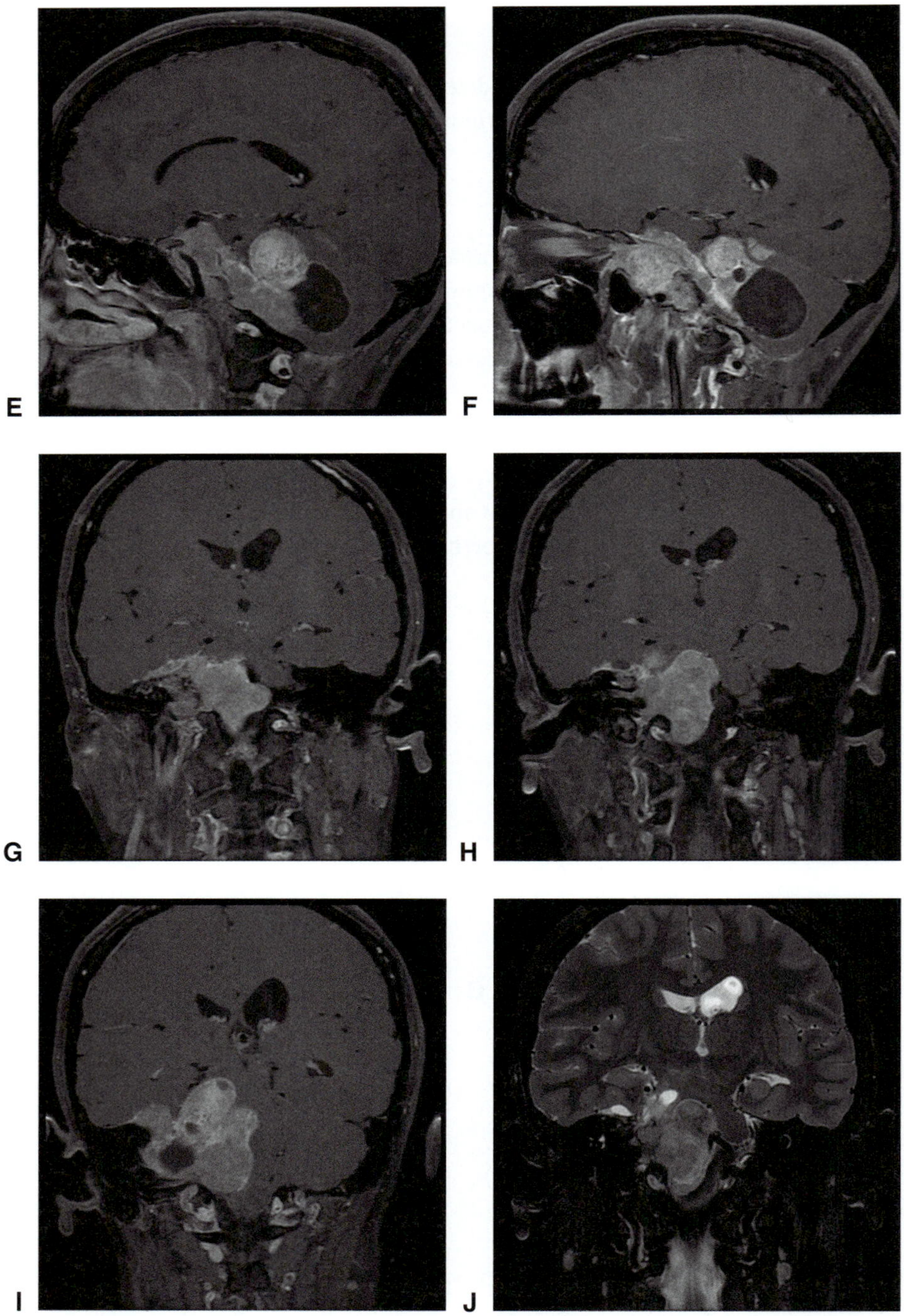

Figure 2.12. ***(continued)*** **D–F.** Sagittal T1 postcontrast: Multicompartmental avidly enhancing masses with irregular border with neighboring brain suggestive of invasion and prominent cystic component. **G–I.** Coronal T1 postcontrast: Multicompartmental avidly enhancing masses with irregular border with neighboring brain suggestive of invasion and prominent cystic component. **J–L.** Coronal T2: Multicompartmental and multilobulated heterogeneously hypointense masses with cystic components.

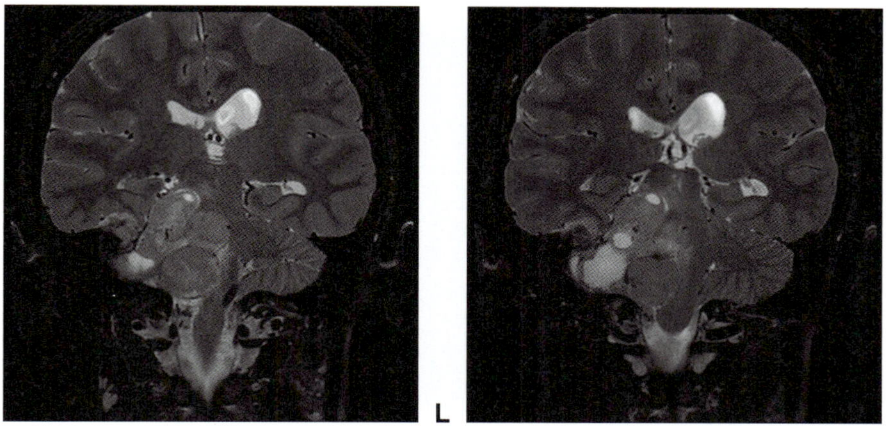

Figure 2.12. ***(continued)***

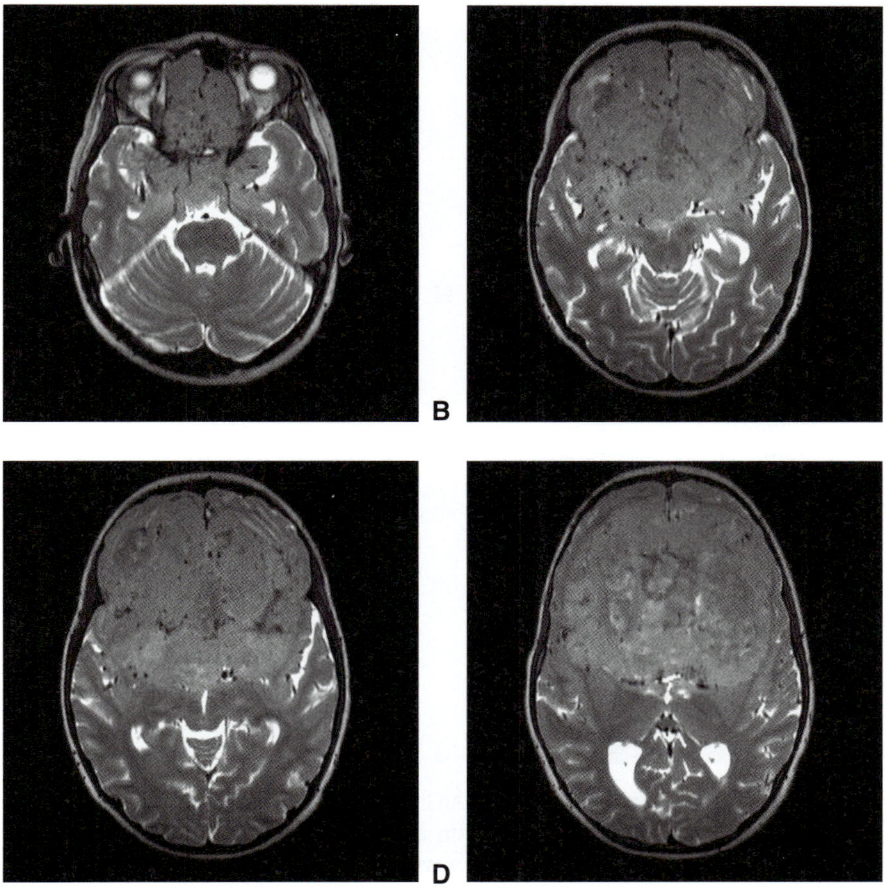

Figure 2.13. Imaging of anaplastic (malignant) meningioma. A–F. Axial T2: Heterogeneously hypointense massive tumor in the anterior cranial fossa spanning from olfactory groove to superior falx.

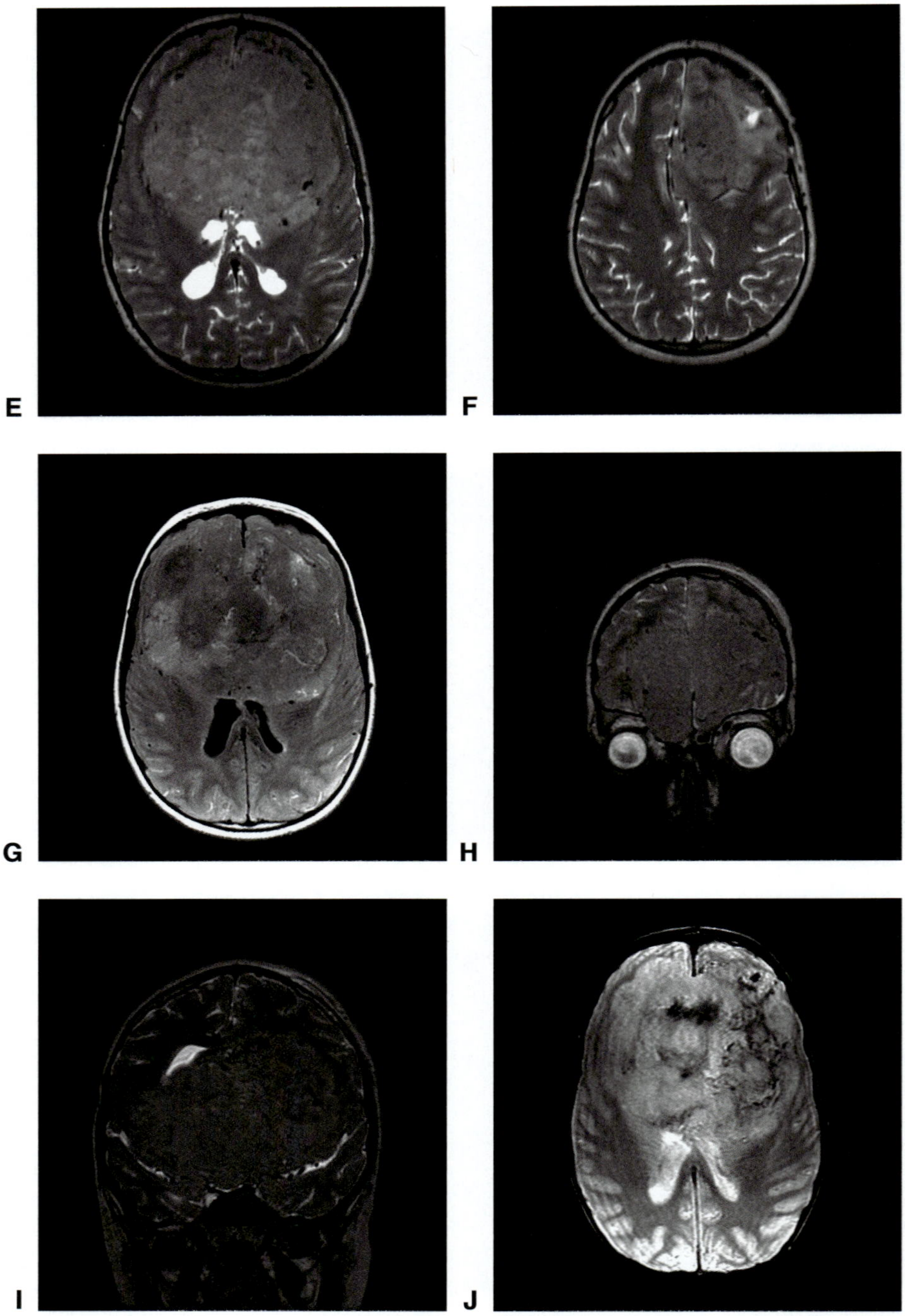

Figure 2.13. ***(continued)*** **G.** Axial FLAIR: Heterogeneous mixed intensity mass. **H.** Coronal T2: Marked expansion of the olfactory groove by the massive tumor. **I.** Coronal T2: Several vessels are seen within and along the perimeter of tumor. **J.** Axial SWI: Heterogeneous multifocal areas of blood products.

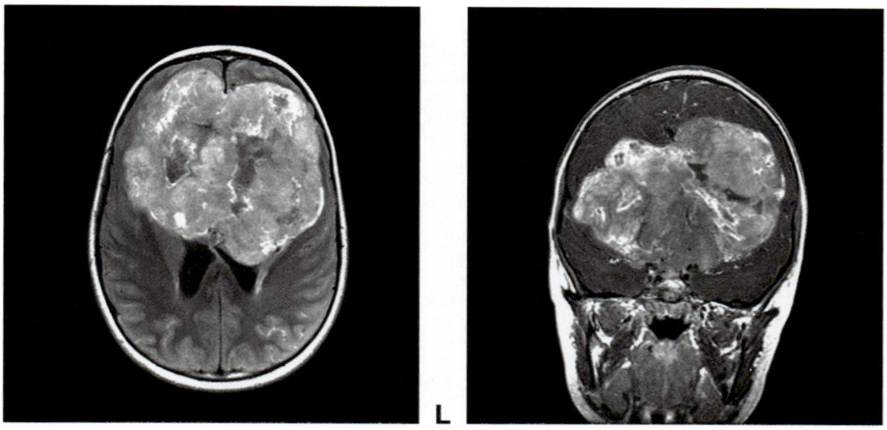

K L

Figure 2.13. ***(continued)*** **K.** Axial T1 postcontrast: Avid but heterogeneous enhancement. **L.** Coronal T1 postcontrast: Avid but heterogeneous enhancement.

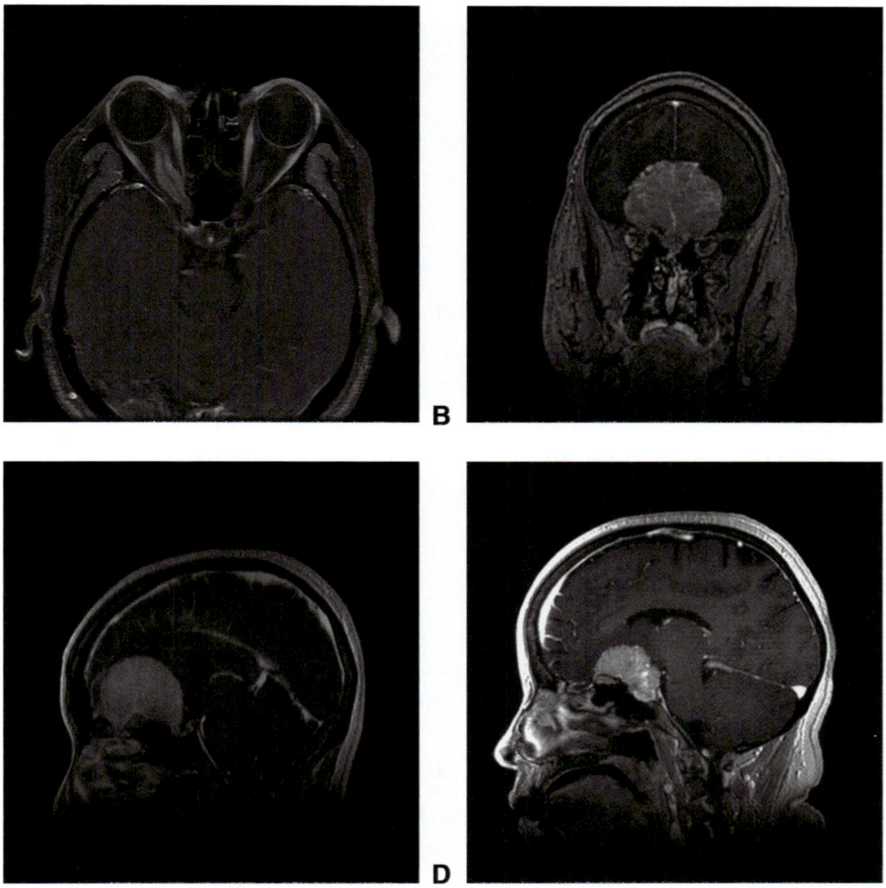

A B C D

Figure 2.14. **Imaging of 15 subtypes of meningioma based on anatomic location.** **A.** Cavernous sinus. **B.** Suprasellar/tuberculum sellae. **C.** Cerebellopontine angle. **D.** Cerebral convexity.

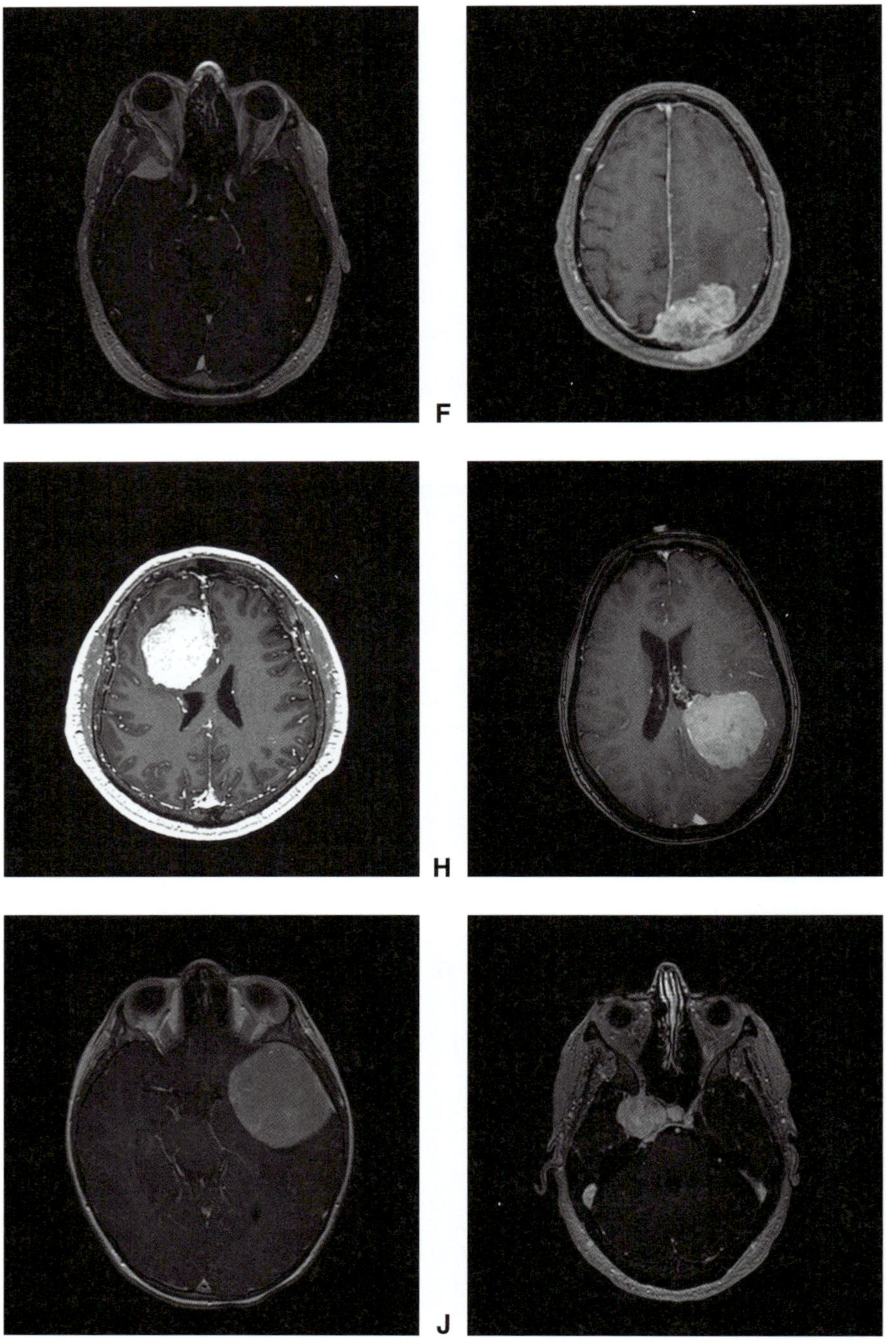

E F G H I J

Figure 2.14. ***(continued)*** **E.** Intraorbital. **F.** Intraventricular. **G.** Olfactory groove. **H.** Parasagittal. **I.** Falcine. **J.** Tentorium.

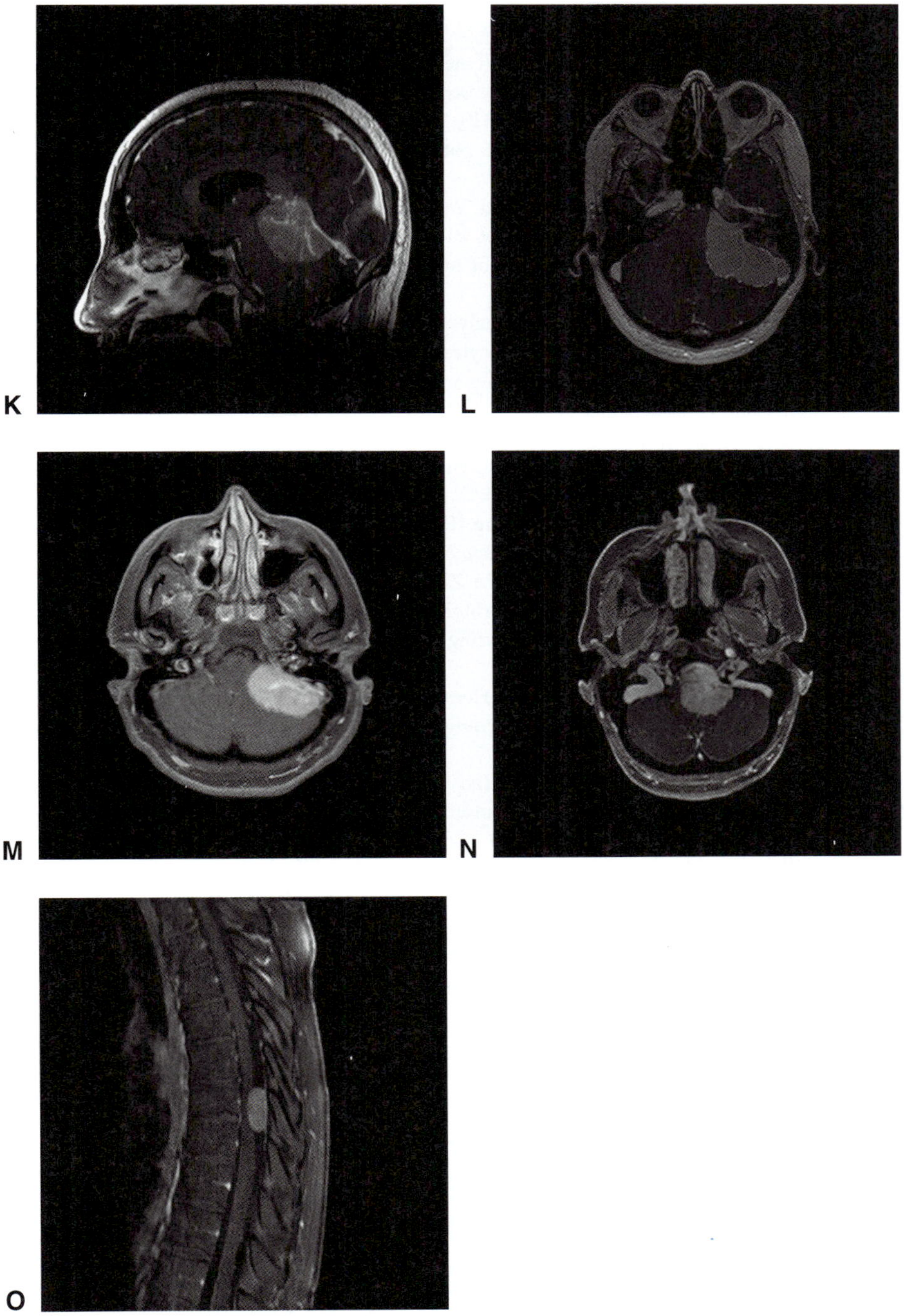

Figure 2.14. ***(continued)*** **K.** Petrous ridge/face. **L.** Posterior fossa. **M.** Sphenoid. **N.** Foramen magnum. **O.** Spinal canal.

Bibliography

Jain D, Sharma MC, Sarkar C, et al. Clear cell meningioma, an uncommon variant of meningioma: a clinicopathologic study of nine cases. *J Neurooncol.* 2007;81:315–321.

Kim EY, Weon YC, Kim ST, Kim HJ, Byun HS, Lee JI, et al. Rhabdoid meningioma: clinical features and MR imaging findings in 15 patients. *AJNR Am J Neuroradiol.* 2007;28(8): 1462–1465.

Kunimatsu A, Kunimatsu N, Kamiya K, et al. Variants of meningiomas: a review of imaging findings and clinical features. *Jpn J Radiol.* 2016:34:459–469.

Lee YS, Lee YS. Molecular characteristics of meningiomas. *J Pathol Transl Med.* 2020;54: 45–63.

Liu JL, Zhou JL, Ma YH, Dong C. An analysis of the magnetic resonance imaging and pathology of intracranial lymphoplasmacyte-rich meningioma. *Eur J Radiol.* 2012;81(5): 968–973.

Liu L, Lu Y, Peng W, et al. Imaging features of intracranial psammomatous meningioma. *J Neuroradiol.* 2017;44:395–399.

Modha A, Gutin PH. Diagnosis and treatment of atypical and anaplastic meningiomas: a review. *Neurosurgery.* 2005; 57:538–550.

Paek SH, Kim SH, Chang KH, Park CK, Kim JE, Kim DG, et al. Microcystic meningiomas: radiological characteristics of 16 cases. *Acta Neurochir (Wien).* 2005;147(9):965–972.

Pond JB, Morgan TG, Hatanpaa KJ, Yetkin ZF, Mickey BE, Mendelsohn DB. Chordoid meningioma: differentiating a rare World Health Organization grade II tumor from other meningioma histologic subtypes using MRI. *AJNR Am J Neuroradiol.* 2015;36(7): 1253–1258.

Regelsberger J, Hagel C, Emami P, Ries T, Heese O, Westphal M. Secretory meningiomas: a benign subgroup causing life-threatening complications. *Neuro Oncol.* 2009;11(6): 819–824.

Wang XQ, Huang MZ, Zhang H, Sun FB, Tao BB, Feng BH, et al. Clear cell meningioma: clinical features, CT, and MR imaging findings in 23 patients. *J Comput Assist Tomogr.* 2014;38(2):200–208.

Wiemels J, Wrensch M, Claus EB. Epidemiology and etiology of meningioma. *J Neurooncol.* 2010;99(3):307–314. http://www.ncbi.nlm.nih.gov/entrez/eutils/elink.fcgi?dbfrom=pubmed&tool=sumsearch.org/cite&retmode=ref&cmd=prlinks&id=20821343.

Yu XR, Jun Z, Zhang BY, Huang WY, Bo Y, Tan WL, et al. Magnetic resonance imaging findings of intracranial papillary meningioma: a study on eight cases. *Clin Imaging.* 2014;38(5):611–615.

3

Mesenchymal Tumors

Overview

Mesenchymal tumors are thought to originate from precursor mesodermal cells that develop into bone, cartilage, or connective tissues, such as fibroblasts, smooth muscle cells, blood vessels, and adipocytes. The central nervous system (CNS) mesenchymal tumors are presumed to arise from the mesodermal cells surrounding the brain parenchyma, and mainly from the meninges, vessels, fibroblasts, and bone.

	Age range (mean)	Female: male	Cell of origin	WHO grade	Molecular/ genetic markers	Prognosis
Solitary fibrous tumor	40–50	1:1.2	Fibroblastic cell type	I	*CD34, NAB2, STAT6*	Favorable
Hemangiopericytoma	40–50	1:1.2	Fibroblastic cell type	II	*CD34, NAB2, STAT6*	Guarded
Hemangioblastoma	Adults (20 yrs, younger in VHL)	1:1	Stromal cell with abundant small vessels	I	*VHL*	Favorable
Inflammatory myofibroblastic tumor	Any age	–	Myofibroblastic-type cell with lymphoplasmacytic infiltrates	I	*ALK, ROS1, PDGFRB, RET*	Favorable
Desmoid-type fibromatosis	Children	–	Myofibroblastic-type cell with collagenous stroma	I	Nuclear beta-catenin	Guarded
Fibrosarcoma	Children	–	Monomorphic spindle cell	IV	-	Guarded
Chondrosarcoma	Adults	–	Hyaline cartilage of low cellularity	III	*SOX9* *NCOA2* gene rearrangement	Guarded
Osteosarcoma	Adolescents, young adults	–	Malignant bone-forming mesenchymal cell	IV	-	Guarded

Solitary Fibrous Tumor and Hemangiopericytoma

Definition: Well-circumscribed tumor originating from fibroblastic cells of the meninges and harbor a genomic inversion at the 12q13 locus fusing the *NAB2* and *STAT6* genes. SFT is considered benign or a lower grade version of hemangiopericytoma (HPC), and both tumor types now fall under the same category but with different WHO gradings.

Epidemiology: Less than 1% of all CNS tumors; peak incidence in the fourth to fifth decades of life; exceedingly rare in the pediatric age group

Molecular and genetic profile: Detection of STAT6 nuclear expression or NAB2-STAT6 fusion related to a genomic inversion at the 12q13 locus is the hallmark feature of SFT and HPC.

Clinical features and standard therapy: Gross total resection of tumor leads to cure for SFT, but in HPC recurrence is not uncommon, especially when there is postoperative residual tumor. For HPC, gross total resection does not necessarily ensure cure because HPC can recur both at the site of original tumor and at a distant site. To minimize local recurrence, adjuvant radiation therapy is often used in HPC, especially when there is any residual tumor, but it does not prevent distant recurrence.

Imaging

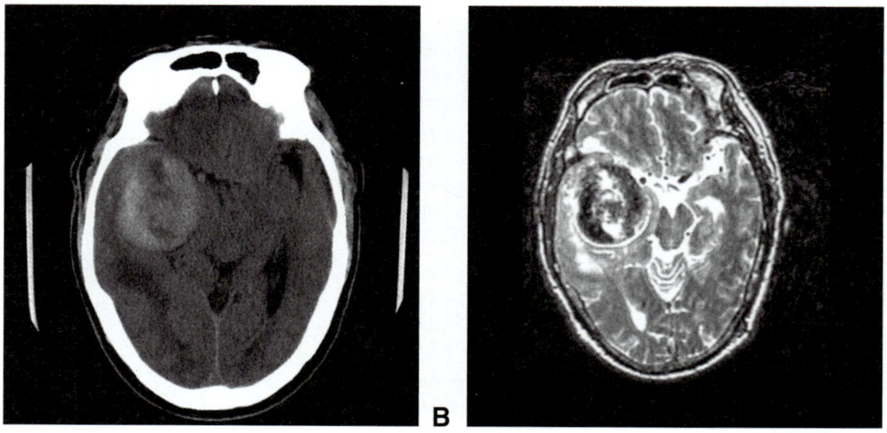

A B

Figure 3.1. Imaging of solitary fibrous tumor. A. Axial unenhanced CT: Hyperdense extra-axial mass. **B.** Axial T2: Marked hypointense periphery and hyperintense core and mild surrounding edema.

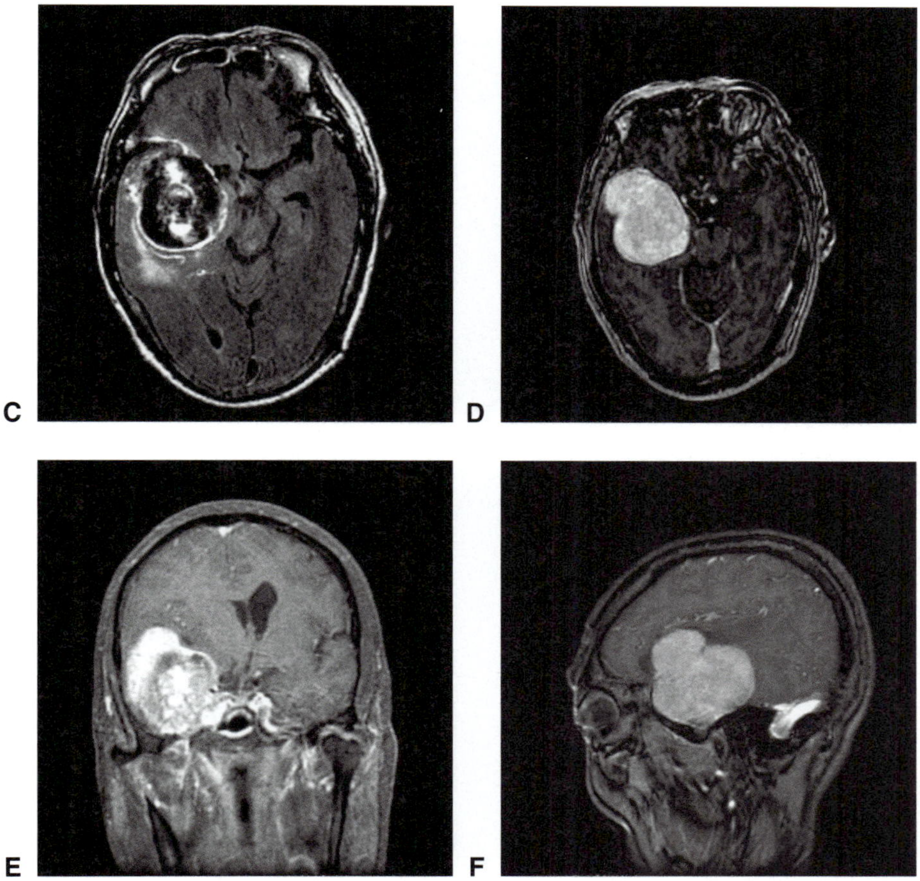

Figure 3.1. ***(continued)*** **C.** Axial Fluid-attenuated inversion recovery (FLAIR): Marked hypointense periphery and hyperintense core and mild surrounding edema. **D.** Axial T1-postcontrast: Avid intratumoral enhancement without distinct dural tail. **E.** Coronal T1-postcontrast: Avid intratumoral enhancement without distinct dural tail. **F.** Sagittal T1-postcontrast: Avid intratumoral enhancement without distinct dural tail.

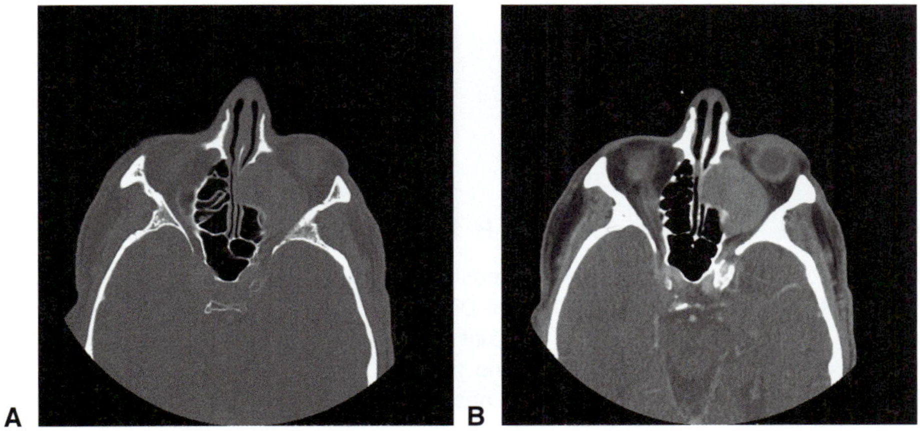

Figure 3.2. **Imaging of orbital solitary fibrous tumor. A.** Axial CT bone window: Medial orbital wall is smoothly eroded and bowed medially by the intraconal soft tissue mass. **B.** Axial CT postcontrast: Mild enhancement associated with the bulky soft tissue mass.

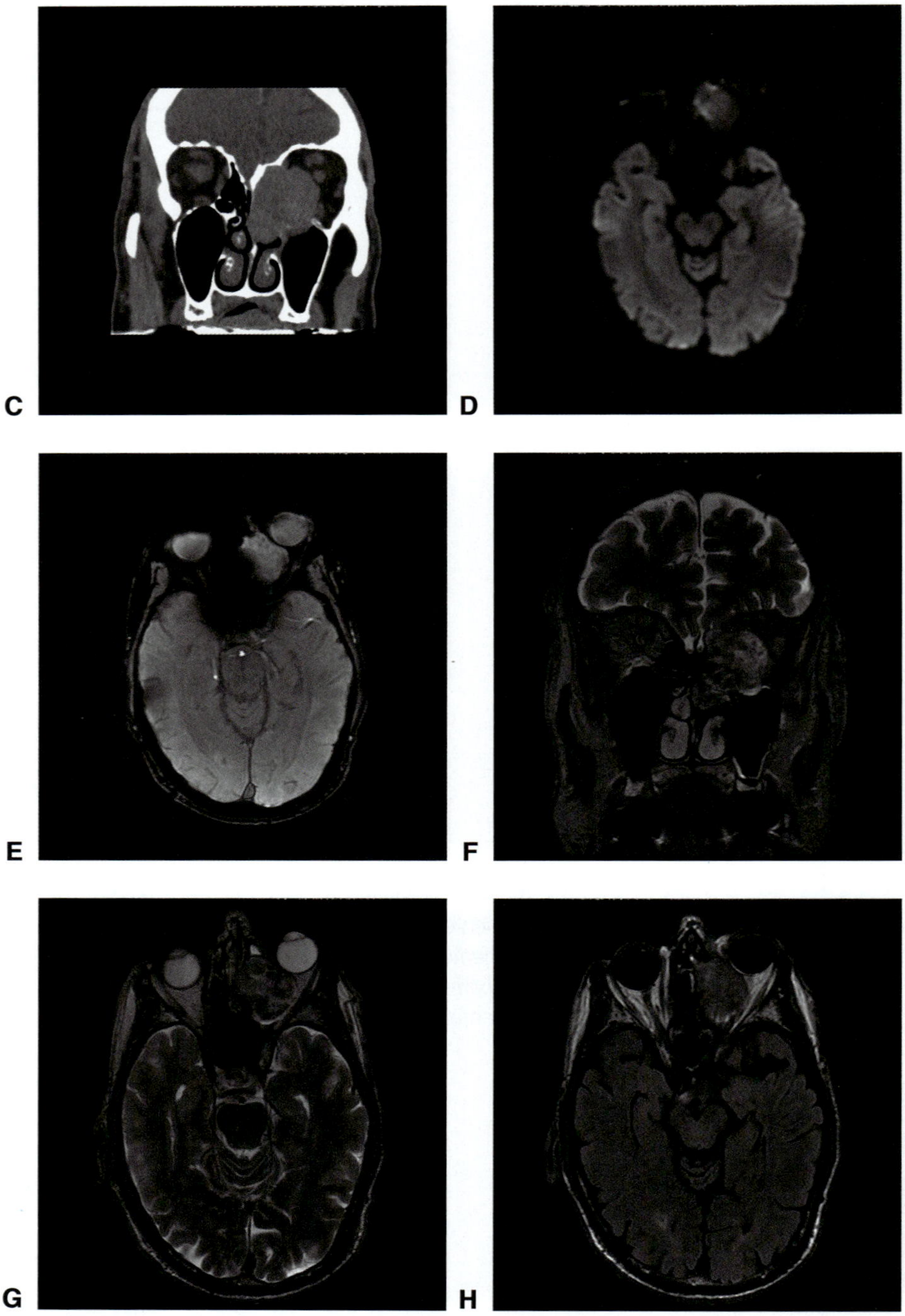

Figure 3.2. ***(continued)*** **C.** Coronal CT postcontrast: Mild enhancement associated with the bulky soft tissue mass. **D.** Axial Diffusion-weighted imaging (DWI): Mildly reduced diffusion within the mass. **E.** Axial Susceptibility-weighted imaging (SWI): No blood products or calcium within the mass. **F.** Coronal T2: Heterogeneously hypointense mass herniating into the nasal cavity. **G.** Axial T2: Circumscribed mass with heterogeneously hypointense signal. **H.** Axial FLAIR: Heterogeneously hypointense mass.

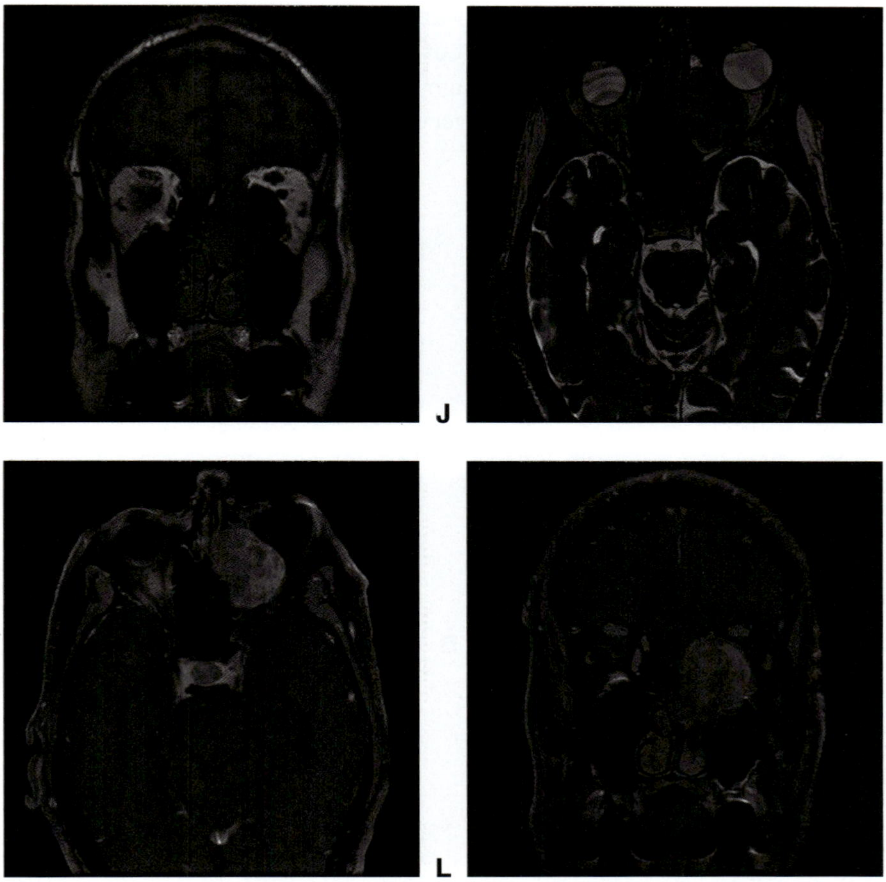

I J K L

Figure 3.2. ***(continued)*** **I.** Coronal T1-precontrast: Homogeneously hypointense mass. **J.** Axial Fast Imaging Employing Steady-state Acquisition (FIESTA): Heterogeneously hypointense mass. **K.** Axial T1-postcontrast: Avid but heterogeneous enhancement within the mass. **L.** Coronal T1-postcontrast: Avid but heterogeneous enhancement within the mass.

▶ Hemangiopericytoma

Definition: Hemangiopericytoma (HPC) is a malignant variant of solitary fibrous tumor (SFT), and HPC/SFT is considered a single entity for sharing common genetic aberration but separated by a three-tiered grading scheme.

Epidemiology: Peak incidence occurs in the fourth to fifth decades of life, with slight male predominance and exceedingly rare in pediatric age group

Molecular and genetic profile: Detection of STAT6 nuclear expression or NAB2-STAT6 fusion related to a genomic inversion at the 12q13 locus is the hallmark feature of SFT and HPC.

Clinical features and standard therapy: Surgical resection is the first line of therapy, and regardless of the extent of resection, adjuvant radiation therapy may be needed because HPC has a high propensity for recurrence, especially when there is residual tumor after surgery.

Imaging

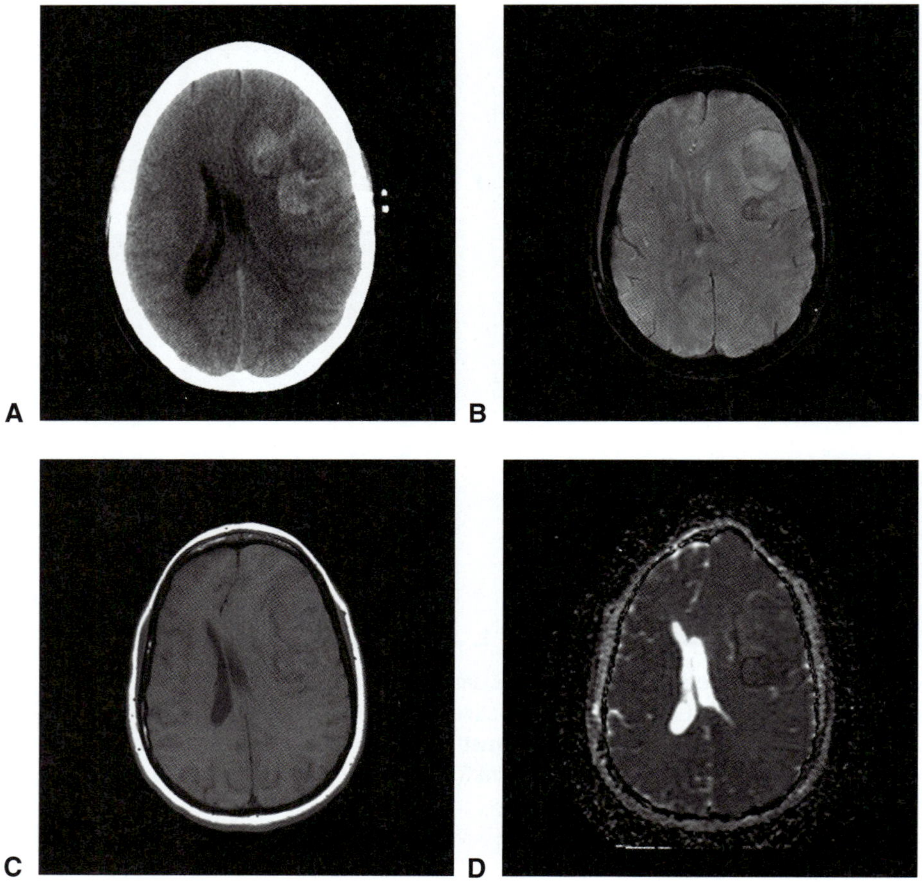

Figure 3.3. Imaging of intracranial hemangiopericytoma. A. Axial CT unenhanced: Hemorrhagic left frontal mass. **B.** Axial SWI: Scattered blood products. **C.** Axial T1 precontrast: Heterogeneously isointense extra-axial mass. **D.** Axial Apparent diffusion coefficient (ADC): Hypointense signal.

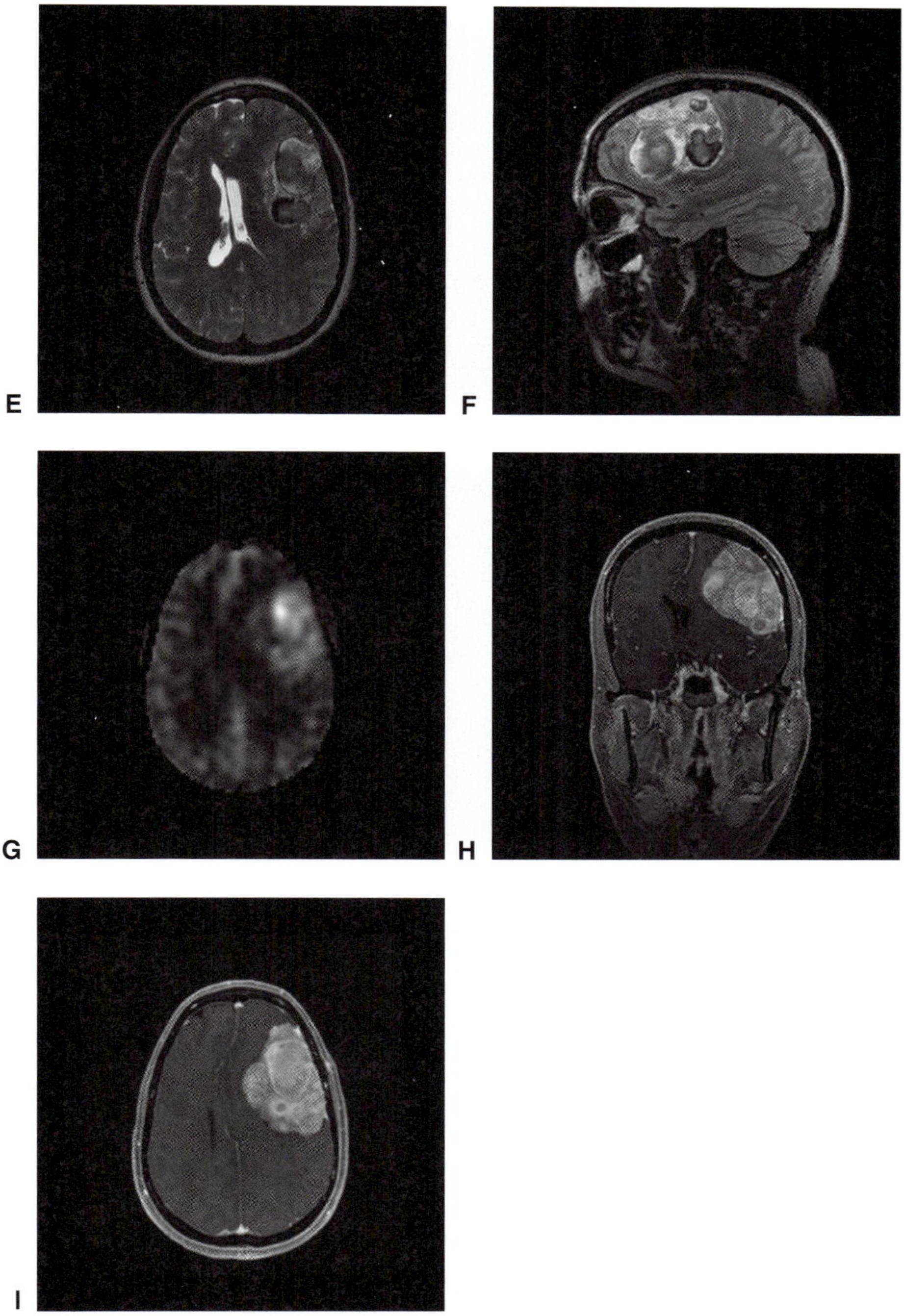

Figure 3.3. ***(continued)*** **E.** Axial T2: Hypointense signal within the areas of hemorrhage. **F.** Sagittal FLAIR: Hypointense signal within the areas of hemorrhage. **G.** Axial Arterial spin labeling (ASL) perfusion: Marked hypervascularity within the tumor. **H.** Coronal T1 postcontrast: Avid but heterogeneous enhancement of tumor. **I.** Axial T1 postcontrast: Avid but heterogeneous enhancement of tumor.

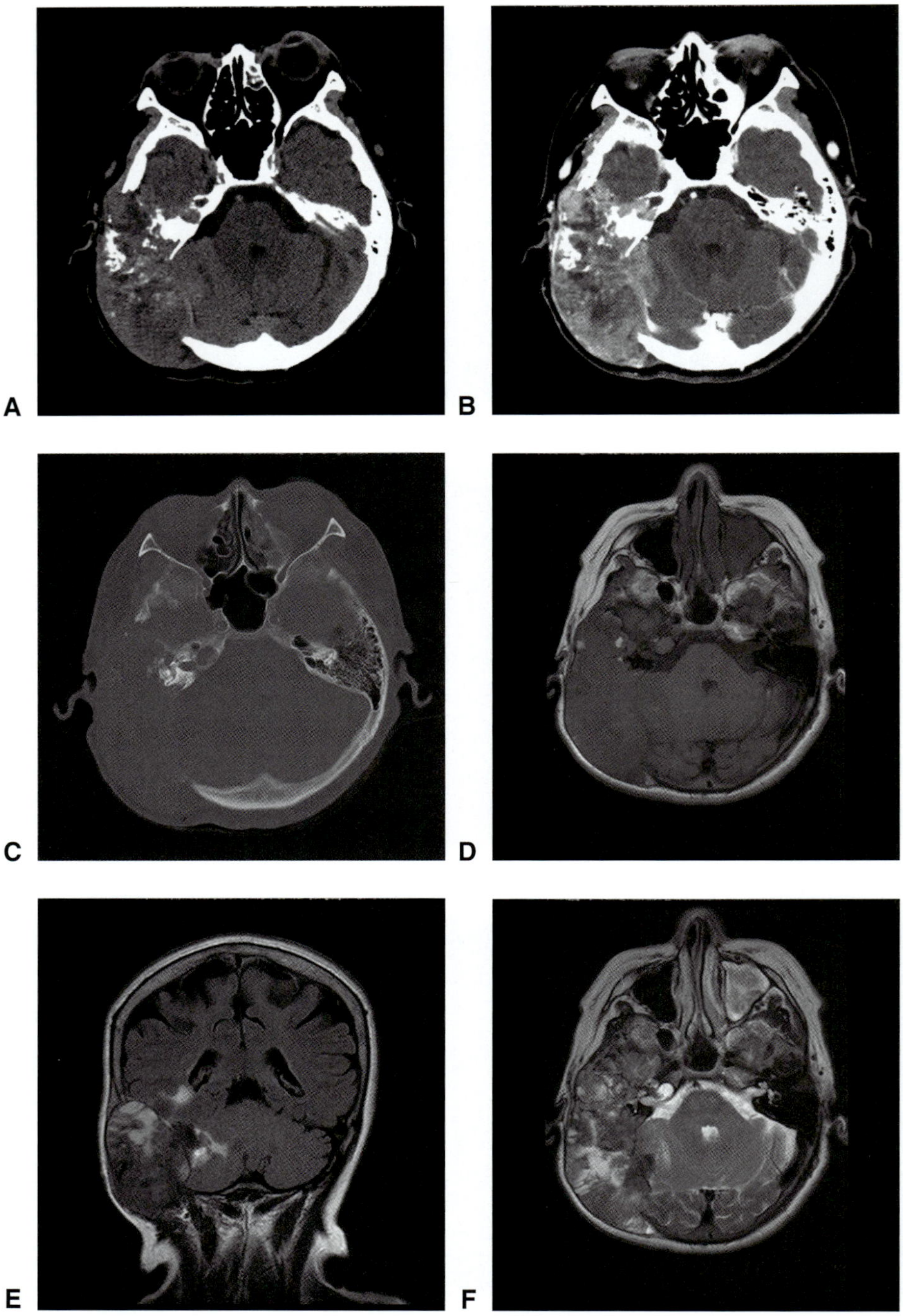

Figure 3.4. Imaging of temporal bone hemangiopericytoma. A. Axial CT precontrast: Large destructive mass centered in the right temporal bone with intracranial and extracranial extension. **B.** Axial CT postcontrast: Heterogeneous enhancement within the mass. **C.** Axial CT bone window: Gross lytic destruction of involved bone is better seen. **D.** Axial T1 precontrast: Homogeneously hypointense mass. **E.** Coronal FLAIR: Heterogeneous mix of signal intensity within the mass. **F.** Axial T2: Heterogeneously hypointense mass with areas of cystic features.

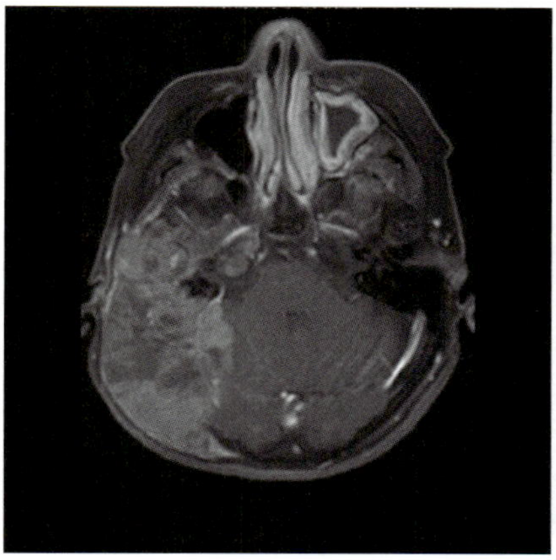

G

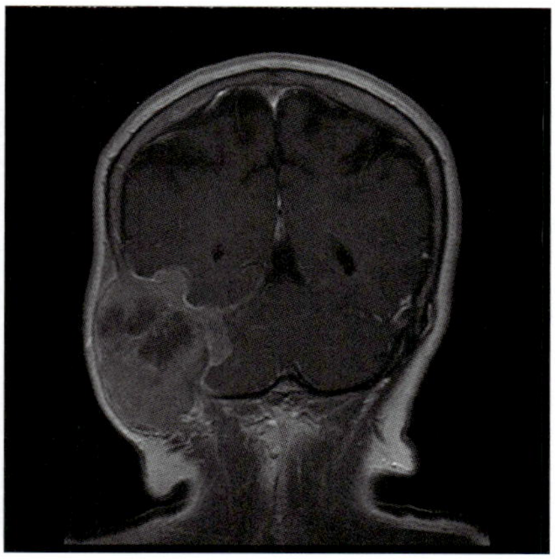

H

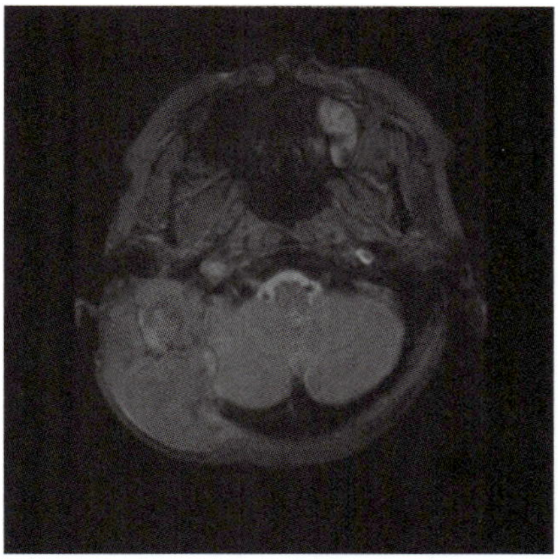

I

Figure 3.4. ***(continued)*** **G.** Axial T1 postcontrast: Avid but heterogeneous enhancement within the mass. **H.** Coronal T1 postcontrast: Avid but heterogeneous enhancement within the mass. **I.** Axial SWI: Minimal blood products within the tumor.

Hemangioblastoma

Definition: Benign slow-growing tumor comprised of neoplastic stromal cells and abundant small vessels.

Epidemiology: Uncommon benign neoplasm that occurs as sporadic lesion and in familial form associated with von Hippel-Lindau (VHL) disease. Adults are more commonly affected, but the average age of patients with hemangioblastoma in VHL is approximately 20 years younger than those affected by sporadic hemangioblastoma. The female-to-male ratio is approximately 1:1.

Molecular and genetic profile: Biallelic inactivation of the VHL gene is a frequent occurrence in familiar hemangioblastomas and can be seen up to 78% in sporadic forms. The VHL tumor suppressor protein forms a ternary complex with Transcription elongation factor B1 (TCEB) and TCEB2 and controls cell cycle regulation. Loss of VHL leads to upregulation of hypoxia-responsive genes, such as those encoding Vascular endothelial growth factor (VEGF) and erythropoietin, despite the absence of tumor hypoxia.

Clinical features and standard therapy: Symptoms of intracranial hemangioblastomas, especially those arising in the posterior fossa, are usually related to impaired cerebrospinal fluid dynamics leading to vasogenic edema or mass effect-related cystic and solid component of tumor. Patients often present with signs and symptoms of increased intracranial pressure or obstructive hydrocephalus. Surgical resection is the primary treatment, and gross total resection leads to cure. There is no effective chemotherapy.

Imaging

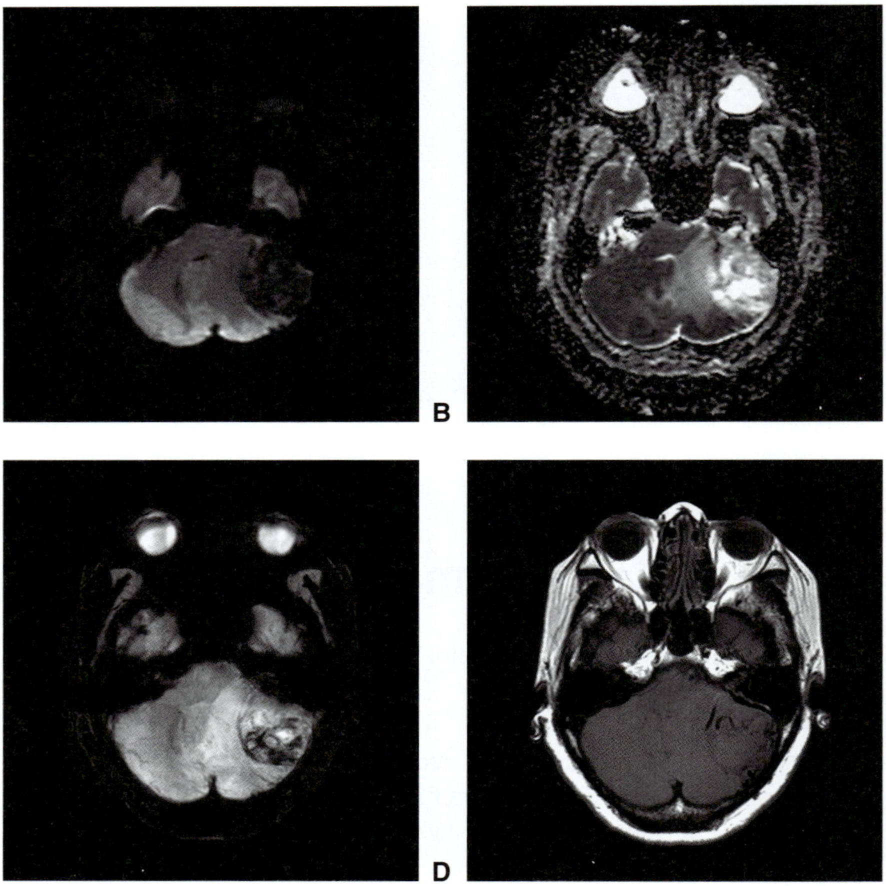

A B C D

Figure 3.5. Imaging of cerebellar hemangioblastoma. A. Axial DWI: Hypointense increased diffusion within the mass. **B.** Axial ADC: Hypointense increased diffusion within the mass. **C.** Axial SWI: Prominent blood products within the mass. **D.** Axial T1 precontrast: Prominent vessels along the deep margin of the mass.

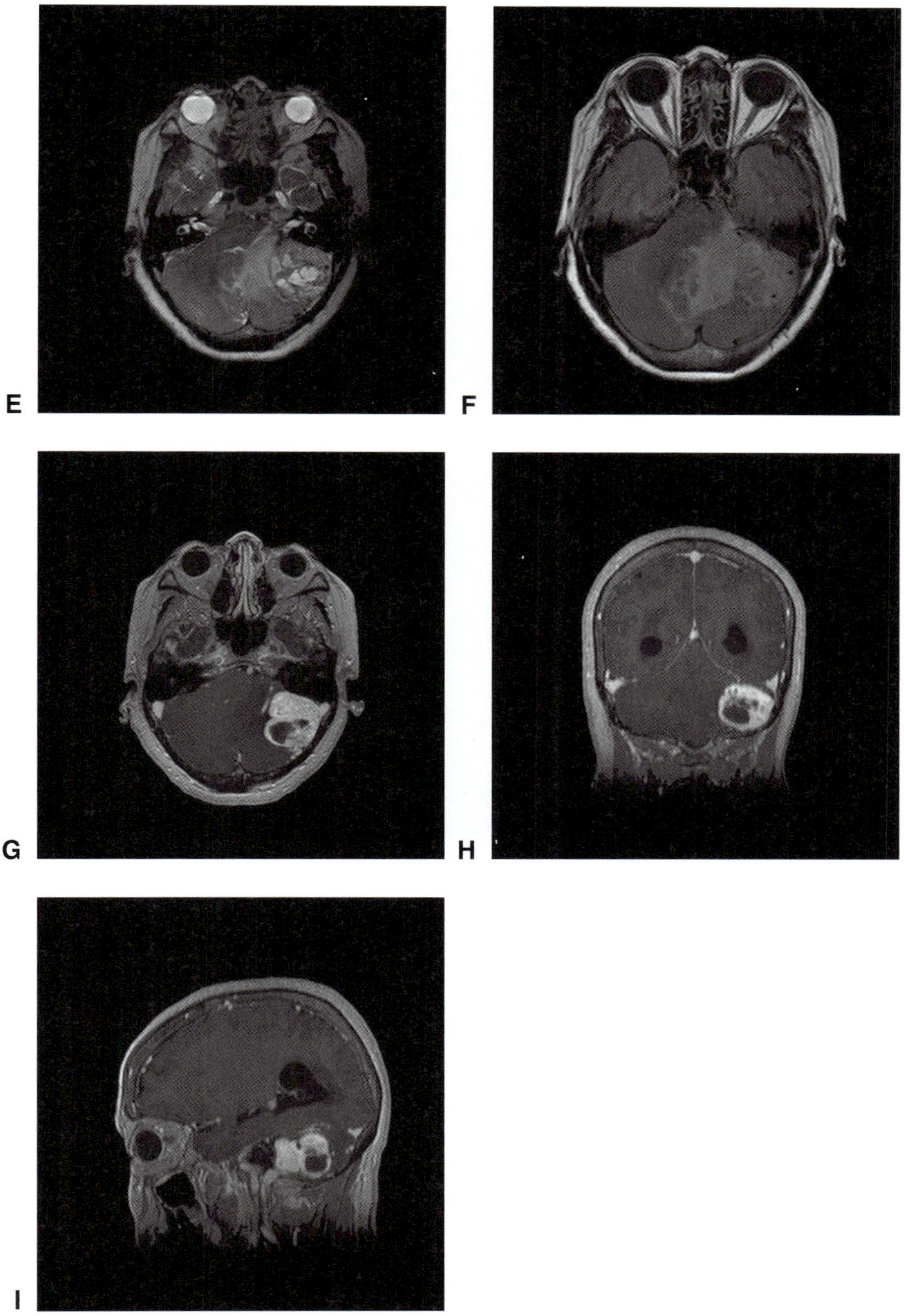

Figure 3.5. ***(continued)*** **E.** Axial T2: Heterogeneously hypointense mass with multiple cystic components and extensive surrounding edema. **F.** Axial FLAIR: Heterogeneously hypointense mass with multiple cystic components and extensive surrounding edema. **G.** Axial T1 postcontrast: Avid and homogeneous enhancement within the solid tumor and no enhancement in the cystic component. **H.** Coronal T1 postcontrast: Avid and homogeneous enhancement within the solid tumor and no enhancement in the cystic component. **I.** Sagittal T1 postcontrast: Avid and homogeneous enhancement within the solid tumor and no enhancement in the cystic component.

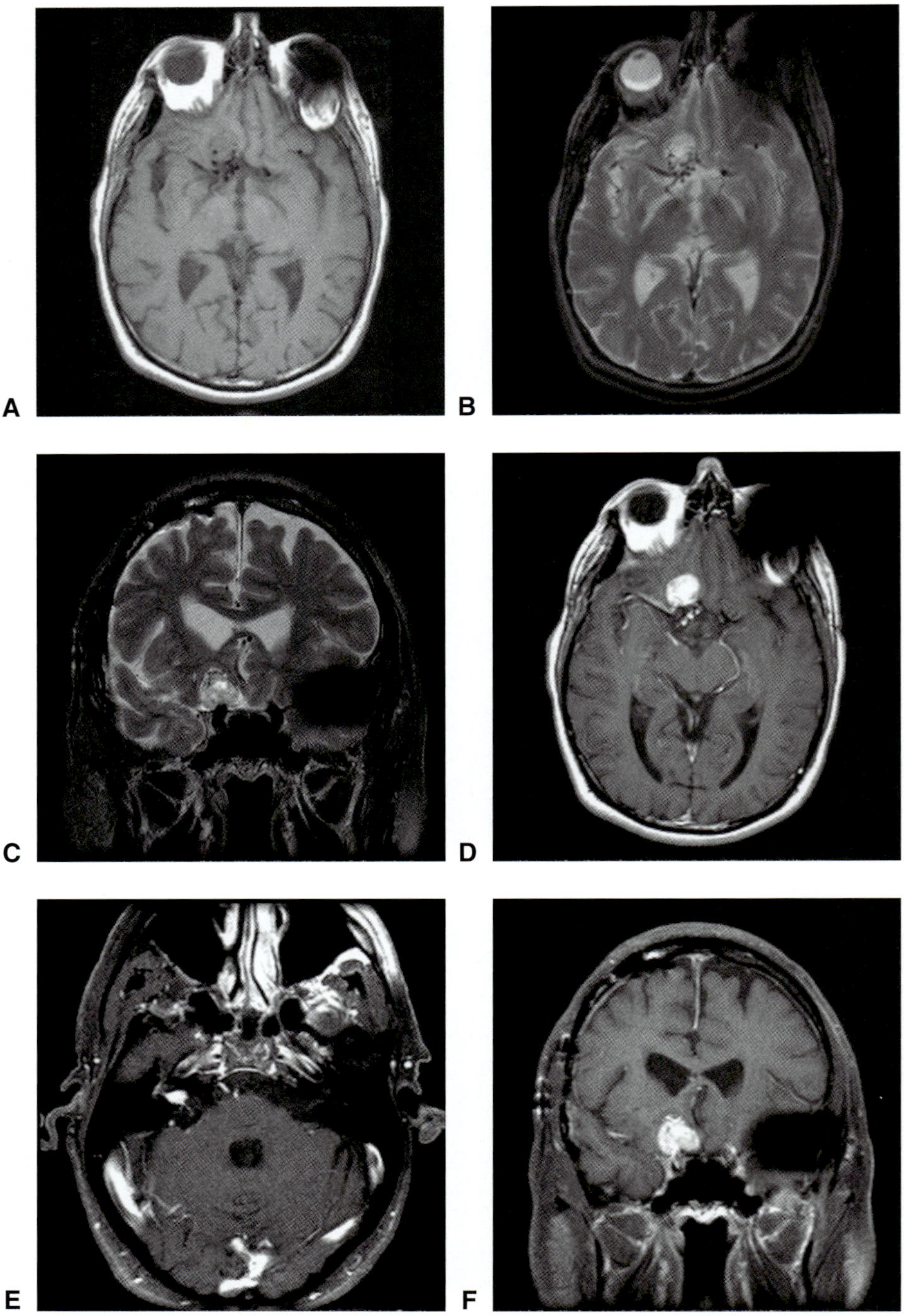

Figure 3.6. Imaging of disseminated hemangioblastoma. A. Axial T1 precontrast: Isointense basal forebrain mass with prominent vessels. **B.** Axial T2: Hyperintense basal forebrain mass with prominent vessels. **C.** Coronal T2: Hyperintense basal forebrain mass with prominent vessels. **D.** Axial T1 postcontrast: Avid and homogeneous enhancement. **E.** Axial T1 postcontrast fat sat: Additional site of enhancing tumor in the right internal auditory canal. **F.** Coronal T1 postcontrast fat sat: Avid and homogeneous enhancement.

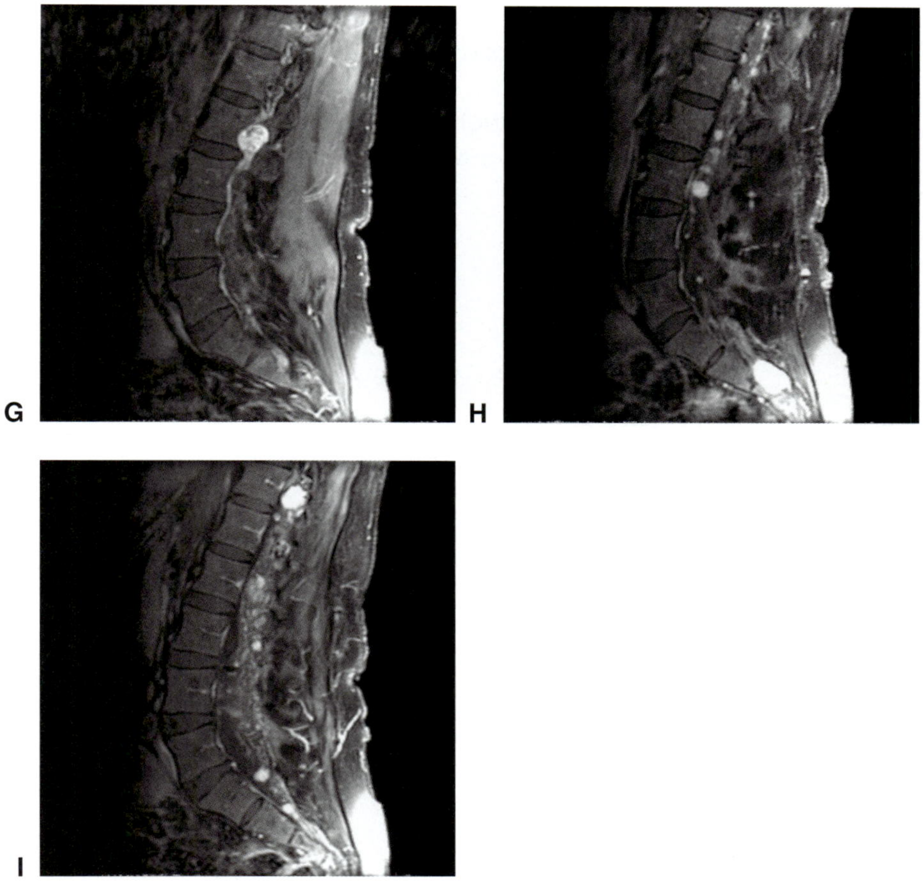

Figure 3.6. ***(continued)*** **G.** Sagittal T1 postcontrast: Heterogeneously enhancing solid mass filling the thecal sac and smoothly remodeling the posterior vertebral body. **H.** Sagittal T1 postcontrast: Innumerable enhancing nodules studded along the cauda equina and filling the distal sacral sac. **I.** Sagittal T1 postcontrast: Innumerable enhancing nodules studded along the cauda equina and conus.

▶ Inflammatory Myofibroblastic Tumor

Definition: Rare tumor composed of bland myofibroblastic-type cells associated with lymphoplasmacytic infiltrates within an edematous stroma.

Epidemiology: Due to its rarity, the exact incidence and demographics of inflammatory myofibroblastic tumor (IMT) are unknown. IMT is very rare and occurs in less than one in one million people, with an estimated 150–200 people diagnosed in the United States annually.

Molecular and genetic profile: Anaplastic lymphoma kinase (ALK) gene rearrangement and Inflammatory myofibroblastic tumor (IMT) harbors frequent anaplastic lymphoma kinase (ALK) and ROS proto-oncogene 1 (ROS1) fusions and rare Novel RET (rearranged during transfection) gene rearrangement.

Clinical features and standard therapy: Surgical gross total resection of the tumor leads to favorable outcomes without recurrence. Chemotherapy or radiation therapy is not indicated.

Imaging

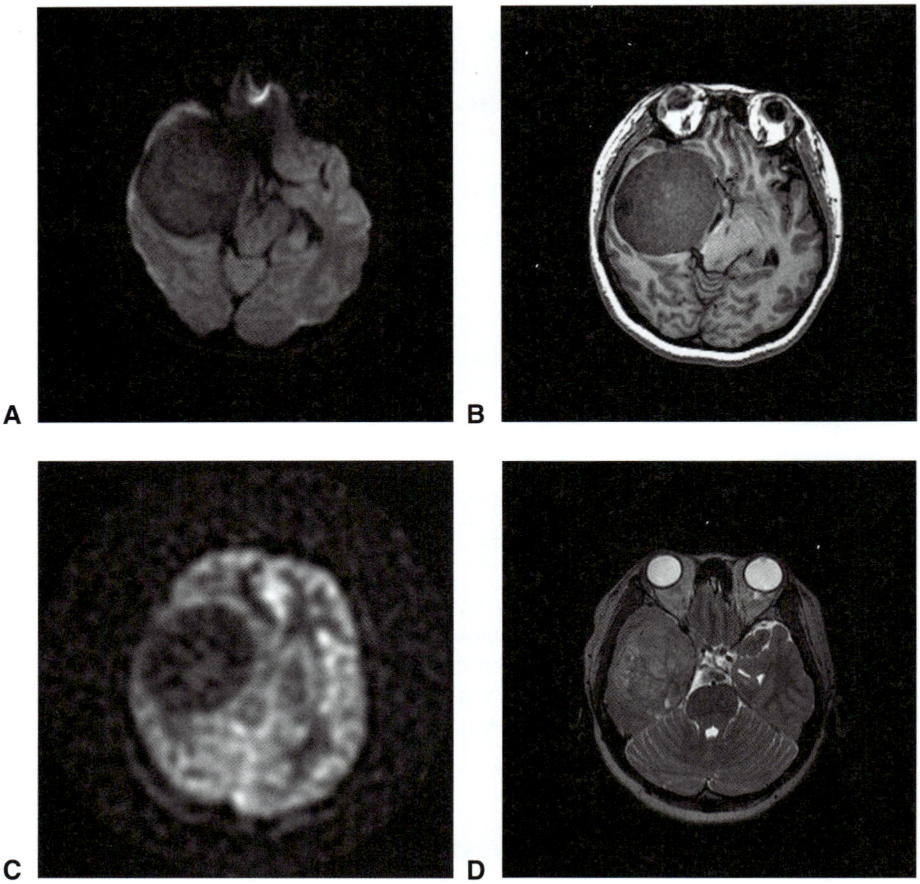

Figure 3.7. Imaging of inflammatory myofibroblastic tumor. A. Axial DWI: Large extra-axial mass with increased diffusion. **B.** Axial T1 precontrast: Hypointense circumscribed mass. **C.** Axial ASL perfusion: Markedly hypovascular mass. **D.** Axial T2: Heterogeneously hypointense mass.

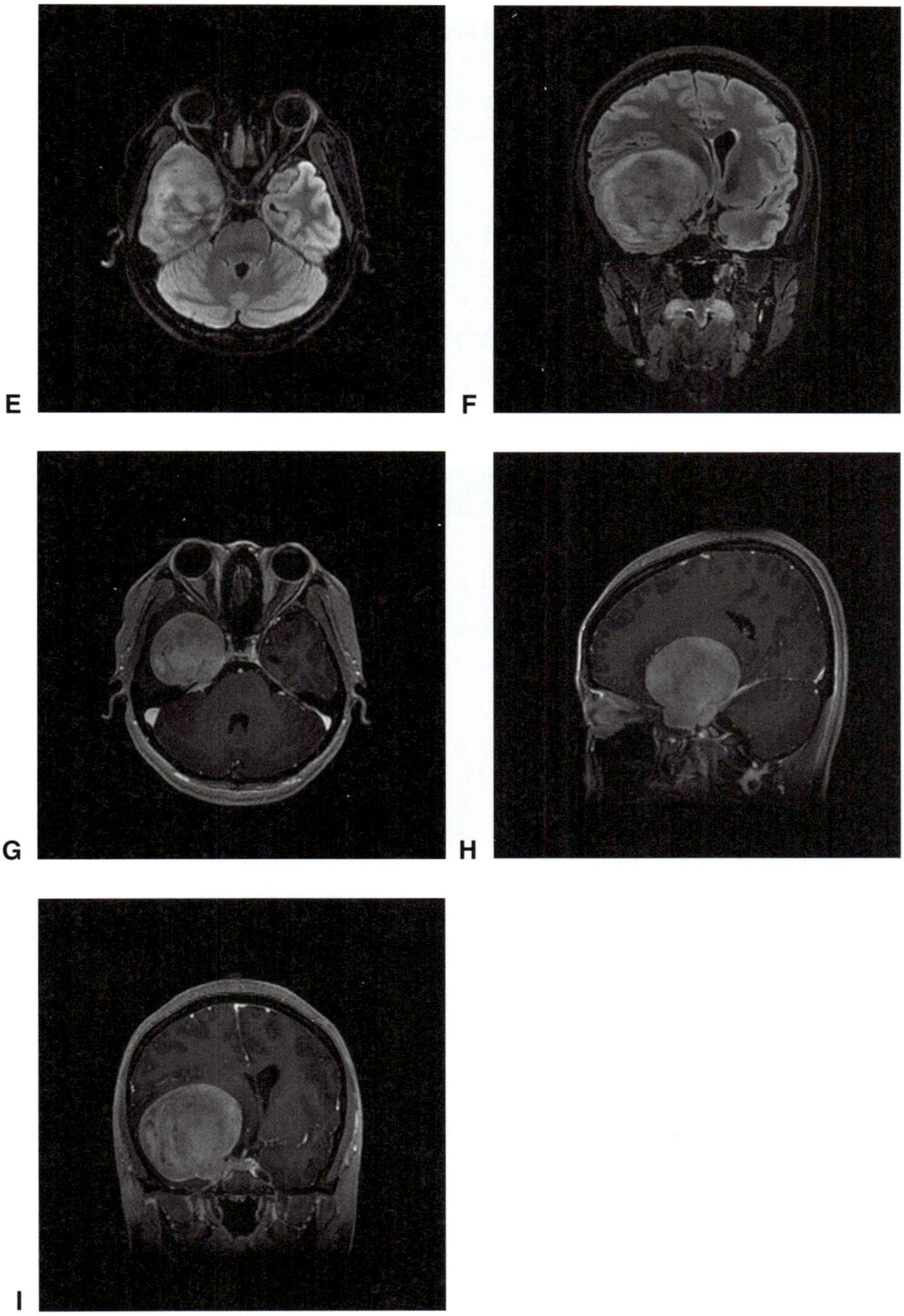

Figure 3.7. ***(continued)*** **E.** Axial FLAIR: Heterogeneously mildly hyper- and hypointense mass. **F.** Coronal FLAIR: Heterogeneously mildly hyper- and hypointense mass. **G.** Axial T1 postcontrast: Avid enhancement and no dural tail. **H.** Sagittal T1 postcontrast: Avid enhancement and no dural tail. **I.** Coronal T1 postcontrast: Avid enhancement and no dural tail.

▶ Desmoid-Type Fibromatosis

Definition: Locally infiltrative but benign clonal fibroblastic neoplasm composed of uniform, myofibroblastic cells in a background of abundant collagenous stroma.

Epidemiology: Due to its rarity of desmoid-type fibromatosis, the exact incidence is unknown but is estimated at 2–4 people per million per year.

Molecular and genetic profile: Presence of nuclear beta-catenin supports the diagnosis.

Clinical features and standard therapy: Due to its infiltrative growth, gross total resection is difficult to achieve without the risk of damaging neighboring structures; locally recurrent but lacks distant metastatic potential.

Imaging

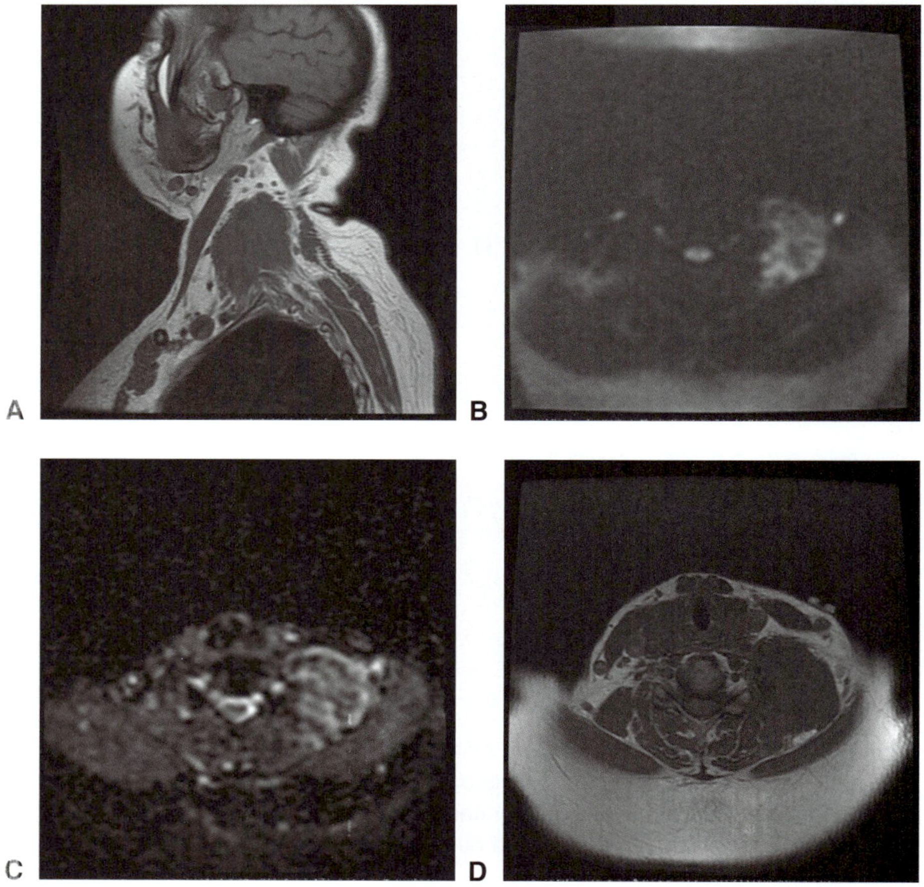

Figure 3.8. Imaging of desmoid-type fibromatosis. A. Sagittal T1 precontrast: Hypointense lateral neck mass. **B.** Axial DWI: Heterogeneously reduced on diffusion. **C.** Axial ADC: Heterogeneously reduced on ADC. **D.** Axial T1 precontrast: Hypointense lateral neck mass.

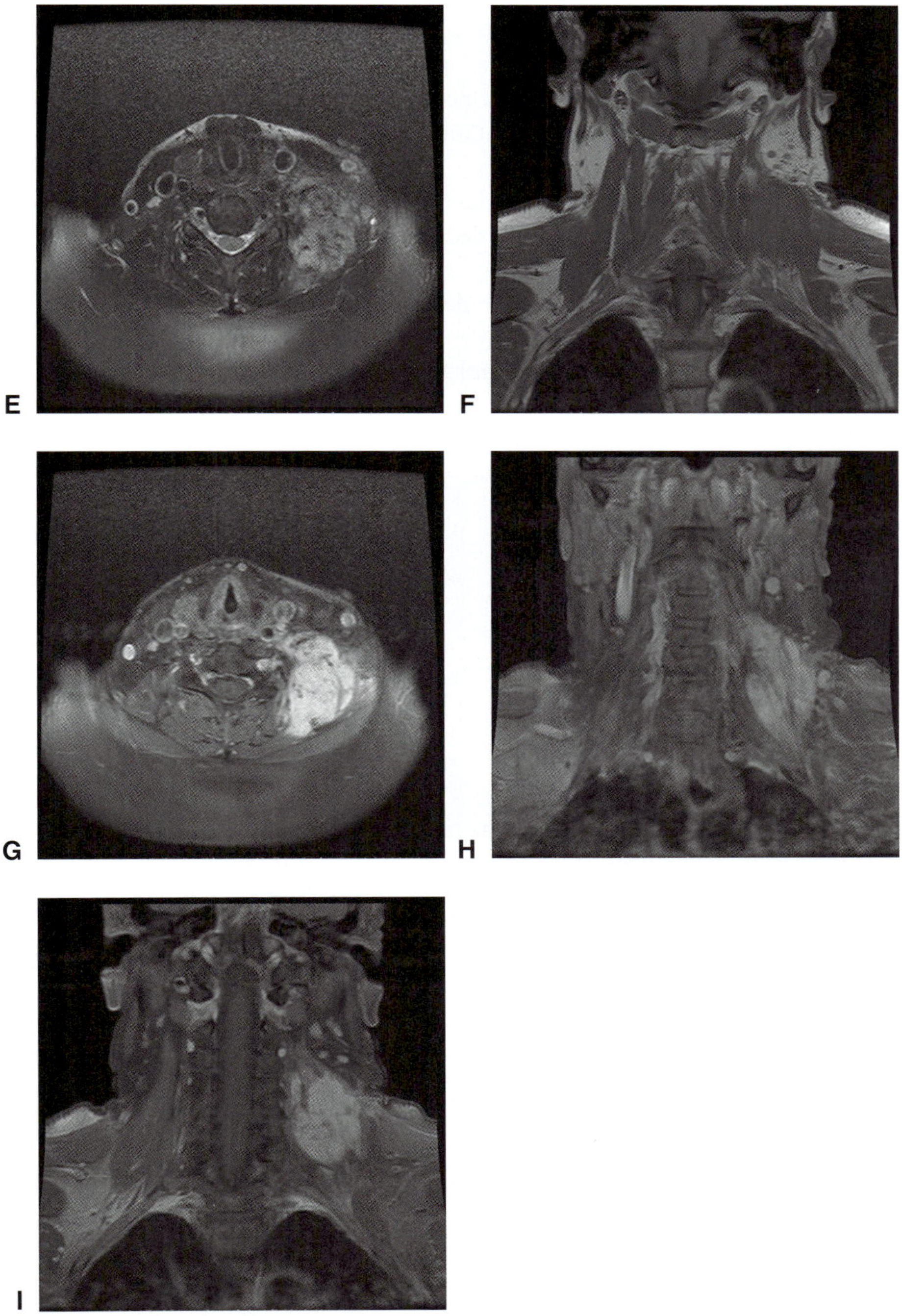

Figure 3.8. ***(continued)*** **E.** Axial T2: Heterogeneously hyperintense lateral neck mass. **F.** Coronal T1 precontrast: Hypointense lateral neck mass. **G.** Axial T1 postcontrast: Avid enhancement. **H.** Coronal T1 postcontrast fat sat: Avid enhancement. **I.** Coronal T1 postcontrast fat sat: Avid enhancement.

▶ Fibrosarcoma

Definition: Malignant mesenchymal neoplasm of fibroblasts or spindle cells with abundant cellularity and can contain hemorrhage or necrosis.

Epidemiology: Rare tumor with less than 50 reported cases with male dominance and in the third to fourth decades of life.

Molecular and genetic profile: Undetermined.

Clinical features and standard therapy: Surgical resection is the mainstay of treatment; local recurrence is common.

Imaging

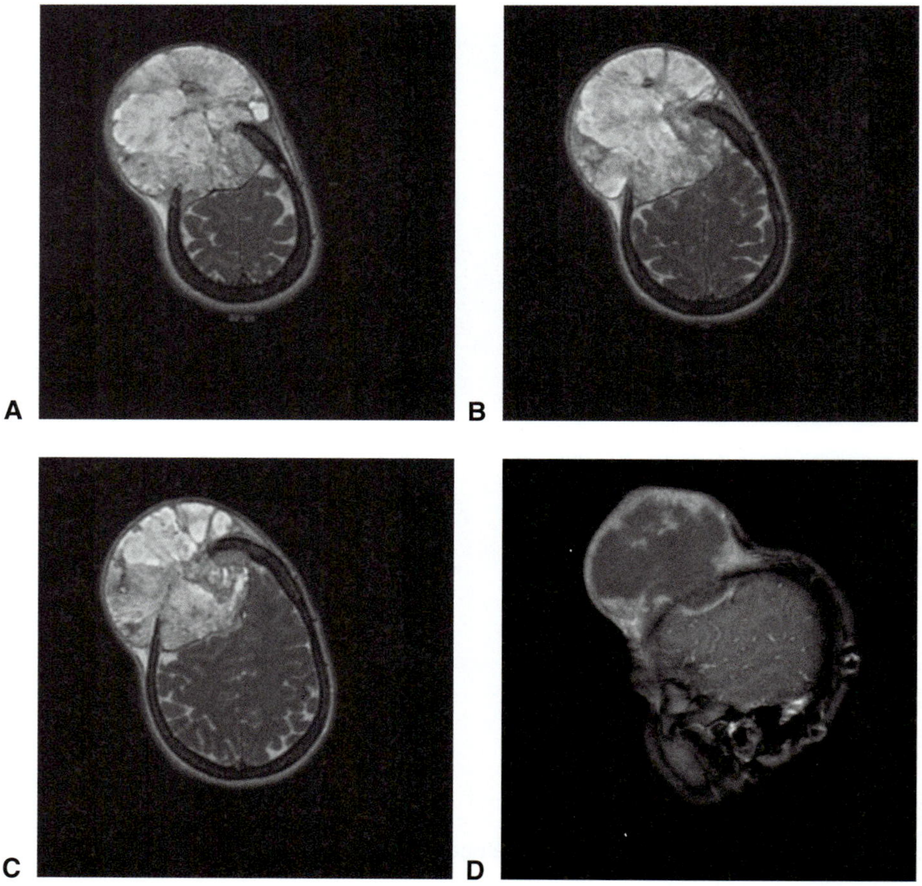

Figure 3.9. Imaging of fibrosarcoma. A. Axial T2: Large heterogeneous hyper- and hypointense mass with intracranial extra-axial and extracranial components and destruction of involved skull. **B.** Axial T2: Large heterogeneous hyper- and hypointense mass with intracranial extra-axial and extracranial components and destruction of involved skull. **C.** Axial T2: Large heterogeneous hyper- and hypointense mass with intracranial extra-axial and extracranial components and destruction of involved skull. **D.** Sagittal T1 postcontrast: Avid enhancement of the peripheral component with large areas of non-enhancing necrotic areas.

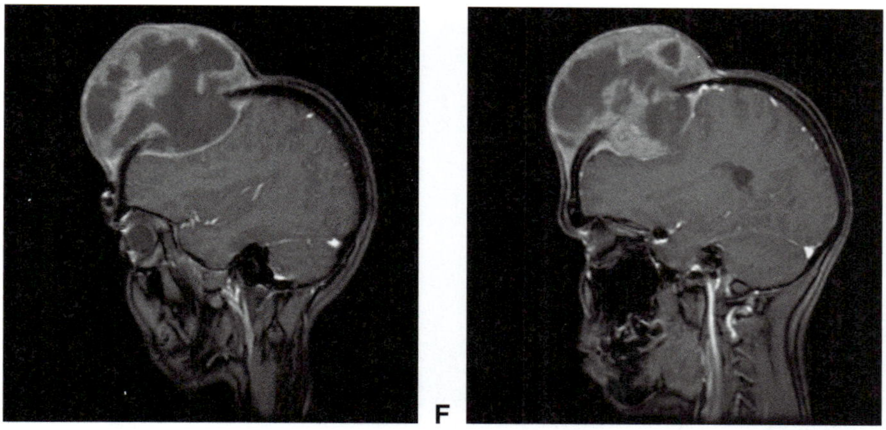

E F

Figure 3.9. ***(continued)*** **E.** Sagittal T1 postcontrast: Avid enhancement of the peripheral component with large areas of non-enhancing necrotic areas. **F.** Sagittal T1 postcontrast: Avid enhancement of the peripheral component with large areas of non-enhancing necrotic areas.

Chondrosarcoma

Definition: Malignant mesenchymal neoplasm with cartilaginous differentiation usually arising de novo within the cartilage cells within the CNS. Two distinct types exist: (1) conventional chondrosarcoma involving the intracranial, extraosseous compartment and (2) mesenchymal chondrosarcoma involving the bones of the skull or spine.

Epidemiology: A rare tumor, about 6% of all skull neoplasms.

Affected age group: Usually affects people in fourth to sixth decades, with female-to-male ratio of 1:1.5.

Molecular and genetic profile: *NCOA2* (nuclear receptor coactivator) gene rearrangement.

Clinical features and standard therapy: Surgery followed by radiation therapy to residual tumor; local recurrence is common.

Imaging

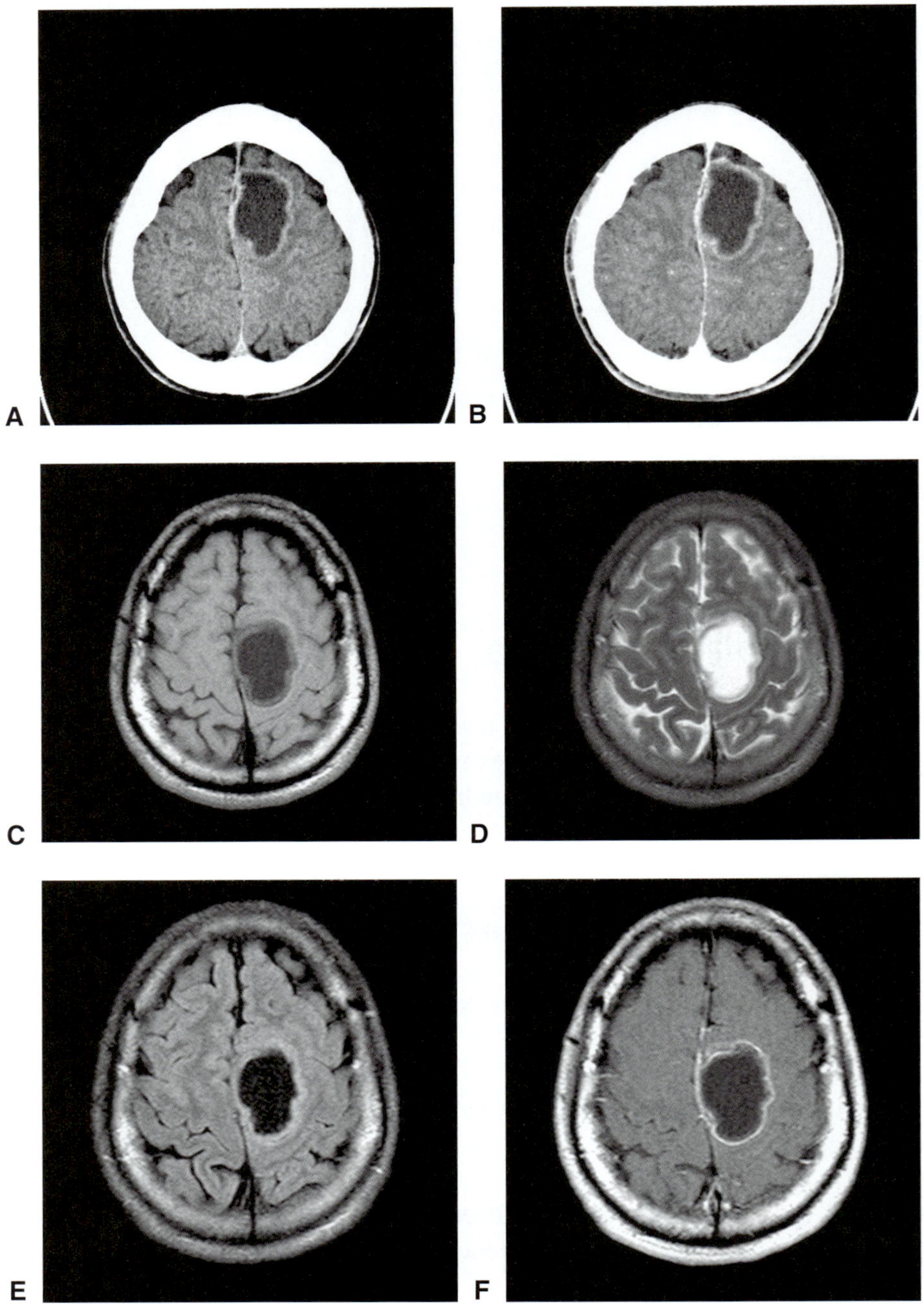

Figure 3.10. Imaging of supratentorial chondrosarcoma. A. Axial CT postcontrast: Extra-axial mass with thin rim of enhancement. **B.** Axial CT postcontrast: Extra-axial mass with thin rim of enhancement. **C.** Axial T1 precontrast: Extra-axial mass with thin rim of hypointense rim of solid tumor. **D.** Axial T2: Homogeneously hyperintense central cystic component. **E.** Axial FLAIR: Homogeneously hypointense central cystic component. **F.** Axial T1 postcontrast: Avid enhancement of the thin rim of solid tumor.

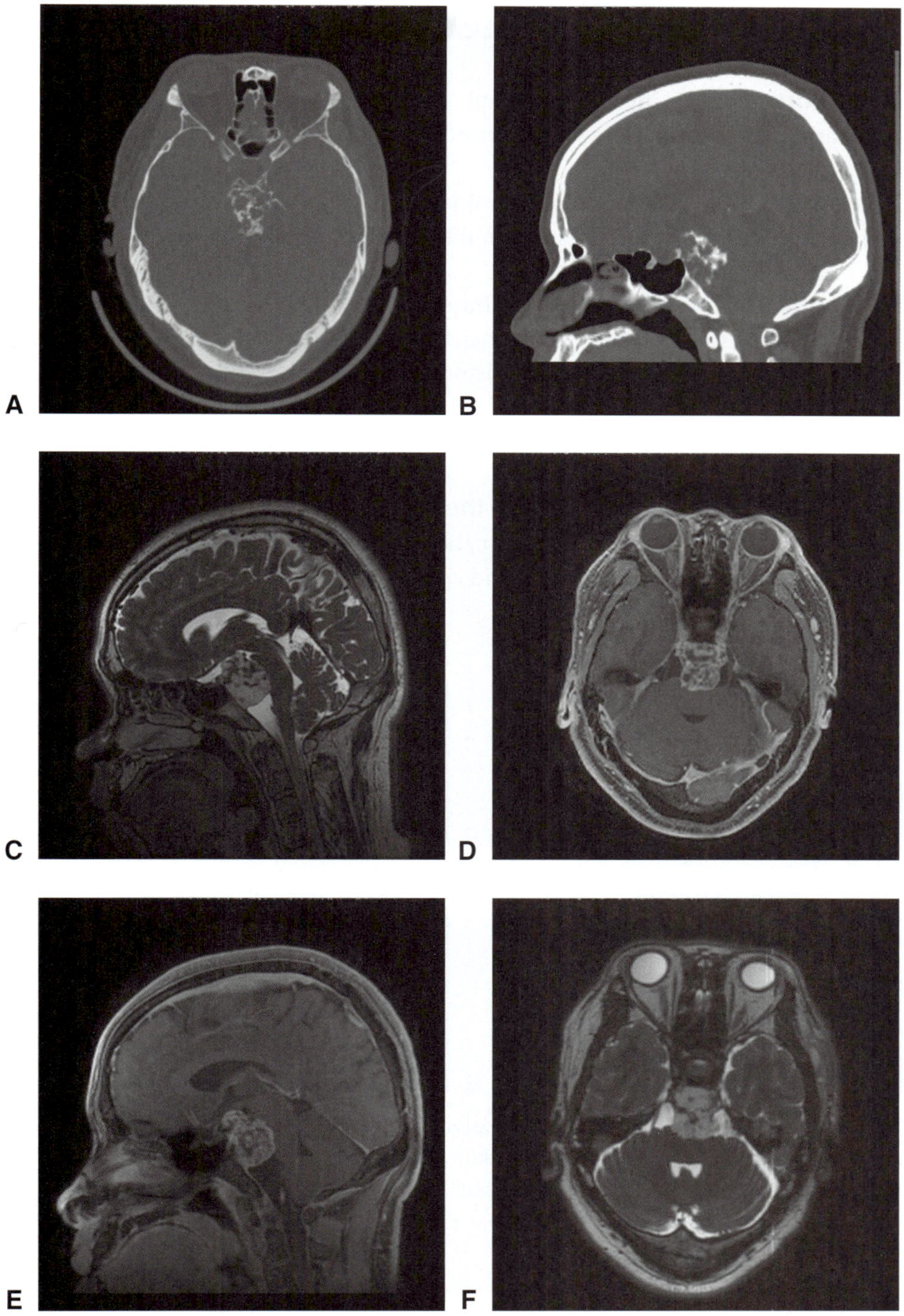

Figure 3.11. Imaging of clival chondrosarcoma. A. Axial CT bone window: Rings and arcs pattern of calcific retroclival mass. **B.** Sagittal CT bone window: Rings and arcs pattern of calcific retroclival mass. **C.** Sagittal T2: Mildly hyperintense solid tumor surrounds the calcific component. **D.** Axial T1 postcontrast: Heterogeneous enhancement with non-enhancement of the calcific component. **E.** Sagittal T1 postcontrast: Heterogeneous enhancement with non-enhancement of the calcific component. **F.** Axial T2: Mildly hyperintense solid tumor surrounds the calcific component.

▶ Primary CNS Osteosarcoma

Definition: Rare primary malignant bone-forming mesenchymal tumor originating from the osseous structures of the cranial vault, face, skull, or spine.

Epidemiology: More commonly seen in adolescents and young adults, with preferred location of skull and spine in the craniospinal axis.

Molecular and genetic profile: Inherited osteosarcomas are seen in the following genetic syndromes with associated key gene mutations: Li–Fraumeni syndrome (p. 53), hereditary retinoblastoma (RB1), Rothmund–Thomson syndrome RecQ Like Helicase 4 (RECQL4), Bloom's syndrome (BLM, RECQL2), and Werner syndrome (WRN, RECQL3).

Clinical features and standard therapy: Surgical resection is the first line of treatment followed by a combination of chemotherapy drugs (cisplatin, doxorubicin, ifosfamide, etoposide, and epirubicin).

Imaging

A B

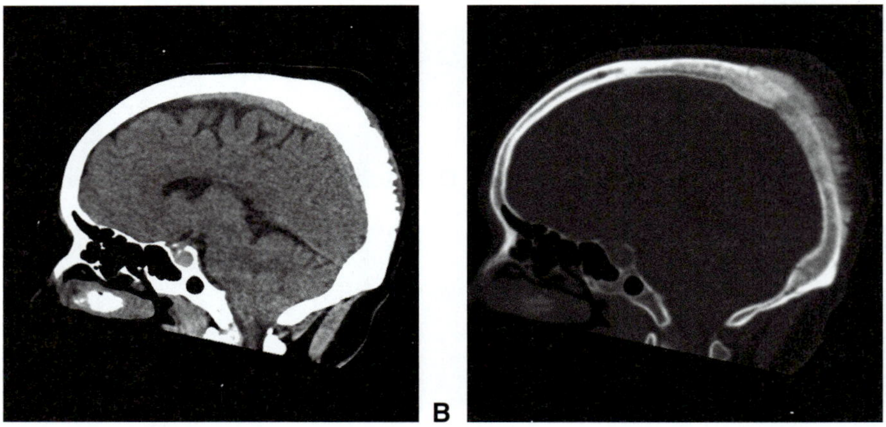

Figure 3.12. Imaging of transcalvarial osteosarcoma. A. Sagittal CT: Diffuse sclerosis and thickening of the parietal skull. **B.** Sagittal CT bone window: Periosteal reaction and permeative destruction of skull.

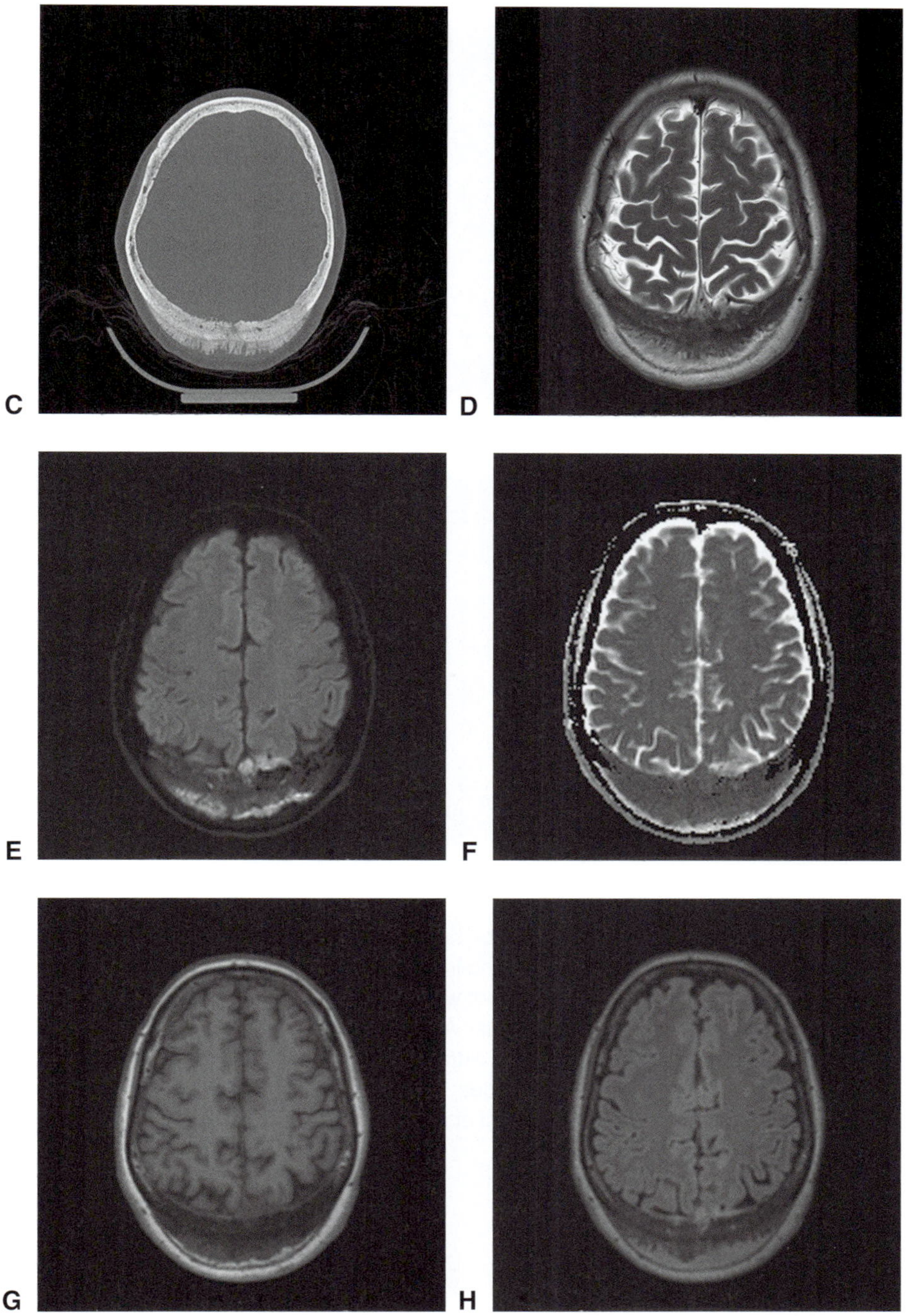

Figure 3.12. ***(continued)*** **C.** Axial CT bone window: Periosteal reaction and permeative destruction of skull. **D.** Axial T2: Diffuse hypointense skull marrow with hyperintense extra-osseous soft tissue component within the scalp. **E.** Axial DWI: Intracranial component and thrombosis of superior sagittal sinus are better seen. **F.** Axial ADC: Diffuse reduced diffusion within the expanded skull. **G.** Axial T1 precontrast: Hypointense intra- and extra-osseous tumor. **H.** Axial FLAIR: Hypointense intraosseous tumor and hyperintense soft tissue tumor.

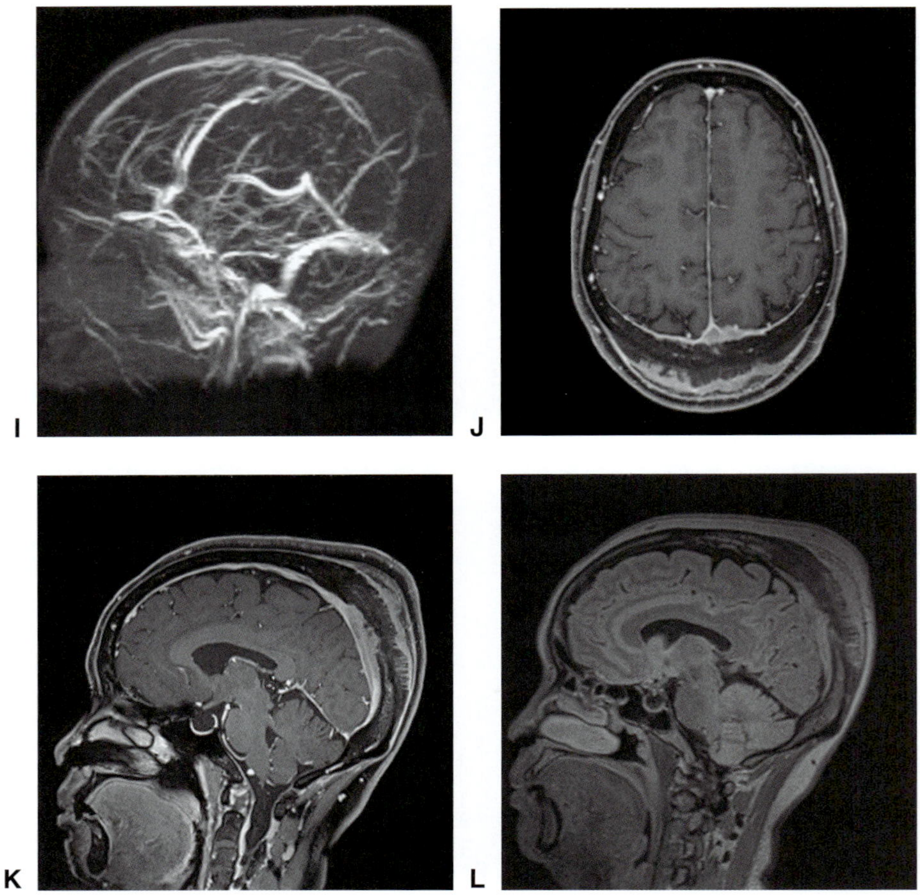

Figure 3.12. ***(continued)*** **I.** Phase contrast Magnetic resonance venogram (MRV): Occlusion of distal one-third of superior sagittal sinus due to tumor. **J.** Axial T1 postcontrast: Avid enhancement within the intracranial dural-based tumor and extra-osseous extracranial soft tissue tumor, but without enhancement within the sclerotic osseous tumor. **K.** Sagittal T1 postcontrast: Avid enhancement within the intracranial dural-based tumor and extra-osseous extracranial soft tissue tumor, but without enhancement within the sclerotic osseous tumor. **L.** Sagittal FLAIR: Hyperintense signal within the occluded distal one-third of superior sagittal sinus and hyperintense extracranial soft tissue tumor.

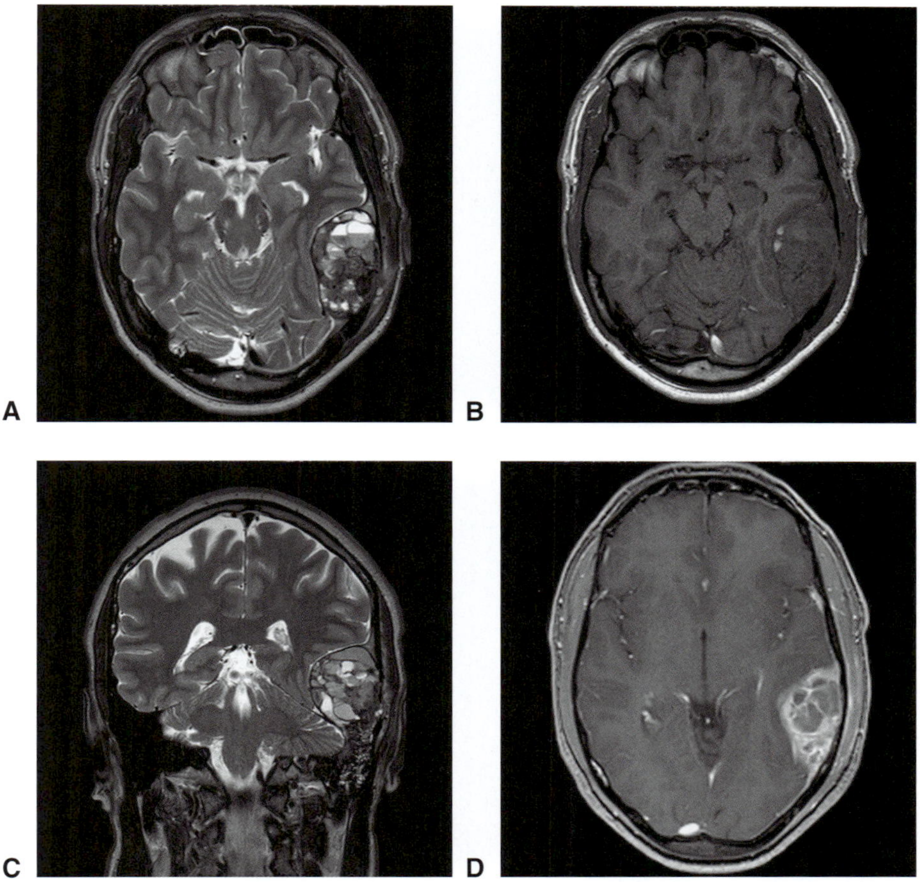

Figure 3.13. Imaging of temporal bone osteosarcoma. A. Axial T2: Heterogeneously hypointense, circumscribed, extra-axial mass with multiple intratumoral cysts with fluid-blood level and containing blood products of varying age. **B.** Axial T1 precontrast: Mostly isointense mass with two discrete areas of T1 shortening, likely blood products, along the deep tumor margin. **C.** Coronal T2: Heterogeneously hypointense extra-axial mass with multiple intratumoral cysts with fluid-blood level and containing blood products of varying age. **D.** Axial T1 postcontrast: Avid but heterogeneous enhancement with non-enhancing cystic areas.

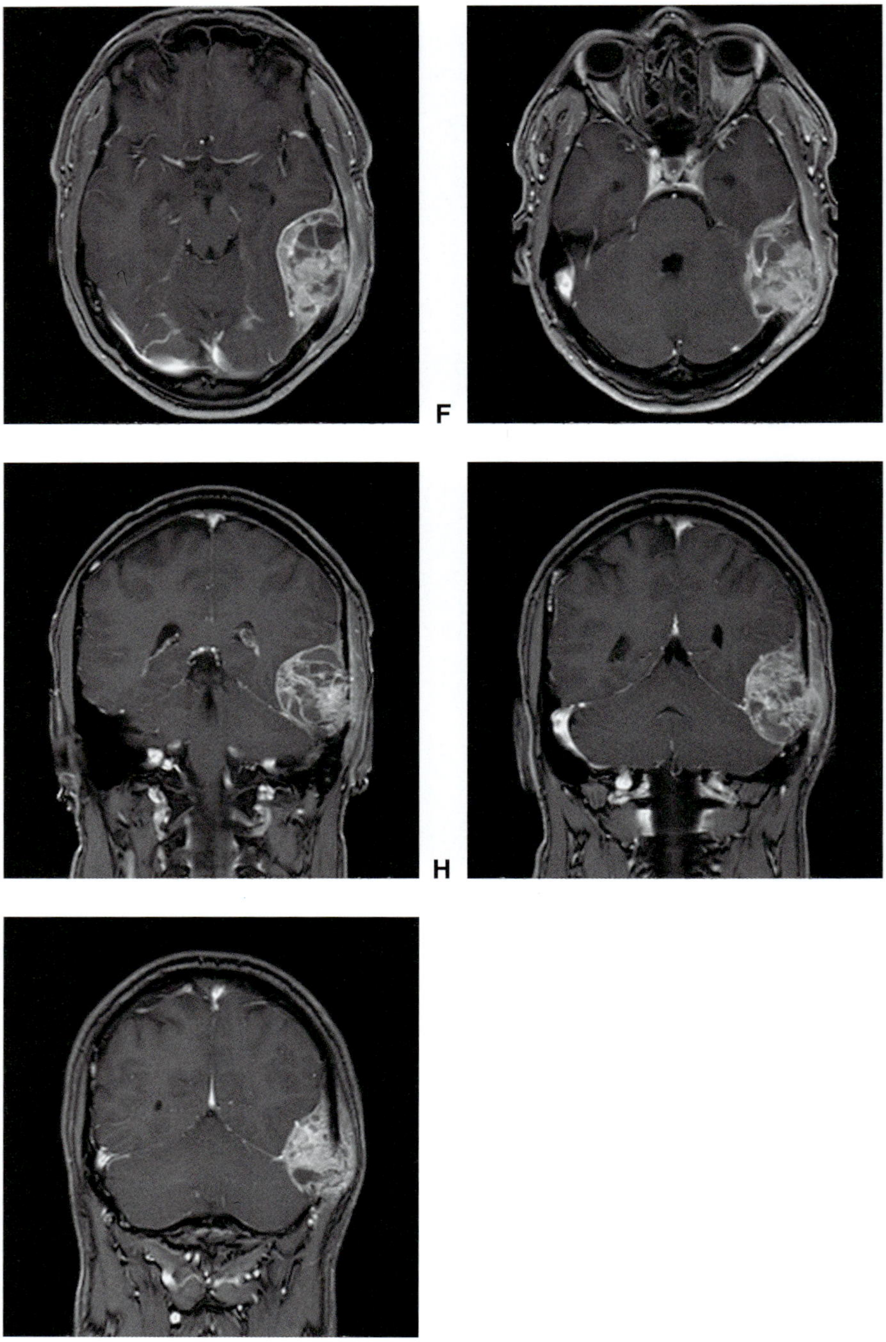

E F G H I

Figure 3.13. ***(continued)*** **E.** Axial T1 postcontrast: Invasion of dura and destruction of skull with extracranial extension of tumor into the scalp tissue. **F.** Axial T1 postcontrast: Invasion of dura and destruction of skull with extracranial extension of tumor into the scalp tissue. **G.** Coronal T1 postcontrast: Avid but heterogeneous enhancement with nonenhancing cystic areas. **H.** Coronal T1 postcontrast: Invasion of dura and destruction of skull with extracranial extension of tumor into the scalp tissue. **I.** Coronal T1 postcontrast: Invasion of dura and destruction of skull with extracranial extension of tumor into the scalp tissue.

Bibliography

Chandler JP, Yashar P, Laskin WB, Russell EJ. Intracranial chondrosarcoma: a case report and review of the literature. *J Neurooncol.* 2004;68:33–39.

Ganeshan D, Menias CO, Pickhardt PJ, et al. Tumors in von Hippel-Lindau syndrome: from head to toe-comprehensive state-of-the-art review. *Radiographics.* 2018;38:849–866.

Hettmer S, Fleischhack G, Hasan C, et al. Intracranial manifestation of osteosarcoma. *Pediatr Hematol Oncol.* 2002;5:347–354.

Kim J-H, Chang K-H, Na DG, et al. Imaging features of meningeal inflammatory myofibroblastic tumor-weighted imaging and dynamic susceptibility contrast-enhanced perfusion-weighted MR imaging. *AJNR Am J Neuroradiol.* 2009;30:1261–1267.

Metellus P, Bouvier C, Guyotat J, et al. Solitary fibrous tumors of the central nervous system: clinicopathological and therapeutic considerations of 18 cases. *Neurosurgery.* 2007;60(4):715–722.

Rhim JH, Kim JH, Moon KC, et al. Desmoid-type fibromatosis in the head and neck: CT and MR imaging characteristics. *Neuroradiology.* 2013;55:351–359.

Schweizer L, Koelsche C, Sahm F, et al. Meningeal hemangiopericytoma and solitary fibrous tumors carry the NAB2-STAT6 fusion and can be diagnosed by nuclear expression of STAT6 protein. *Acta Neuropathol.* 2013;125(5):651–658.

She D, Yang X, Xing Z, Cao D. Differentiating hemangioblastomas from brain metastases using diffusion-weighted imaging and dynamic susceptibility contrast-enhanced perfusion-weighted MR imaging. *AJNR Am J Neuroradiol.* 2016;37:1844–1850.

Weon YC, Kim EY, Kim HJ, Byun HS, Park K, Kim JH. Intracranial solitary fibrous tumors: imaging findings in 6 consecutive patients. *AJNR Am J Neuroradiol.* 2007;28(8):1466–1469.

4 CNS Lymphomas

Overview

CNS lymphomas are extranodal, non-Hodgkin's lymphomas confined to the brain and spine comprised of malignant lymph tissues. Vast majority (~90%) are diffuse large B-cell lymphomas arising inside the central nervous system (CNS) without systemic disease, and the remaining 10% are a heterogeneous group made up of mucosa-associated lymphoid tissue (MALT) lymphoma of the dura, intravascular large B-cell lymphoma, anaplastic large cell lymphoma, and immunodeficiency-associated lymphoma.

	Age range in years (mean)	Female: Male	Cell of origin	WHO Grade	Molecular/ genetic markers	Prognosis
Diffuse large B-cell lymphoma	52–77 (67)	1:0.8	Large B-cell	NA	*CD20, PAX5, CD79a*	Guarded
Extranodal marginal zone or MALT lymphoma of the dura	60–70 (65)	1.5:1	Marginal zone B-cell	NA	*BIRC3*, *MALT1*	Favorable
Intravascular lymphoma	60–79	1:1	Large B-cell	NA	Unknown	Poor
Anaplastic large cell lymphoma	20–30	1:3	T-cell	NA	*CD30* *ALK*+ (young) *ALK*− (older)	Guarded to poor
Immunodeficiency-associated lymphoma	32–42 (37) in HIV 42–62 (52) in transplant	1:11	Large B-cell	NA	*EBV*	Poor
Lymphomatosis cerebri	41–72 (63)	1:1	Large B cell	NA	Unknown	Poor

Diffuse Large B-cell CNS Lymphoma

Definition: Malignant neoplasm comprised of mature large B-cell lymphocytes confined to the CNS at presentation and commonly referred to as primary CNS lymphoma (PCNSL) or diffuse large B-cell CNS lymphoma (DLBCL).

Epidemiology: Up to 3% of all brain tumors primarily affecting older adults with peak incidence during the fifth to seventh decades of life, median patient age of 56 years, and the female-to-male ratio of 2:3.

Molecular and genetic profile: The pathogenesis of PCNSL remains largely unclear, but aberrant somatic hypermutation has a major impact on the pathogenesis of PCNSL with the expression of the following genes—*BCL6*, *BCL2*, *MYC*, *PIM1*, *PAX5*, *RHOH*, *KLHL14*, *OSBPL10*, and *SUSD2*.

CSF markers: The presence of lymphoma cells in cerebrospinal fluid (CSF) is sufficient to diagnose PCNSL without the need for brain biopsy. Immunophenotyping using flow cytometric analysis and polymerase chain reaction (PCR) analysis of CSF can aid in distinguishing malignant and reactive lymphocytes in CSF.

Clinical features and standard therapy: Clinical presentation of PCNSL depends on the location of tumor, but patients most commonly present with signs and symptoms of mass effect or seizure. The current standard therapy for newly diagnosed PCSNL is high-dose intravenous methotrexate (antifolate and antimetabolite)-based chemotherapy with additional agents including temozolomide, rituximab, etoposide, and cytarabine.

Prognosis: With prompt diagnosis and treatment, there is a trend toward a survival increase in more recent years, especially in those patients enrolled in clinical trials with aggressive multidrug chemotherapy regimens. However, the prognosis of patients with PCNSL is guarded, with overall survival at 53%, 38%, and 26% at 1, 2, and 5 years after diagnosis, respectively.

Imaging of Primary CNS Lymphoma or Diffuse Large B-cell CNS Lymphoma

PCNSL usually presents as single or multiple solid, avidly enhancing, and homogeneously intraparenchymal masses with exuberant surrounding vasogenic edema and mass effect.

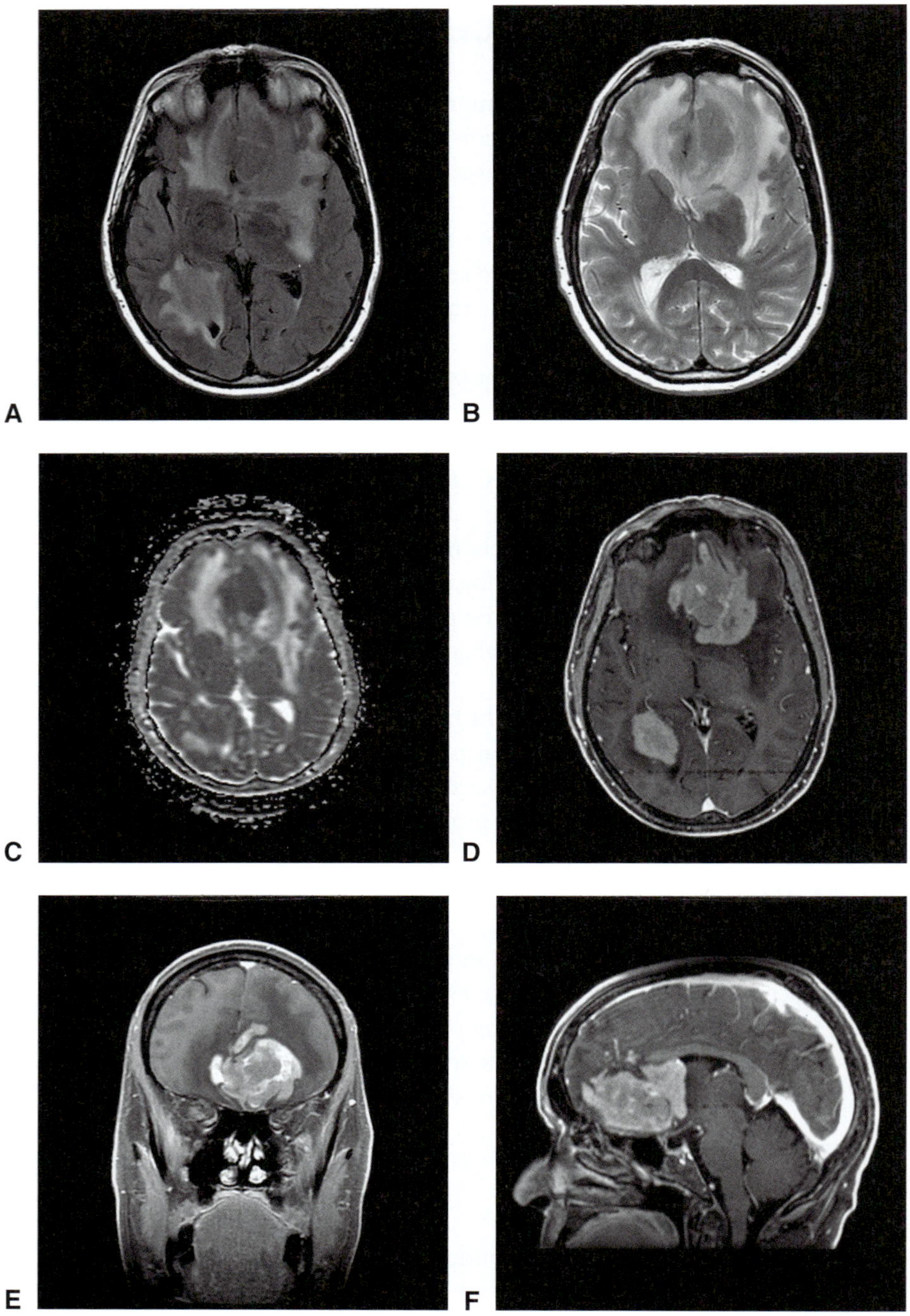

Figure 4.1. Imaging of CNS lymphoma. A. Axial Fluid-attenuated inversion recovery (FLAIR): Two large hypointense masses—anterior frontal midline and right intraventricular—with surrounding edema. **B.** Axial T2: Hypointense tumor. **C.** Axial Apparent diffusion coefficient (ADC): Marked reduced diffusion. **D.** Axial T1 postcontrast: Avid but heterogeneous enhancement within both tumors. **E.** Coronal T1 postcontrast: Avid but heterogeneous enhancement within both tumors. **F.** Sagittal T1 postcontrast: Avid but heterogeneous enhancement within both tumors.

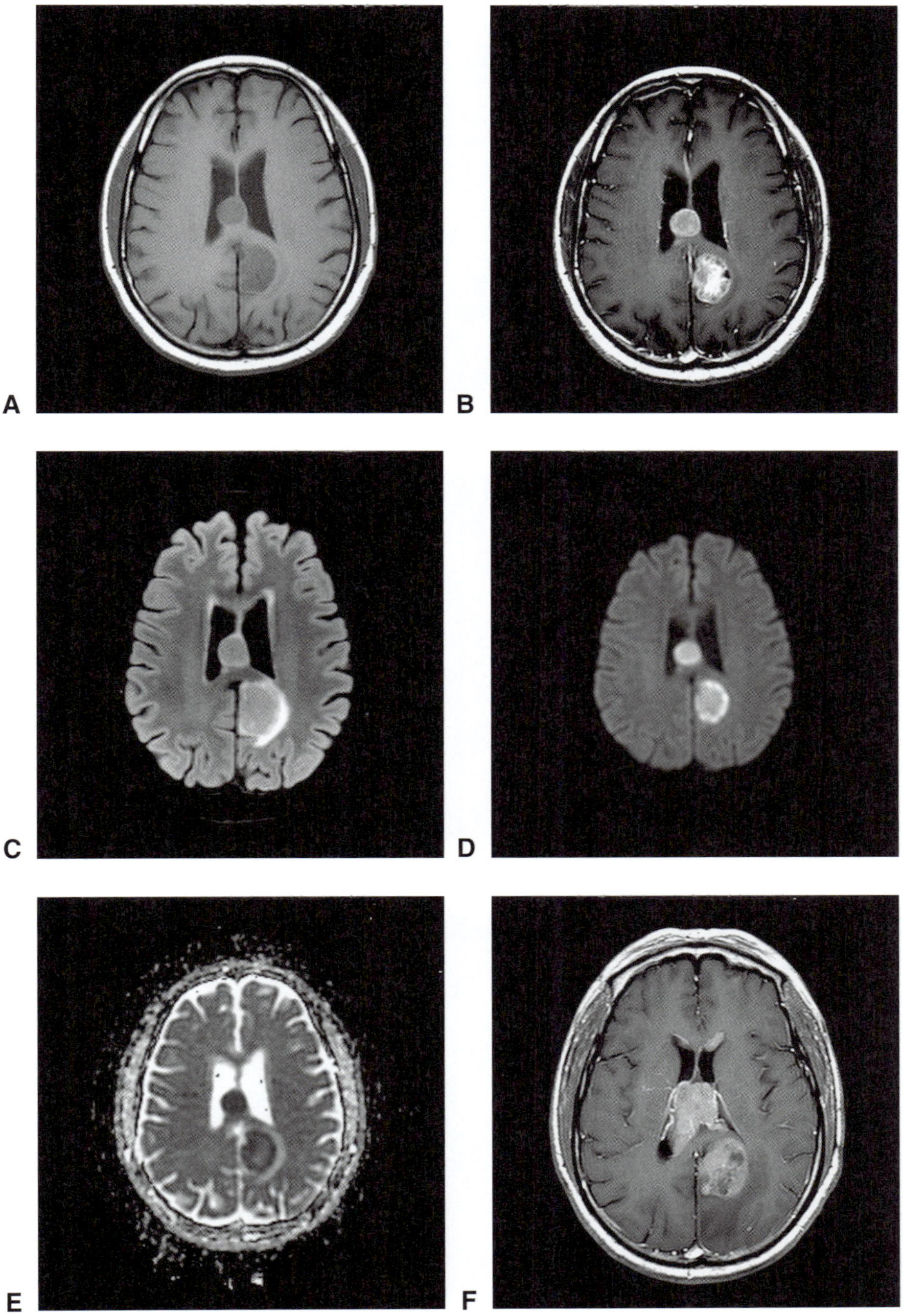

Figure 4.2. Imaging of CNS lymphoma. A. Axial T1 precontrast: Hypointense two solid masses. **B.** Axial T1 postcontrast: Avid but heterogeneous enhancement. **C.** Axial FLAIR: Hypointense solid masses. **D.** Diffusion-weighted imaging (DWI): Homogeneously high-signal intensity on DWI. **E.** ADC: Homogeneously reduced on ADC map. **F.** Axial T1 postcontrast (4 months follow-up): Growth of two solid masses and bifrontal subependymal spread of tumor.

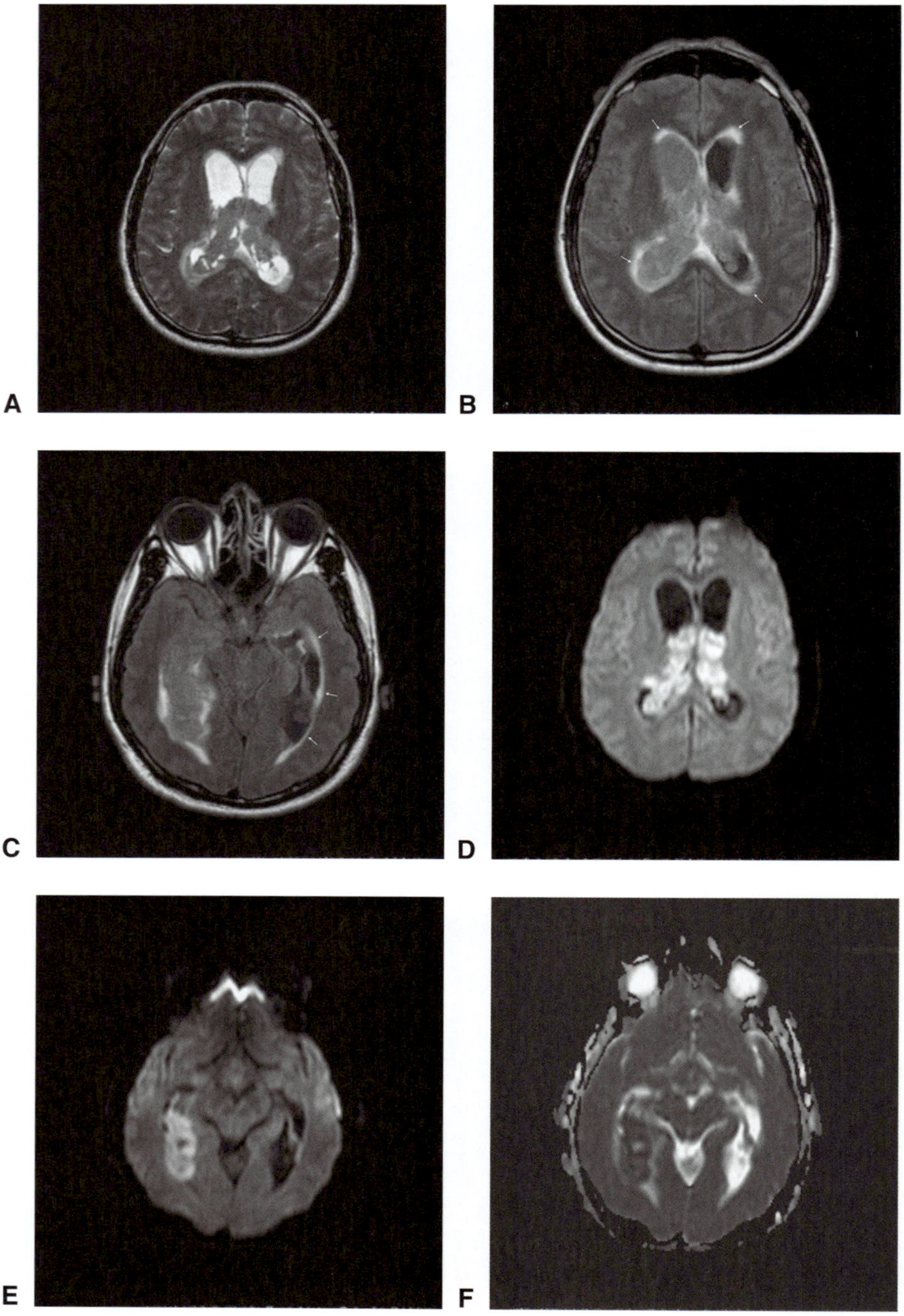

Figure 4.3. Imaging of CNS lymphoma. A. Axial T1 precontrast: Hypointense two solid masses. **B.** Axial T1 postcontrast: Avid but heterogeneous enhancement. **C.** Axial FLAIR: Hypointense solid masses. **D.** DWI: Homogeneously high-signal intensity on DWI. **E.** ADC: Homogeneously reduced on ADC map. **F.** Axial T1 postcontrast (4 months follow-up): Growth of two solid masses and bifrontal subependymal spread of tumor.

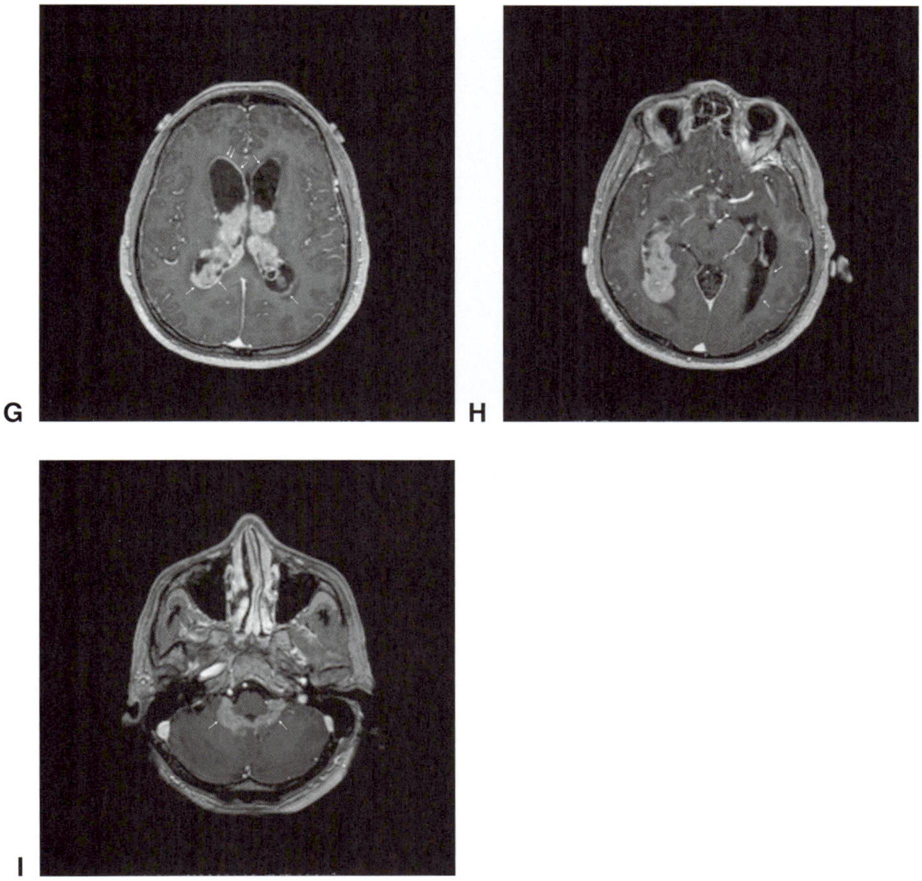

Figure 4.3. ***(continued)*** **G, H.** Axial T1 postcontrast: Nodular intraventricular enhancing masses filling the lateral ventricles and diffuse linear subependymal enhancement (arrows) coating the ventricular surface. **I.** Axial T1 postcontrast: Bulky enhancing masses filling bilateral foramina of Luschka (arrows).

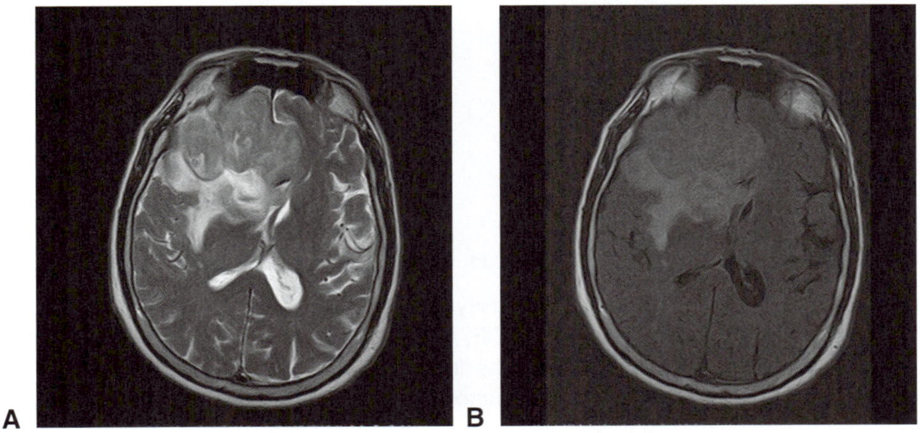

Figure 4.4. Imaging of CNS lymphoma. A. Axial T1 precontrast: Hypointense two solid masses. **B.** Axial T1 postcontrast: Avid but heterogeneous enhancement.

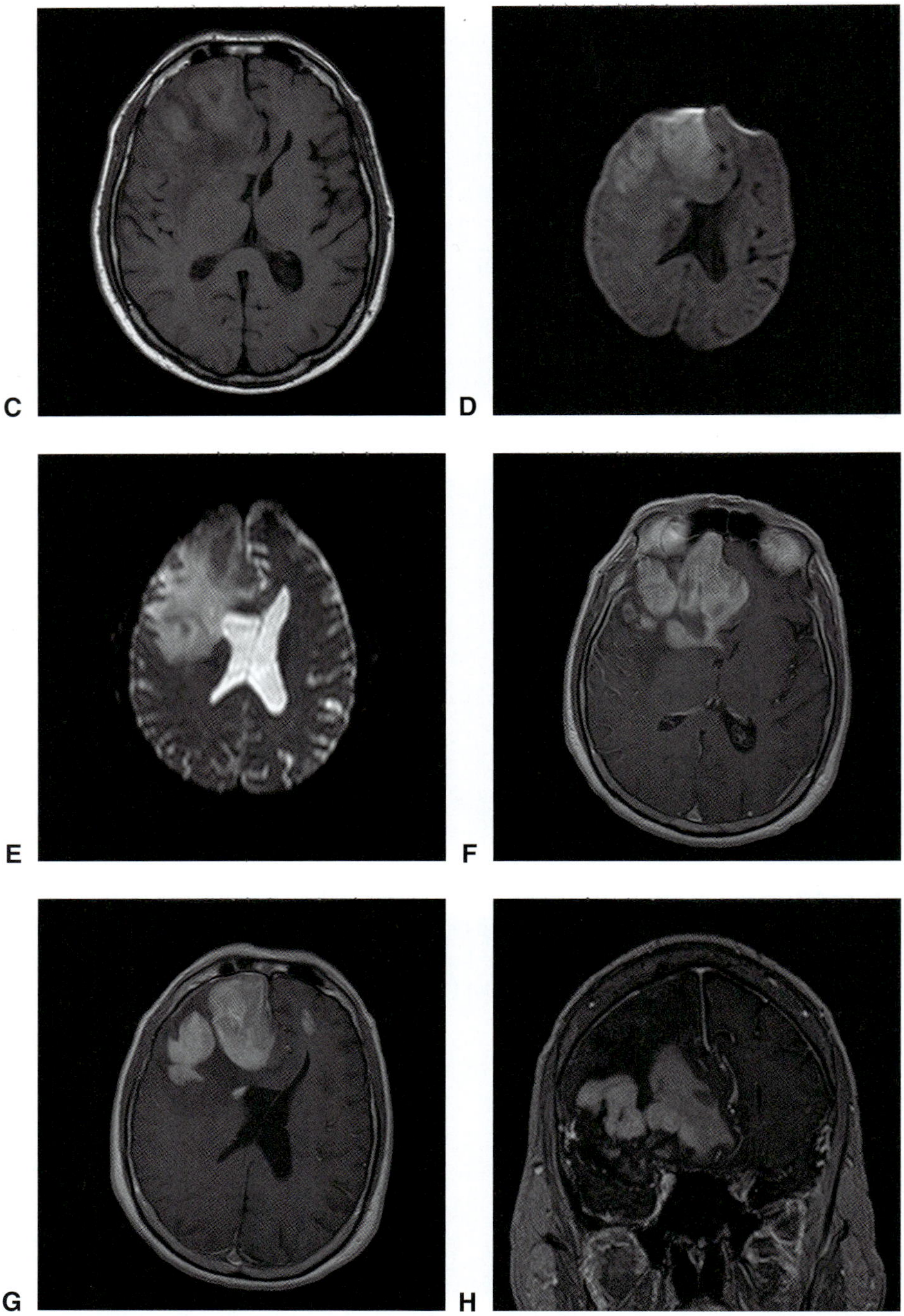

Figure 4.4. ***(continued)*** **C.** Axial FLAIR: Hypointense solid masses. **D.** DWI: Homogeneously high-signal intensity on DWI. **E.** ADC: Homogeneously reduced on ADC map. **F.** Axial T1 postcontrast (4 months follow-up): Growth of two solid masses and bifrontal subependymal spread of tumor. **G–I.** Axial T1 (G), coronal T1 (H), and sagittal T1 (I) postcontrast images: Bulky solid masses with avid enhancement; the largest conglomerate mass in the right inferior frontal gyrus and additional subependymal and left frontal tumor.

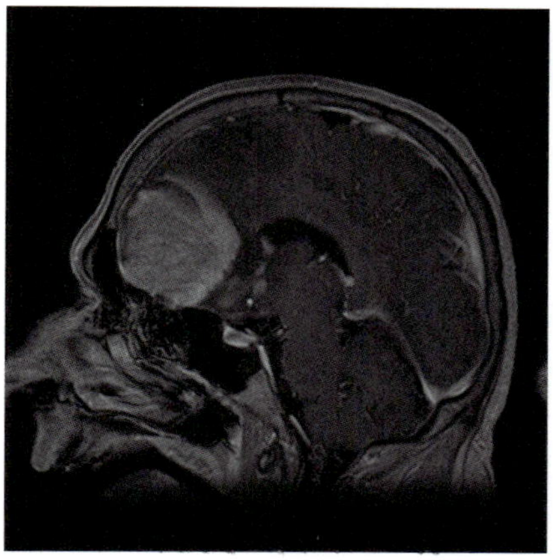

I

Figure 4.4. ***(continued)***

Mucosa-Associated Lymphoid Tissue Lymphoma of the Dura

Definition: A biologically distinct subtype of lymphoma arising from the dura mater and comprised of low-grade B-cell marginal zone lymphoma (MZL), which is an indolent non-Hodgkin lymphoma that occurs more frequently in the gastrointestinal tract, where it has been called the "mucosa-associated lymphoid tissue (MALT)" lymphoma. Characteristically, MALT lymphoma in the brain almost exclusively involves the dura and spares the brain parenchyma.

Epidemiology: Less than 3% of all PCNSLs with a predilection for late-middle-aged women, in contrast to brain parenchyma PCNSL, which has a slight male and elderly predilection.

Molecular and genetic profile: Lack of CD10, CD5, and CD23.

CSF markers: No specific markers have been identified.

Clinical features and standard therapy: Patients with MALT lymphoma of the dura have better prognosis than those with parenchymal PCNSL with 5-year overall survival rate greater than 86%.

Imaging

MALT lymphoma of the dura presents as extra-axial enhancing mass that can involve both subdural and subarachnoid spaces.

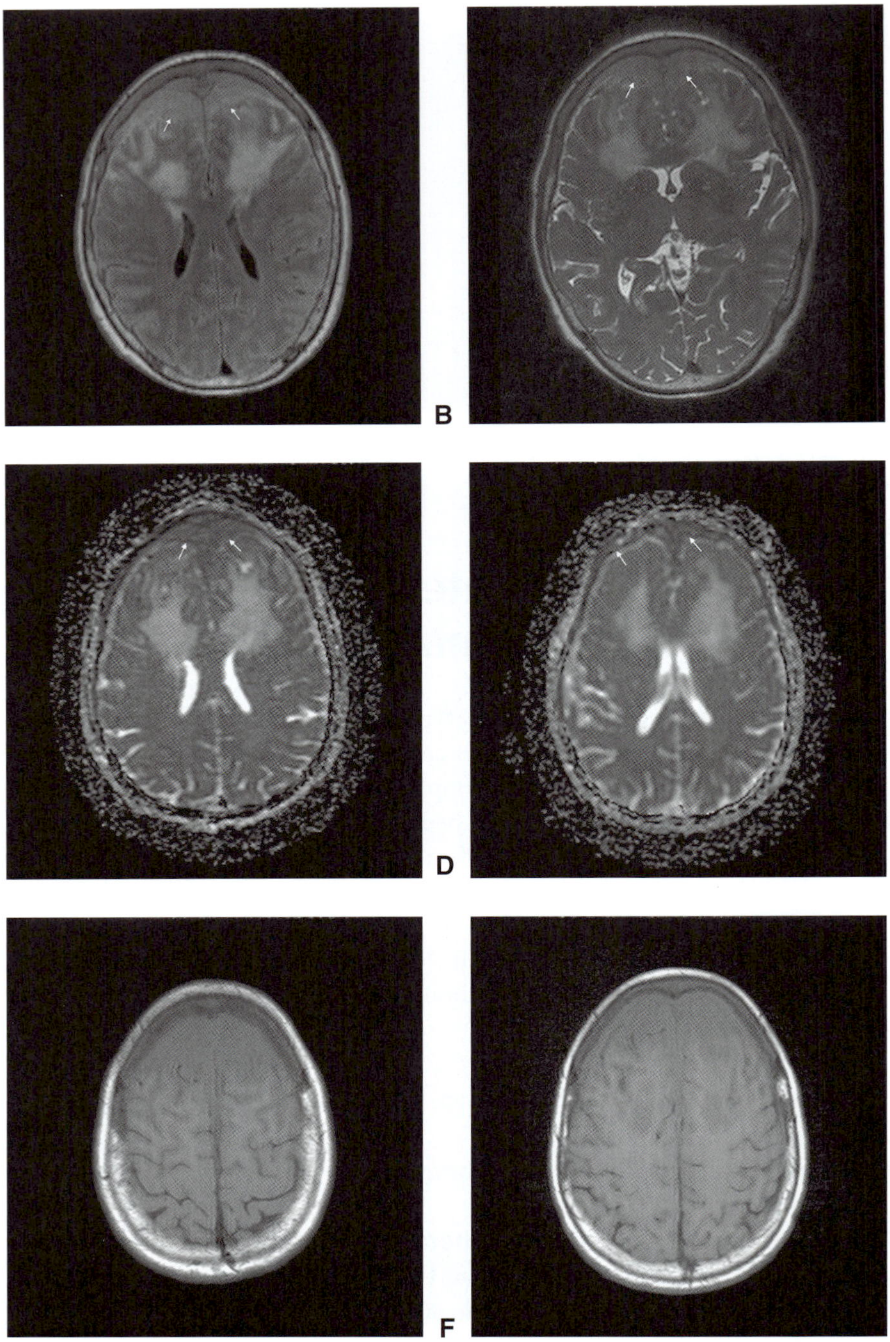

A B C D E F

Figure 4.5. Imaging MALT lymphoma. A. Axial Fluid-attenuated inversion recovery (FLAIR): Mildly hyperintense mass in the bilateral frontal extra-axial space (arrows). **B.** Axial T2 Fast spin echo (FSE): Heterogeneously hypointense mass in the bilateral frontal extra-axial space (arrows). **C.** Axial Apparent diffusion coefficient (ADC): Reduced diffusion with the mass (arrows). **D.** Axial Apparent diffusion coefficient (ADC): Reduced diffusion with the mass (arrows). **E.** Axial T1 precontrast: Homogeneously hypointense dural based mass. **F.** Axial T1 precontrast: Homogeneously hypointense dural based mass.

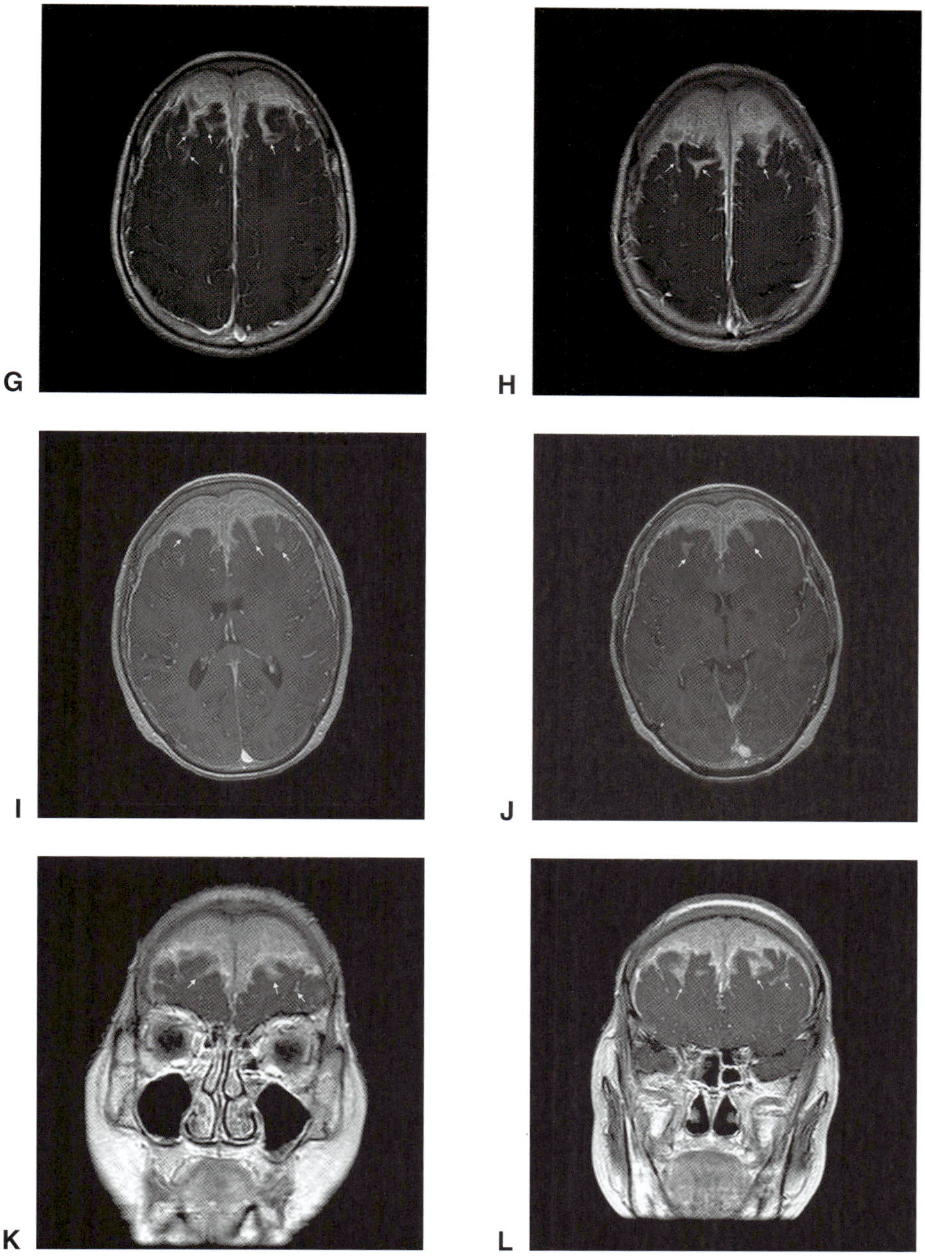

Figure 4.5. ***(continued)*** **G.** Axial T1 postcontrast: Avid enhancement within the dural based mass with extension into the adjacent subarachnoid space (arrows). **H.** Axial T1 postcontrast: Avid enhancement within the dural based mass with extension into the adjacent subarachnoid space (arrows). **I.** Axial T1 postcontrast: Avid enhancement within the dural based mass with extension into the adjacent subarachnoid space (arrows). **J.** Axial T1 postcontrast: Avid enhancement within the dural based mass with extension into the adjacent subarachnoid space (arrows). **K.** Coronal T1 postcontast: Avid enhancement within the dural based mass with extension into the adjacent subarachnoid space (arrows). **L.** Coronal T1 postcontast: Avid enhancement within the dural based mass with extension into the adjacent subarachnoid space (arrows).

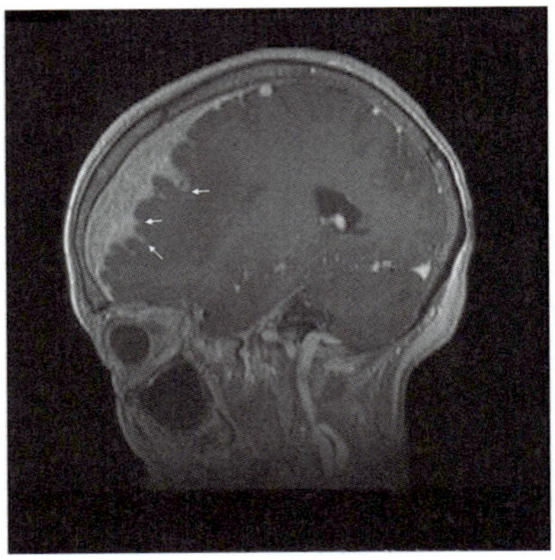
M

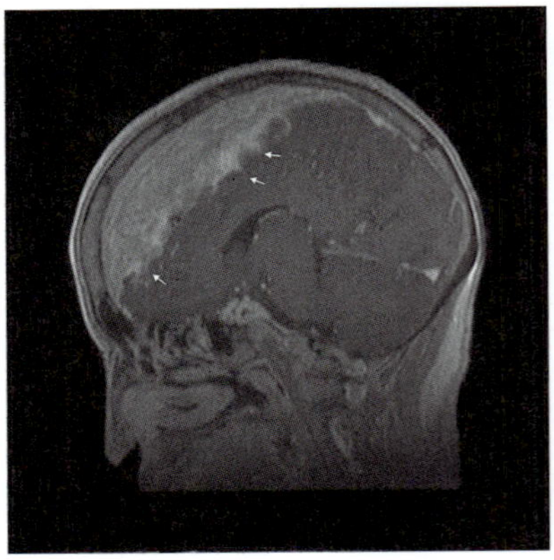
N

Figure 4.5. ***(continued)*** **M.** Sagittal T1 postcontast: Avid enhancement within the dural based mass with extension into the adjacent subarachnoid space (arrows). **N.** Sagittal T1 postcontast: Avid enhancement within the dural based mass with extension into the adjacent subarachnoid space (arrows).

▶ Intravascular Lymphoma

Definition: A distinct and rare subtype of extranodal non-Hodgkin's diffuse large B-cell lymphoma characterized by the proliferation of clonal lymphocytes within the intravascular compartment, especially arterioles and capillaries, of the brain and rarely involving the spinal cord.

Epidemiology: Intravascular lymphoma (IVL) is rare and has an estimated incidence of 0.095 cases/1,000,000) with the median age at diagnosis of 70 years and slight male predominance.

Molecular and genetic profile: There is scant information on tissue analysis of IVL due to the paucity of available brain tissue biopsy. Diagnosis of IVL is often delayed due to neurologic clinical presentation simulating stroke that leads to cerebrovascular disease workup.

CSF markers: Due to its growth confined within the intravascular lumen, IVL is not usually detectable on CSF analysis.

Clinical features and standard therapy: Patients with IVL often present with focal neurological symptoms, including motor and sensory deficits, hemiparesis, altered mental status, cognitive decline, seizure, or transient ischemic attack-like symptoms. Dementia and seizure outnumber stroke-like clinical presentation.

Diagnosis of IVL is often delayed or missed because of the clinical presentation that mimics stroke, dementia, or nonspecific neurodegenerative pattern of symptoms. Diagnosis at autopsy is not infrequent. Currently, there is no standard-of-care therapy, but rituximab-containing chemotherapies with or without radiotherapy have been tried without much success in prolonging survival.

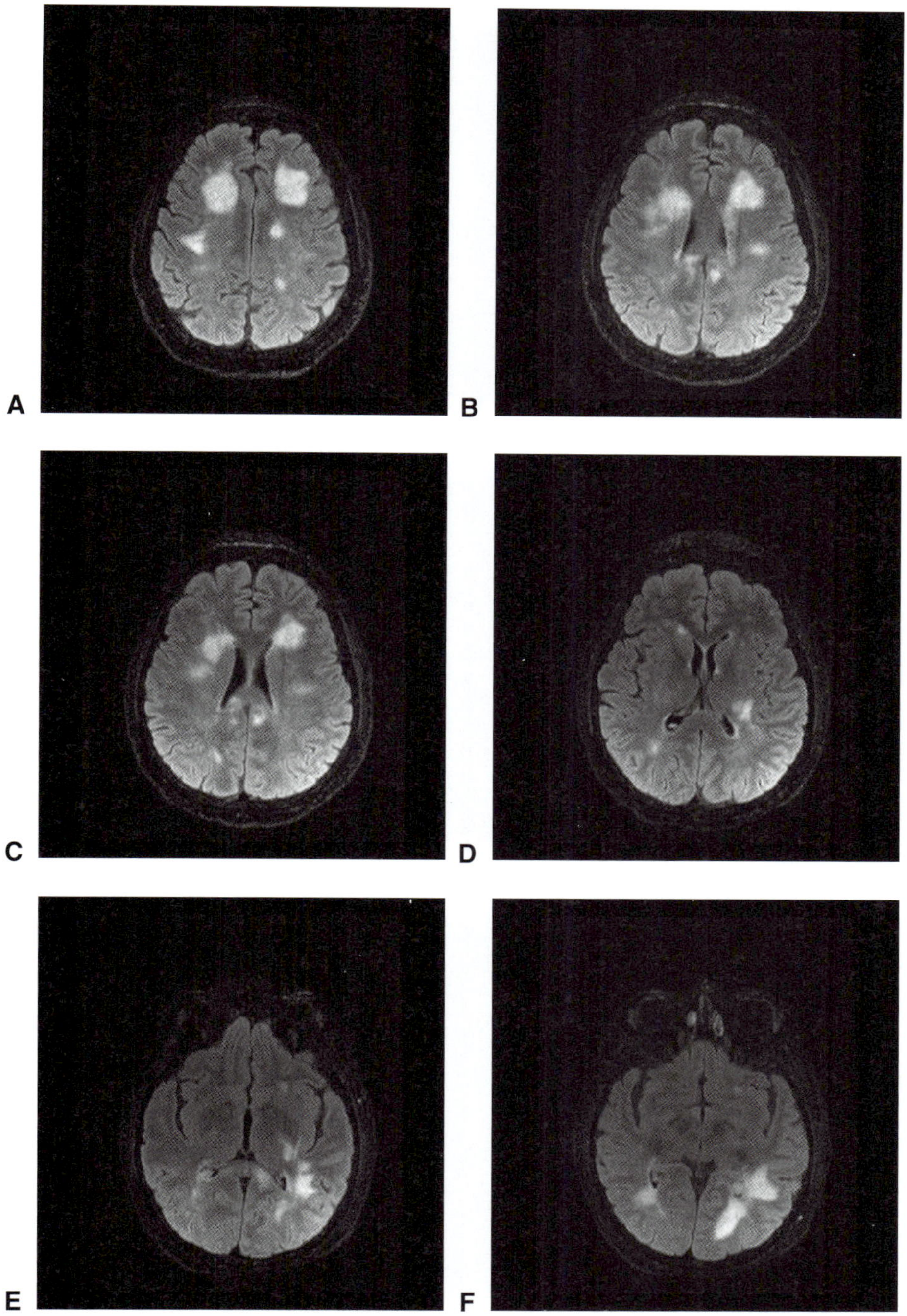

Figure 4.6. Imaging of intravascular lymphoma. A–F. Axial FLAIR: Multiple foci of periventricular or deep white matter hyperintense lesions with the largest ones in the bilateral frontal lobes and left peri-atrial white matter.

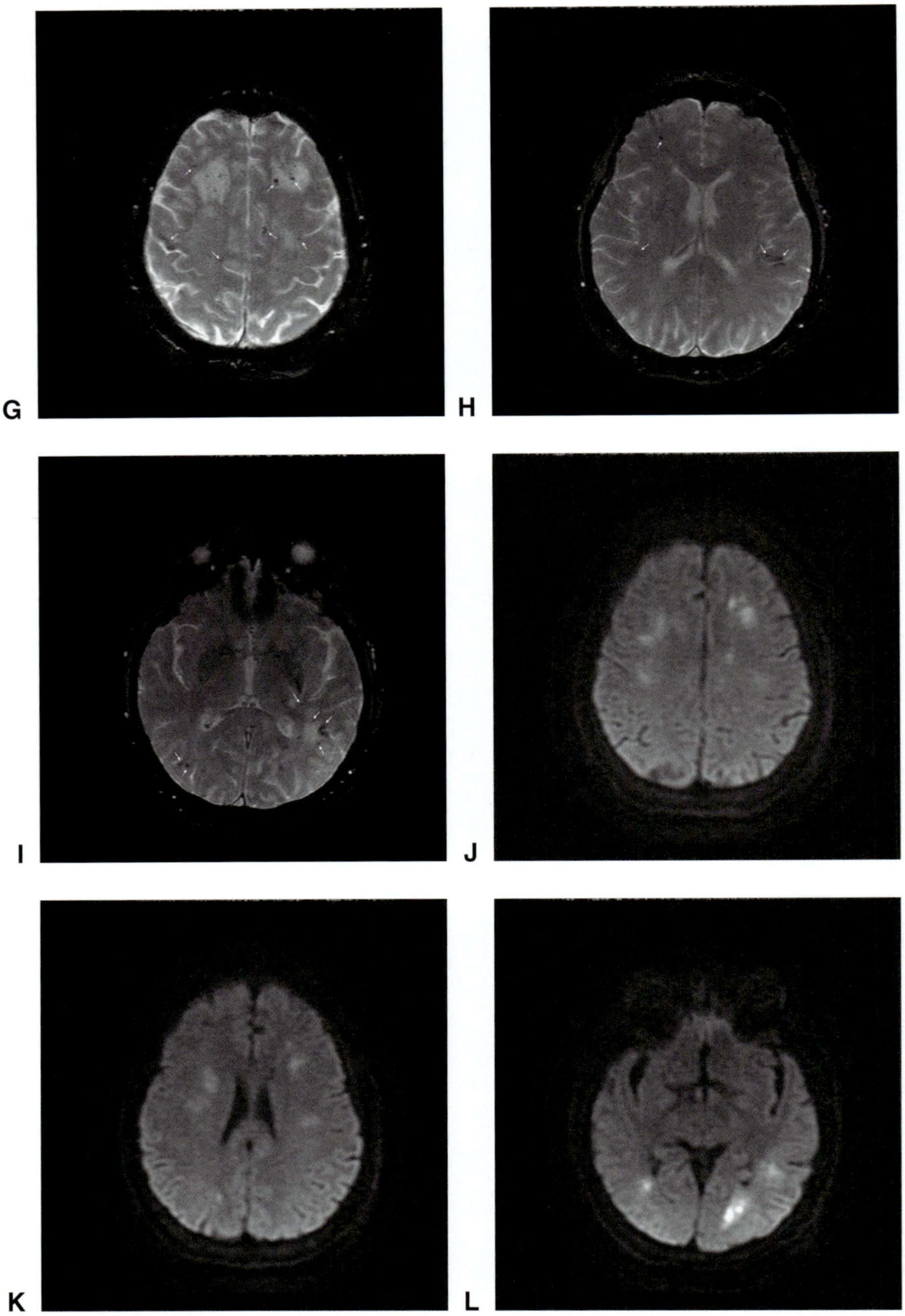

Figure 4.6. ***(continued)*** **G–I.** Axial SWI: Numerous punctate or gyriform susceptibility lesions (arrows) with or without underlying FLAIR abnormality are seen. **J–L.** Axial DWI: Reduced diffusion associated with multiple foci of periventricular or deep white matter hyperintense lesions.

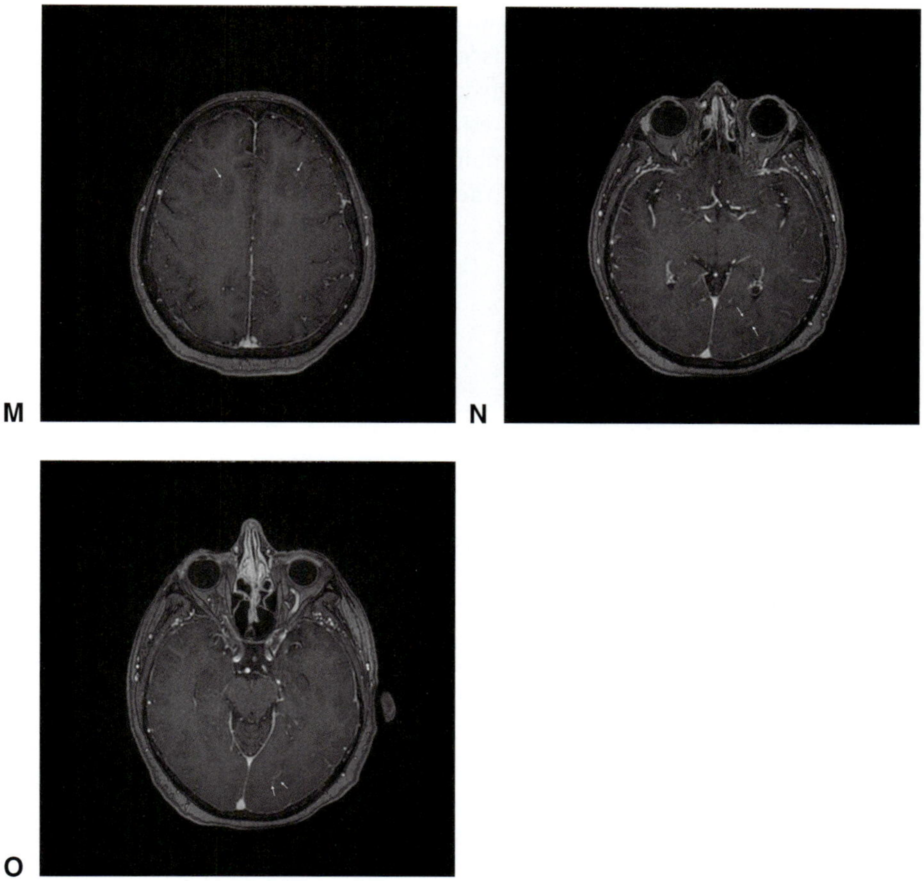

Figure 4.6. ***(continued)*** **M–O.** Axial T1 postcontrast: Patchy or curvilinear enhancement (arrows) associated with the larger bilateral frontal and left peri-atrial white matter lesions.

Anaplastic Large Cell Lymphoma

Definition: An aggressive T-cell lymphoma, a rare distinct subtype of CNS lymphoma, that frequently expresses anaplastic lymphoma kinase (ALK) and characteristically involves the leptomeningeal compartment of the brain.

Epidemiology: Less than 10% of PCNSL affecting much younger age group, usually the first to third decades of life, without gender predilection. There are two clinicopathologic groups: ALK-positive ALCL occurring in young patients (mean, 13 years) and ALK-negative ALCL occurring in older patients (mean, 43 years).

Molecular and genetic profile: Anaplastic large cell lymphoma refers to a group of CD30-positive and anaplastic lymphoma kinase (ALK)-positive T-cell non-Hodgkin lymphomas.

Clinical features and standard therapy: Due to frequent leptomeningeal involvement, patients with anaplastic large cell lymphoma (ALCL) can present with symptoms and signs of viral or mycobacterial meningoencephalitis. Standard therapy for ALCL has not been established mainly because of the great rarity of this lymphoma variant. A combination of methotrexate-based chemotherapies is considered the first line of therapy.

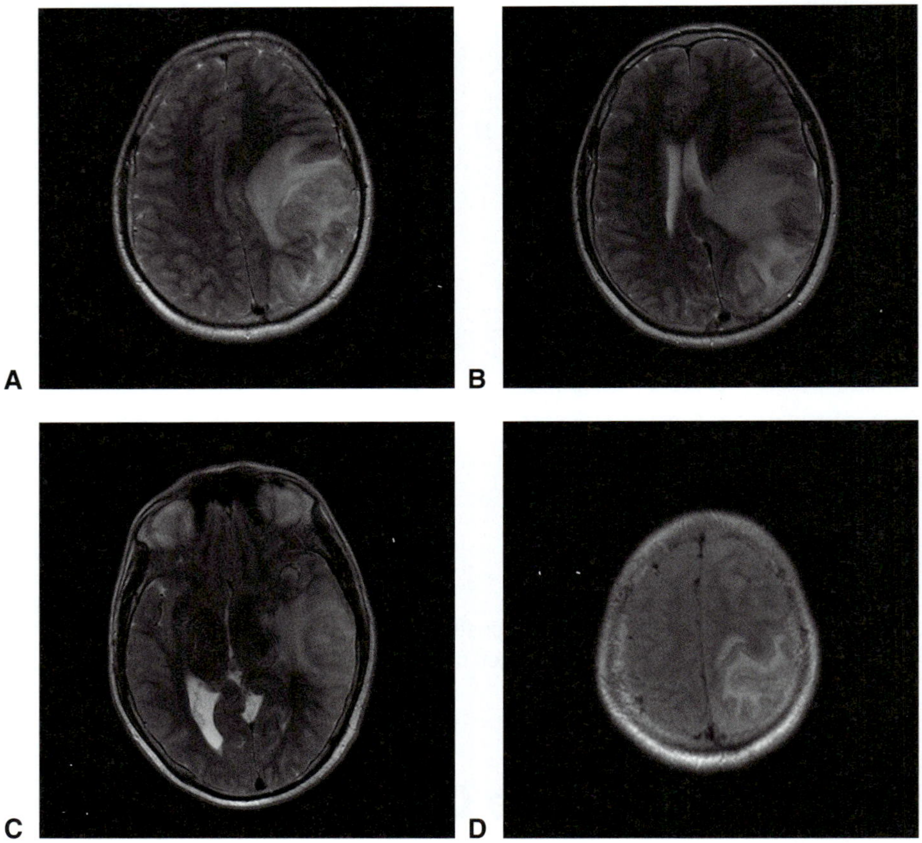

Figure 4.7. **Imaging of anaplastic large cell lymphoma. A–C.** Axial T2: Lobular hypointense mass in the right parietal and temporal lobes associated with surrounding edema and mass effect. **D–F.** Axial FLAIR: Lobular hypointense masses in the right frontal and temporal lobes associated with surrounding edema and mass effect.

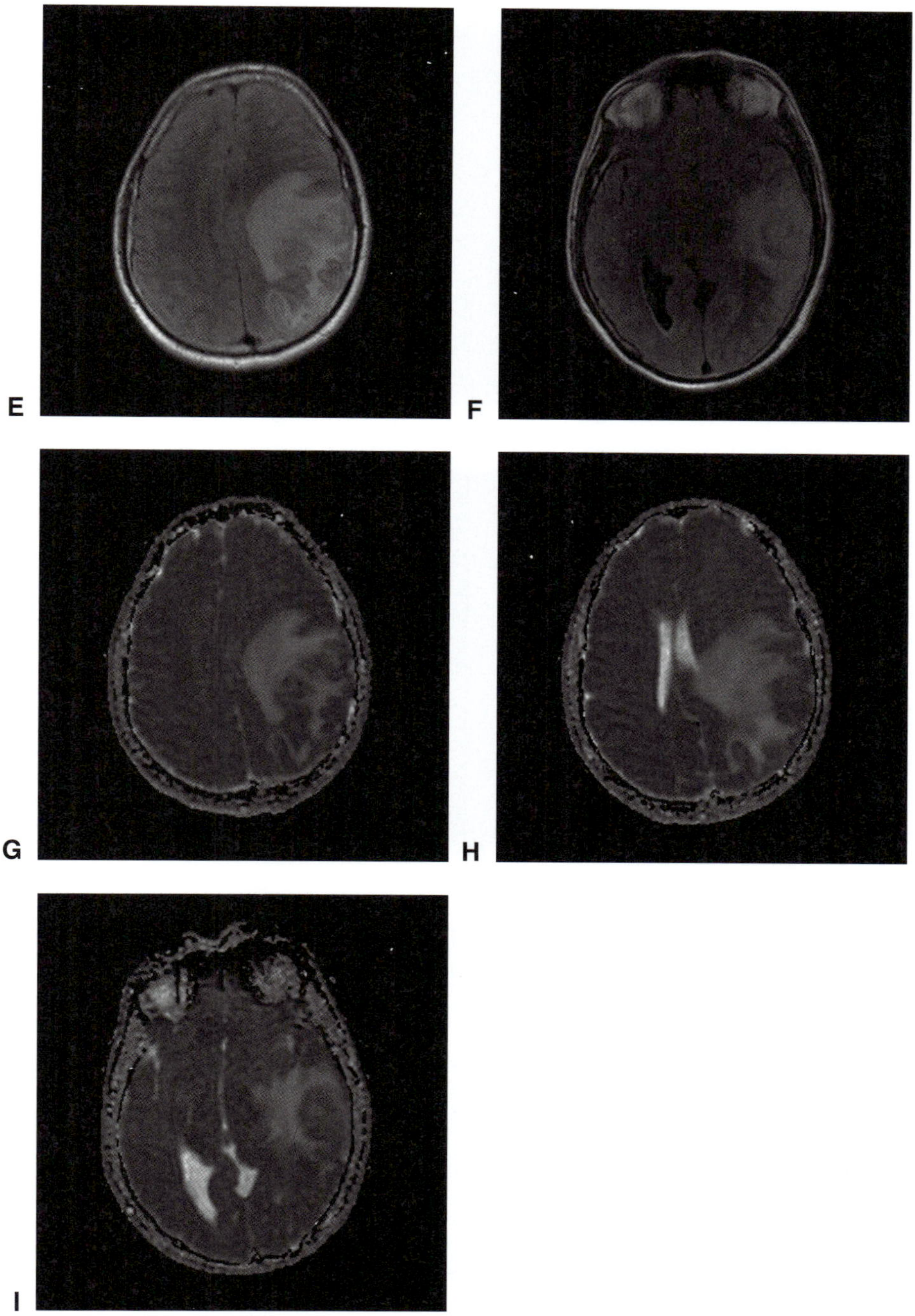

Figure 4.7. ***(continued)*** **G–I.** Axial ADC: Reduced diffusion within the hypointense mass.

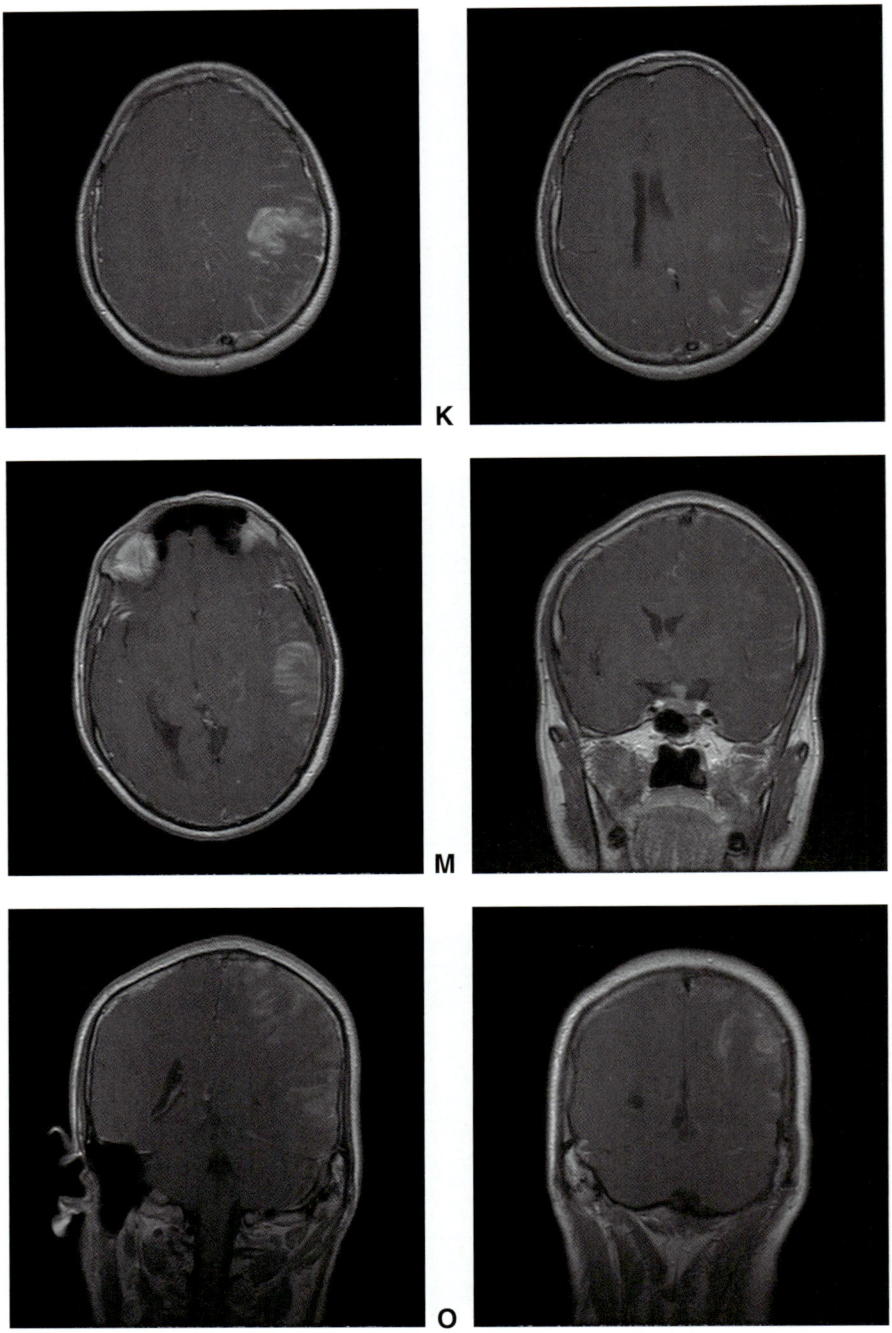

J K L M N O

Figure 4.7. ***(continued)*** **J–L.** Axial T1 postcontrast: Avid enhancement of the right frontal and temporal masses associated with extensive neighboring leptomeningeal enhancement. **M–O.** Coronal T1 postcontrast: Diffuse leptomeningeal enhancement is noted in the left frontal and temporal convexities.

Immunodeficiency-Associated CNS Lymphoma

Definition: CNS lymphoma occurring in individuals with inherited or acquired immunodeficiency syndromes.

Epidemiology: HIV infection was largely responsible for the significant increase in the incidence of CNS lymphoma in the 1980s, but it is suspected that the rates are increasing among immunocompetent individuals. The median age of lymphoma in HIV-infected individuals is 37; it is 52 in transplant recipients and 67 in immunocompetent patients.

Molecular and genetic profile: Immunosuppression-associated CNS lymphoma is Epstein-Barr Virus (EBV) related and, hence, the lymphoma cell expresses Epstein-Barr Nuclear Antigen (EBNA1–6), Latent membrane protein (LMP1), Epstein-Barr virus (EBV)-encoded RNA (EBER1), and EBER2.

Clinical features and standard therapy: First-line therapy is high-dose intravenous methotrexate along with combination antiretroviral therapy (ART).

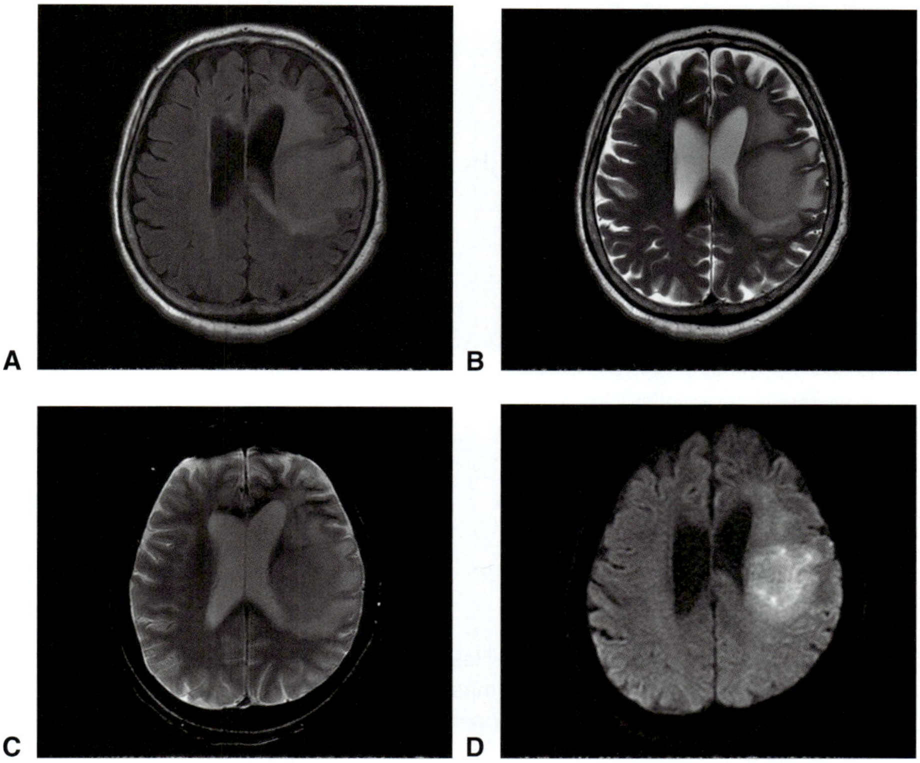

Figure 4.8. Imaging of immunodeficiency-associated CNS lymphoma. A. Axial FLAIR: Round mass isointense to normal brain centered in the left frontal periventricular white matter with surrounding edema. **B.** Axial T2: Round mass isointense to normal brain centered in the left frontal periventricular white matter with surrounding edema. **C.** Axial SWI: No blood products within the mass. **D.** Axial DWI: Heterogeneously hyperintense primarily around the peripheral margin of the mass.

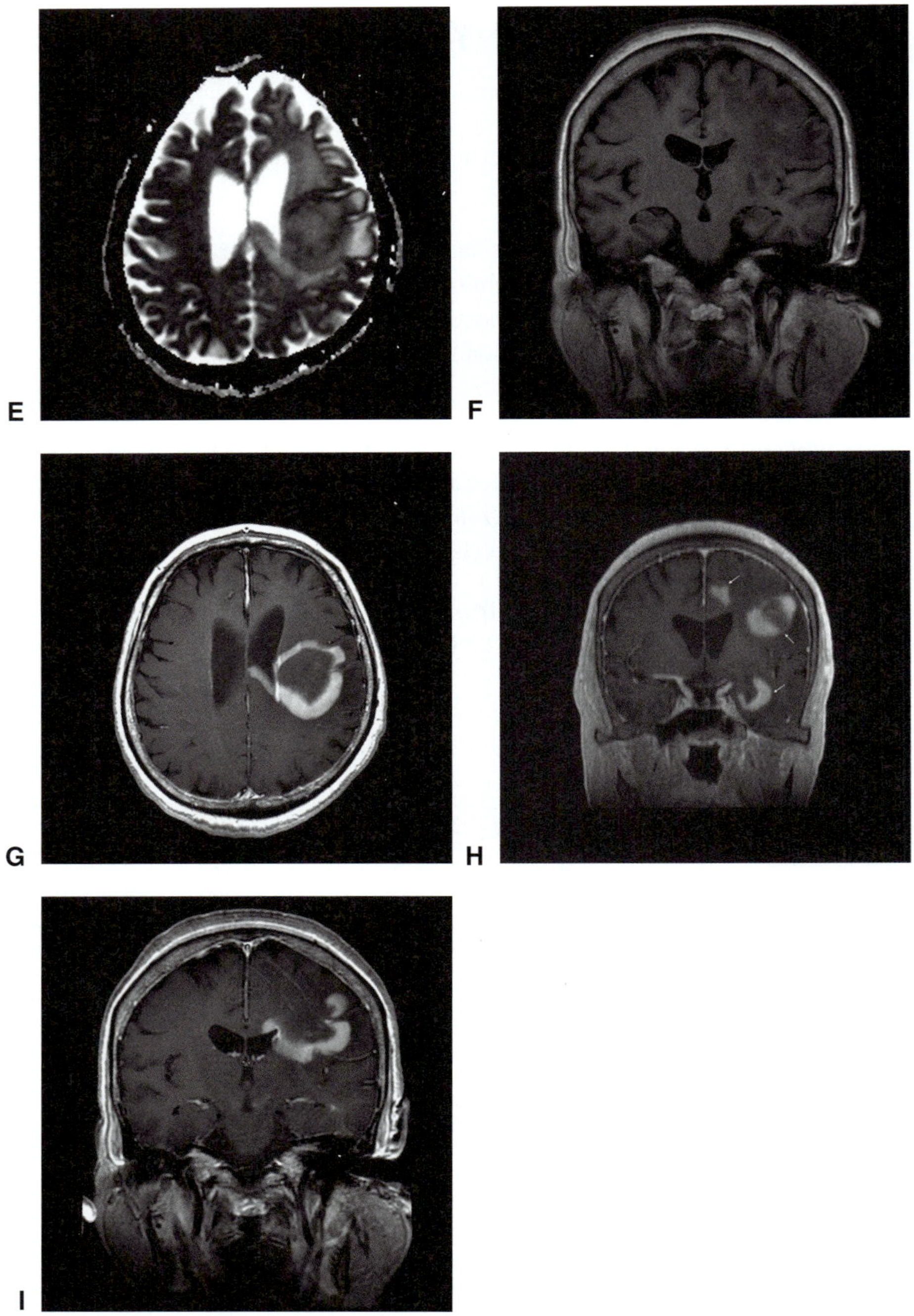

Figure 4.8. ***(continued)*** **E.** Axial ADC: Heterogeneously reduced diffusion primarily around the peripheral margin of the mass. **F.** Axial T1 precontrast: Thick rind of enhancement with large central area of necrosis. **G.** Axial T1 postcontrast: Thick rim enhancing mass with central necrosis. **H.** Coronal T1 postcontrast: Three discrete discontiguous enhancing masses (arrows). **I.** Coronal T1 postcontrast: Incomplete rim of enhancement within the dominant mass.

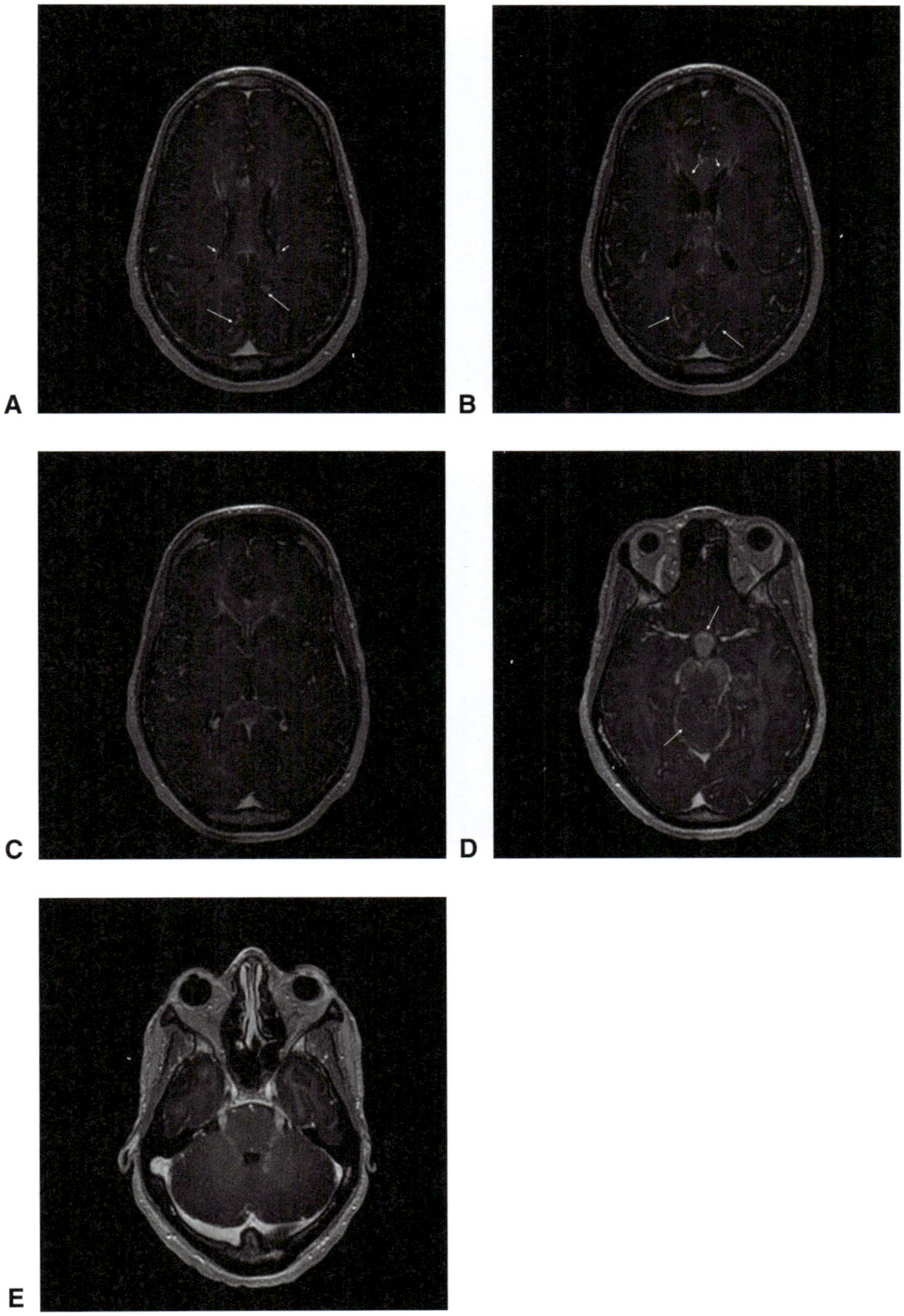

Figure 4.9. Imaging of immunodeficiency-associated leptomeningeal CNS lymphoma. A–E. Axial T1-postcontrast: Bilateral diffuse leptomeningeal (long white arrows), subependymal (short white arrows), and perivascular (short black arrows) enhancing disease.

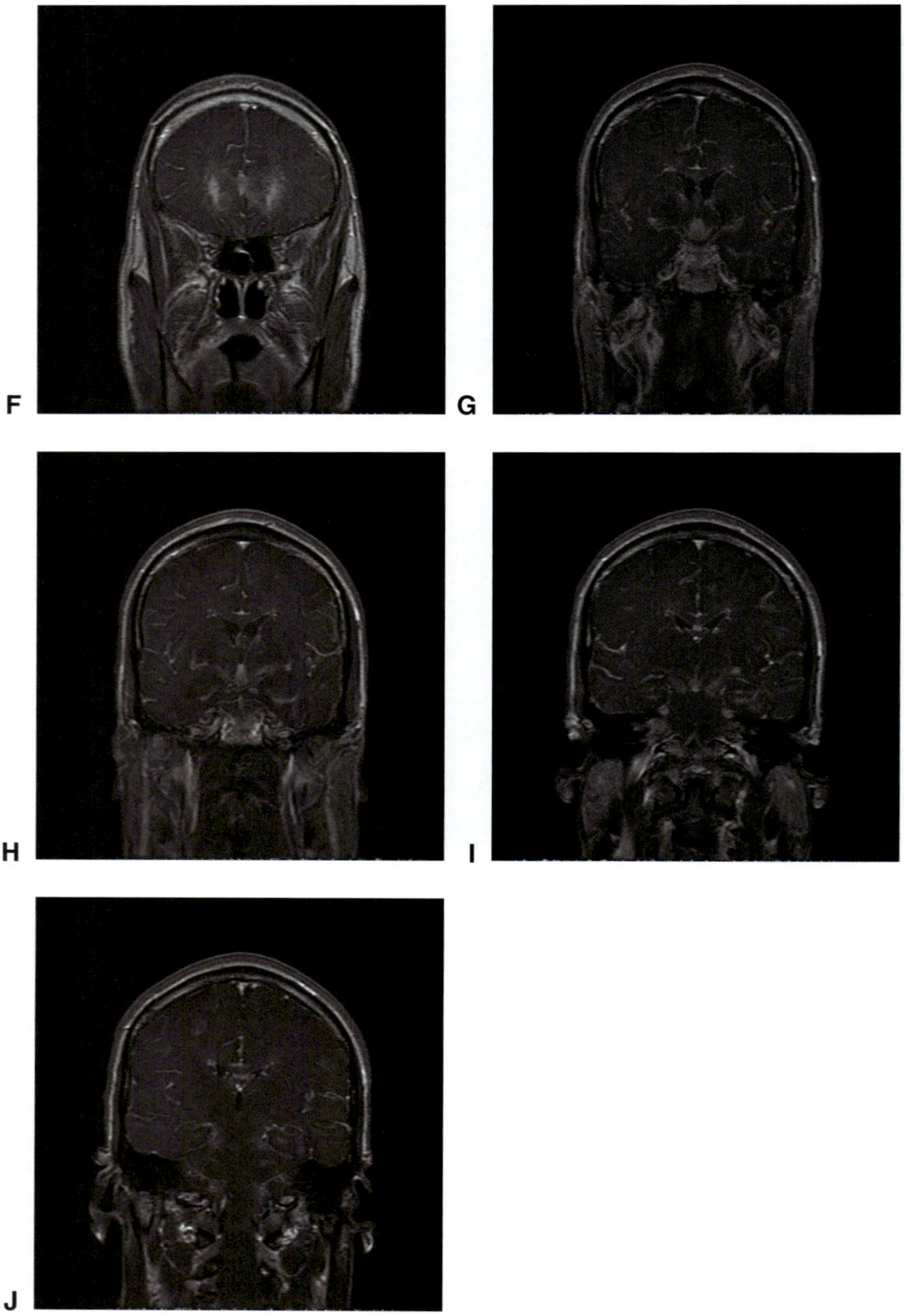

Figure 4.9. ***(continued)*** **F–J.** Coronal T1-postcontrast: Bilateral diffuse leptomeningeal, subependymal, and perivascular enhancing disease.

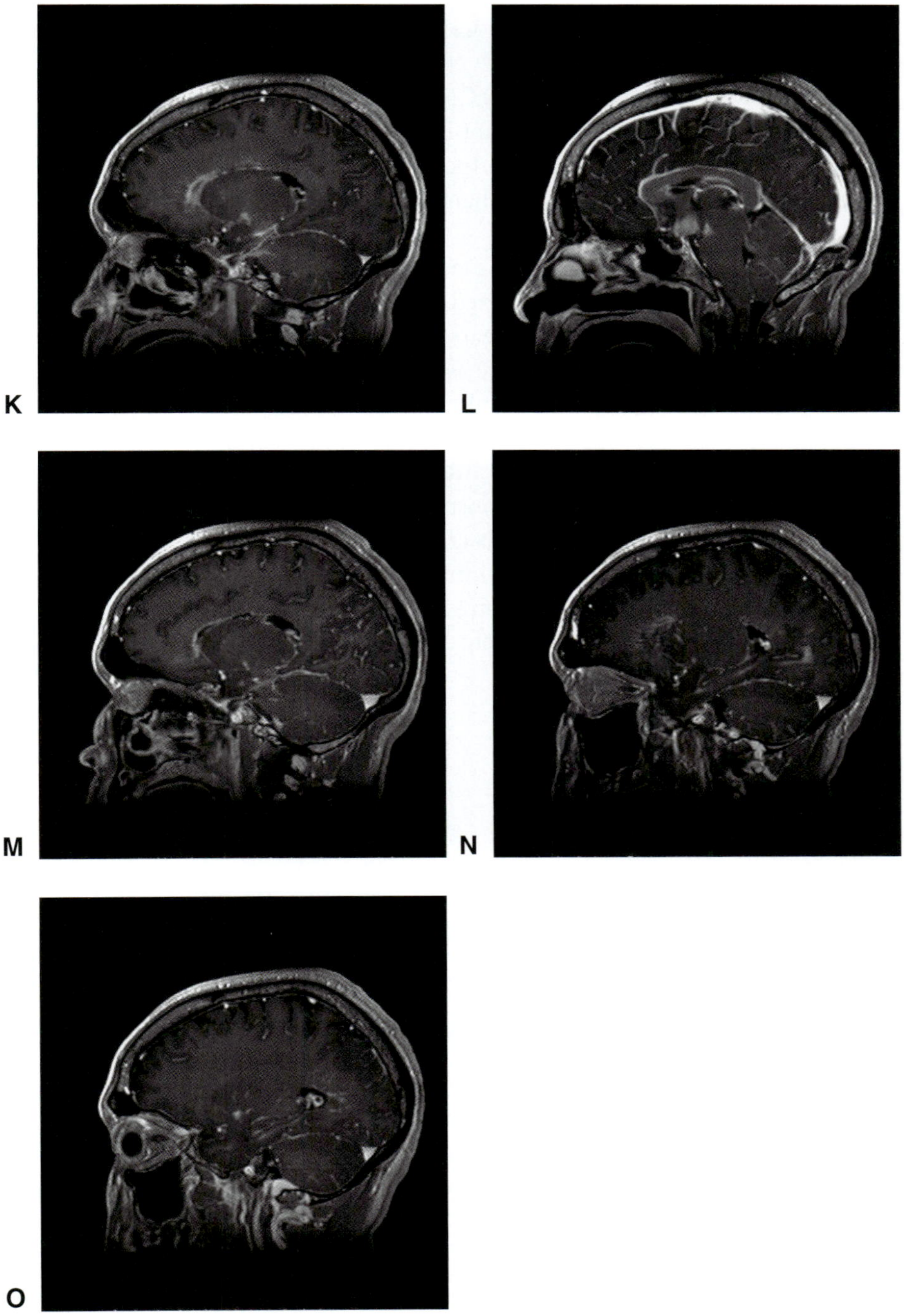

Figure 4.9. ***(continued)*** **K–O.** Sagittal T1-postcontrast: Bilateral diffuse leptomeningeal, subependymal, and perivascular enhancing disease.

Lymphomatosis Cerebri

Definition: A rare subtype of primary CNS lymphoma characterized by diffuse lymphomatous infiltration of malignant B-cells in the brain parenchyma without the formation of a discrete mass. Increased tumor cellularity in the white matter without apparent destructive changes.

Epidemiology: Due to its rarity, the exact incidence of lymphomatosis cerebri (LC) is unknown. Based on 16 reported cases of LC, the mean patient age is 62.6 years with the age range 41–72 years with equal gender distribution.

Molecular and genetic profile: Unknown.

Clinical features and standard therapy: Clinical symptoms and signs related to LC can be insidious and nonspecific, rendering early accurate diagnosis difficult. Early tissue diagnosis is critical for prompt initiation of specific therapy and intervention. High-dose intravenous methotrexate and rituximab are the starting chemotherapy regimen given to patients with LC, with overall prognosis remaining poor due to widely disseminated disease.

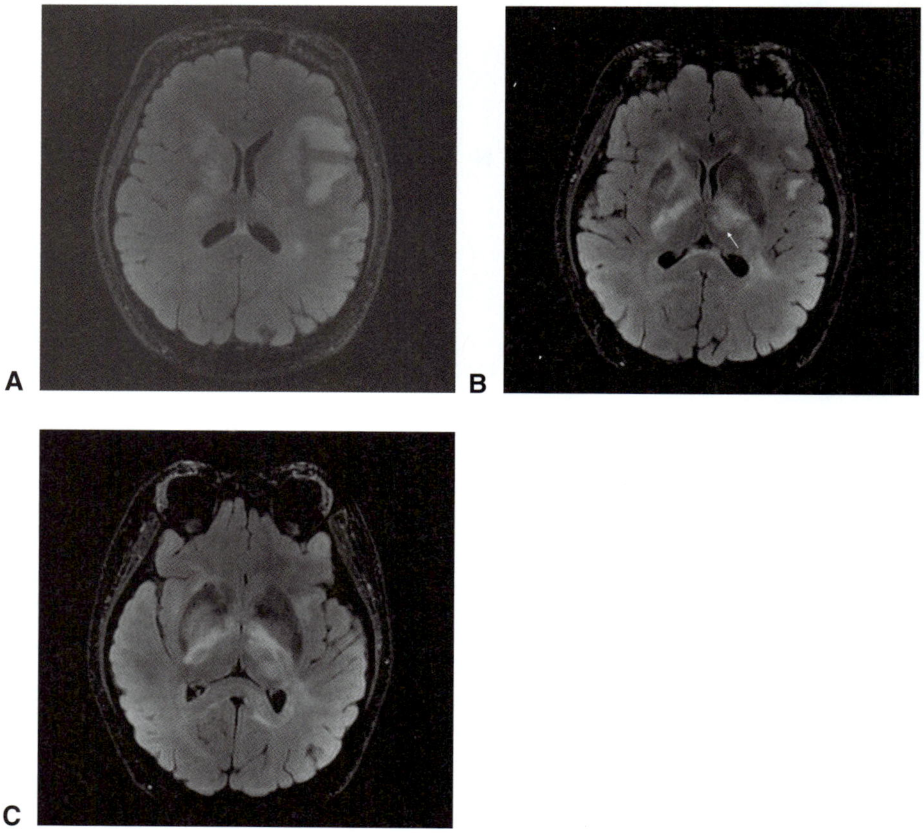

Figure 4.10. Imaging of lymphomatosis cerebri. A–C. Axial FLAIR: Bilateral infiltrative pattern of hyperintense lesion involving white and gray matter including thalamus (white arrow).

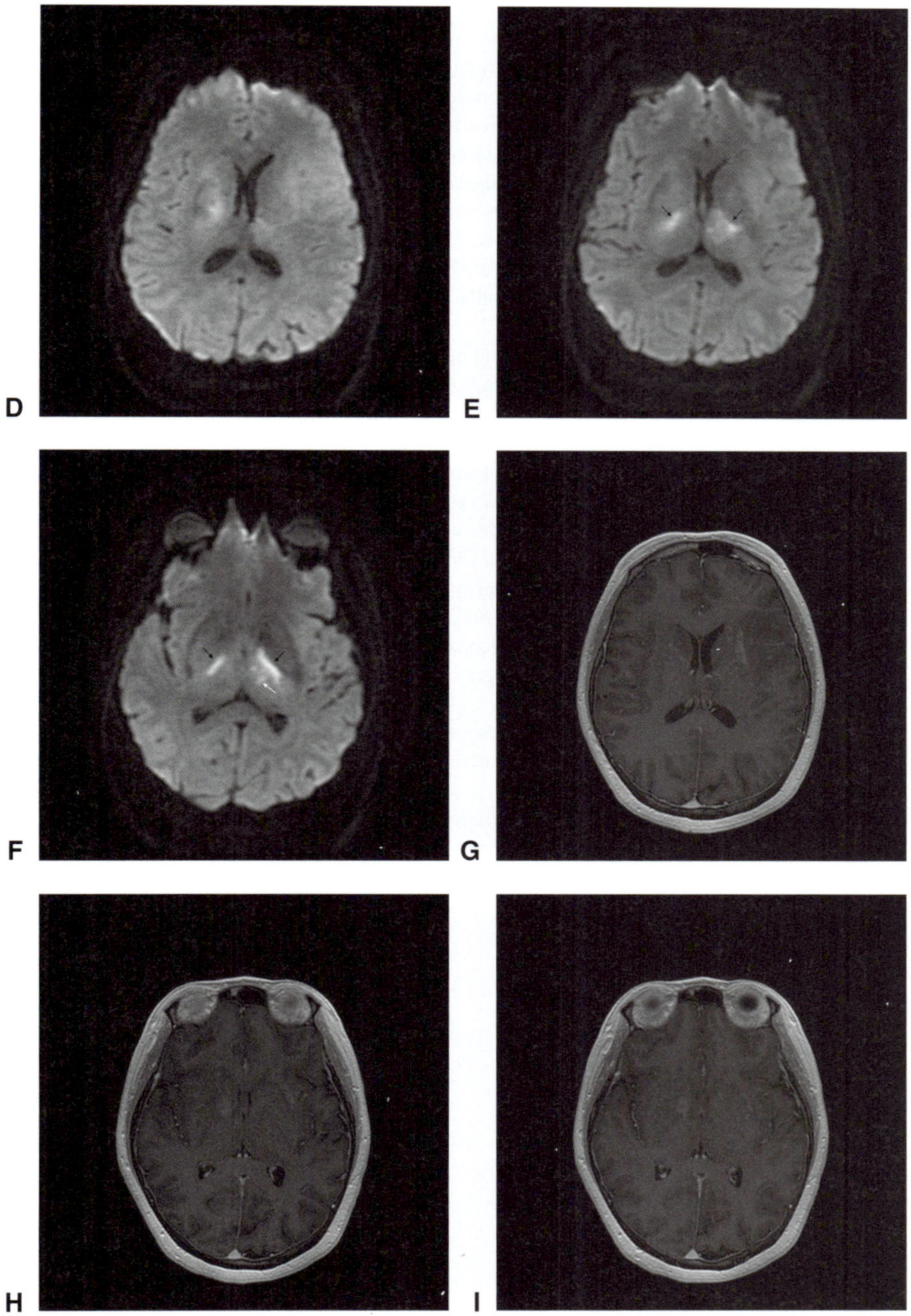

Figure 4.10. ***(continued)*** **D–F.** Axial DWI: Mildly reduced diffusion in the white matter lesions and prominently reduced diffusion in the bilateral posterior limb of the internal capsules (arrows). **G–I.** Axial T1-postcontrast: Punctate, patchy, or ill-defined pattern of enhancement.

Bibliography

Barajas RF Jr, Rubenstein JL, Chang JS, Hwang J, Cha S. Diffusion-weighted MR imaging derived apparent diffusion coefficient is predictive of clinical outcome in primary central nervous system lymphoma. *AJNR Am J Neuroradiol.* 2010;31:60–66.

Corti M, Villafañe F, Trione N, et-al. Primary central nervous system lymphomas in AIDS patients. *Enferm Infecc Microbiol Clin.* 2004;22(6): 332–336.

Fonkem E, Dayawansa S, Stroberg E, et al. Neurological presentations of intravascular lymphoma: meta-analysis of 654 patients. *BMC Neurol.* 2016;16:9.

George DH, Scheithauer BW, Aker FV, et al. Primary anaplastic large cell lymphoma of the central nervous system: prognostic effect of ALK-1 expression. *Am J Surg Pathol.* 2003;27:487–493.

Haldorsen IS, Espeland A, Larsson EM. Central nervous system lymphoma: characteristic findings on traditional and advanced imaging. *AJNR Am J Neuroradiol.* 2011;32(6): 984–992.

Kulkarni KM, Sternau L, Dubovy SR, et al. Primary dural lymphoma masquerading as a meningioma. *J Neuroophtalmol.* 2012;32(3):240–242.

Li L, Rong J-H, Feng J. Neuroradiological features of lymphomatosis cerebri: A systemic review of the English literature with a new case report. *Oncol Lett.* 2018;16:1463–1474.

Nomura M, Narita Y, Miyakita Y, et al. Clinical presentation of anaplastic large-cell lymphoma in the central nervous system. *Mol Clin Oncol.* 2013;4:655–660.

Rollins KE, Kleinschmidt-DeMasters BK, Corby JR, et al. Lymphomatosis cerebri as a cause of white matter dementia. *Hum Pathol.* 2005;36:282–290.

Tu PH, Giannini C, Judkins AR, et al. Clinicopathologic and genetic profile of intracranial marginal zone lymphoma: a primary low grade CNS lymphoma that mimics meningioma. *J Clin Oncol.* 2005;23:5718–5727.

Ueba T, Okawa M, Abe H, et al. Central nervous system marginal zone B-cell lymphoma of mucosa-associated lymphoid tissue type involving the brain and spinal cord parenchyma. *Neuropathology.* 2013;33(3):306–311.

Yamaura G, Ogasawara A, Ito T, et al. Pathologically proven gadolinium-enhanced MRI lesions in the bilateral corticospinal tracts in lymphomatosis cerebri. *Intern Med.* 2020;59:2931–2934.

5

Histiocytic Tumors

Overview

Histiocytic tumors are a rare heterogeneous group of tumor of the hematopoietic and lymphoid tissues and broadly classified into two categories: Langerhans cell histiocytosis and non-Langerhans histiocytosis.

Tumor Subtypes

- Langerhans Cell Histiocytosis
- Erdheim-Chester Disease
- Rosai-Dorfman Disease
- Histiocytic Sarcoma

	Age range (mean)	Female:male ratio	Cell of origin	WHO grade	Molecular/ genetic markers	Prognosis
Langerhans cell histiocytosis	0–15 (1.5)	1:1	Langerhans cell histiocyte	NA	*BRAF* V600E *MAP2K1*	Variable
Erdheim-Chester disease	40–60 (50)	1:1.5	Non-Langerhans cell histiocyte	NA	CD68	Variable
Rosai-Dorfman disease	20–30 (25)	–	Non-Langerhans cell histiocyte	NA	MAPK/ERK	Favorable
Histiocytic sarcoma	18–96 (63)	1:1.5	Malignant mature histiocyte	IV	Unknown	Guarded

▸ Langerhans Cell Histiocytosis

Definition: An immune-mediated disorder characterized by a clonal proliferation of immature Langerhans cells resulting in formation of granulomas throughout the body, especially in the skin, lymph nodes, lungs, liver, bone marrow, and brain and spine.

Epidemiology: Mostly affects children, with an annual incidence of 0.5 cases per 100,000 individuals aged <15 years, with a mean age of 1.5 years.

Molecular and genetic profile: A clonal proliferation of Langerhans cell histiocytes expresses *CD1a*, *langerin (CD207)*, and *S100 protein*. *BRAF* 600E mutations seen in up to half of all cases; in *BRAF*-wildtype, up to half can harbor *MAP2K1* mutations.

Clinical features and standard therapy: Clinical presentation depends on which part of the central nervous system (CNS) is involved but two of the most common signs and symptoms of Langerhans cell histiocytosis (LCH) are diabetes insipidus and hypothalamic dysfunction due to frequent involvement of the pituitary infundibulum and hypothalamus. Asymptomatic lytic skull lesions are not uncommon, as is complete marrow replacement of spine leading to vertebra plana.

Imaging

The imaging hallmark of LCH is proliferation and accumulation of Langerhans histiocytes primarily within the bone but also in the brain, both in the intra-axial and extra-axial compartments. Computed tomography is better suited for characterization of lytic or expansile osseous lesion and assessment of cortical breakthrough. Magnetic resonance is superior in assessment of extent of marrow involvement, soft tissue component, dural or brain invasion, and unsuspected additional lesions.

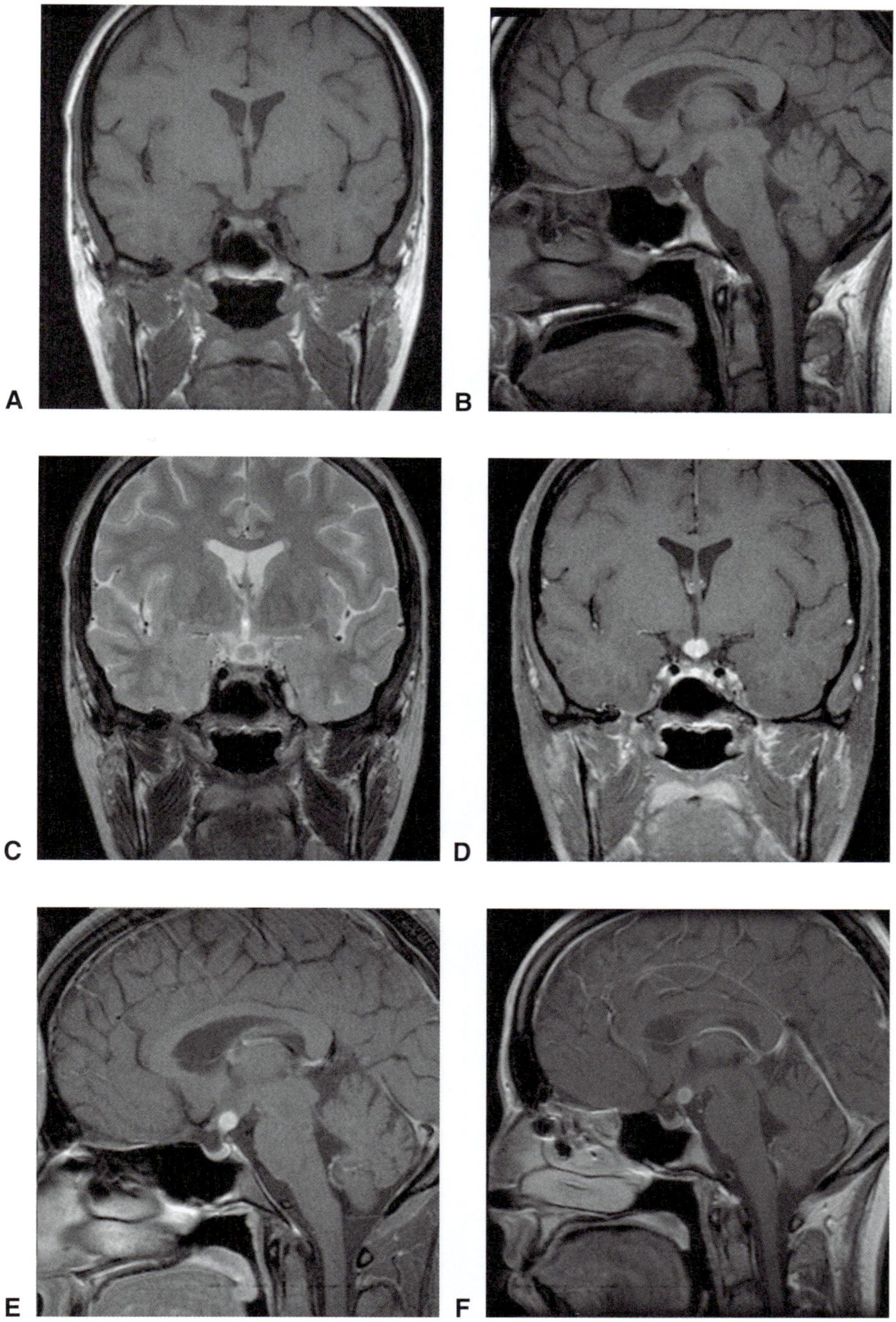

Figure 5.1. Imaging of Langerhans cell histiocytosis of pituitary infundibulum and temporal bone. A. Coronal T1-precontrast: Soft tissue pituitary infundibular mass isointense signal to the neighboring optic chiasm. **B.** Sagittal T1-precontrast: Soft tissue pituitary infundibular mass isointense signal to the neighboring optic chiasm. **C.** Coronal T2-FSE: Soft tissue pituitary infundibular mass isointense signal to the white matter of the brain. **D.** Coronal T1-postcontrast: Avid enhancement of the soft tissue pituitary infundibular mass. **E.** Sagittal T1-postcontrast: Avid enhancement of the soft tissue pituitary infundibular mass. **F.** Axial CT: Lytic destructive lesion centered in the left mastoid temporal bone.

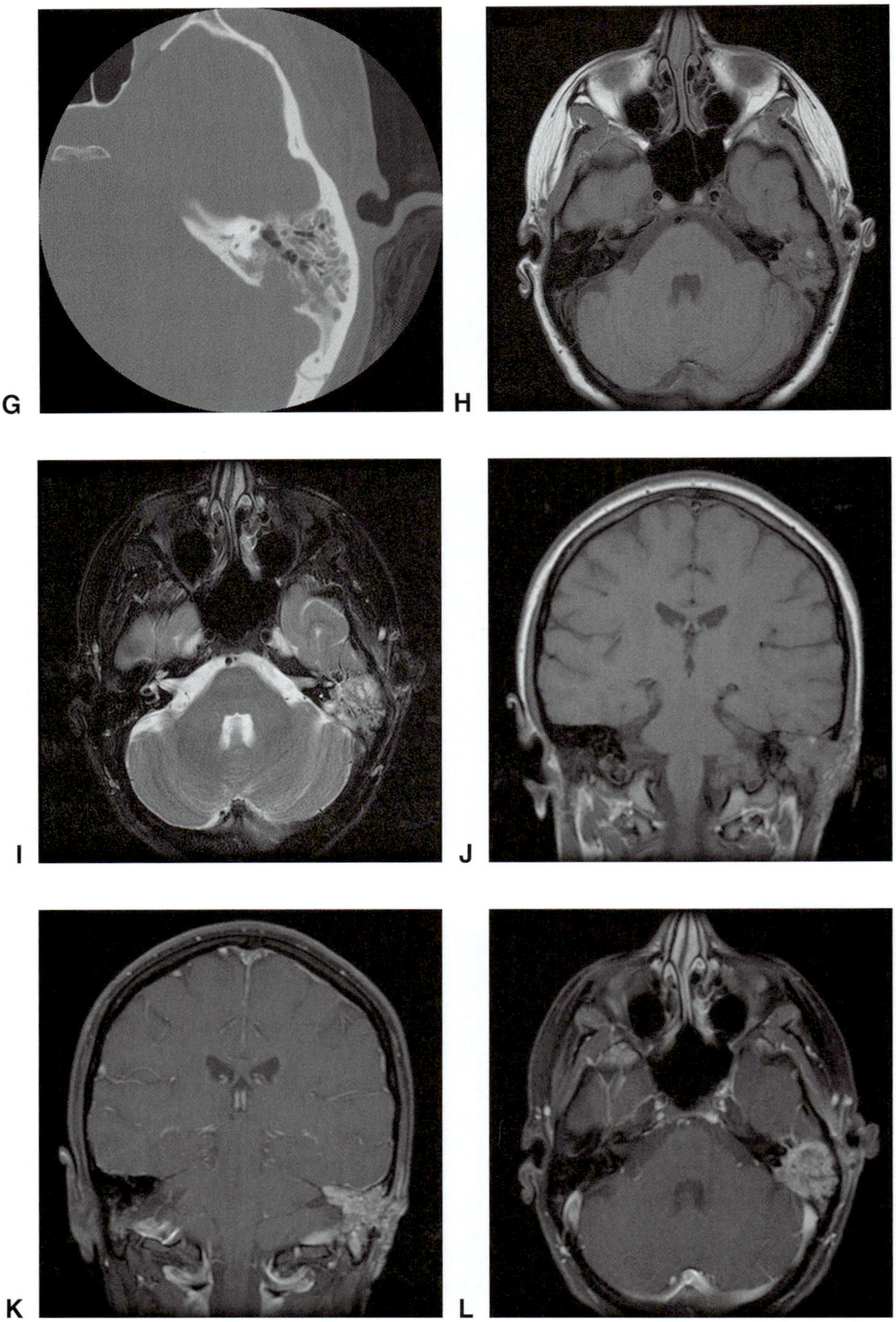

Figure 5.1. ***(continued)*** **G.** Axial T1-precontrast: Mass isointense to the brain within the left mastoid temporal bone. **H.** Axial T2 FSE: Heterogeneous signal of the mass filling the left mastoid temporal bone. **I.** Coronal T1-precontrast: Mass isointense to the brain within the left mastoid temporal bone. **J.** Coronal T1-postcontrast. **K.** Sagittal T1-postcontrast. **L.** Axial T1-postcontrast.

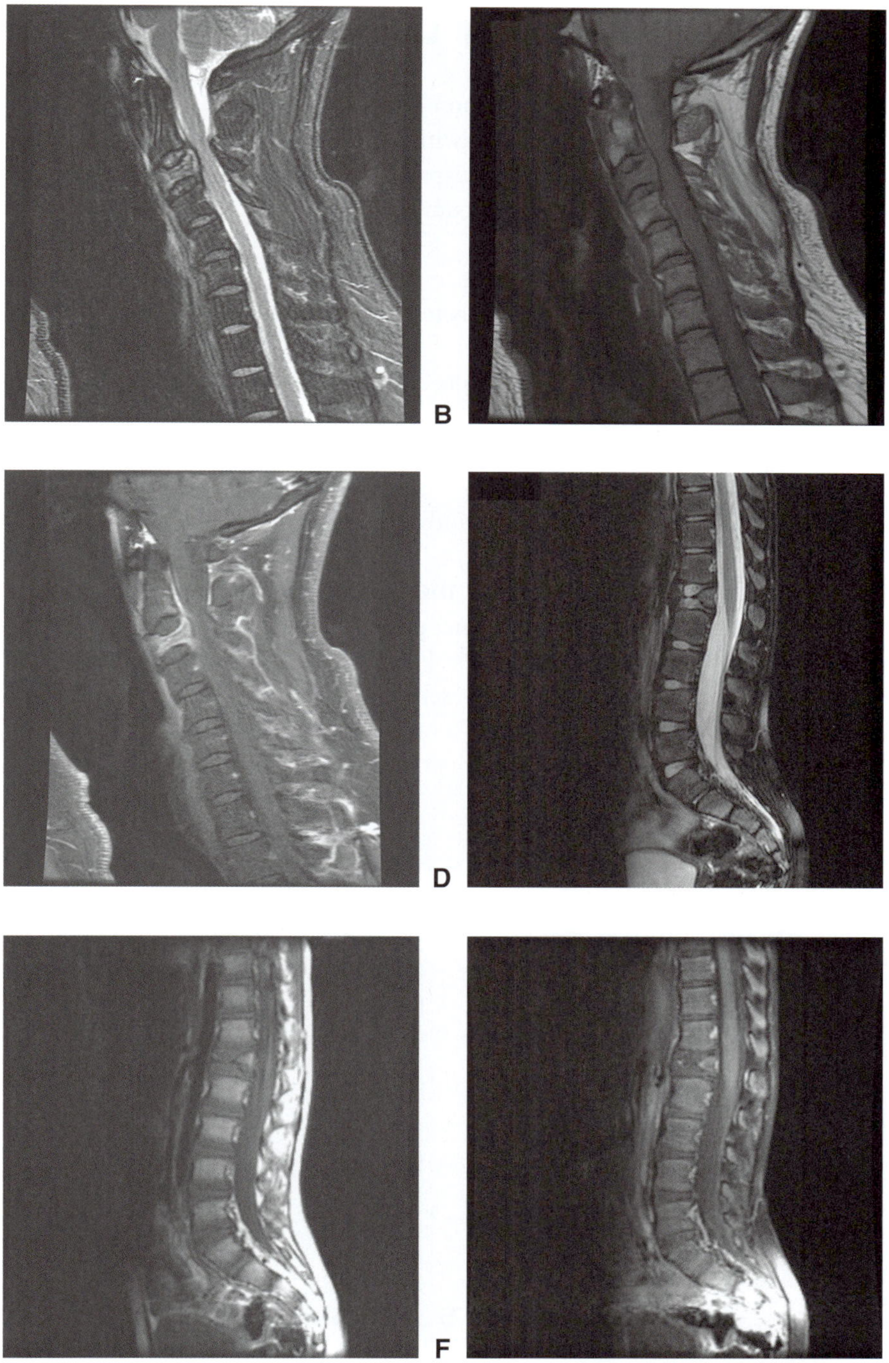

A B C D E F

Figure 5.2. Imaging of spinal LCH. A. Sagittal T2: Hyperintense signal replacing the marrow of collapsed C3 vertebral body. **B.** Sagittal T1-precontrast: Hypointense signal replacing the marrow of collapsed C3 vertebral body. **C.** Sagittal T1-postcontrast: Avid but heterogeneous enhancement of C3. **D.** Sagittal T2: Vertebra plana of L1. **E.** Sagittal T1-precontrast: Complete collapse of anterior half of L1 vertebral body. **F.** Sagittal T1-postcontrast: No enhancement within the collapsed L1 vertebral body.

▶ Erdheim-Chester Disease

Definition: A rare type of sporadic non-Langerhans cell histiocytic neoplasm comprised of lipid-laden histiocytes with multiorgan involvement including CNS involvement, manifested as widespread infiltrative parenchymal lesions, dural thickening, orbital lesions, or a combination thereof.

Epidemiology: The exact prevalence of Erdheim-Chester disease (ECD) is unknown but more than 500 affected individuals worldwide have been described in the medical literature.

ECD most commonly affects adults ages 40 to 60, with a mean age of 53, although it can occur at any age.

Molecular and genetic profile: At least 50% of patients with ECD carry *BRAF* V600E mutations, 17% *NRAS*, and 12% *PIK3CA* mutations.

Clinical features and standard therapy: Due to predilection of ECD lesions in the posterior fossa and spine, patients most often present with cerebellar signs or pyramidal syndromes. Patients can present with nonspecific symptoms such as seizures, headaches, sensory deficits, neurocognitive deficits, or cranial neuropathies.

Imaging

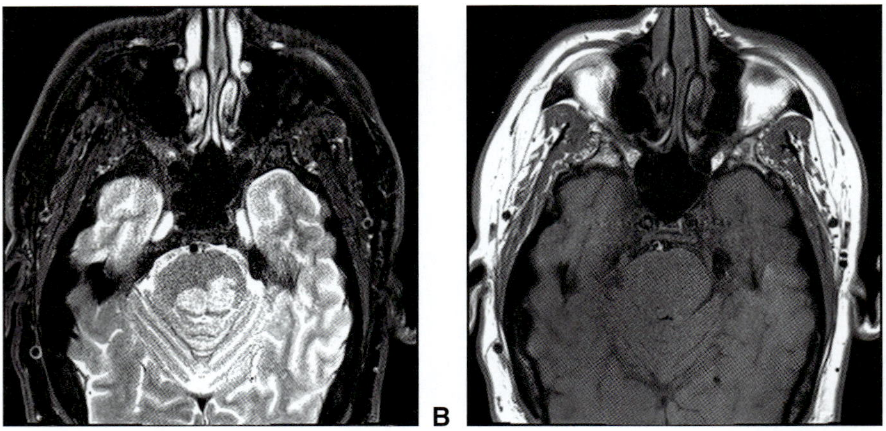
A B

Figure 5.3. **Erdheim-Chester disease of pons. A.** Axial T2: Hyperintense lobulated lesion in the pons with minimal mass effect. **B.** Axial T1-precontrast: Pontine lesion is isointense to normal pons and not clearly seen.

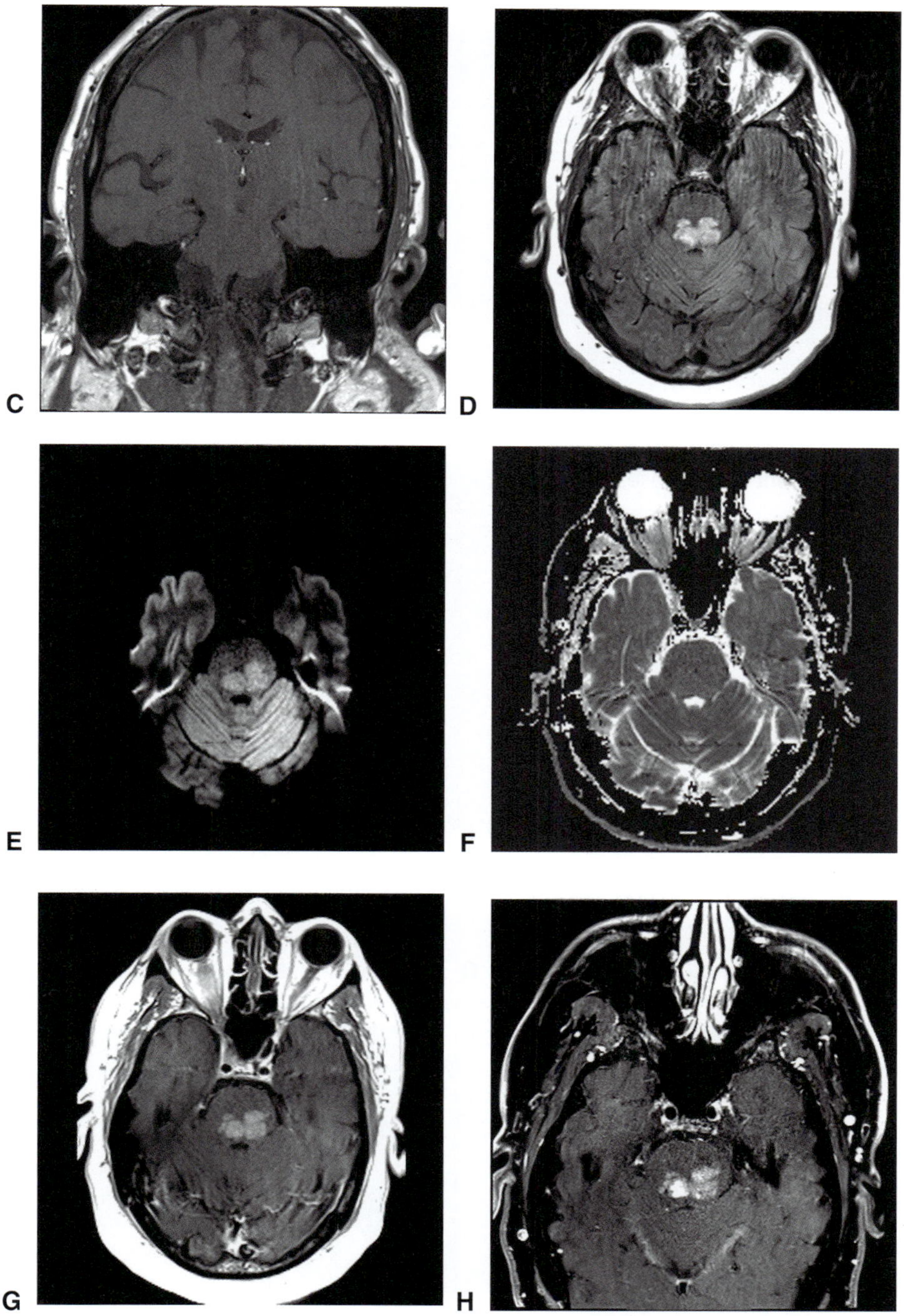

Figure 5.3. ***(continued)*** **C.** Coronal T1-precontrast: Pontine lesion is isointense to normal pons and not clearly seen. **D.** Axial FLAIR: Hyperintense lobulated lesion in the pons with minimal mass effect. **E.** Axial diffusion-weighted imaging (DWI): Hyperintense due to T2 shine through. **F.** Axial apparent diffusion coefficient (ADC): Isointense to normal pons and not clearly seen. **G.** Axial T1-postcontrast: Avid and homogeneous enhancement within the lesion. **H.** Axial T1-postcontrast fat-sat: Avid and homogeneous enhancement within the lesion.

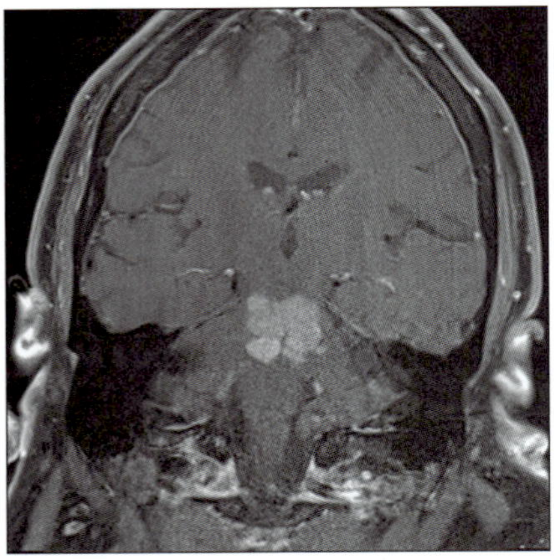

I

Figure 5.3. ***(continued)*** **I.** Coronal T1-postcontrast fat-sat: Avid and homogeneous enhancement within the lesion.

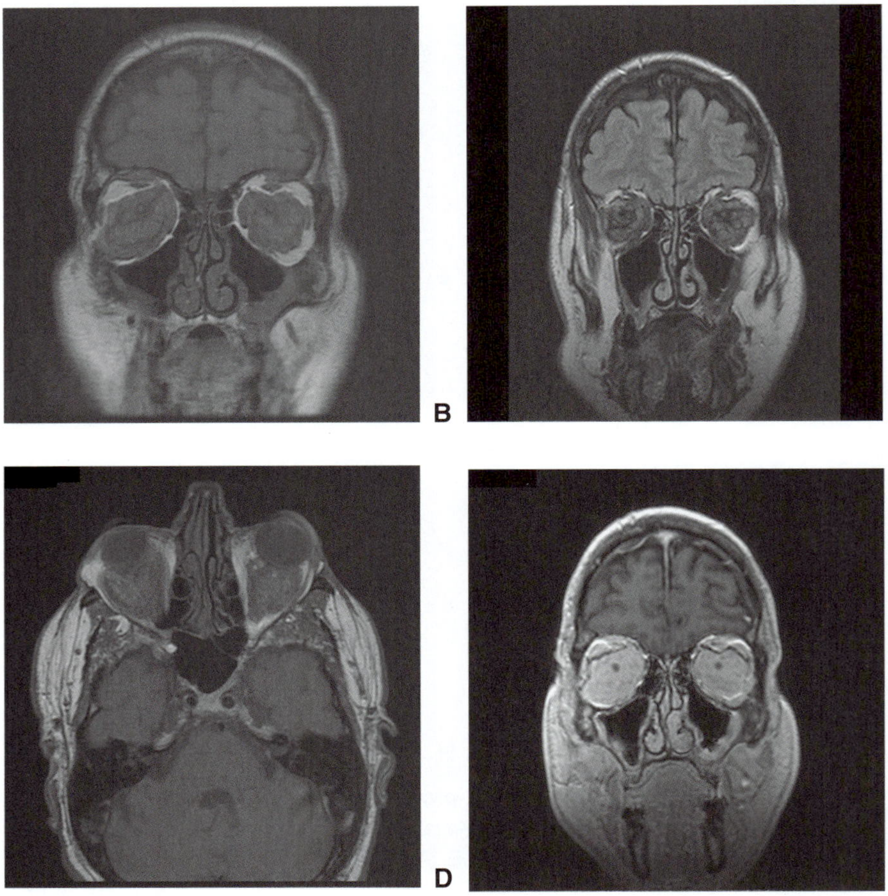

A B C D

Figure 5.4. Erdheim-Chester disease of orbits. A. Coronal T1-precontrast: Bulky soft tissue mass with isointense signal to extraocular muscle filling the orbit bilaterally. **B.** Coronal fluid attenuated inversion recovery (FLAIR): Heterogeneously hypointense FLAIR signal intensity of the mass. **C.** Axial T1-preconstrast: Bulky soft tissue mass with isointense signal to extraocular muscle filling the orbit bilaterally. **D.** Coronal T1-postcontrast: Avid and homogeneous enhancement of the mass.

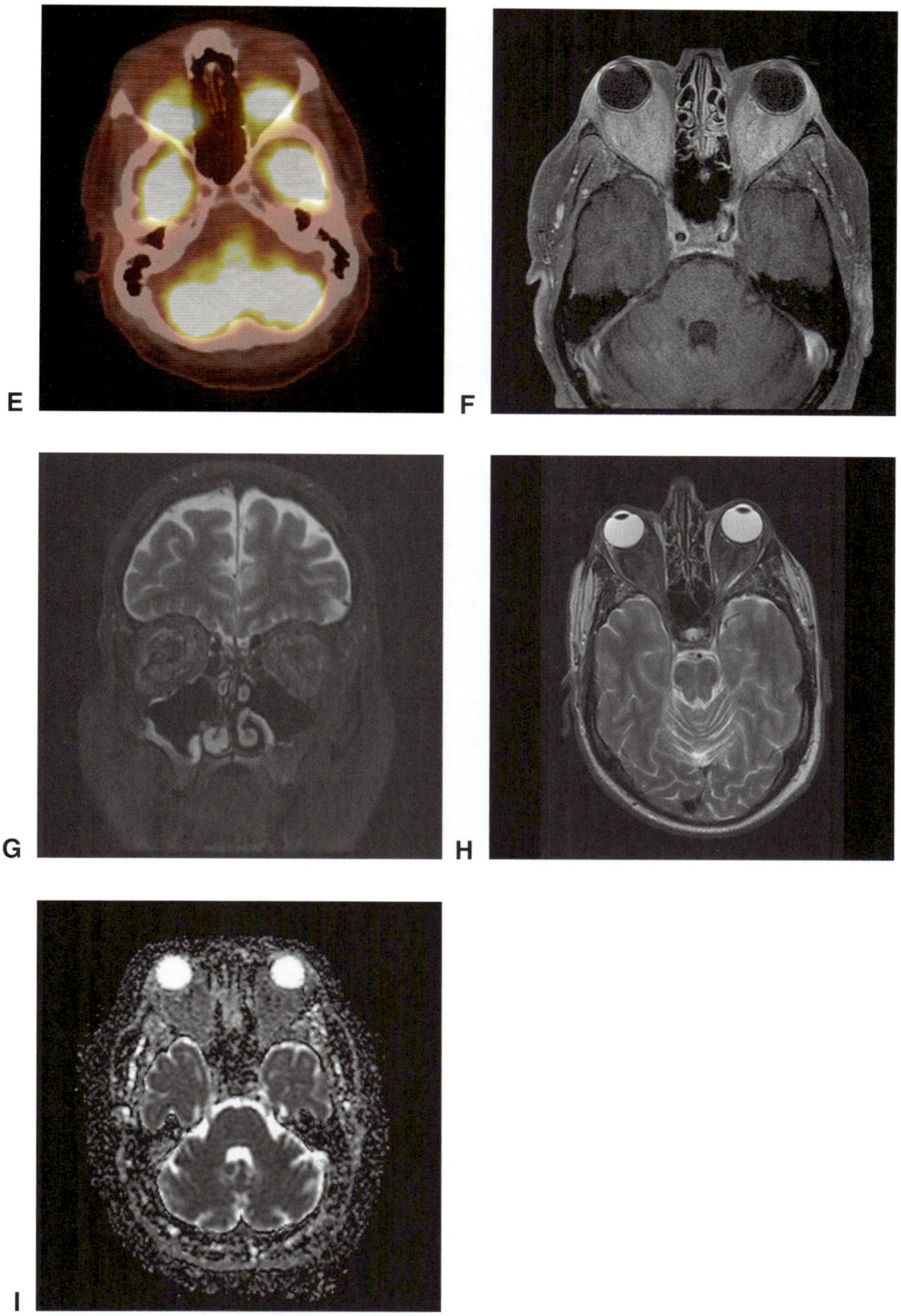

Figure 5.4. ***(continued)*** **E.** Axial fluorodeoxyglucose-positron emission tomography (FDG-PET) CT: Marked FDG-avidity of the mass. **F.** Axial T1-postcontrast fat-sat: Avid and homogeneous enhancement of the mass. **G.** Coronal T2 fat-sat: Heterogeneously hypointense T2 signal intensity of the mass. **H.** Axial T2: Heterogeneously hypointense T2 signal intensity of the mass. **I.** Axial ADC: Heterogeneously hypointense ADC signal intensity of the mass.

Rosai-Dorfman Disease

Definition: Rosai-Dorfman disease (RDD), also known as sinus histiocytosis with massive lymphadenopathy, is a rare, mostly self-limiting disorder caused by proliferation of non-Langerhans cell histiocytes within lymph nodes. Although there is no lymphatic system in the CNS, RDD can be seen in the CNS and in the extranodal sites as solid masses. CNS RDD can mimic disseminated tumor or metastatic disease due to multifocal involvement.

Epidemiology: This rare disorder affects primarily the older teenagers or young adults, with a mean age of 21 years and slight male predominance.

Molecular and genetic profile: No known characteristics or molecular or genetic aberrations have been identified.

Clinical features and standard therapy: Clinical presentation at initial diagnosis depends on the location of lesions in the CNS but most patients present with nonspecific constitutional symptoms such as fever, malaise, night sweats, weight loss, headache, nausea, vomiting, dizziness, or seizure and cervical lymphadenopathy. When RDD involves pituitary infundibulum or hypothalamus, diabetes insipidus and hypopituitarism can be seen.

In many cases, patients experience spontaneous remission without any intervening therapy over months to years. Careful follow-up and clinical observation are the mainstay unless there is worsening or difficulty in controlling the symptoms. Various treatment options are targeted to the management of symptoms rather than eradication of tumor. Surgical resection is an option, especially for large lesions causing mass effect; various drug regimens have been, used including steroids, alpha interferon, and chemotherapy with variable success.

Imaging

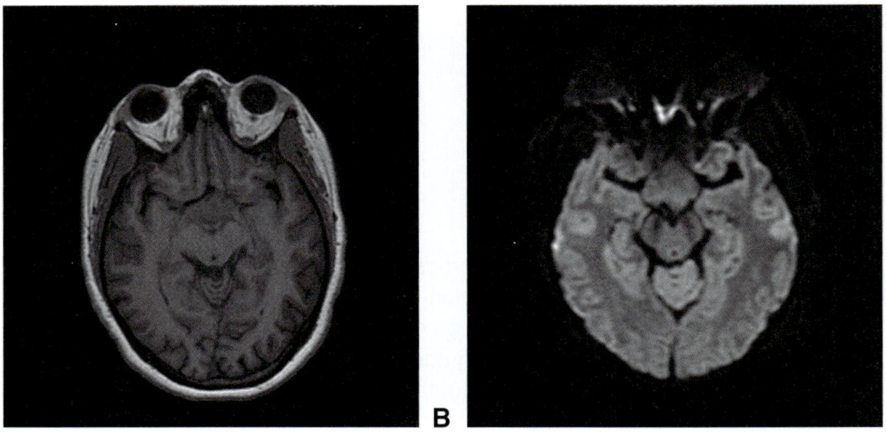

A B

Figure 5.5. Imaging of CNS Rosai-Dorfman disease. A. Axial T1-precontrast: Hypointense suprasellar mass. **B.** Axial DWI: Isointense to surrounding brain.

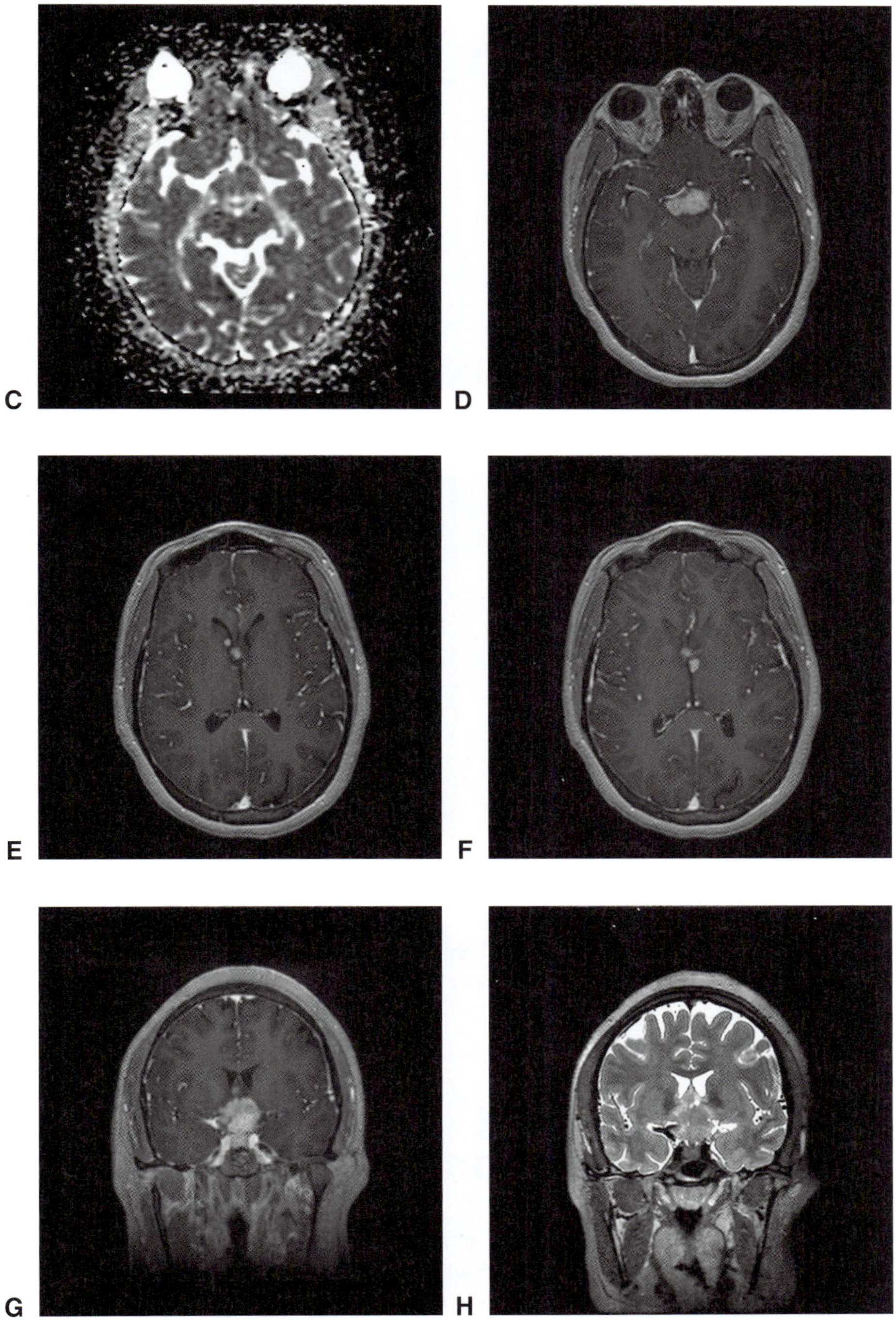

Figure 5.5. ***(continued)*** **C.** Axial ADC: Isointense to surrounding brain. **D.** Axial T1-postcontrast: Avid and homogeneous enhancement of suprasellar mass. **E.** Axial T1-postcontrast: Multiple small enhancing nodules in and around foramen of Monro. **F.** Axial T1-postcontrast: Multiple small enhancing nodules in and around foramen of Monro. **G.** Coronal T1-postcontrast: Avid and homogeneous enhancement of suprasellar mass. **H.** Coronal T2: Hypointense T2 signal of the mass.

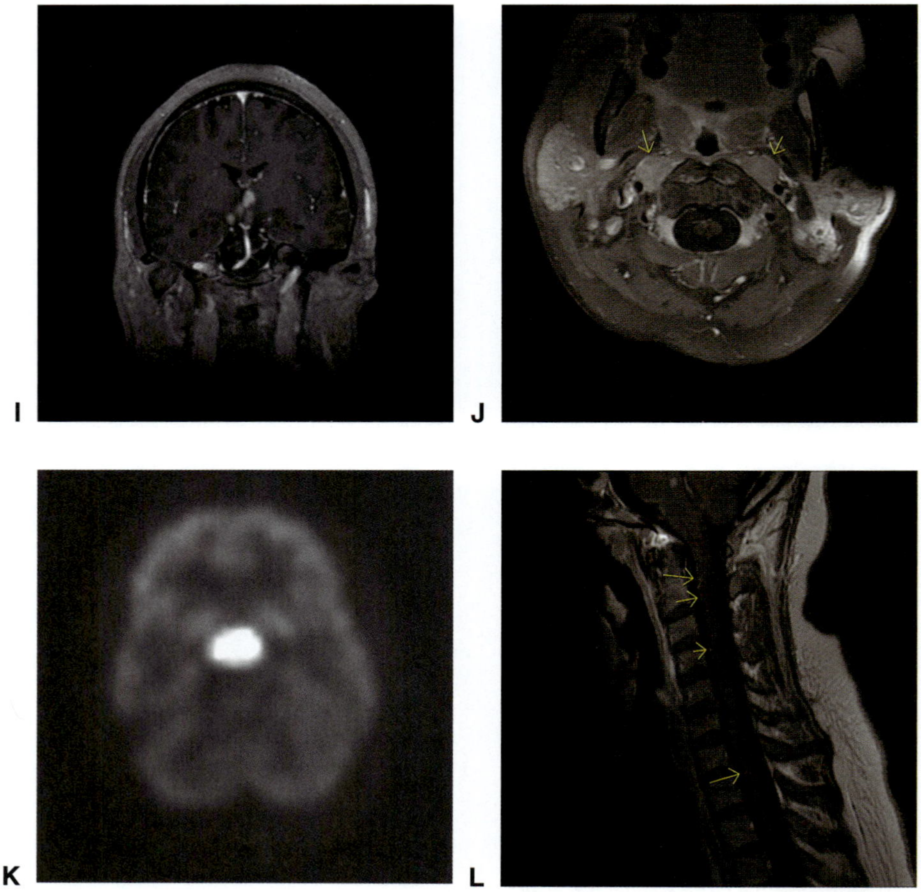

Figure 5.5. ***(continued)*** **I.** Coronal T1-postcontrast: Multiple small enhancing nodules in and around third ventricle. **J.** Axial T1-postcontrast: Bilateral enlarged lateral retropharyngeal nodes (arrows). **K.** Axial FDG-PET: Marked FDG avidity of the mass. **L.** Sagittal T1-postcontrast: Multiple small nodules (arrows) along the pial surface of the cord.

Histiocytic Sarcoma

Definition: Histiocytic sarcoma is a rare malignant tumor arising from mature histiocytes, characterized by high cellularity, mitotically active histiocytes with abundant eosinophilic cytoplasm, and prominent background of reactive inflammation.

Epidemiology: The exact prevalence of histiocytic sarcoma is unknown due to its extreme rarity but isolated cases of radiation-associated side effects have been reported. Histiocytic sarcoma can be seen in any age group but the mean reported patient age in case series is 52 years.

Molecular and genetic profile: No specific marker has been described.

Clinical features and standard therapy: Clinical presenting symptoms are related to mass effect caused by the tumor or surrounding edema. Surgical resection of the mass is the primary strategy because there are no known effective therapeutic options. Both radiotherapy and chemotherapy are ineffective in controlling recurrence or spread of tumor elsewhere in the CNS.

Imaging

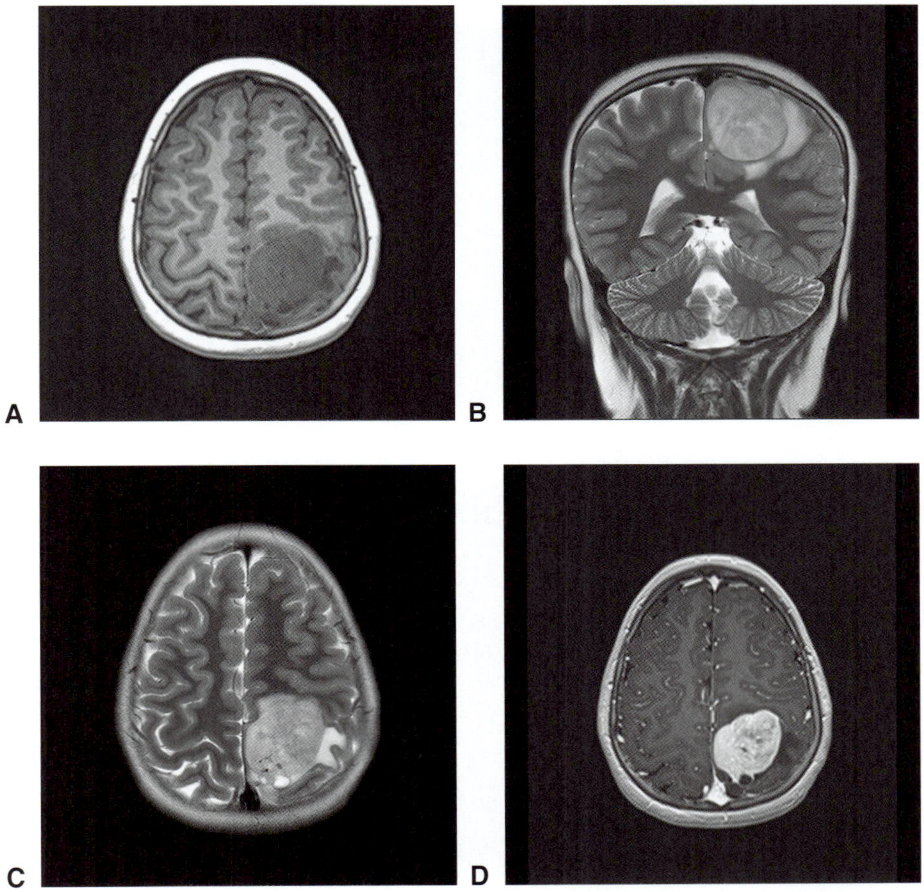

Figure 5.6. **Imaging of CNS histiocytic sarcoma. A.** Axial T1-precontrast: Hypointense circumscribed mass. **B.** Coronal T2: Heterogeneous hyperintense circumscribed mass. **C.** Axial T2: Heterogeneous hyperintense circumscribed mass. **D.** Axial T1-postcontrat: Avid enhancement.

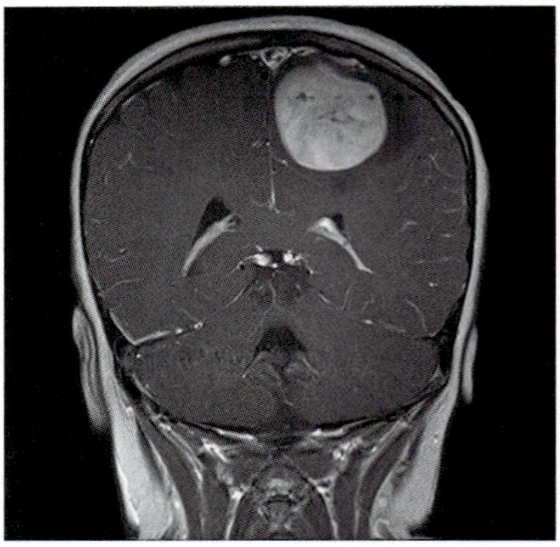

E

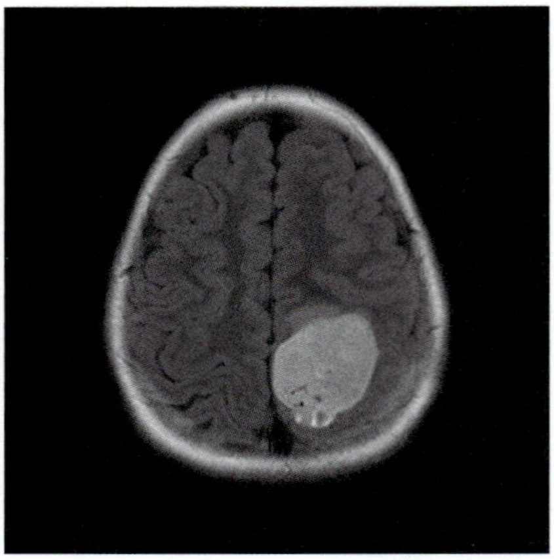

F

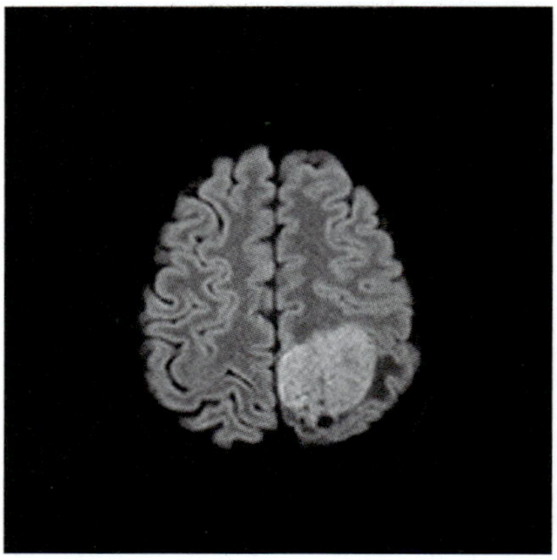

G

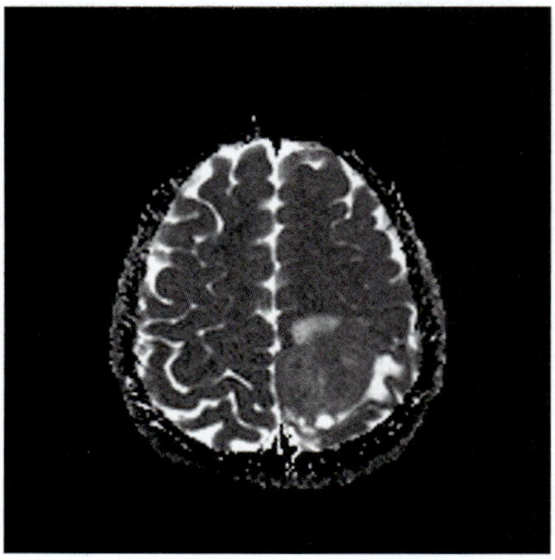

H

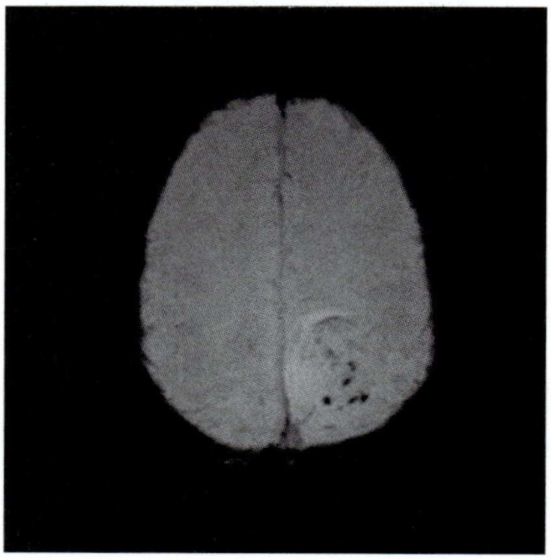

I

Figure 5.6. ***(continued)*** **E.** Coronal T1-postcontrast: Avid enhancement. **F.** Axial FLAIR: Hyperintense mass. **G.** Axial DWI: Homogeneously reduced. **H.** Axial ADC: Homogeneously reduced. **I.** Axial gradient echo: Few punctate blood products within the mass.

Bibliography

Drier A, Haroche J, Savatovsky J, et al. Cerebral, facial, and orbital involvement in Erdheim-Chester disease: CT and MR imaging findings. *Radiology*. 2010;255:586–594.

Johnson MD, Aulino JP, Jagasia M, et al. Erdheim-Chester disease mimicking multiple meningiomas syndrome. *AJNR Am J Neuroradiol.* 2004;25:134–137.

Konishi E, Ibayashi N, Yamamoto S, et al. Isolated intracranial Rosai-Dorfman disease (sinus histiocytosis with massive lymphadenopathy). *AJNR Am J Neuroradiol.* 2003;24:515–518.

May JM, Waddle MR, Miller DH, et al. Primary histiocytic sarcoma of the central nervous system: a case report with platelet derived growth factor receptor mutation and PD-L1/PD-L2 expression and literature review. *Radiat Oncol.* 2018;13:167.

Raslan OA, Schellingerhout D, Fuller GN, Ketonen LM. Rosai-Dorfman disease in neuroradiology: imaging findings in a series of 10 patients. *AJR Am J Roentgenol.* 2011 Feb;196:187–193.

Wang E, Anzai Y, Paulino A, et al. Rosai-Dorfman disease presenting with isolated bilateral orbital masses: report of two cases. *AJNR Am J Neuroradiol.* 2001;22:1386–1388.

Zaveri J, La Q, Yarmish G, Neuman J. More than just Langerhans cell histiocytosis: a radiologic review of histiocytic disorders. *Radiographics*. 2014;34:2008–2024.

6 Germ Cell Tumors

Overview

Germ cell tumors (GCTs) are a heterogeneous group of central nervous system (CNS) tumors with morphologic, immunophenotypic, and genetic homologs of gonadal and other extra-CNS germ cell neoplasm but with distinct clinical behavior and possibly in their cellular origin. There are six main histologic variants of CNS GCTs: germinoma, teratoma, yolk sac tumor, embryonal carcinoma, choriocarcinoma, and mixed cell type. CNS GCTs likely develop through combined genetic and epigenetic mechanisms from a common ancestral cell and share identical somatic mutations in the *MAPK/PI3K* pathway. GCTs are one of the more common solid tumors of childhood and occur more frequently in young adolescent males living in Japan and other Asian countries than in North America and Europe.

	Age range (mean)	Female: male ratio	Cell of origin	Serum/ CSF tumor markers	Molecular/ genetic markers	Prognosis
Germinoma	7–30 (19.2)	Overwhelming gender majority is males, with ratio of 1:15	Primordial germ cell; syncytiotrophoblastic giant cells	HCG, PLAP	PLAP, KIT/ RAS AKT/ mTOR	Good
Teratoma	0–20 (13)		Somatic tissues derived from germ layers (ectoderm, endoderm, mesoderm)	–	–	Intermediate
Mixed germ cell tumor	0–20 (14)		Several germ cell components			
Yolk sac tumor	8–23		Primitive germ cell	AFP	AFP	Poor
Embryonal carcinoma	8–23		Large epithelioid cells of embryonic germ disc	–	CD30 CK AE1/3	Poor
Choriocarcinoma	8–23		Non-germinomatous malignant germ cell	HCG	HCG	Poor

AFP, alpha-fetoprotein; ASK, arabidopsis skp-like; CD, cluster of differentiation; CK, cytokeratin, pan antibody; CSF, cerebrospinal fluid; HCG, human chorionic gonadotropin; KIT, KIT proto-oncogene, receptor tyrosine kinase; PLAP, placental-like alkaline phosphatase; RAS, rat sarcoma; TOR, target of rapamycin.

Germ Cell Tumors of the Central Nervous System

Definition: Germ cell tumors (GCTs) of the central nervous system (CNS) are a heterogeneous group of neoplasms with the morphologic, immunophenotypic, and genetic homologs of gonadal and other extraneuraxial GCTs. However, CNS GCTs differ from their gonadal and extraneuraxial GCTs in many aspects, including morphology, clinical behavior, and possibly their cell of origin. CNS GCTs are broadly classified as germinomatous and non-germinomatous GCTs on the basis of clinicopathological and laboratory findings and serum and CSF tumor markers.

Epidemiology: GCTs primarily affect children and adolescents, male more frequently than female, with much higher geographic prevalence in eastern Asia (e.g., Japan, Taiwan, China, Korea) than in Europe or the United States. GCTs represent up to 15% of all pediatric brain tumors in these regions. Pure germinomas outnumber other histologic subtypes and comprise about 40% of all GCTs.

Affected age group: Bimodal distribution of CNS GCT incidence shows a small peak for infants less than 2 years of age and a larger peak for adolescents (13–19 years). The vast majority of patients with GCT are younger than 25 years of age, with peak incidence coinciding with the onset of puberty. Males are more frequently affected than females, except for infantile GCT, which is more common in females. There is a large gender difference in GCTs arising in the pineal region and diagnosed in the age group of 10–19 years, where the male-to-female ratio can be higher than 9:1. It remains speculative as to why there is such great male gender predominance in GCTs in the pineal region and the young adolescent age group, but the physiological and hormonal changes in male puberty appear to favor neoplastic transformation in the male pineal region and during the height of pubescent growth. Patients with teratoma or choriocarcinoma tend to present with symptoms when they are about 10 years younger, while pure germinomas are more commonly seen in older age group, usually in the second decade. Choriocarcinomas are the rarest, most malignant CNS GCTs with elevated serum and CSF b-HCG levels.

Molecular and genetic profile: Each histologic subtype of GCT has its own unique molecular and genetic alteration.

Clinical features and standard therapy: The most common location of central nervous system (CNS) GCTs is the pineal region (45%), and the second most common location is the suprasellar region (30%). Basal ganglia location is rare but well described in published reports. The signs and symptoms of CNS GCTs depend on the location of the tumor. Patients with pineal region GCTs often present with signs and symptoms of raised intracranial pressure, diplopia, and hydrocephalus related to compression of tectum and cerebral aqueduct, respectively. Patients with suprasellar region GCTs often present with hormonal deficiencies, most commonly diabetes insipidus caused by antidiuretic hormone deficiency, and chronic protracted prodrome lasting months to years.

Imaging

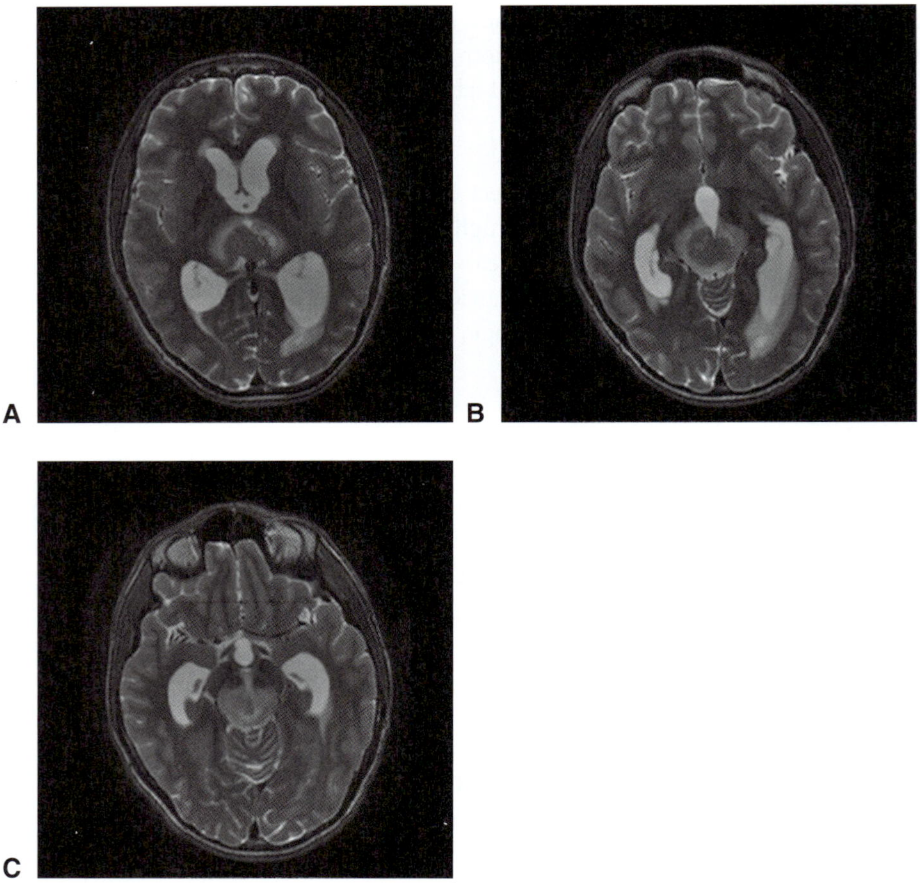

Figure 6.1. Imaging of germinoma of the pineal region. A–C. Axial T2: Homogeneously low-signal intensity pineal mass with mild surrounding edema.

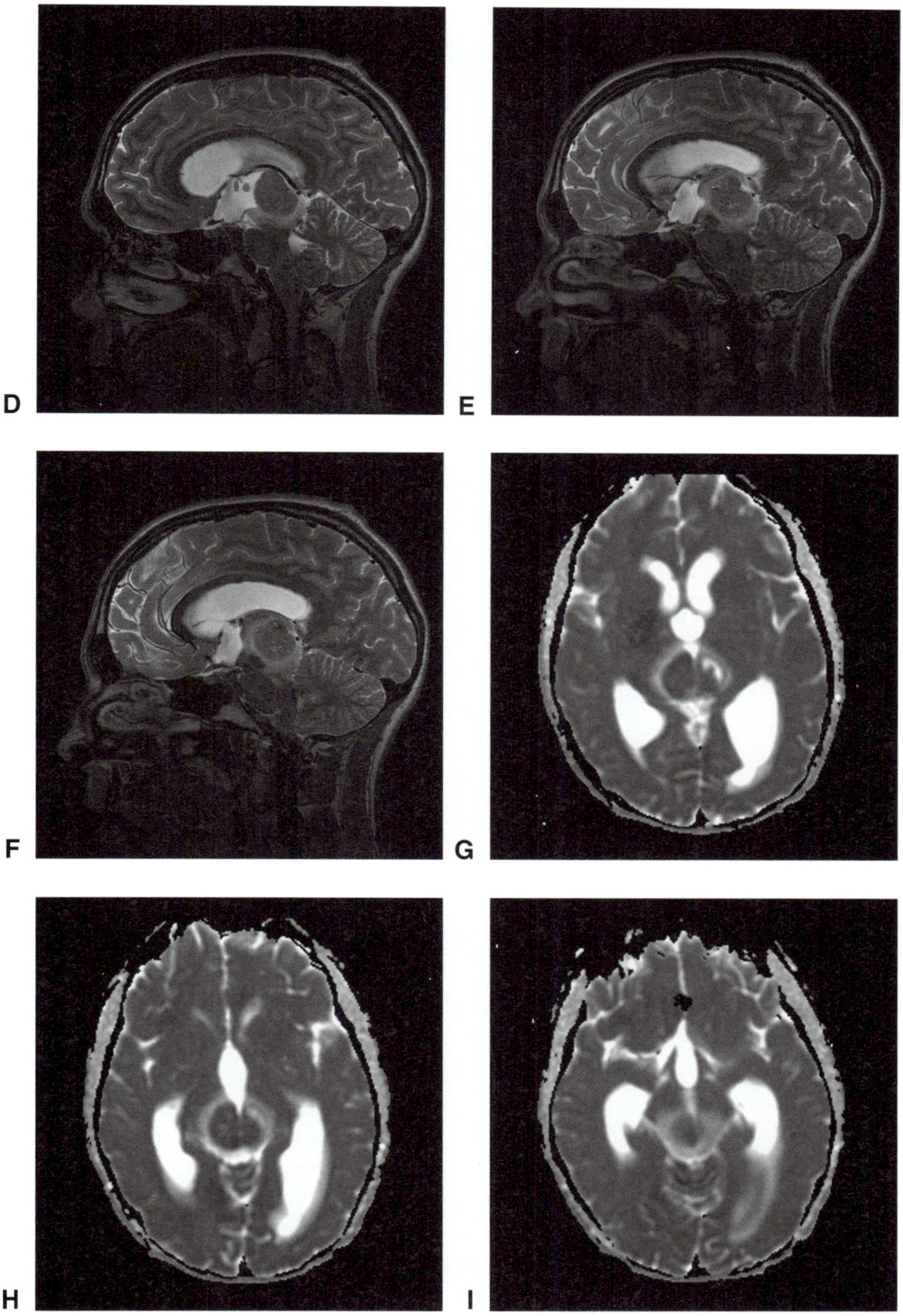

Figure 6.1. ***(continued)*** **D–F.** Sagittal T2: Homogeneously low-signal intensity pineal mass with mild surrounding edema. **G–I.** Axial apparent diffusion coefficient (ADC): Homogeneously reduced diffusion within the pineal mass.

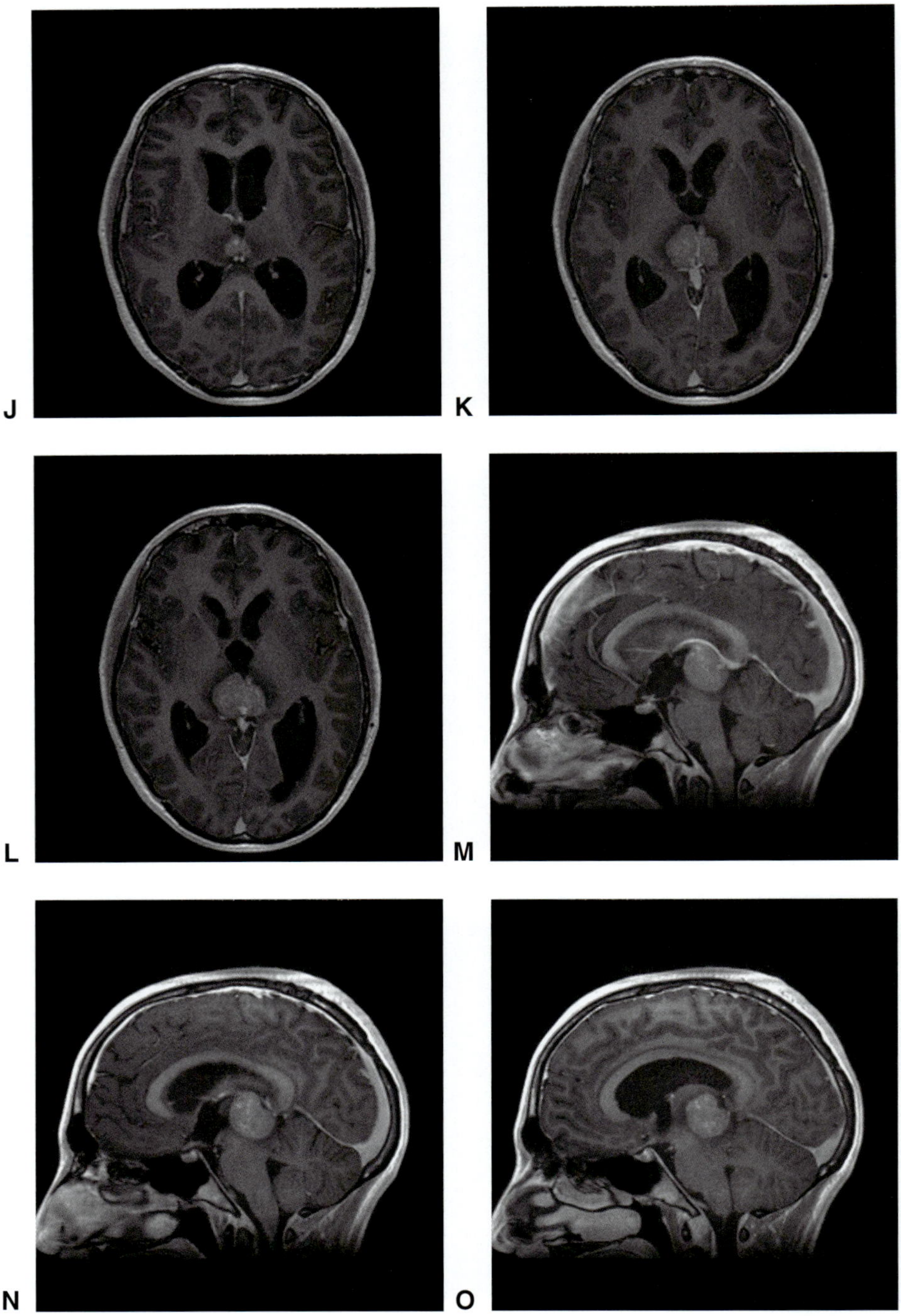

Figure 6.1. ***(continued)*** **J–L.** Axial T1-postcontrast: Avid but heterogeneous enhancement within the mass. **M–O.** Sagittal T1-postcontrast: Avid but heterogeneous enhancement within the circumscribed pineal mass.

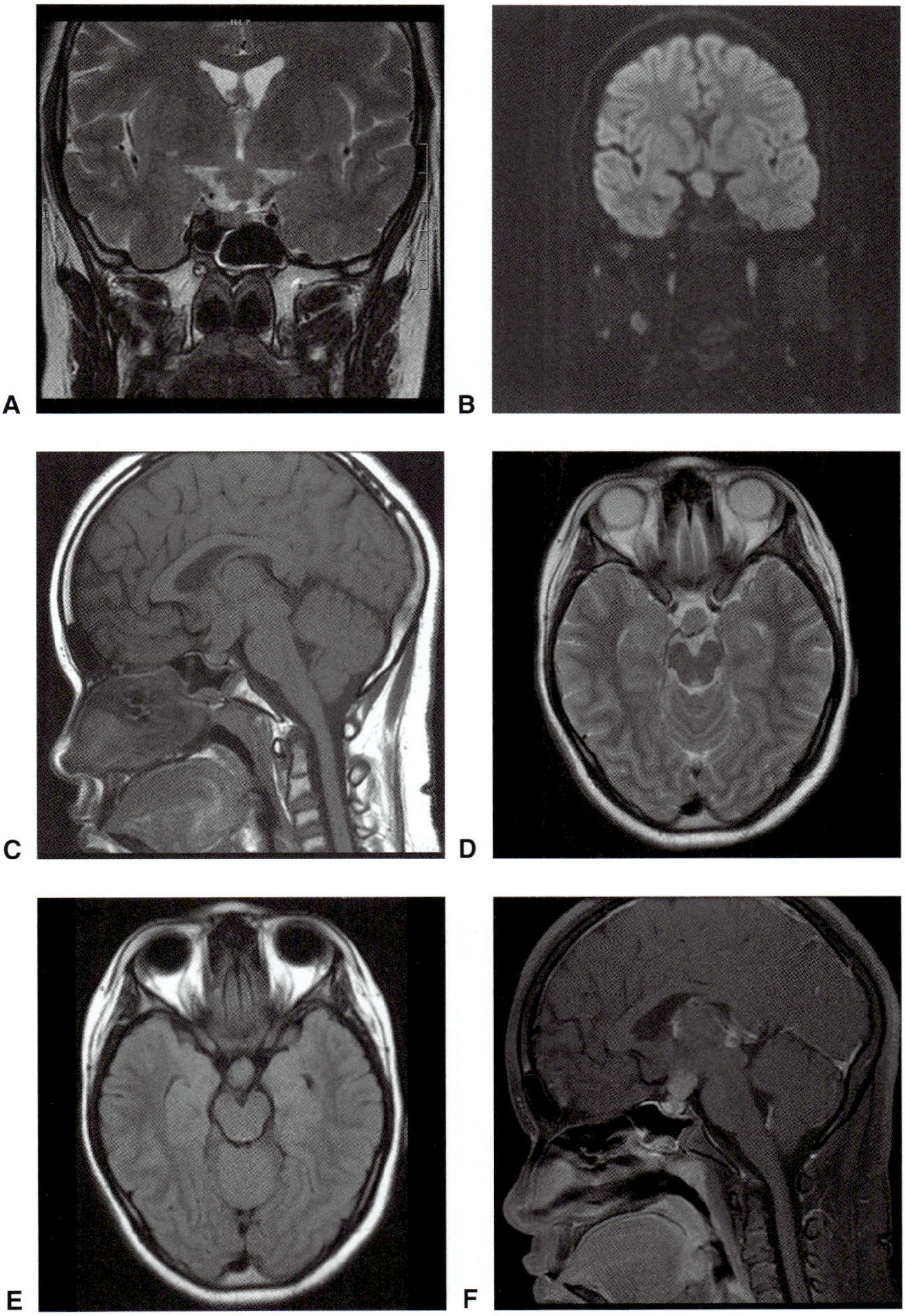

Figure 6.2. Imaging of germinoma of the suprasellar region. A. Coronal T2: Homogeneously low-signal intensity suprasellar mass. **B.** Coronal diffusion-weighted imaging (DWI): No reduced diffusion within the mass. **C.** Sagittal T1-precontrast: Homogeneously isointense signal intensity of the mass to normal brain. **D.** Axial T2: Homogeneously low-signal intensity suprasellar mass. **E.** Axial fluid attenuated inversion recovery (FLAIR): Homogeneously isointense signal intensity of the mass to the normal brain. **F.** Coronal T1-postcontrast: Heterogeneous enhancement of the suprasellar mass within the intrasellar extension.

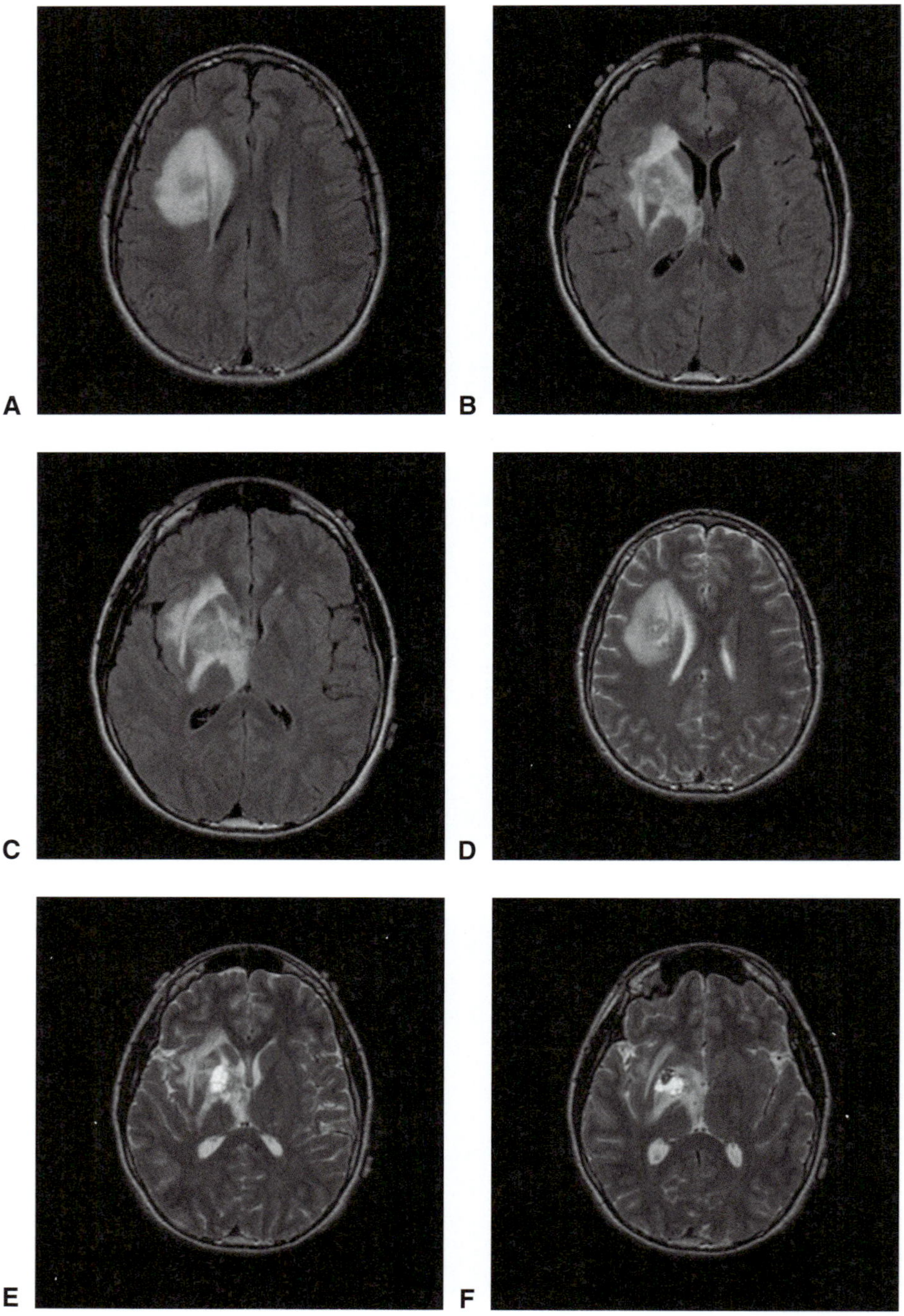

Figure 6.3. Imaging of germinoma of the basal ganglia. A–C. Axial FLAIR: Heterogeneously low-signal intensity mass with prominent surrounding edema. **D–F.** Axial T2: Heterogeneously low-signal intensity mass with prominent surrounding edema.

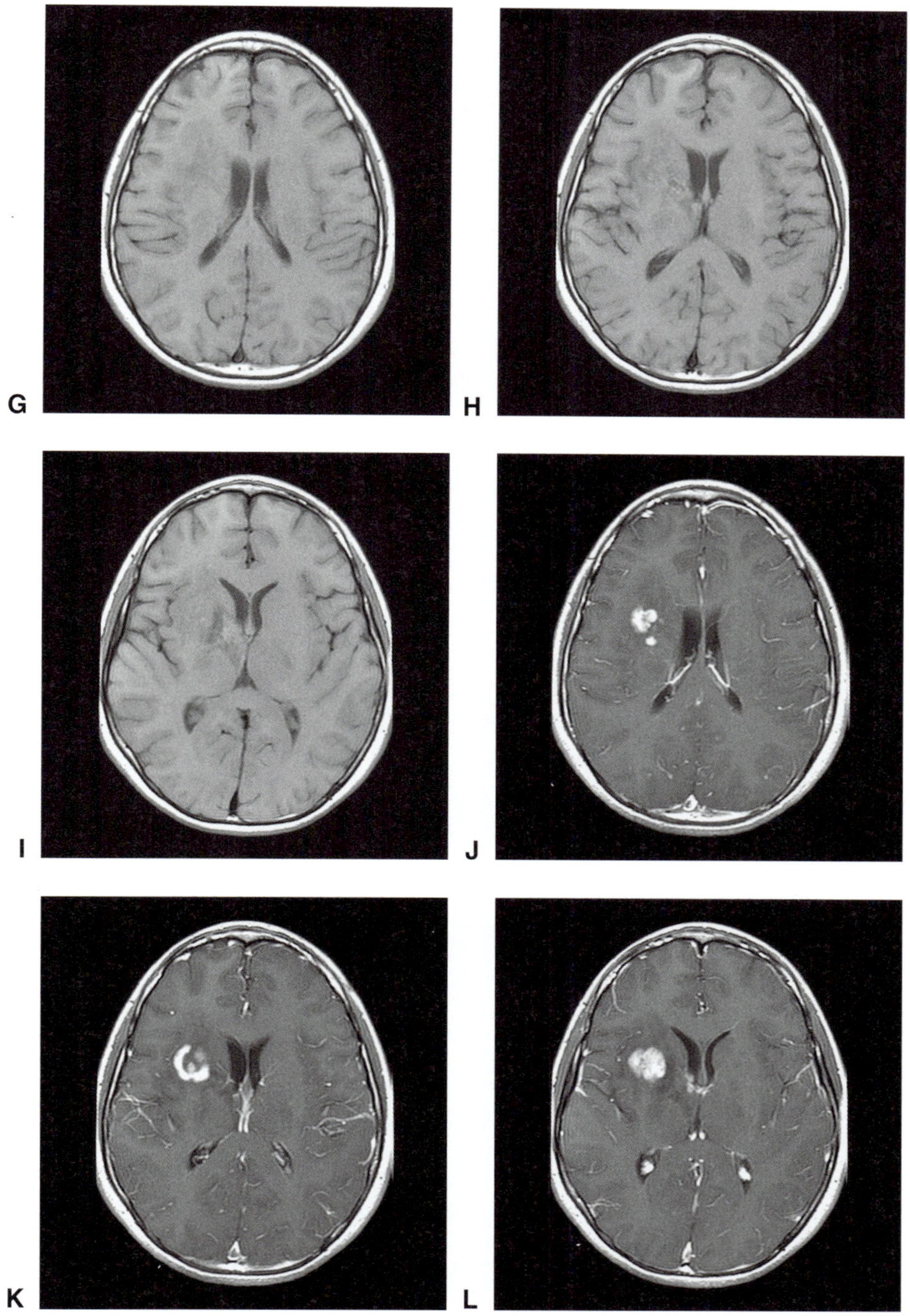

Figure 6.3. ***(continued)*** **G–I.** Axial T1-precontrast: Heterogeneously low-signal intensity mass. **J–L.** Axial T1-postcontrast: Avid and heterogeneous enhancement within the mass.

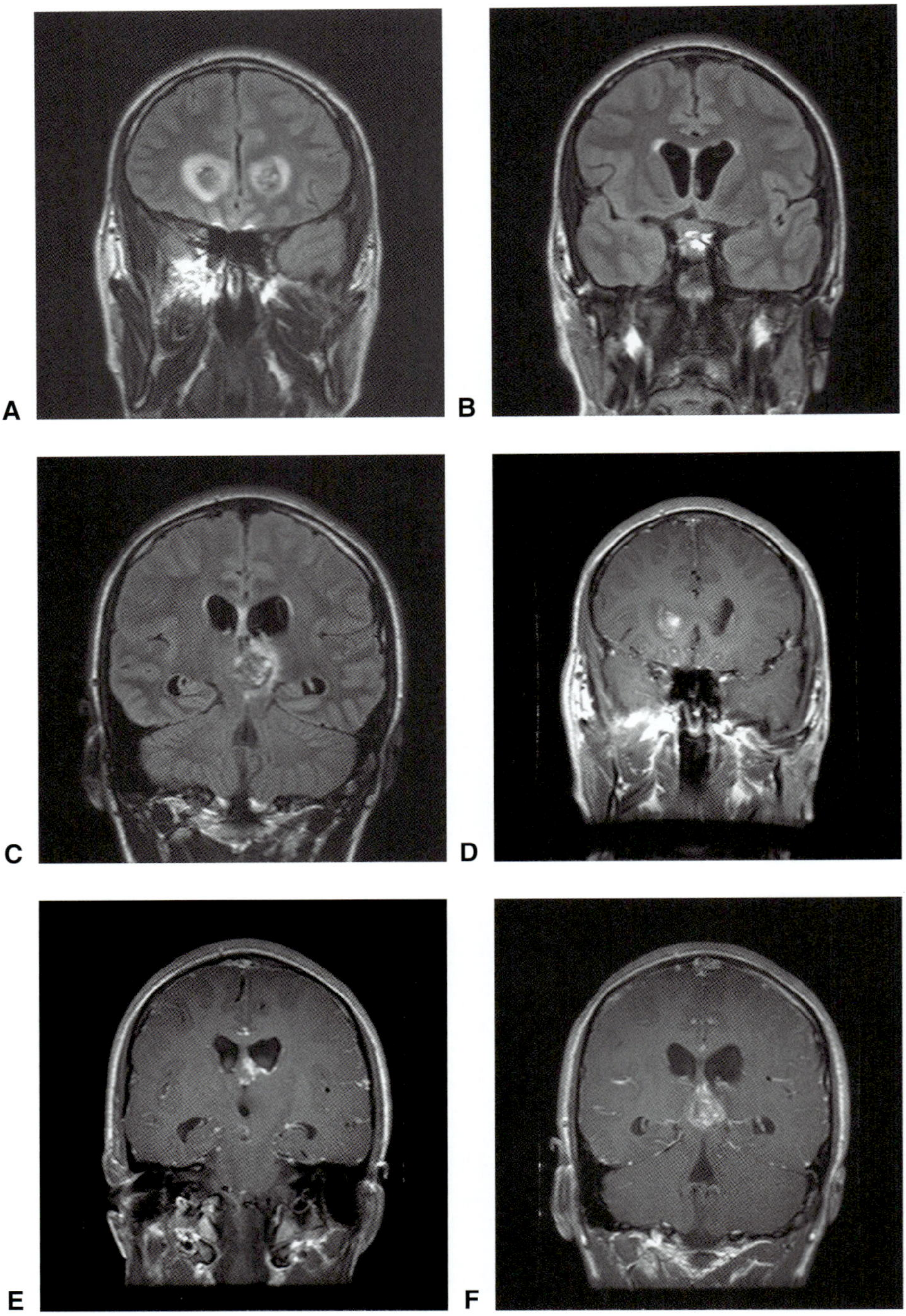

Figure 6.4. Imaging of disseminated germinoma at diagnosis. A–C. Coronal FLAIR. **D–F.** Coronal T1-postcontrast.

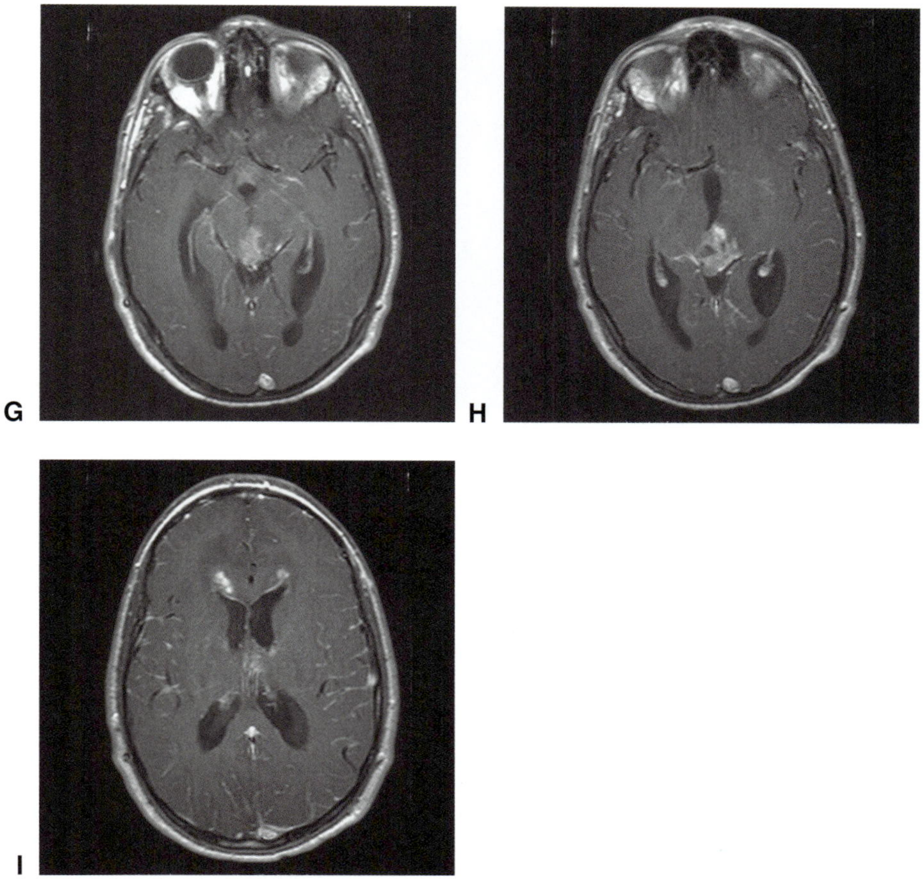

Figure 6.4. ***(continued)*** **G–I.** Axial T1-postcontrast.

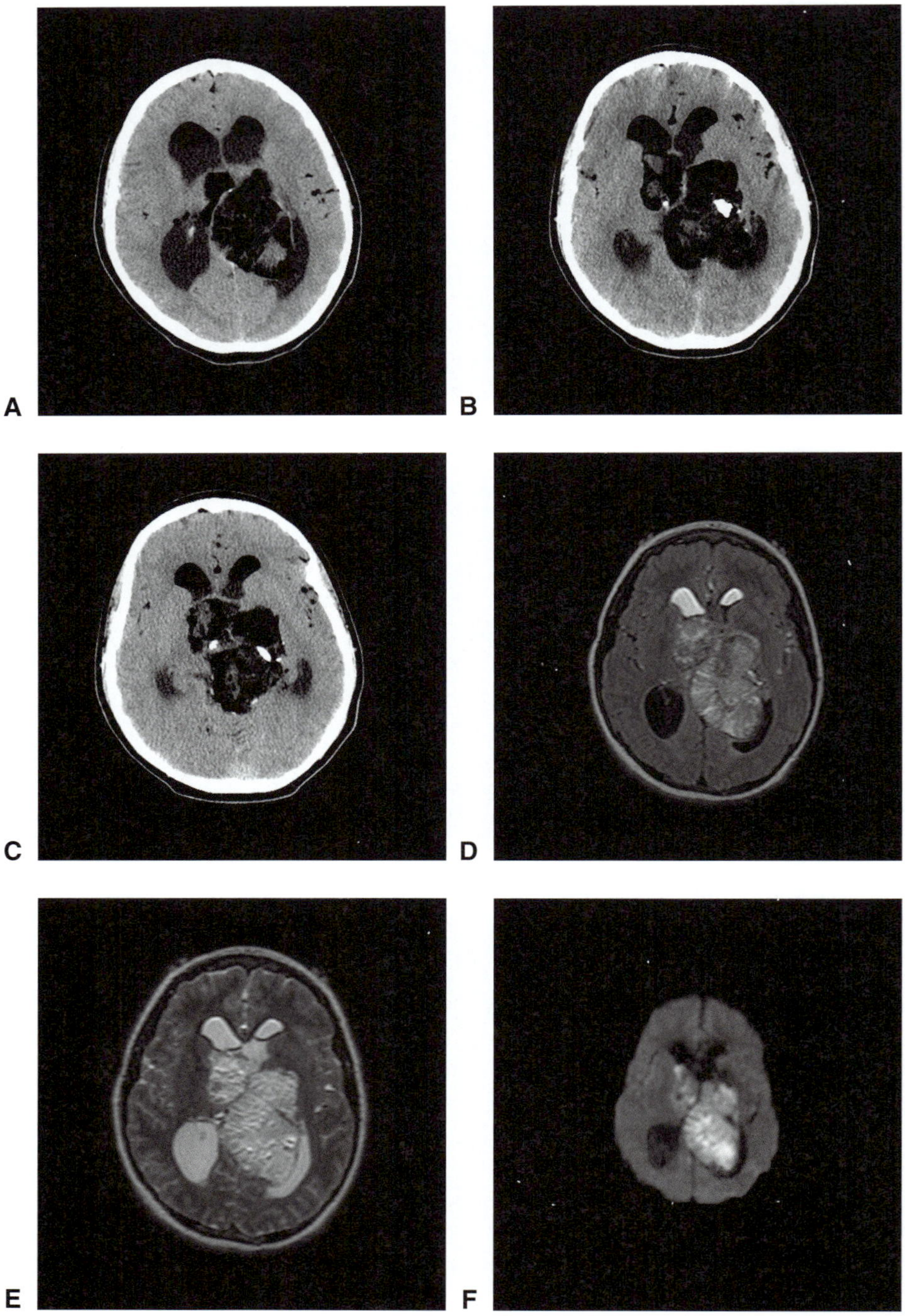

Figure 6.5. Imaging of teratoma arising within a dermoid. A–C. Axial CT: Large lobulated fat density mass within the left lateral ventricle with scattered areas of calcium. **D.** Axial FLAIR: Heterogeneously high-signal intensity within the mass with layering fatty material within the bilateral frontal horns. **E.** Axial T2: Heterogeneously high-signal intensity within the mass with layering fatty material within the bilateral frontal horns. **F.** Axial DWI: Heterogeneously high-signal intensity within the mass.

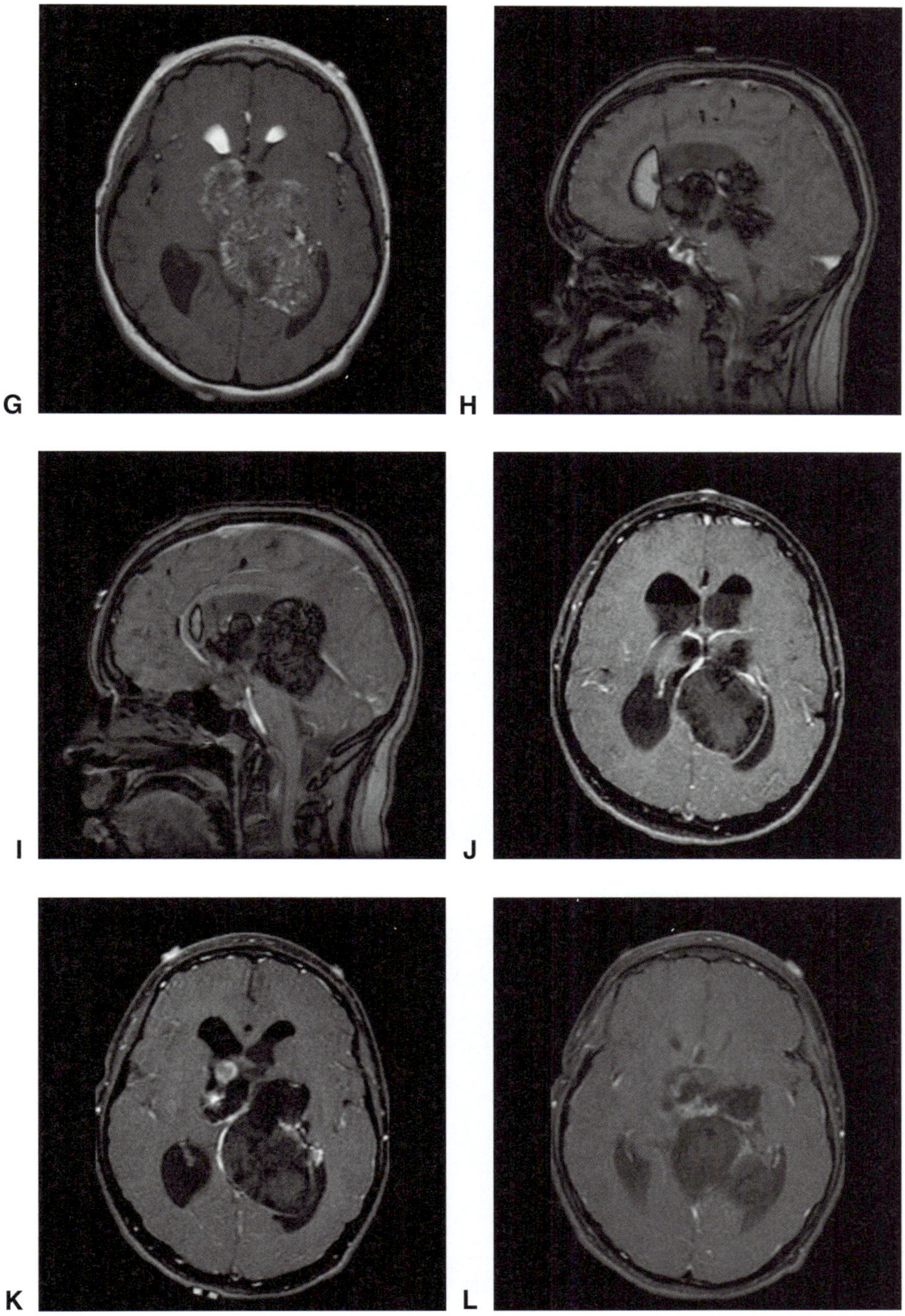

Figure 6.5. ***(continued)*** **G.** Axial T1-precontrast: Heterogeneously high-signal intensity within the mass with layering fatty material within the bilateral frontal horns. **H and I.** Sagittal gradient echo T1-precontrast: Layering fatty material within the bilateral frontal horns with prominent chemical shift artifact. **J–L.** Axial T1-postcontrast, fat-saturated: Uniform suppression of fat within the dermoid except for the enhancing teratoma in the right frontal horn.

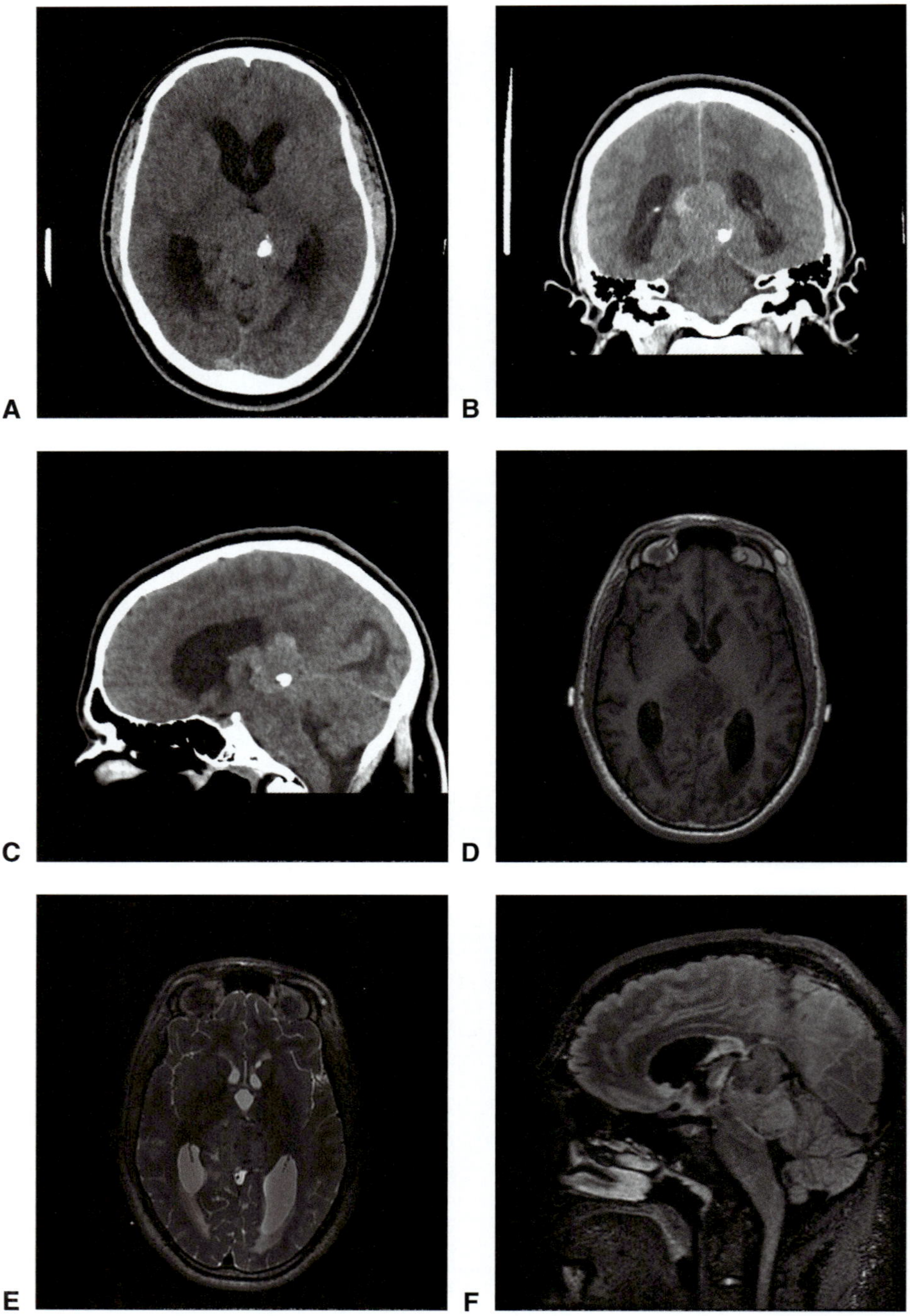

Figure 6.6. Imaging of embryonal carcinoma. A. Axial CT unenhanced: Slightly hyperdense pineal mass with focal area of chunky calcium on the left. **B.** Coronal CT unenhanced: Slightly hyperdense pineal mass with focal area of chunky calcium on the left. **C.** Sagittal CT unenhanced: Slightly hyperdense pineal mass with focal area of chunky calcium on the left. **D.** Axial T1-precontrast: Homogeneously low-signal intensity mass. **E.** Axial T2: Heterogeneously low-signal intensity mass with minimal surrounding edema. **F.** Sagittal FLAIR: Bilobed mass with superior low-signal intensity component and inferior high-signal intensity component.

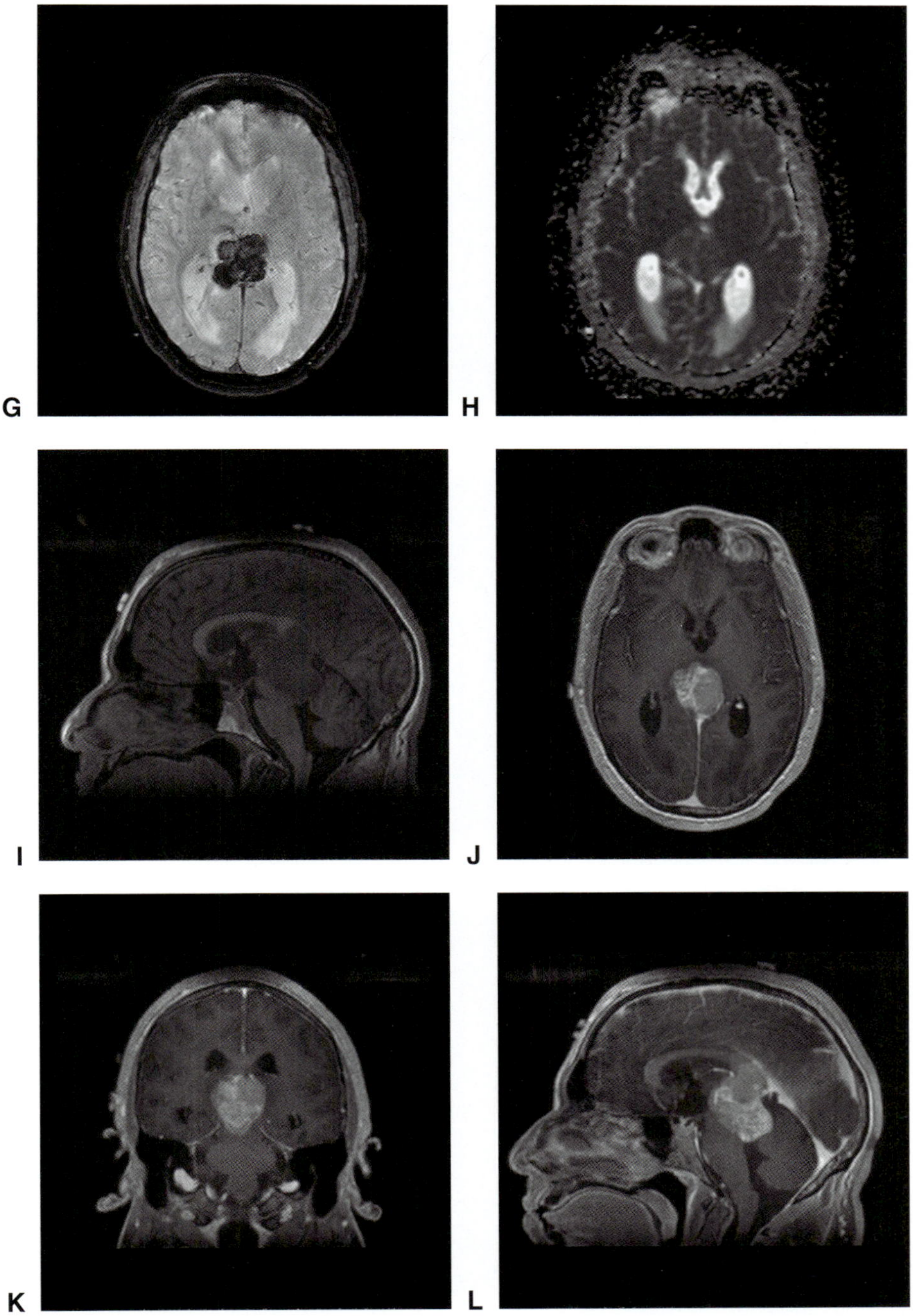

Figure 6.6. ***(continued)*** **G.** Axial susceptibility-weighted imaging (SWI): Marked susceptibility signal throughout the entire mass. **H.** Axial ADC: Mildly reduced signal intensity within the mass. **I.** Sagittal T1-precontrast: Heterogeneously low-signal intensity. **J.** Axial T1-postcontrast: Heterogeneous enhancement with more avid enhancement in the right half of the tumor. **K.** Coronal T1-postcontrast: Heterogeneous enhancement with more avid enhancement in the right half of the tumor. **L.** Sagittal T1-postcontrast: Heterogeneous enhancement with less avid enhancement in the superior component of the tumor.

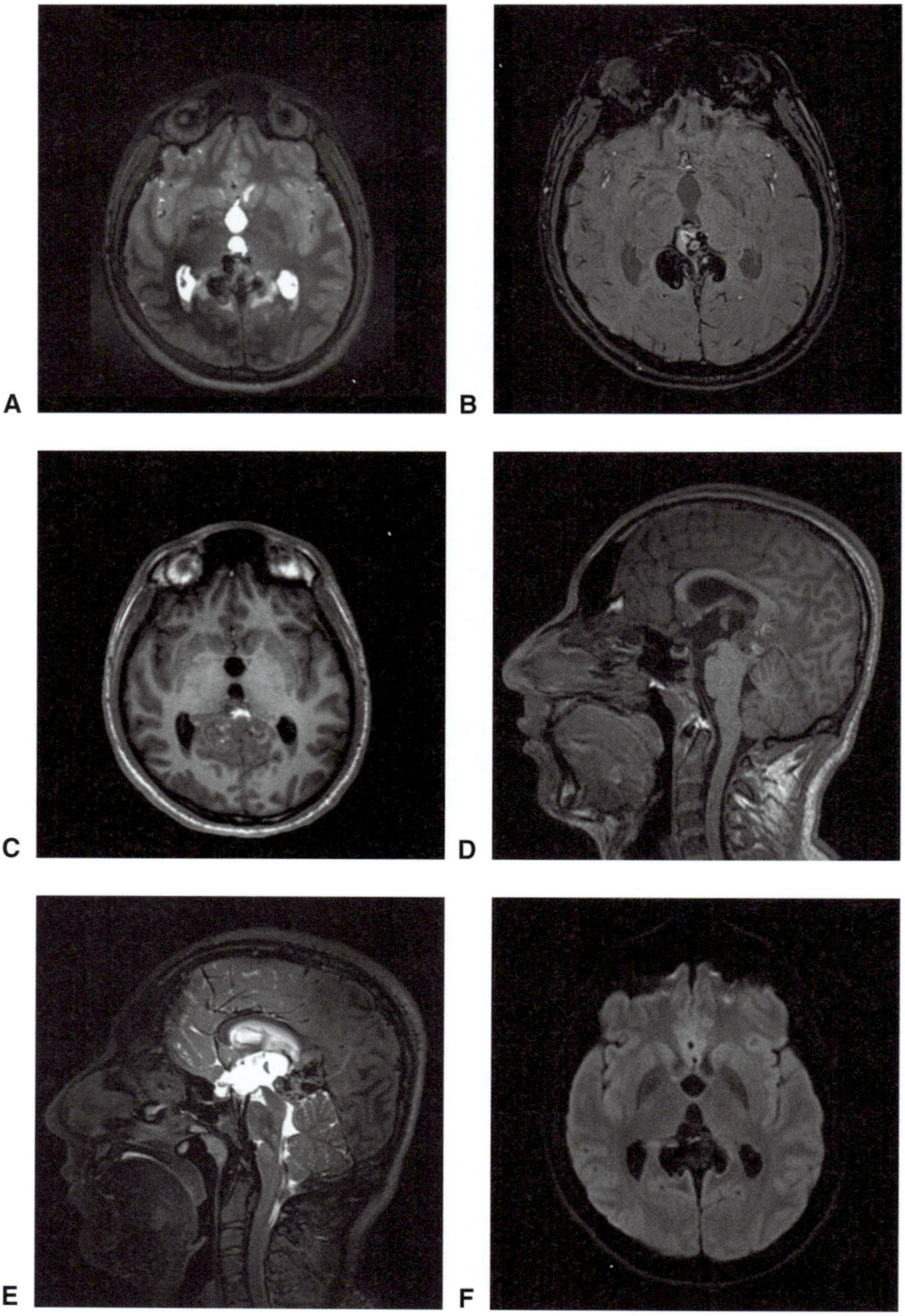

Figure 6.7. **Imaging of choriocarcinoma. A.** Axial T2: Heterogeneously low-signal intensity pineal mass with areas of marked hypointensity. **B.** Axial SWI: Marked susceptibility signal within the mass. **C.** Axial T1-precontrast: Heterogeneously low-signal intensity mass. **D.** Sagittal T1-precontrast: Heterogeneously low-signal intensity mass. **E.** Sagittal T2: Heterogeneously low-signal intensity mass with areas of marked hypointensity. **F.** Axial DWI: Homogeneously low-signal intensity.

G
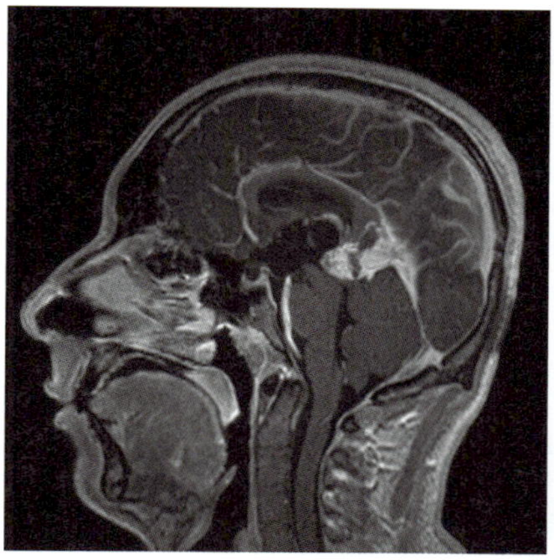

H
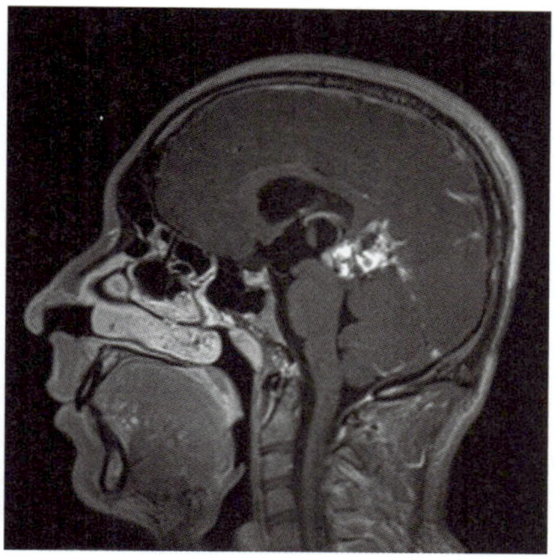

I
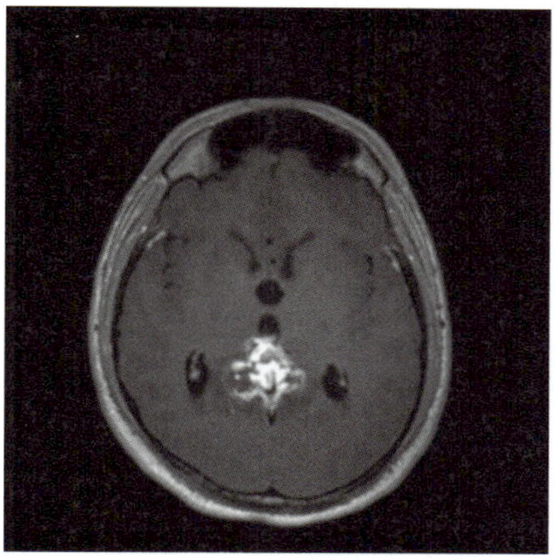

Figure 6.7. ***(continued)*** **G.** Sagittal T1-postcontrast: Heterogeneous enhancement with central tumor areas of non-enhancement. **H.** Sagittal T1-postcontrast: Heterogeneous enhancement with central tumor areas of non-enhancement. **I.** Axial T1-postcontrast: Heterogeneous enhancement with central tumor areas of non-enhancement.

Bibliography

Huang X, Zhang R, Mao Y, Zhou L-F, Zhang C. Recent advances in molecular biology and treatment strategies for intracranial germ cell tumors. *World J Pediatr.* 2016;12: 275–282.

Lee SM, Kim I-O, Choi YH, et al. Early imaging findings in germ cell tumors arising from the basal ganglia. *Pediatr Radiol.* 2016;46:719–726.

Liu Z, Lv X, Wang W, et al. Imaging characteristics of primary intracranial teratoma. *Acta Radiol.* 2014;55:874–881.

Lv X-F, Qui Y-W, Zhang X-L, et al. Primary intracranial choriocarcinoma: MR imaging findings. *Am J Neuroradiol.* 2010;31:1994–1998.

Villano JL, Propp JM, Porter KR et al. Malignant pineal germ-cell tumors: an analysis of cases from three tumor registries. *Neuro Oncol.* 2008;10:121–130.

Wang L, Yamaguchi S, Burstein MD, et al. Novel somatic and germline mutations in intracranial germ cell tumours. *Nature.* 2014;511:241–245.

Wang M, Zhou P, Zhang, S et al. Clinical features, radiologic findings, and treatment of pediatric germ cell tumors involving the basal ganglia and thalamus: a retrospective series of 15 cases at a single center. *Child Nerv Syst.* 2018;34:423–430.

7

Melanocytic Tumors

Overview

Primary melanocytic tumors of the central nervous system (CNS) are rare tumors, distinct and unrelated to systemic melanoma, that can be focal or diffuse and arise from the leptomeningeal melanocytes. There are four types of meningeal melanocytic tumors: two diffuse subtypes—meningeal melanocytosis and melanomatosis—and two focal subtypes—meningeal melanocytoma and melanoma. Lesions can present as diffuse dissemination within the subarachnoid space or as solid masses and can be benign or malignant. There is no concurrent presence of systemic melanoma.

	Age range (mean)	Female: male ratio	Cell of origin	WHO grade	Molecular/ genetic markers	Prognosis
Meningeal melanocytosis	Any age	1:1	Melanocytes of leptomeninges (neuroectodermal origin)	NA	—	Guarded
Meningeal melanomatosis	Any age	1:1		NA	—	Guarded
Meningeal melanocytoma	45–50	1.5:1		NA	*GNAQ/ GNA11*	Favorable
Meningeal melanoma	15–71	1:1		NA	*GNAQ/ GNA11*	Guarded

Meningeal Melanocytosis

Definition: Melanocytic tumors are a rare variant of primary central nervous system (CNS) melanomas that comprise two distinct phenotypes: diffuse melanocytosis and melanomatosis to well-differentiated melanocytoma and melanoma. Diffuse melanocytosis is confined to the subarachnoid space, but melanomatosis can extend into the perivascular spaces with a superficial invasion of the neighboring brain.

Epidemiology: The estimated incidence of meningeal melanocytic tumors is 0.9 per 10 million and can affect any age group. Gender predilection is not known because of its rarity.

Clinical features and standard therapy: Although histologically benign, meningeal melanocytosis can be clinically and biologically aggressive. Complete surgical resection is curative for most cases. Radiation therapy is used after incomplete resection of tumor because recurrence rate is high in residual tumor.

Imaging

Meningeal melanocytosis is a diffuse tumor that infiltrates leptomeninges but remains within the subarachnoid space. Diffuse enhancement of the leptomeninges on imaging can mimic subarachnoid hemorrhage, pus, or metastatic tumor.

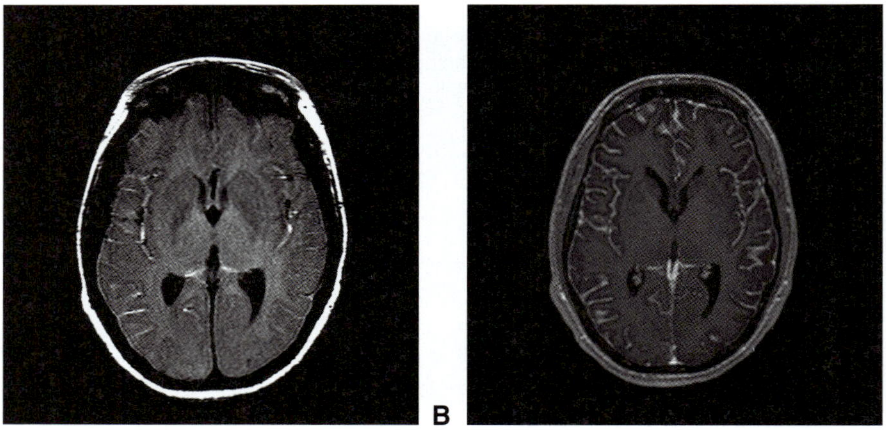

A B

Figure 7.1. **Meningeal melanocytosis. A.** Axial T1-precontrast: Linear T1 shortening diffusely filling the subarachnoid space. **B.** Axial T1-postcontrast: Avid enhancement of subarachnoid tumor without focal nodularity or mass-like feature.

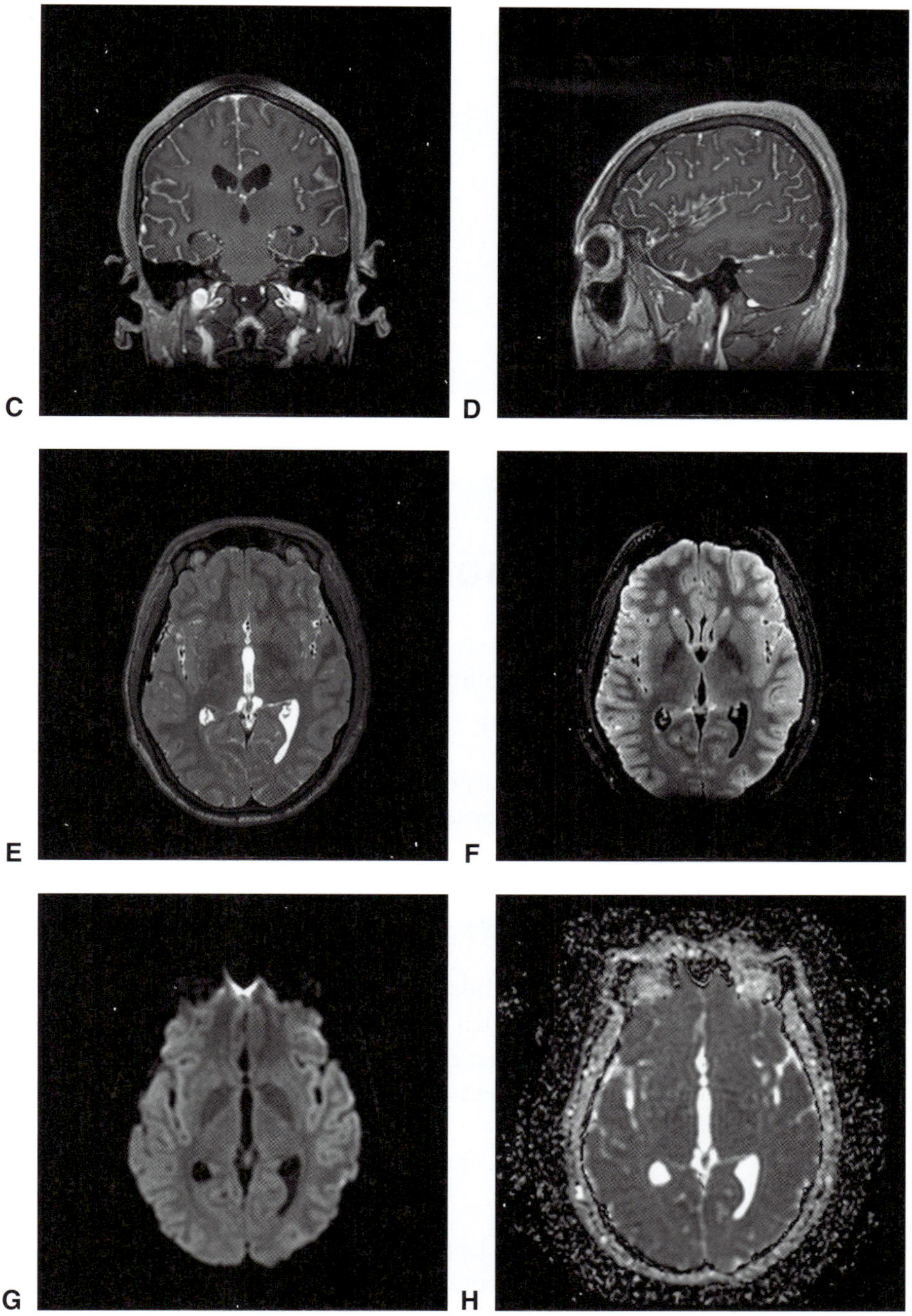

C D E F G H

Figure 7.1. ***(continued)*** **C.** Coronal T1-postcontrast: Avid enhancement of subarachnoid tumor without focal nodularity or mass-like feature. **D.** Sagittal T1-postcontrast: Avid enhancement of subarachnoid tumor without focal nodularity or mass-like feature. **E.** Axial T2 FSE: Diffuse subarachnoid tumor is barely visible. **F.** Axial FLAIR: Slight hyperintensity within the diffuse subarachnoid tumor. **G.** Diffusion-weighted imaging (DWI): Diffuse subarachnoid tumor is barely visible. **H.** Apparent diffusion coefficient (ADC): Diffuse subarachnoid tumor is barely visible.

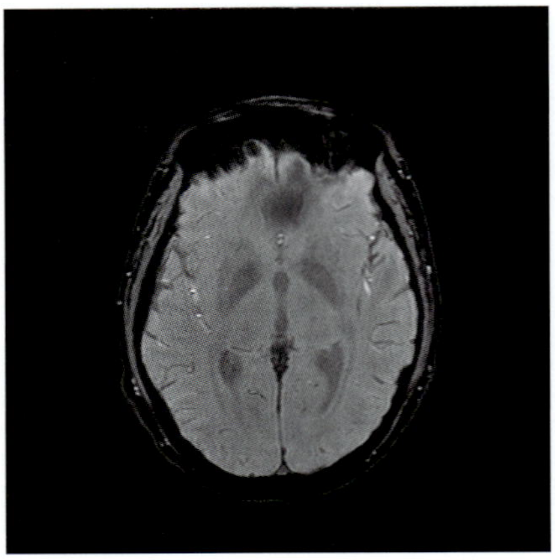

I

Figure 7.1. *(continued)* **I.** Susceptibility-weighted imaging (SWI): Diffuse subarachnoid tumor is barely visible.

Meningeal Melanomatosis

Definition: Meningeal melanomatosis is a malignant tumor with diffuse meningeal growth that infiltrates leptomeninges and subarachnoid space and can invade the perivascular spaces.

Epidemiology: The estimated incidence of meningeal melanocytic tumors is 0.9 per 10 million and can affect any age group. Gender predilection is not known because of its rarity.

Molecular and genetic profile: None.

Clinical features and standard therapy: Due to extensive infiltration of the subarachnoid space, the patient often presents with signs and symptoms of hydrocephalus or localized mass effect. Surgical resection is not feasible, and there is no effective chemotherapy agent. Radiation therapy is given as a palliative measure.

Imaging

Meningeal melanomatosis is a diffuse leptomeningeal tumor that can be bulky and invade the perivascular space and the neighboring brain.

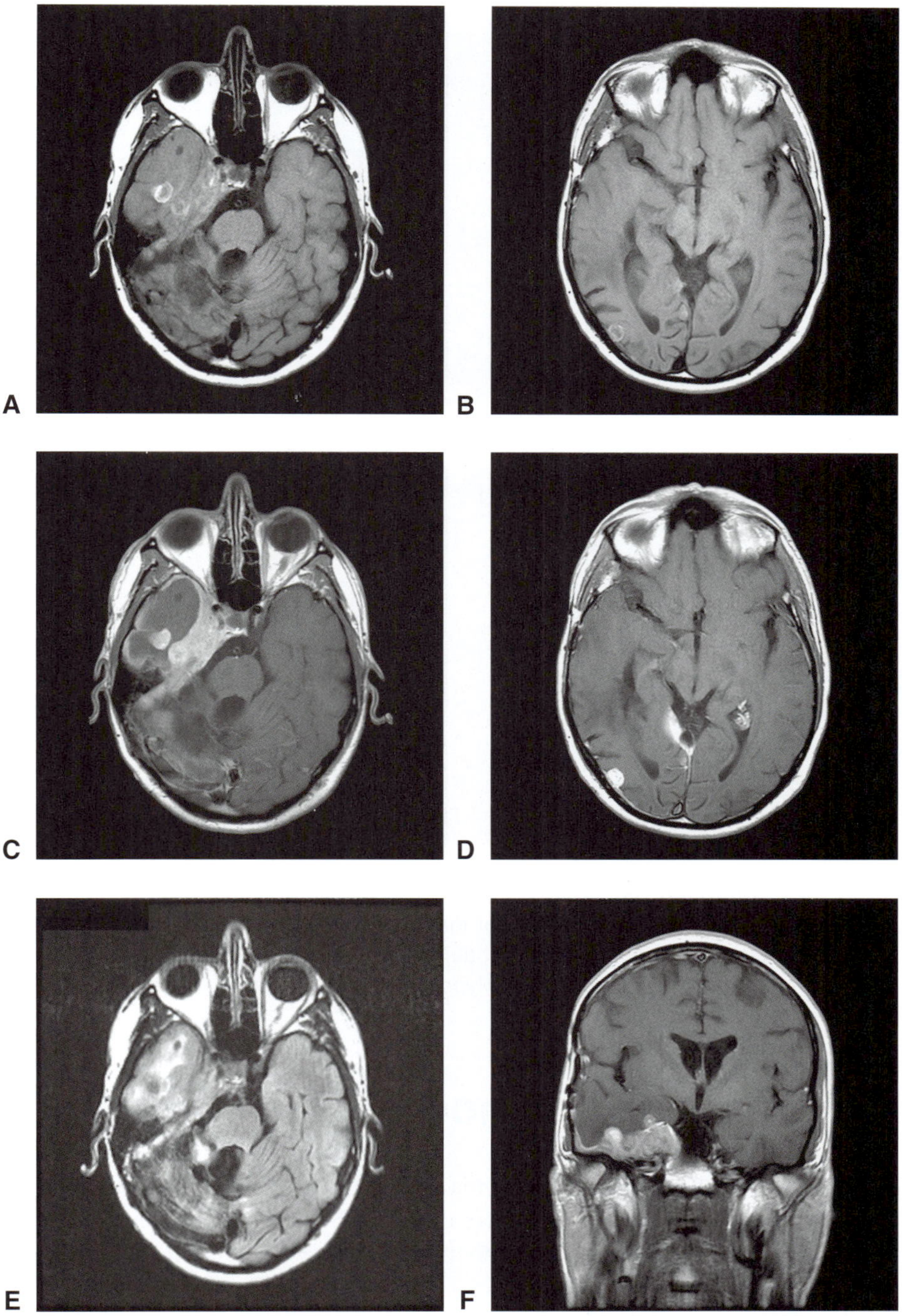

Figure 7.2. Recurrent meningeal melanomatosis. A. Axial T1-precontrast: Multifocal areas of T1 shortening within the right temporal lobe and along the right cavernous sinus and tentorium. **B.** Axial T1-precontrast: Nodular mass with T1 shortening along the right lateral occipital convexity. **C.** Axial T1-postcontrast: Avid enhancement of right temporal lobe and along the right cavernous sinus and tentorium. **D.** Axial T1-postcontrast: Avid enhancement of the nodular mass along the right lateral occipital convexity. **E.** Axial FLAIR: Isointense. **F.** Coronal T1-postcontrast: Avid enhancement of nodular and dural-based mass along the floor of the right middle cranial fossa.

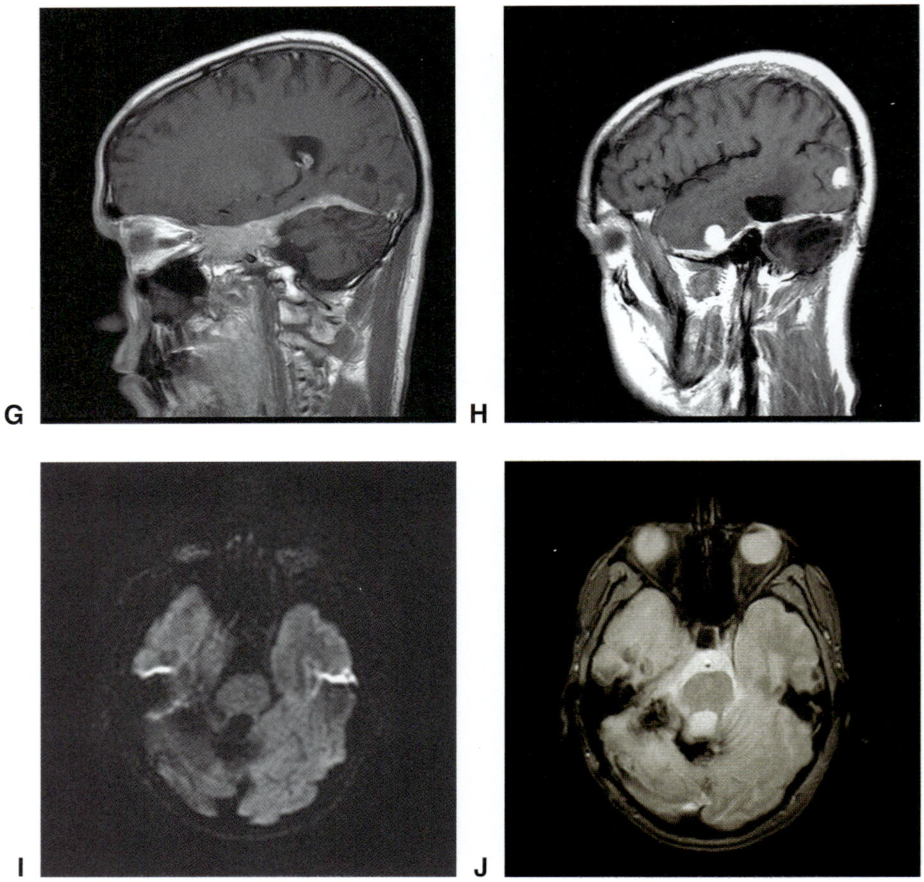

Figure 7.2. ***(continued)*** **G.** Sagittal T1-postcontrast: Avid enhancement of nodular and dural-based mass along the floor of the right middle cranial fossa. **H.** Sagittal T1-postcontrast: Additional enhancing nodules adjacent to the temporal and occipital lobes. **I.** DWI: Hypointense. **J.** SWI: Hypointense due to underlying melanin and blood products.

Meningeal Melanocytoma

Definition: Meningeal melanocytoma is a solitary, well-circumscribed, melanocytic tumor occurring anywhere in the CNS but with a predilection to spinal canal and posterior fossa, with no invasion of the surrounding structures.

Epidemiology: The estimated incidence of meningeal melanocytic tumors is 0.9 per 10 million and usually affects adults in the age range of 45 to 50 years, with a slight female predilection.

Molecular and genetic profile: Characteristic hotspot mutations of *GNAQ* or *GNA11*, most often involving codon 209, can be seen in meningeal melanocytoma.

Clinical features and standard therapy: Patients usually present with symptoms and signs related to local mass effect or hydrocephalus caused by the solitary mass.

Imaging

Meningeal melanocytoma is a solitary, circumscribed subarachnoid mass with no features of invasion.

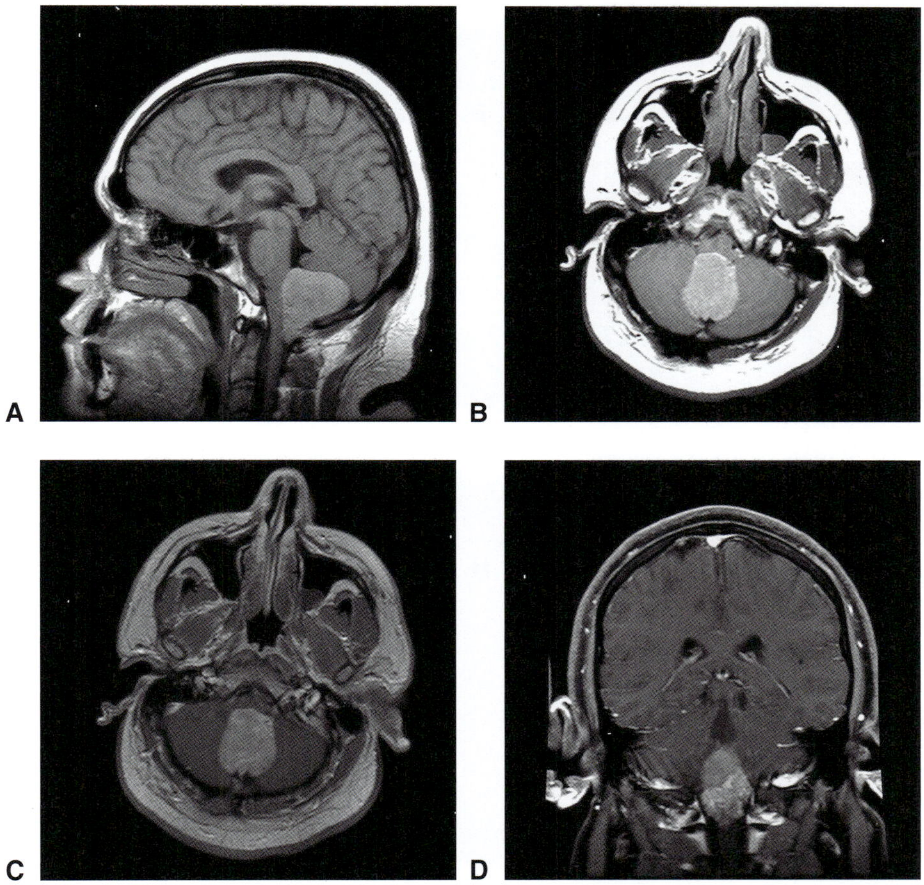

Figure 7.3. **Meningeal melanocytoma, posterior fossa. A.** Sagittal T1-precontrast: Circumscribed subarachnoid mass with intrinsic T1 shortening. **B.** Axial T1-precontrast: Homogeneous enhancement. **C.** Axial T1-postcontrast: Homogeneous enhancement. **D.** Coronal T1-postcontrast: Homogeneous enhancement.

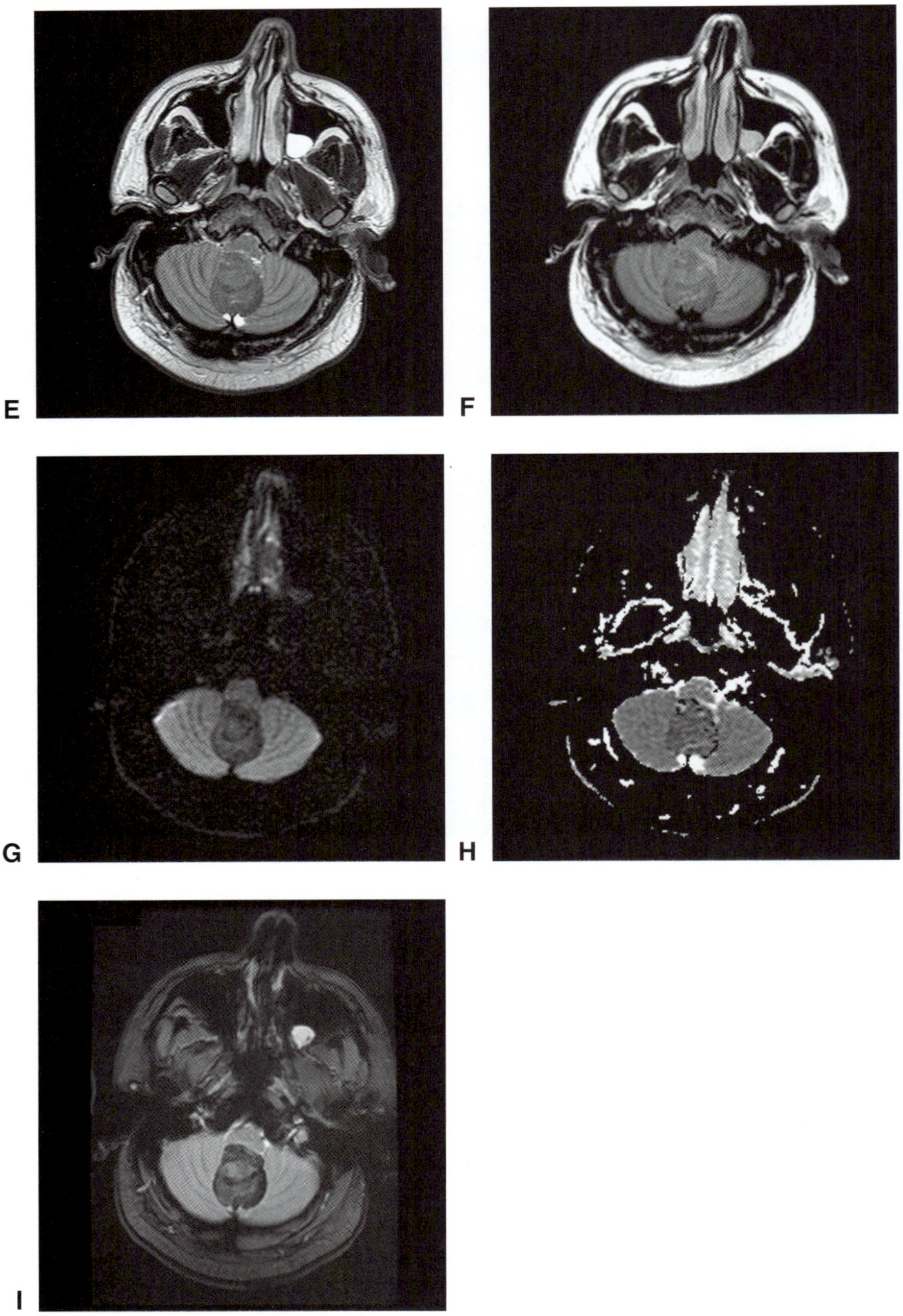

Figure 7.3. ***(continued)*** **E.** Axial T2 FSE: Hypointense. **F.** Axial FLAIR: Hypointense. **G.** DWI: Markedly hypointense. **H.** ADC: Hypointense. **I.** SWI: Hypointense.

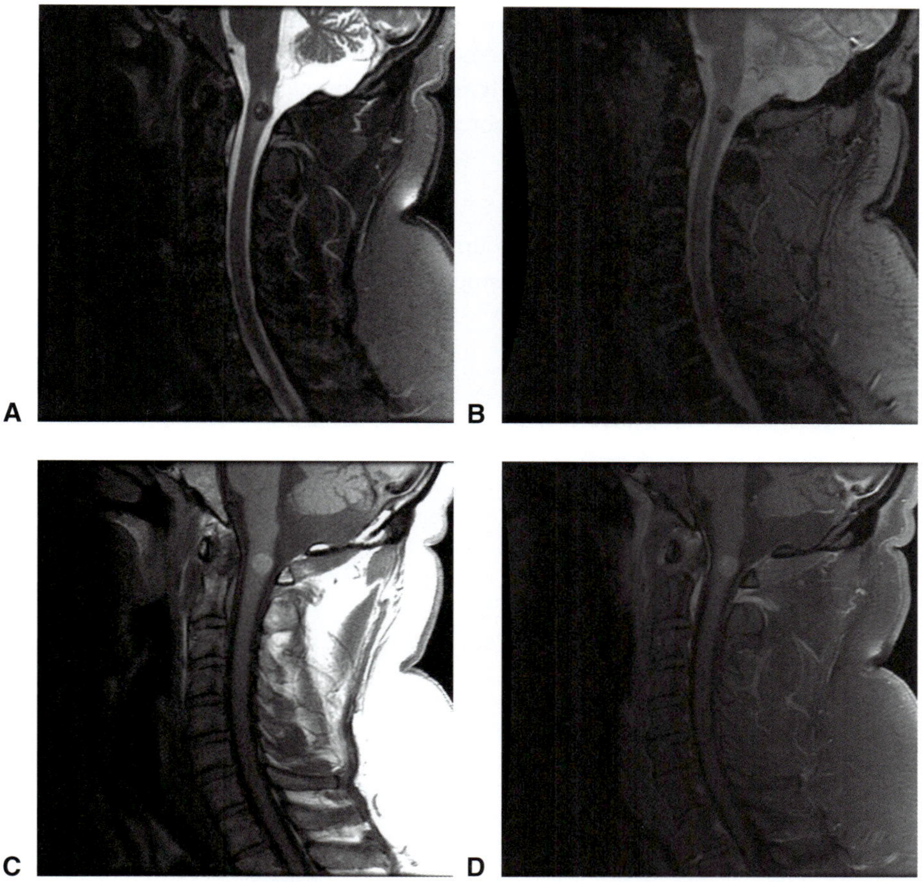

Figure 7.4. Meningeal melanocytoma, spinal cord. A. Sagittal T2: Homogeneous enhancement. **B.** Sagittal gradient echo: Homogeneous enhancement. **C.** Sagittal T1-precontrast: Circumscribed subarachnoid mass with intrinsic T1 shortening. **D.** Sagittal T1-postcontrast: Homogeneous enhancement.

Meningeal Melanoma

Definition: Meningeal melanoma is a primary malignant melanoma of the CNS arising from the leptomeningeal melanocytes. Distinct from melanocytomas, meningeal melanomas have higher cellular density, cellular pleomorphism, and nuclear atypia.

Epidemiology: The estimated incidence of meningeal melanocytic tumors is 0.9 per 10 million, affecting a wide range of age groups of 15 to 71 years without gender predilection. Primary meningeal melanoma accounts for <1% of all melanomas.

Molecular and genetic profile: Characteristic hotspot mutations of *GNAQ* or *GNA11*, most often involving codon 209, can be seen in meningeal melanomas but not as frequently as seen in meningeal melanocytomas.

Clinical features and standard therapy: Surgical resection is the primary treatment, and there is no effective chemotherapy or targeted agents. There is a higher recurrence rate for incompletely resected tumor, and adjuvant radiation therapy is needed to control local tumor growth.

Imaging

Meningeal melanoma is a solitary, circumscribed, extra-axial mass with higher propensity for brain invasion and causing brain edema.

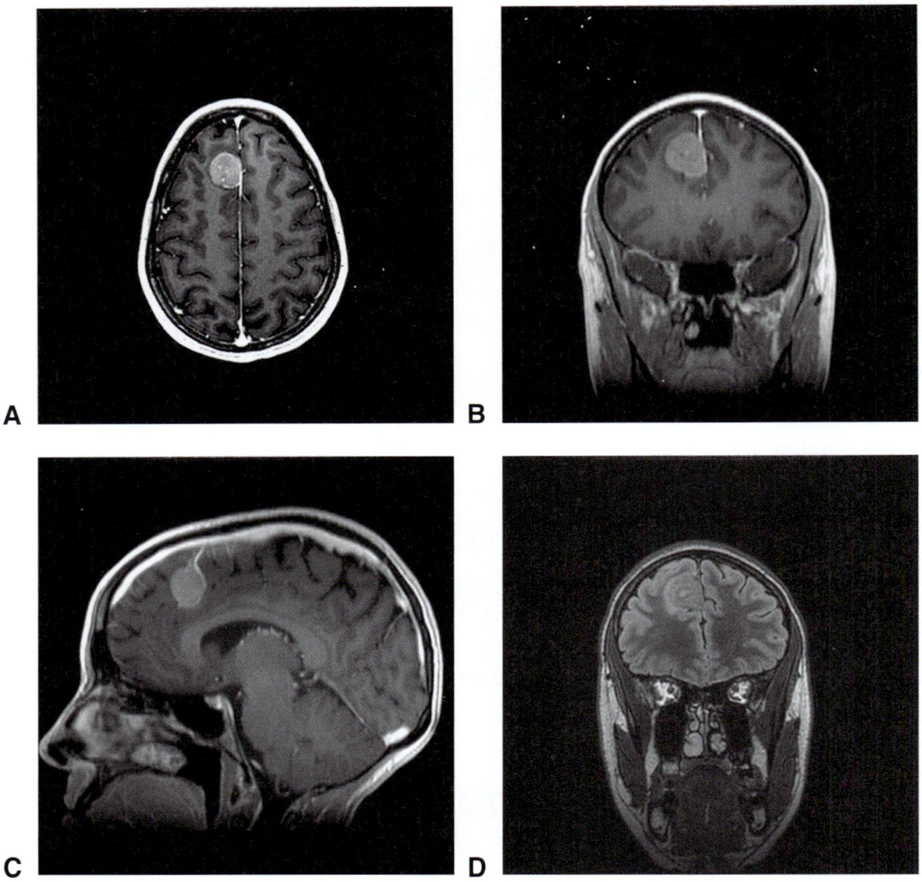

Figure 7.5. Meningeal melanoma. A. Axial T1-postcontrast: Avid enhancement of the right falcine mass. **B.** Coronal T1-postcontrast: Avid enhancement of the right falcine mass. **C.** Sagittal T1-postcontrast: Avid enhancement of the right falcine mass. **D.** Coronal FLAIR: Isointense to brain.

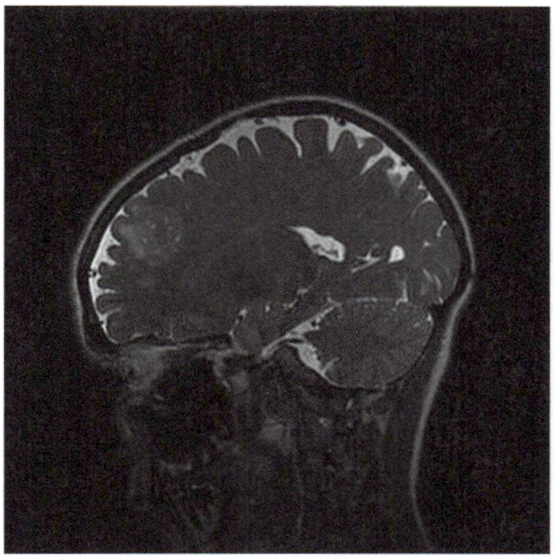

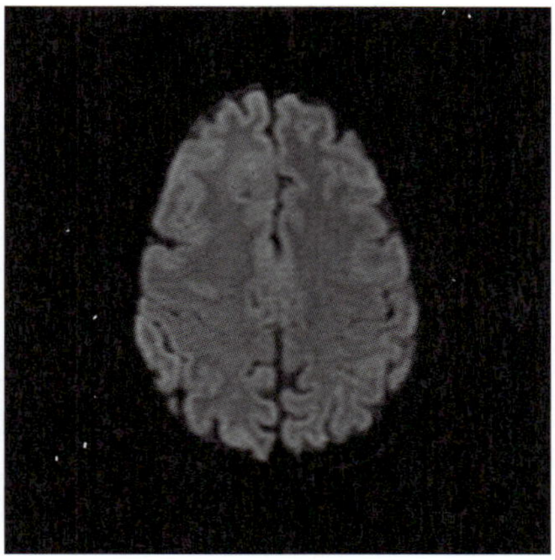

Figure 7.5. ***(continued)*** **E.** Sagittal T2 FSE: Isointense to brain with mild edema. **F.** Axial DWI: Isointense to brain; no reduced diffusion.

Bibliography

Arias M, Alberte-Woodward M, Arias S, Dapena D, Prieto A, Suarez-Penaranda JM. Primary malignant meningeal melanomatosis: a clinical, radiological and pathologic case study. *Acta Neurol Belg*. 2011;111:228–231.

Jaiswal S, Vij M, Tungria A, Jaiswal AK, Srivastava AK, Behari S. Primary melanocytic tumors of the central nervous system: a neuroradiological and clinicopathological study of five cases and brief review of literature. *Neurol India*. 2011;59:413–419.

Liubinas SV, Maartens N, Drummond KJ. Primary melanocytic neoplasms of the central nervous system. *J Clin Neurosci*. 2010;17:1227–1232.

Pirini MG, Mascalchi M, Salvi F, Tassinari CA, Zanella L, Bacchini P, et al. Primary diffuse meningeal melanomatosis: radiologic-pathologic correlation. *AJNR Am J Neuroradiol*. 2003;24:115–118.

Smith AB, Rushing EJ, Smirniotopoulos JG. Pigmented lesions of the central nervous system: radiologic-pathologic correlation. *Radiographics*. 2009;29:1503–1524.

8 Tumors of the Cranial and Paraspinal Nerves

Overview

Tumors of the cranial and paraspinal nerves are usually benign, slow-growing neoplasms composed of one or more elements of a nerve cell (Schwann cell, perineural cells, fibroblasts, mast cells, ganglion cells, myxoid/collagenous matrix, and axons). The most common nerve tumor is schwannoma in the general population and in the setting of neurofibromatosis type 2; neurofibromas including plexiform subtype are most commonly seen in the setting of neurofibromatosis type 1.

	Age range (mean)	Female: male ratio	Cell of origin	WHO grade	Molecular/ genetic markers	Prognosis
Schwannoma	40–60	1:1	Schwann cell	I	Loss of merlin (*NF2* gene)	Favorable
Neurofibroma	0–40	1:1	Schwann cell	I	*NF1*	Favorable
Plexiform neurofibroma	0–40	1:1	Schwann cell	I	*NF1*	Favorable
Malignant peripheral nerve sheath tumor	28–36 (*NF1*) 40–44 (sporadic)	1:1	Schwann cell	II	*NF1*	Guarded

▶ Schwannoma

Definition: Schwannoma is a globular, circumscribed, and encapsulated benign nerve sheath tumor composed of well-differentiated Schwann cells and comprise three main types: conventional, cellular, and plexiform.

Epidemiology: This is the most common peripheral nerve neoplasm, often solitary (90%) but can be multiple in the setting of neurofibromatosis type 2 (4%). It accounts for 8% of all intracranial tumors, 85% of cerebellopontine angle tumors, and 30% of spinal nerve root tumors. No gender predilection has been noted.

Affected age group: Patients of any age are affected, but this tumor is distinctly rare in the pediatric age group. Cerebral intraparenchymal schwannomas are more common in the younger age group, with male dominance.

Molecular and genetic profile: Multiple schwannomas often occur in the setting of two tumor syndromes: neurofibromatosis 2 (*NF2*) and schwannomatosis. A mosaic pattern of *SMARCB1* (*INI1*) expression is seen in 93% of familial schwannomatosis, 55% of sporadic schwannomatosis, 83% of *NF2*-associated schwannomas, and only 5% of solitary, sporadic schwannomas.

Clinical features and standard therapy: Clinical presentation depends on the location and type of involved nerve, and incidental detection is common, especially in the peripherally situated schwannomas. Patients with schwannoma involving cranial nerves, such as vestibulocochlear nerve or trigeminal nerve, may present with insidious onset of hearing loss or trigeminal neuralgia, respectively. If resected completely, schwannomas usually do not recur; however, incomplete resection can lead to slow regrowth. Radiation therapy, including ablative radiotherapy such as gamma knife radiosurgery and cyberknife radiotherapy, has been used to treat residual tumors or tumors not amenable to surgery. There is no effective chemotherapy but bevacizumab has been used with mixed response.

Imaging

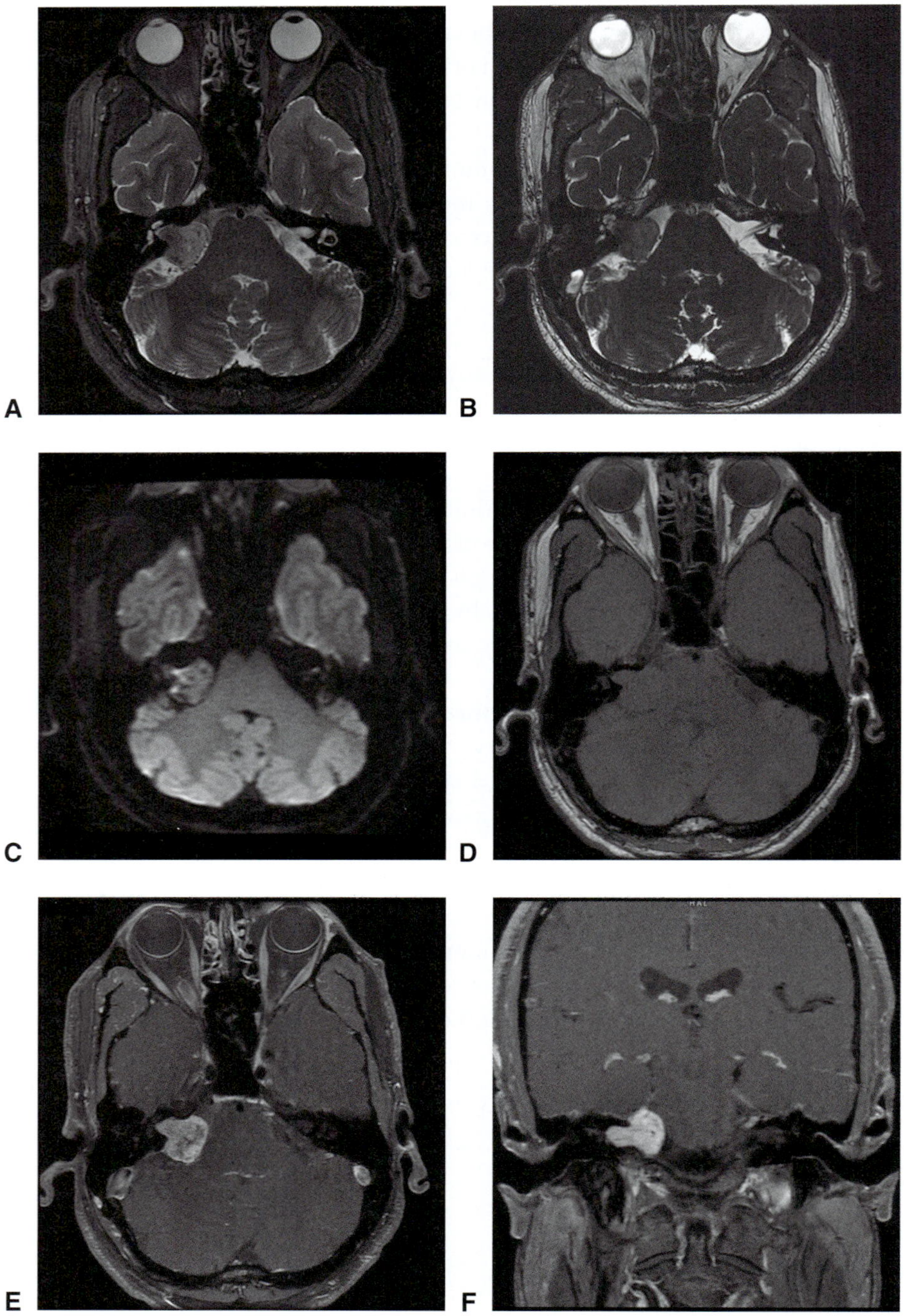

Figure 8.1. Imaging of right vestibular schwannoma. A. Axial T2: Heterogeneous hypointense mass in the right internal auditory canal and cerebellopontine angle cistern. **B.** Axial FIESTA: Homogeneous hypointense mass. **C.** Axial diffusion-weighted imaging (DWI): Heterogeneous isointense mass. **D.** Axial T1 precontrast: Heterogeneous isointense mass. **E.** Axial T1 postcontrast: Heterogeneous but avidly enhancing mass. **F.** Coronal T1 postcontrast: Heterogeneous but avidly enhancing mass.

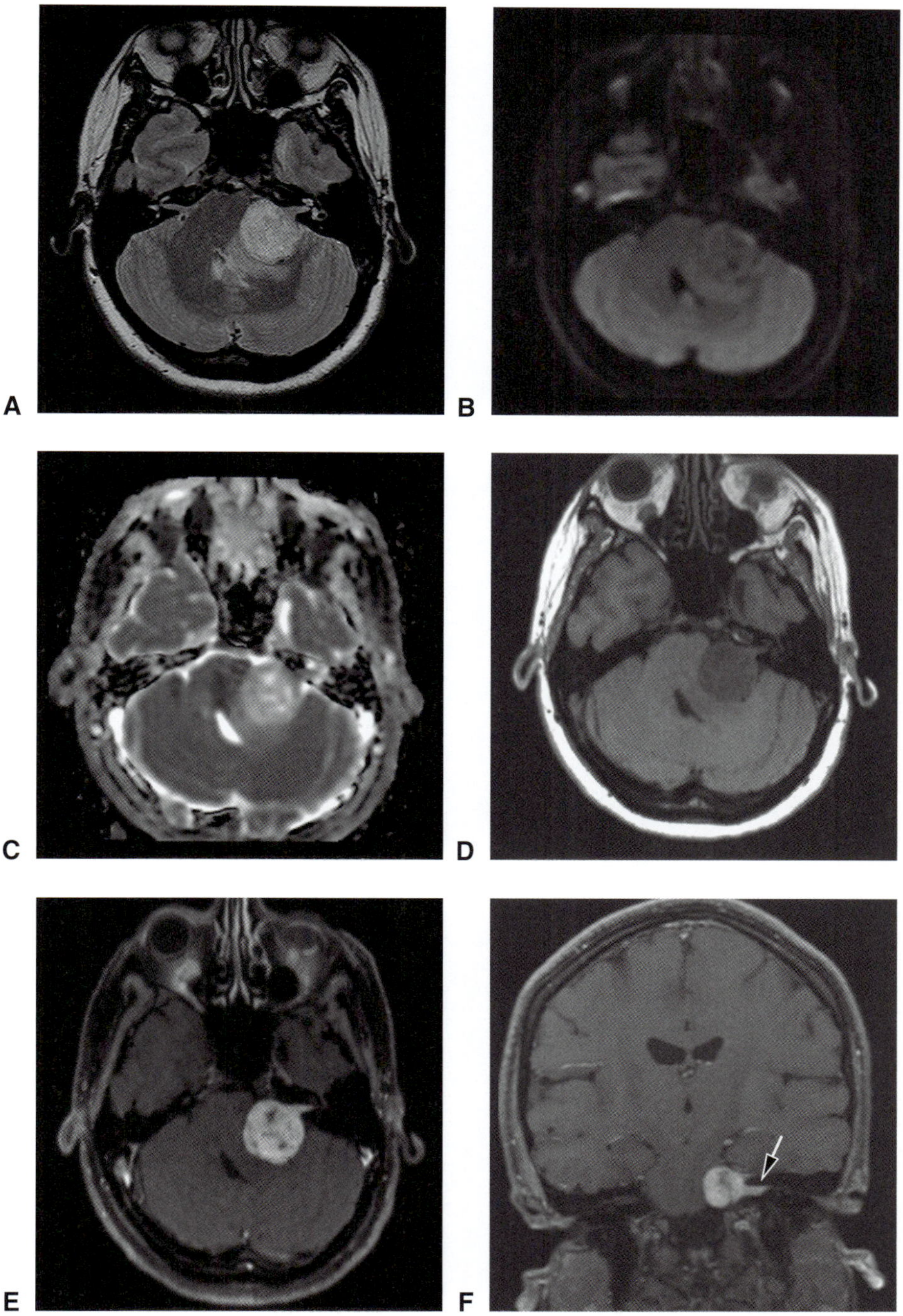

Figure 8.2. Imaging of left vestibular schwannoma. A. Axial T2: Heterogeneous hyperintense mass in the left IAC and CP angle cistern. **B.** Axial DWI: Heterogeneous isointense mass. **C.** Axial apparent diffusion coefficient (ADC): Heterogeneous hyperintense mass. **D.** Axial T1 precontrast: Hypointense mass. **E.** Axial T1 postcontrast: Heterogeneous and avidly enhancing mass. **F.** Coronal T1 postcontrast: Heterogeneous and avidly enhancing mass-dominant component in CP angle and smaller component in the left internal auditory canal (IAC) (arrow).

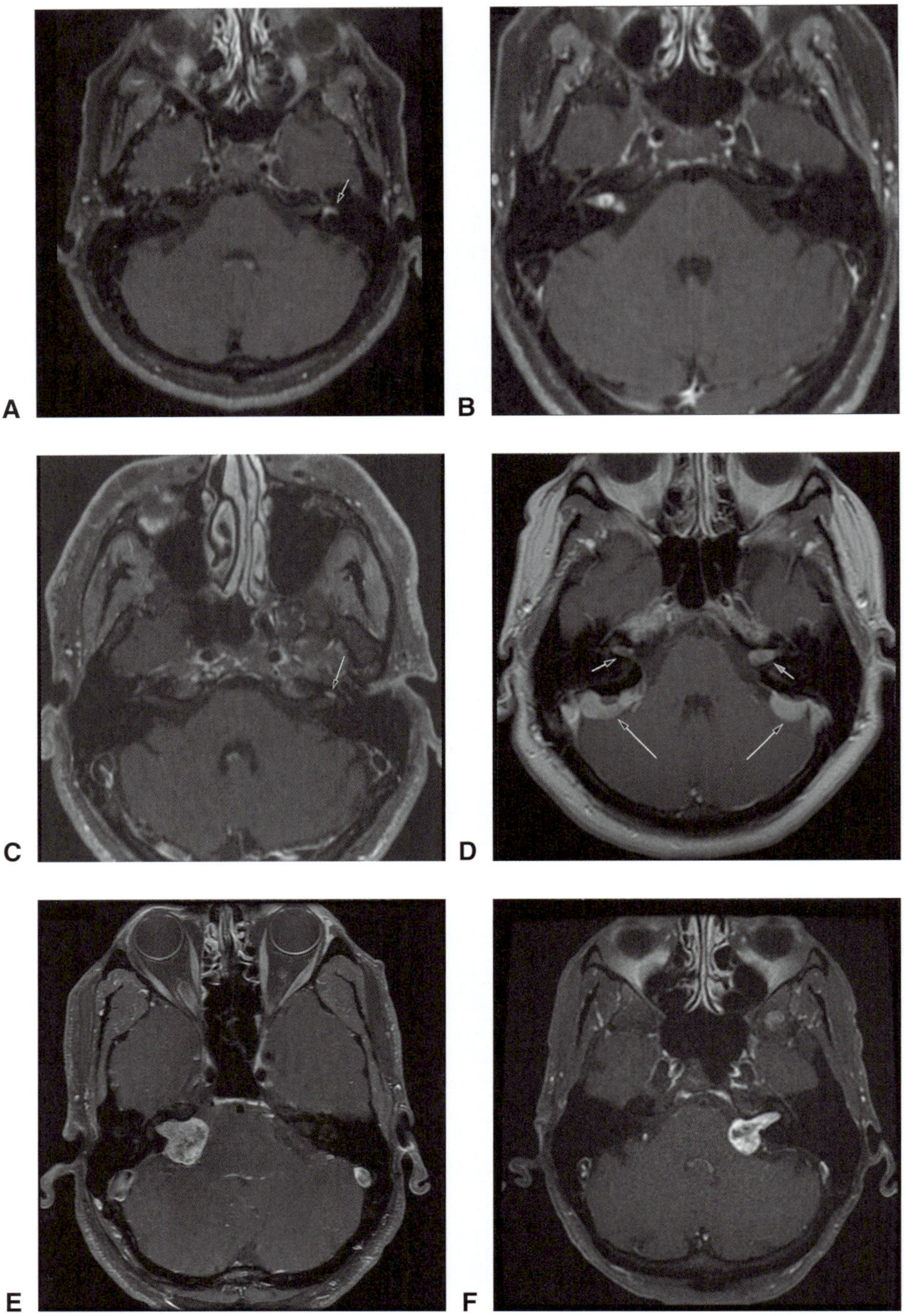

Figure 8.3. Imaging of vestibular or cochlear schwannomas, 12 differentpatients, axial T1 postcontrast images. A. Left vestibular schwannoma involving vestibule and lateral semicircular canal (arrow). **B.** Right intracanalicular schwannoma. **C.** Left cochlear schwannoma (arrow). **D.** NF type 2 patient: Bilateral internal auditory canal schwannomas (small arrows) and bilateral petrous face meningiomas (long arrows). **E.** Right IAC and cerebellopontine angle cistern vestibular schwannoma. **F.** Left IAC and cerebellopontine angle cistern vestibular schwannoma.

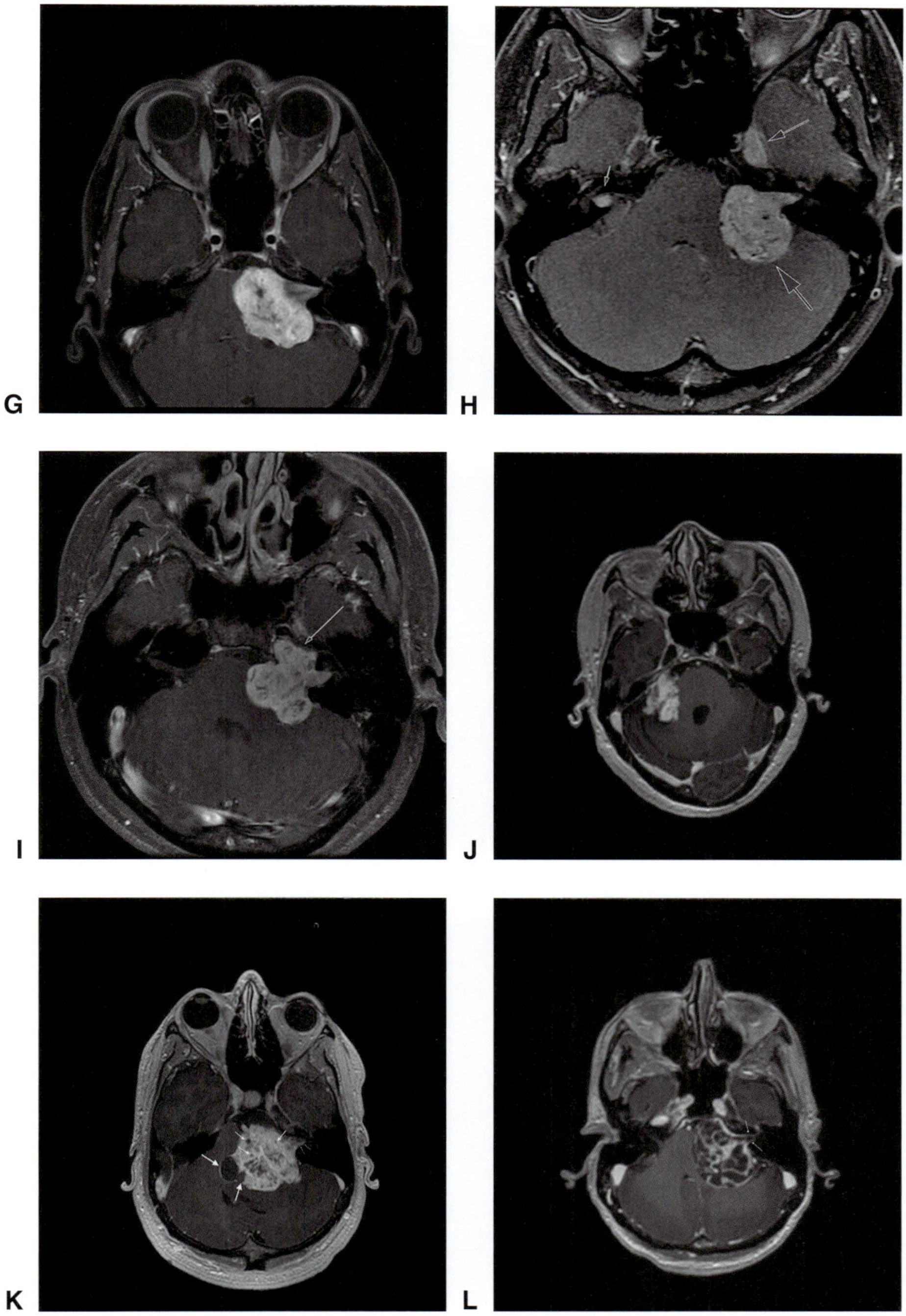

Figure 8.3. ***(continued)*** **G.** Left IAC and large cerebellopontine angle cistern vestibular schwannoma. **H.** NF type 2 patient: Left IAC and large cerebellopontine angle cistern vestibular schwannoma, left Meckel's cave trigeminal schwannoma, and right intracanalicular vestibular schwannoma. **I.** Left IAC and CP angle vestibular schwannoma with anterior extension (arrow). **J.** Lobular contour solid enhancing mass in the right CP angle. **K.** Large heterogeneous, mostly solid left CP angle mass with peripheral (long arrows) and central (short arrows) cystic changes. **L.** Large heterogeneous, mostly cystic left CP angle mass with internal septations.

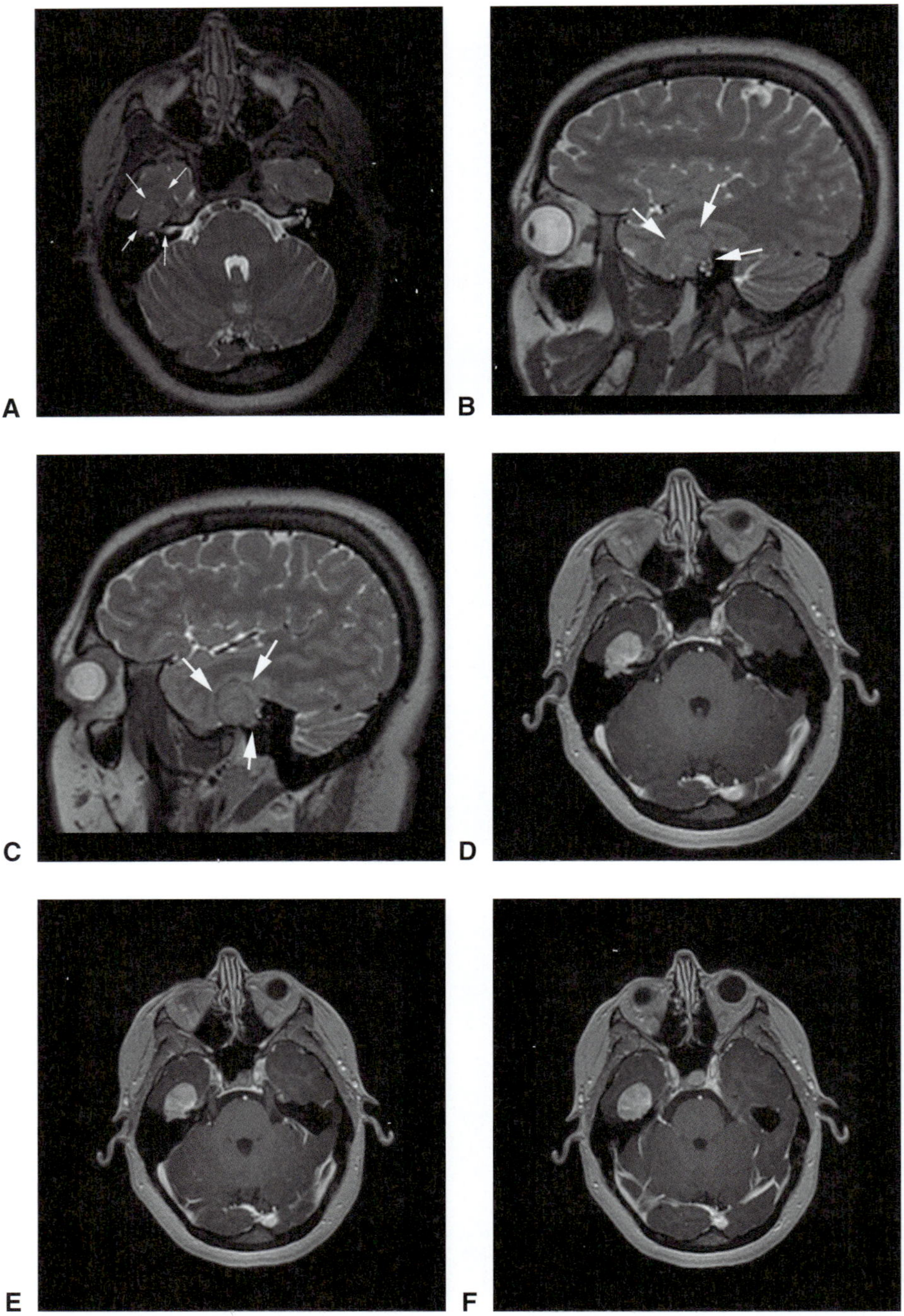

Figure 8.4. **Imaging of facial nerve schwannoma. A–C.** Axial (A) and sagittal T2 (B,C): Isointense expansile mass (arrows) in the right geniculate ganglion. **D–F.** Axial T1 postcontrast: Avid enhancement within the mass.

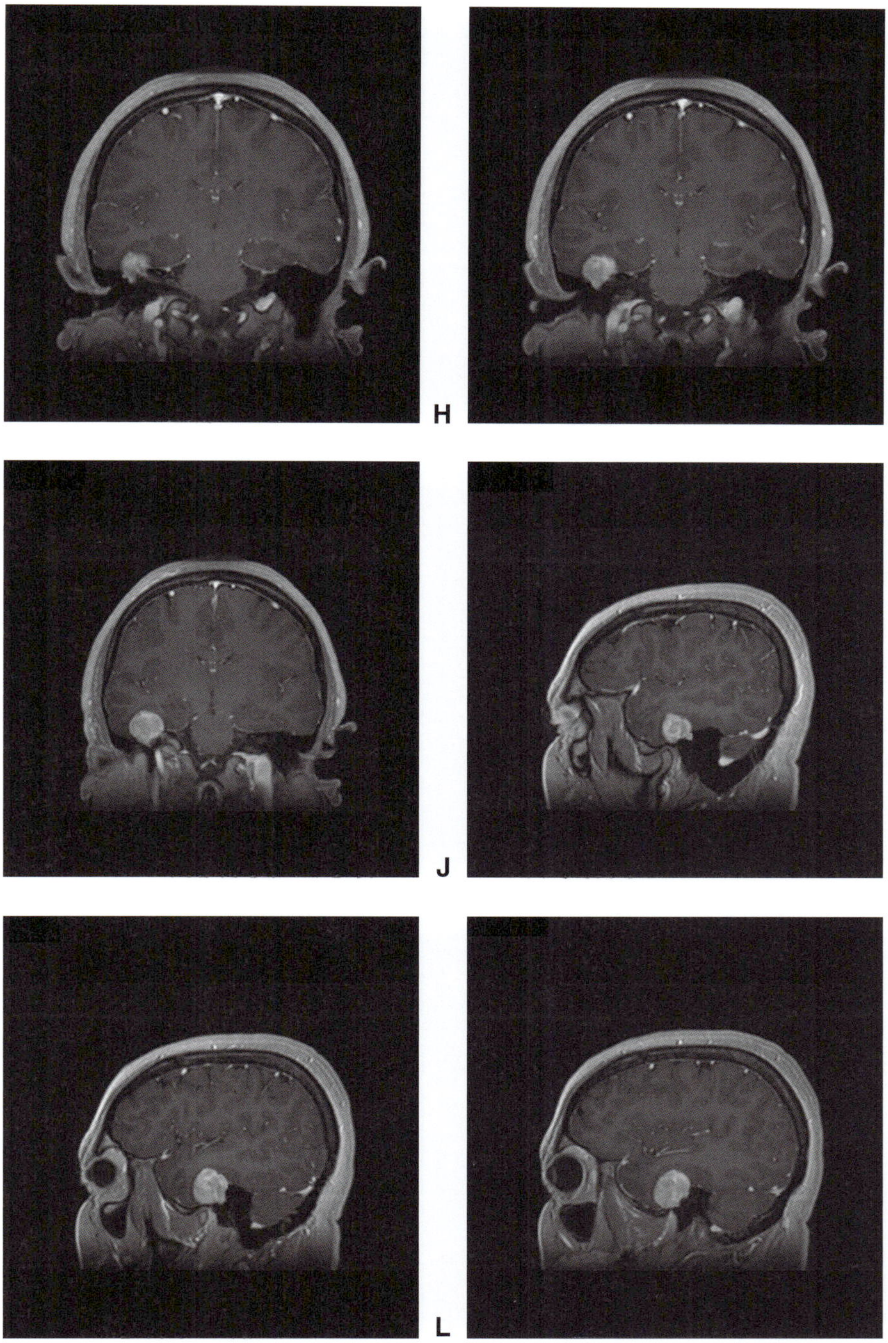

G H I J K L

Figure 8.4. ***(continued)*** **G–I.** Coronal T1 postcontrast: Avid enhancement within the mass. **J–L.** Sagittal T1 postcontrast: Avid enhancement within the mass.

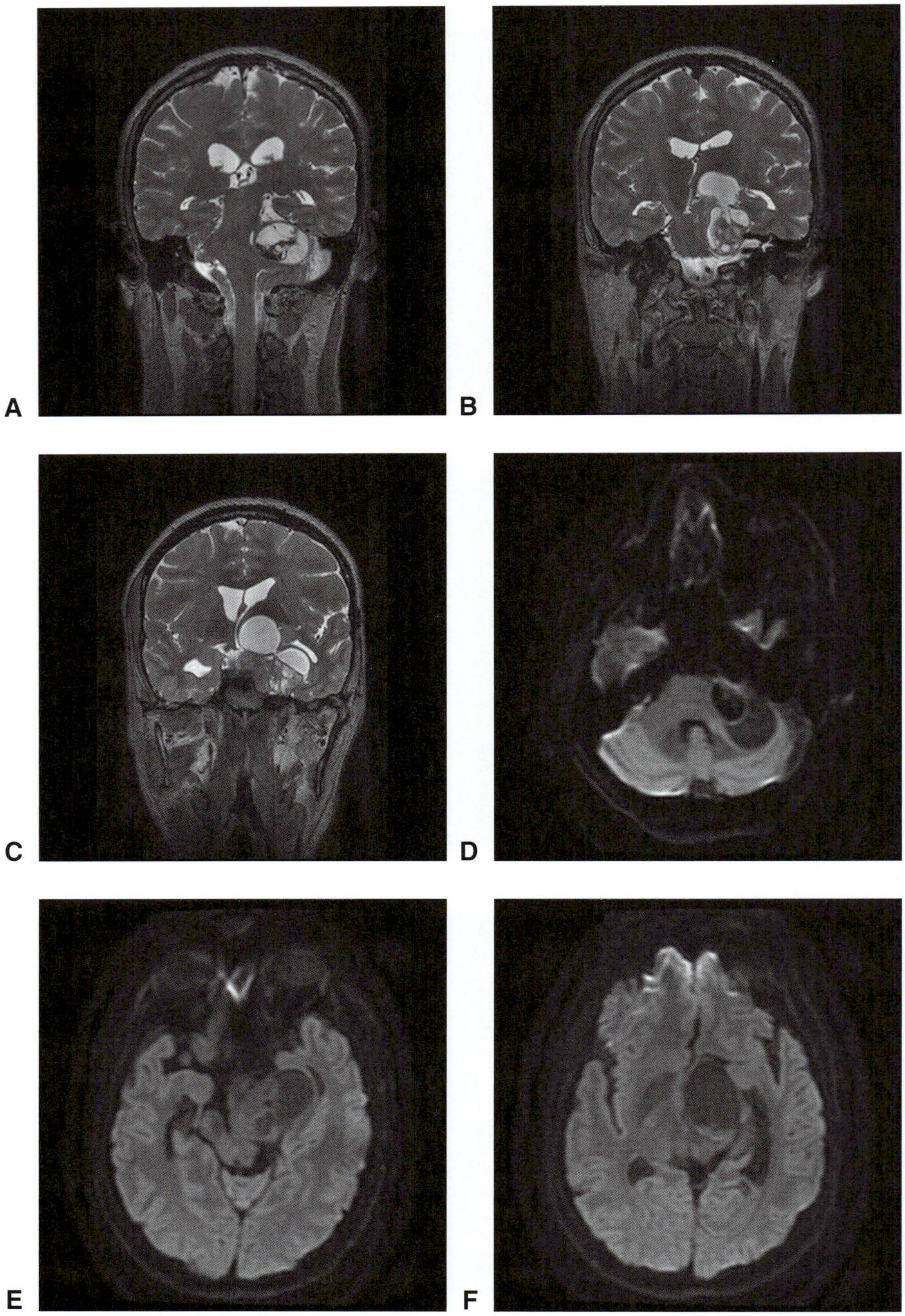

Figure 8.5. Imaging of trigeminal schwannoma. A–C. Coronal T2: Cystic and solid mass in the left cerebellopontine angle cistern and Meckel's cave. **D–F.** Axial DWI: Increased diffusion within the cystic components (long arrow) and lack of reduced diffusion within the solid components (short arrow).

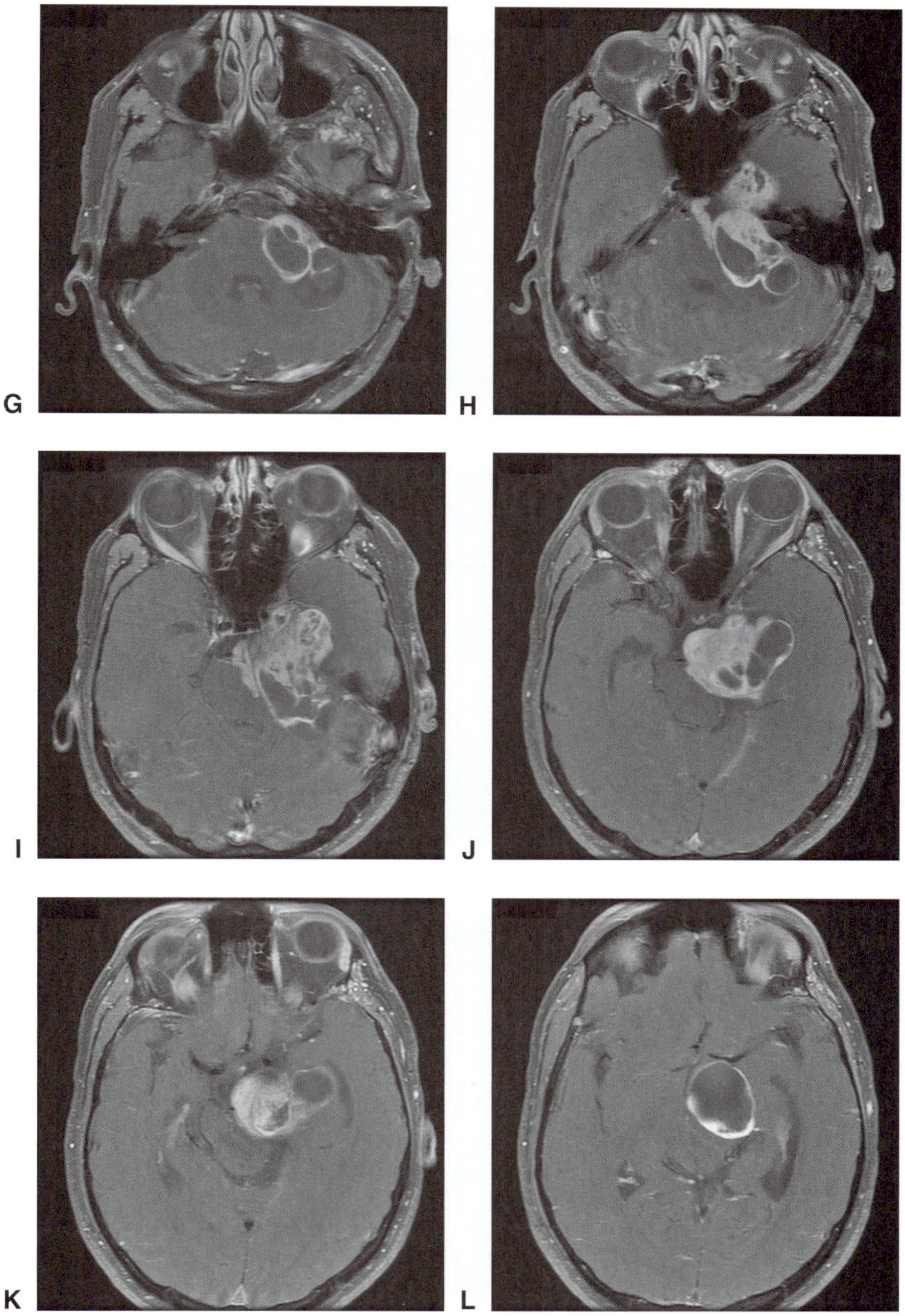

Figure 8.5. ***(continued)*** **G–L.** Axial T1 postcontrast: Heterogeneously enhancing solid and cystic mass spanning from CP angle (long arrows), Meckel's cave (medium arrows), and crural cistern (small arrows).

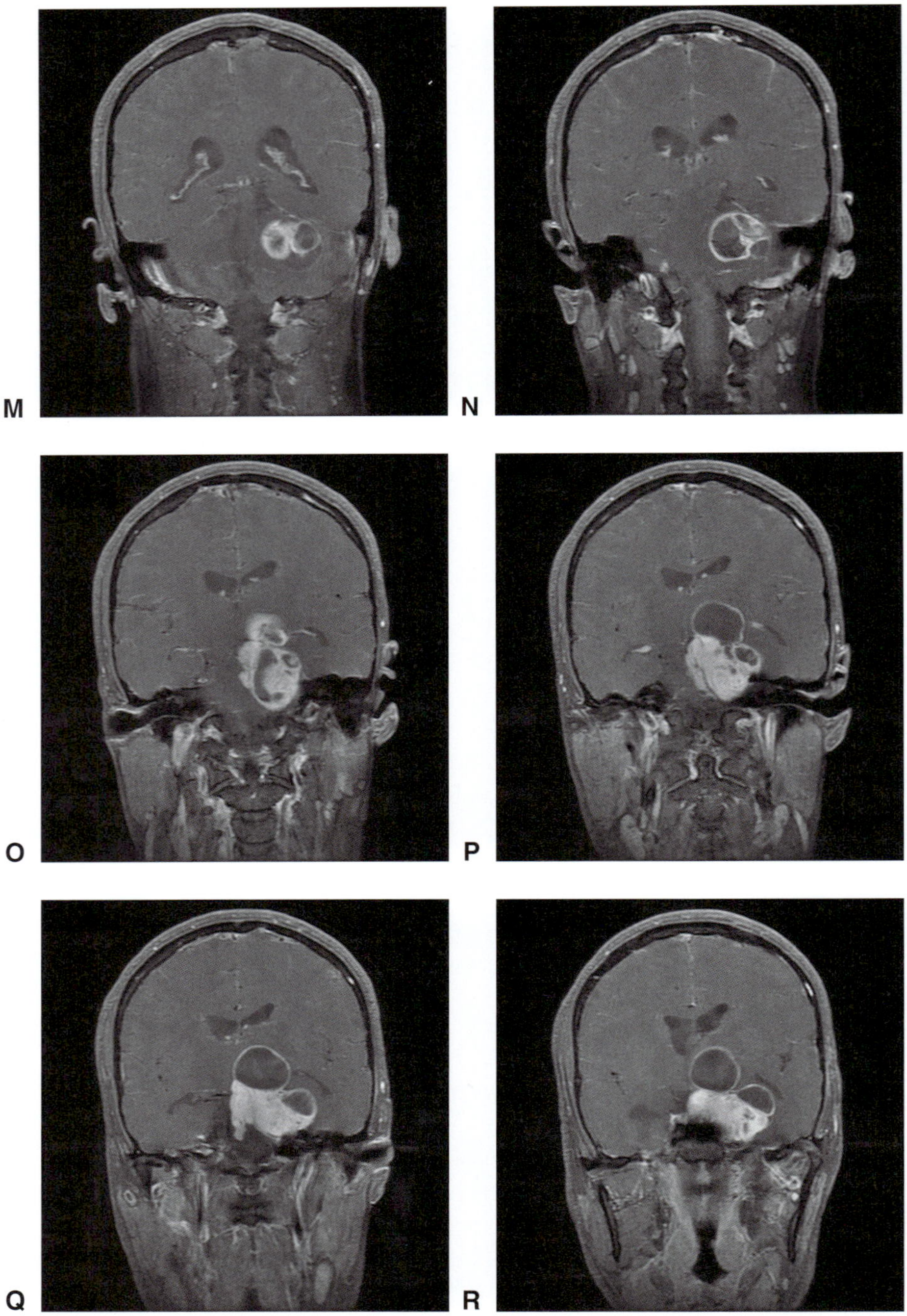

Figure 8.5. ***(continued)*** **M–R.** Coronal T1 postcontrast: Heterogeneously enhancing solid and cystic mass spanning from CP angle (long arrows), Meckel's cave (medium arrows), and crural cistern (small arrows).

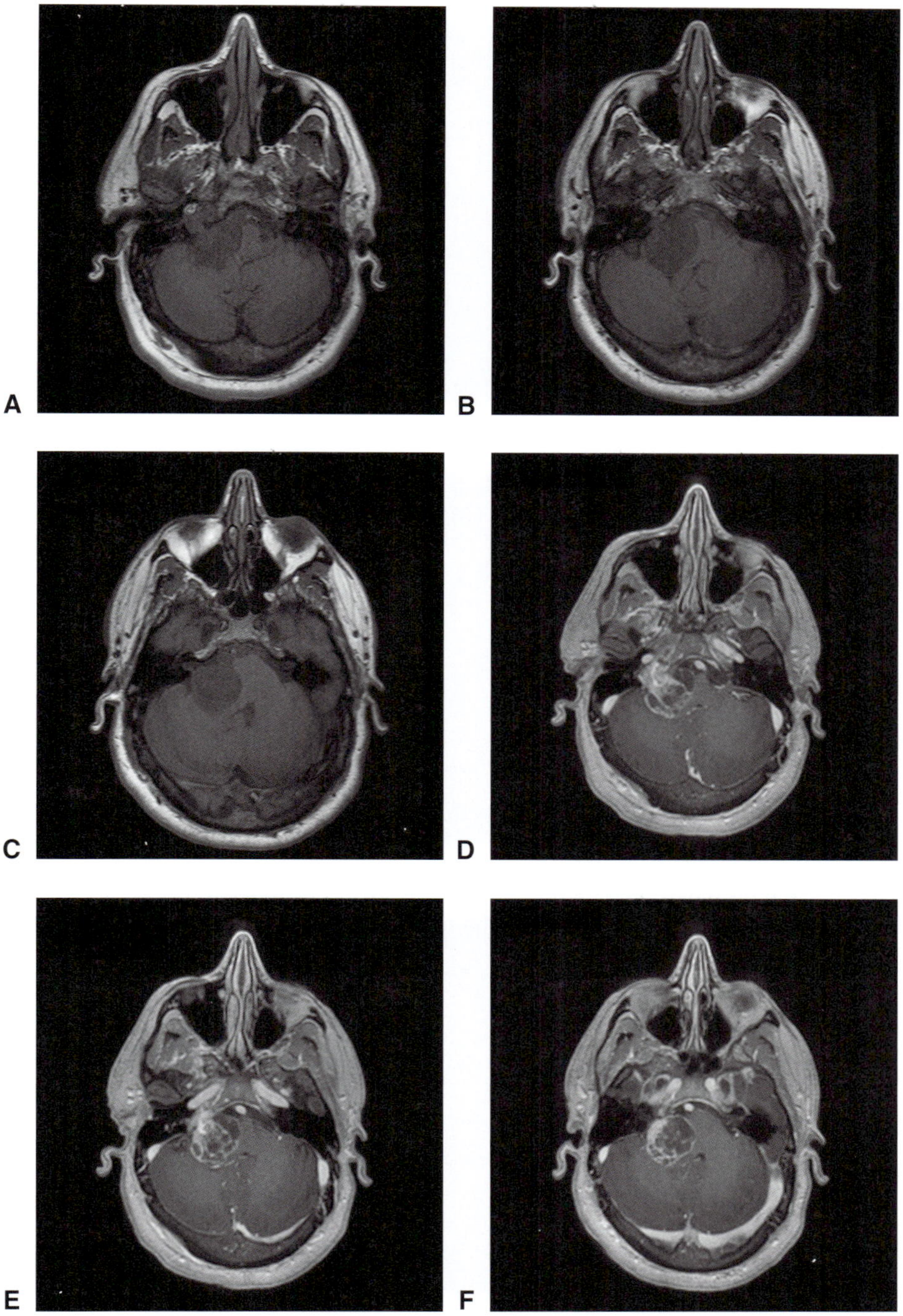

Figure 8.6. Imaging of glossopharyngeal schwannoma. A–C. Axial T1 precontrast: Homogeneously low-intensity mass in the right medullary cistern and jugular foramen. **D–F.** Axial T1 postcontrast: Heterogeneously enhancing, multiloculated cystic mass centered in the right medullary cistern and no extension into the internal auditory canal.

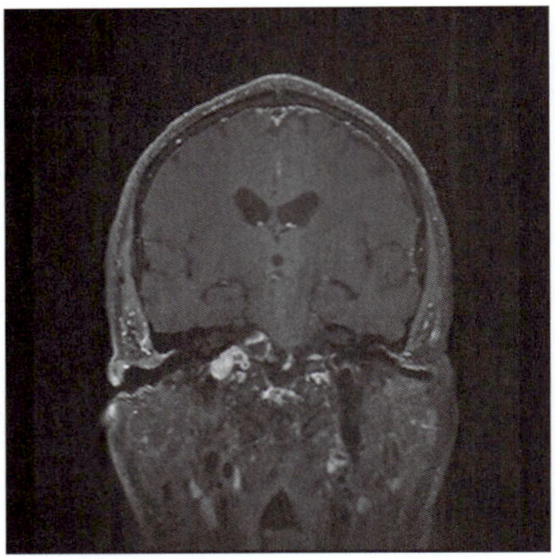

G

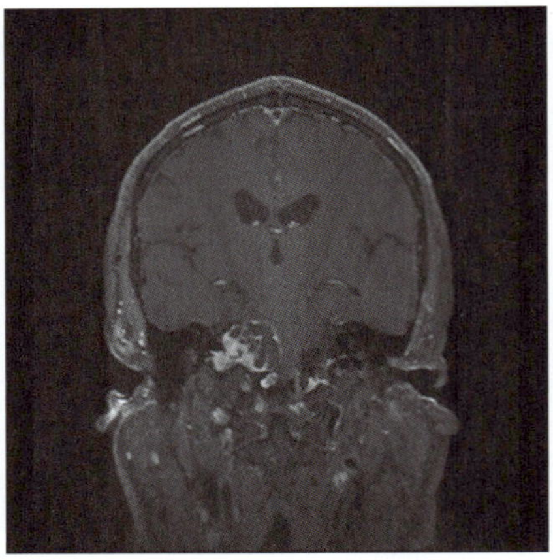

H

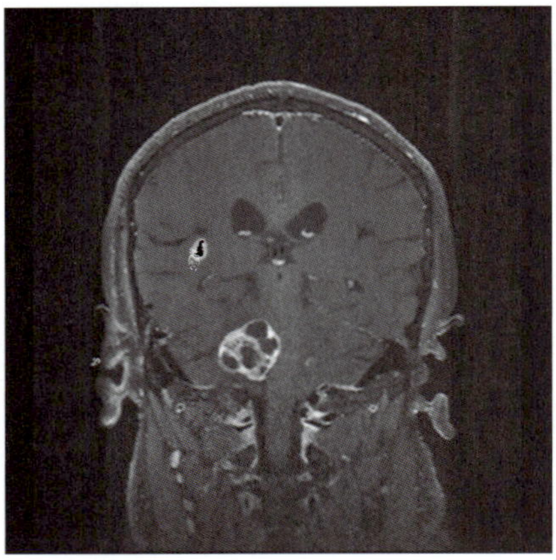

I

Figure 8.6. ***(continued)*** **G–I.** Coronal T1 postcontrast: Heterogeneously enhancing, multiloculated cystic mass centered in the right medullary cistern and no extension into the internal auditory canal.

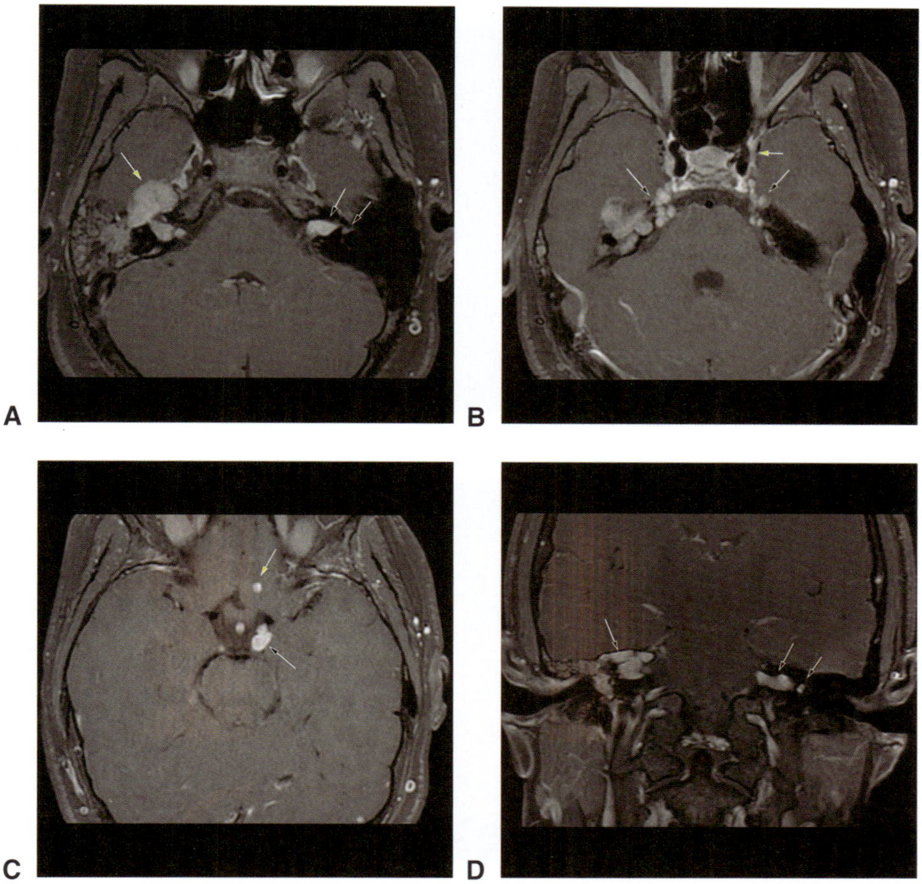

Figure 8.7. Imaging of schwannomatosis. A. Axial T1 postcontrast: Avidly enhancing bilateral vestibular schwannoma involving internal auditory canals and extending into left vestibule (black arrows) and bulky enhancing facial schwannoma centered in the geniculate ganglion of right facial nerve (arrow). **B.** Axial T1 postcontrast: Bilateral cisternal trigeminal schwannomas (black arrows) and extension into the left foramen rotundum on the left (yellow arrow). **C.** Axial T1 postcontrast: Left oculomotor schwannoma (black arrow) and left olfactory schwannoma (yellow arrow). **D.** Coronal T1 postcontrast: Bilateral vestibular schwannoma and right facial schwannoma.

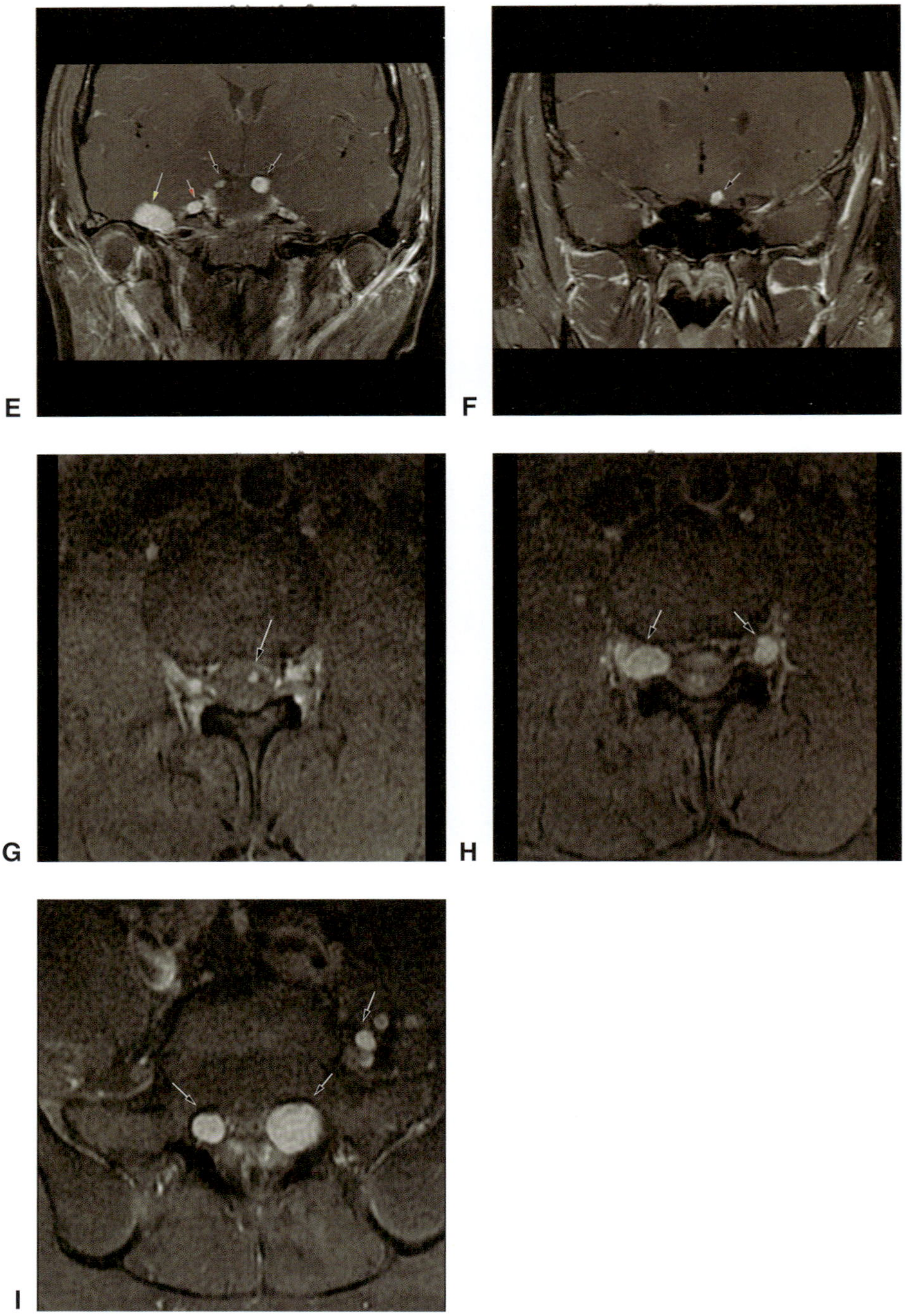

Figure 8.7. ***(continued)*** **E.** Coronal T1 postcontrast: Bilateral oculomotor schwannomas (black arrows), right trigeminal schwannoma (red arrow), and right facial schwannoma (yellow arrow). **F.** Coronal T1 postcontrast: Left olfactory schwannoma (black arrow). **G.** Axial T1 postcontrast: Intrathecal left L2 schwannoma (black arrow). **H.** Axial T1 postcontrast: Bilateral L3 lumbar dorsal root ganglion schwannomas (black arrows). **I.** Axial T1 postcontrast: Bilateral S1 lumbar dorsal root ganglion schwannomas (black arrows) and left L5 extraforaminal schwannoma.

Neurofibroma

Definition: Neurofibroma is a benign, well-circumscribed nerve sheath neoplasm arising from intraneural or diffusely infiltrative extraneural nerve sheath and composed of well-differentiated Schwann cells intermixed with nonneoplastic elements, including fibroblasts, mast cells, myxoid or collagenous matrix, and residual axons or ganglion cells.

Epidemiology: Neurofibroma affects patients of any age, race, or gender and commonly occurs as sporadic solitary or multiple masses or less frequently in the setting of neurofibromatosis type 1 (*NF1*).

Molecular and genetic profile: Neurofibromas with S100-positive Schwann cells can show allelic loss of the *NF1* gene region of 17q. Downstream effects of *NF1* loss include activation of the rat sarcoma/mitogen-activated protein kinase (*RAS/MAPK*) and AKT/mammalian target of rapamycin (*AKT/mTOR*) pathways. Chromosomal losses can be seen in 19p, 19q, and 22q in *NF1*-associated neurofibromas and in 19q and 22q in sporadic neurofibromas. Neurofibromas are exceedingly rare in *NF2* and schwannomatosis.

Clinical features and standard therapy: Surgical resection is the primary treatment, and there is no effective chemotherapy or targeted agents. If totally resected, recurrence rate is low, but due to frequently infiltrative growth, gross total resection is often not feasible without causing functional compromise and chronic morbidity.

Imaging

A B

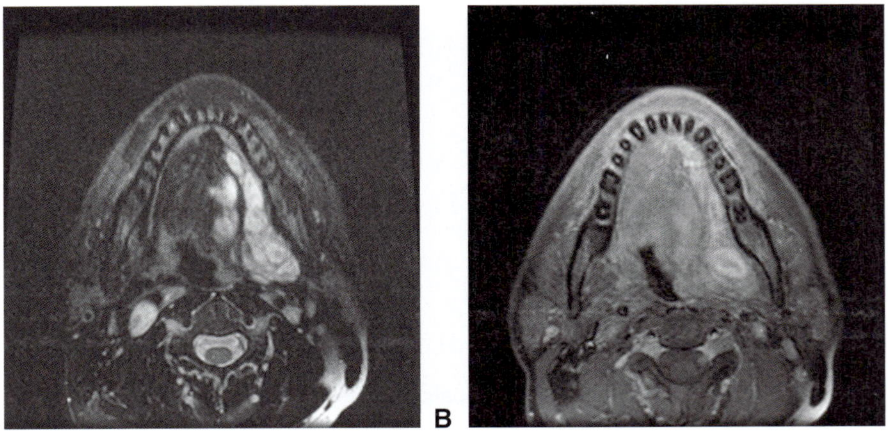

Figure 8.8. **Imaging of neurofibromas. A.** Axial T2: Heterogeneously high-signal intensity of the left sublingual neurofibroma. **B.** Axial T1 postcontrast: Heterogeneously enhancement of the left sublingual neurofibroma.

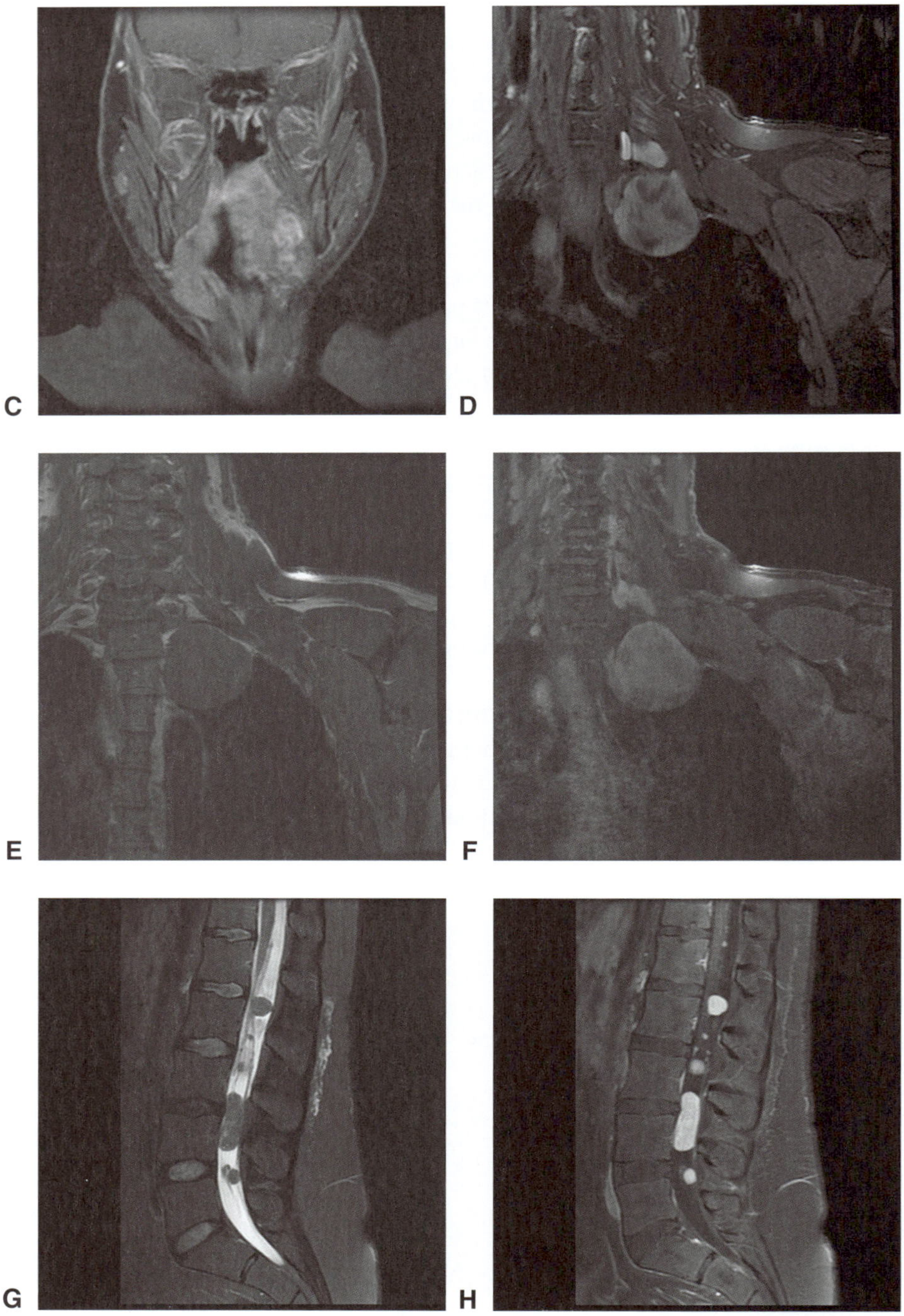

Figure 8.8. ***(continued)*** **C.** Coronal T1 postcontrast: Heterogeneously enhancement of the left sublingual neurofibroma. **D.** Coronal T2: Heterogeneously high-signal intensity of the left T1 nerve root neurofibroma. **E.** Coronal T1 precontrast: Homogeneously low-signal intensity of the left T1 nerve root neurofibroma. **F.** Coronal T1 postcontrast: Heterogeneous enhancement of the left T1 nerve root neurofibroma. **G.** Sagittal T2: Homogeneously low-signal intensity multiple neurofibromas along the nerve roots of cauda equina. **H.** Sagittal T1 postcontrast: Homogeneously enhancing multiple neurofibromas along the nerve roots of cauda equina.

I

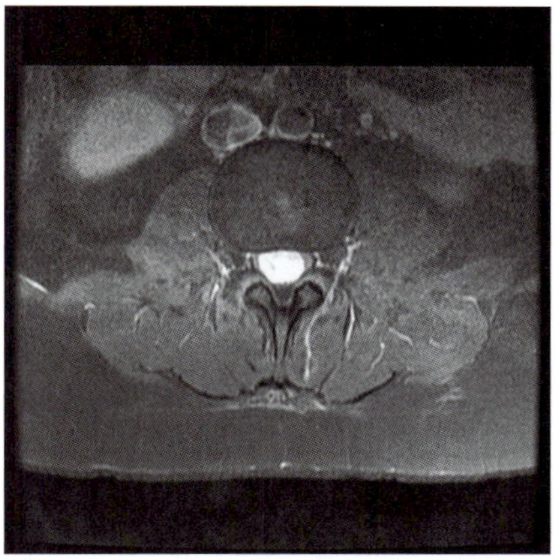

Figure 8.8. ***(continued)*** **I.** Axial T1 postcontrast: Homogeneously enhancing L4 neurofibroma filling the spinal canal.

Plexiform Neurofibroma

Definition: Plexiform Neurofibroma is a variant of neurofibroma growing in a plexiform, multinodular, or expansile pattern, involving multiple nerve fascicles, nerve plexus, and/or collagen, occurring primarily in the head and neck, deep face or orbit, or back and usually in the setting of *NF1*. This benign tumor is prone to local recurrence but has no malignant or metastasizing potential despite often rapid growth, high cellularity, increased mitotic activity, and large size.

Epidemiology: Plexiform neurofibromas (PNs) occur in 20% to 50% of all patients with *NF1* and can be a major source of morbidity. There is no gender or race predilection. PNs may undergo transformation to malignant nerve sheath tumors (MPNST) in 8% to 13% of NF1 patients during their lifetime, although some of the MPNST can occur in the absence of pre-existing PNs.

Molecular and genetic profile: Plexiform schwannomas express strong and diffuse expression of S100 protein, *SOX10*, *LEU7*, and calretinin and may focally express glial fibrillary acidic protein (GFAP). *NF2* gene and the merlin protein (a.k.a. schwannomin) expression are hallmarks of schwannoma associated with *NF2*.

Clinical features and standard therapy: Presenting symptoms depend on the location of neurofibroma, and imaging is needed to precisely localize and evaluate neurofibromas. Treatment usually is not needed for a single, small, and non-symptomatic lesions and involves monitoring with serial imaging and surgical intervention when there is clear growth with new or worsening symptoms.

Imaging

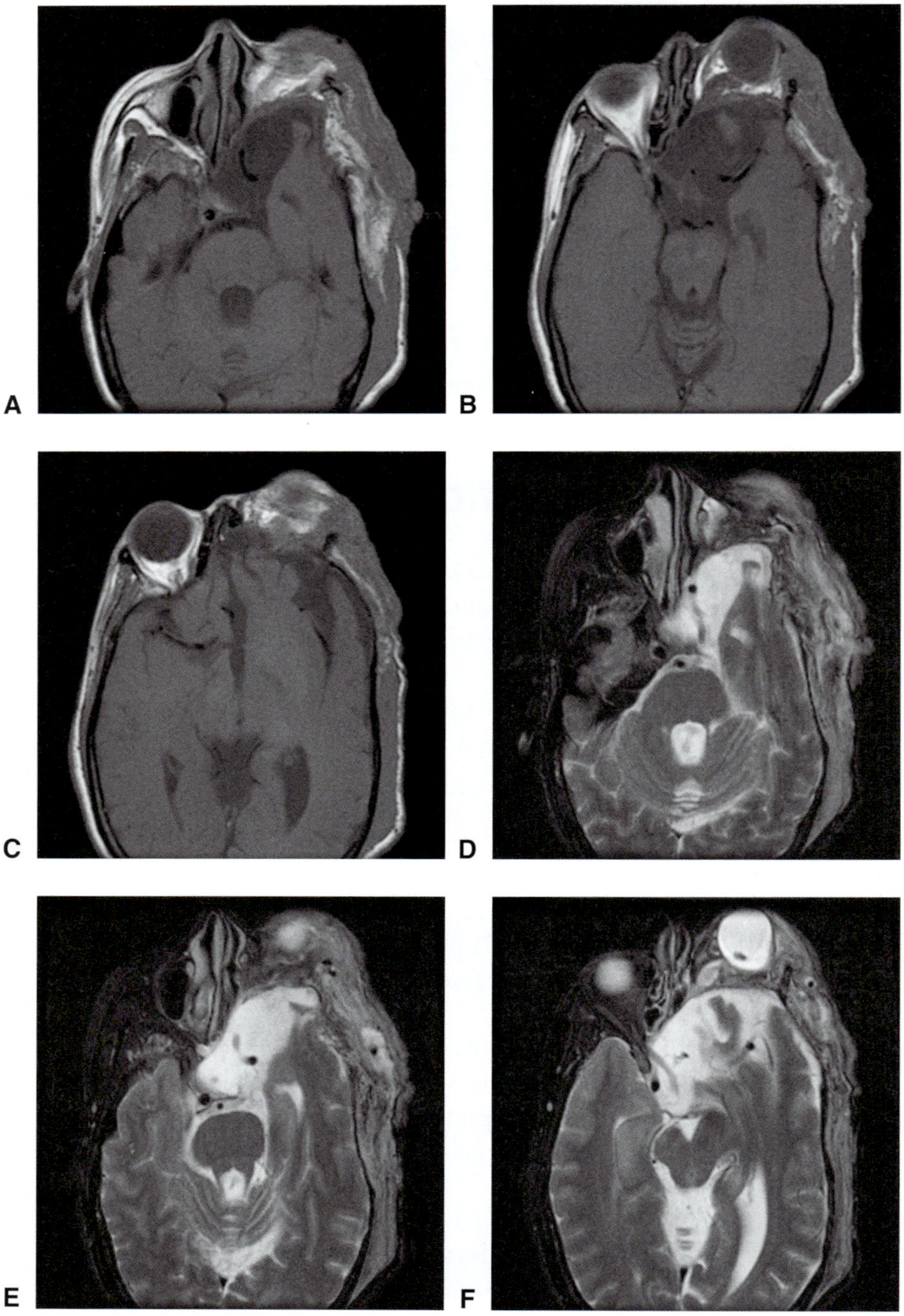

Figure 8.9. Imaging of plexiform neurofibroma. A–C. Axial T1 precontrast: Homogeneously low-signal intensity infiltrative mass along the left peri- and intraorbital soft tissue and entire left hemispheric scalp and dural ectasia with dilated posterior orbital subarachnoid space causing left proptosis. **D–F.** Axial T2: Homogeneously mixed low- and high-signal intensity infiltrative mass along the left peri- and intraorbital soft tissue and entire left hemispheric scalp and dural ectasia with dilated posterior orbital subarachnoid space causing left proptosis.

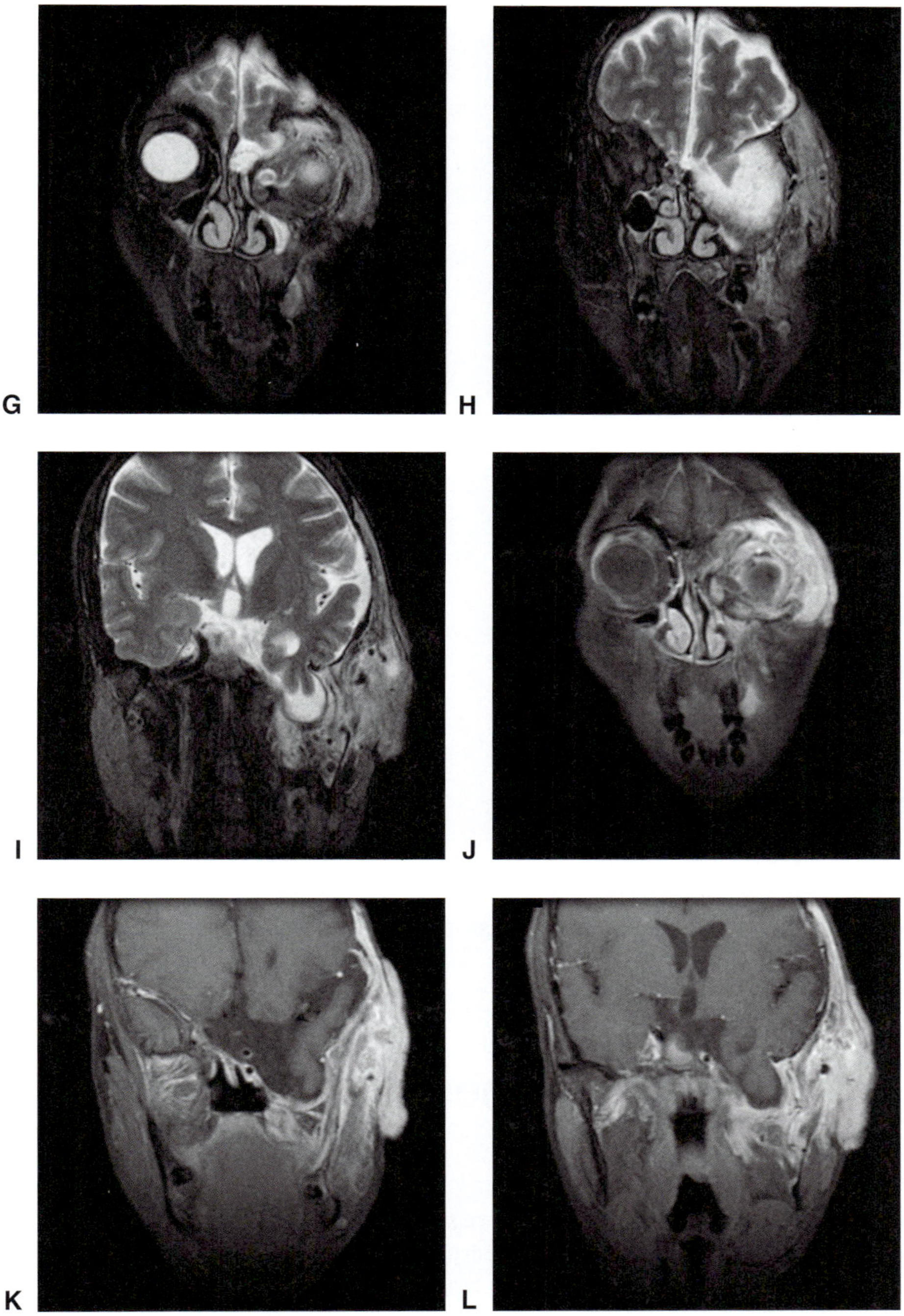

Figure 8.9. ***(continued)*** **G–I**. Coronal T2: Homogeneously mixed low- and high-signal intensity infiltrative mass along the left peri- and intraorbital soft tissue and entire left hemispheric scalp and extension into the left masticator space. **J–L.** Coronal T1 postcontrast: Heterogeneous but avid enhancement of the infiltrative scalp mass invading the left orbit and masticator space.

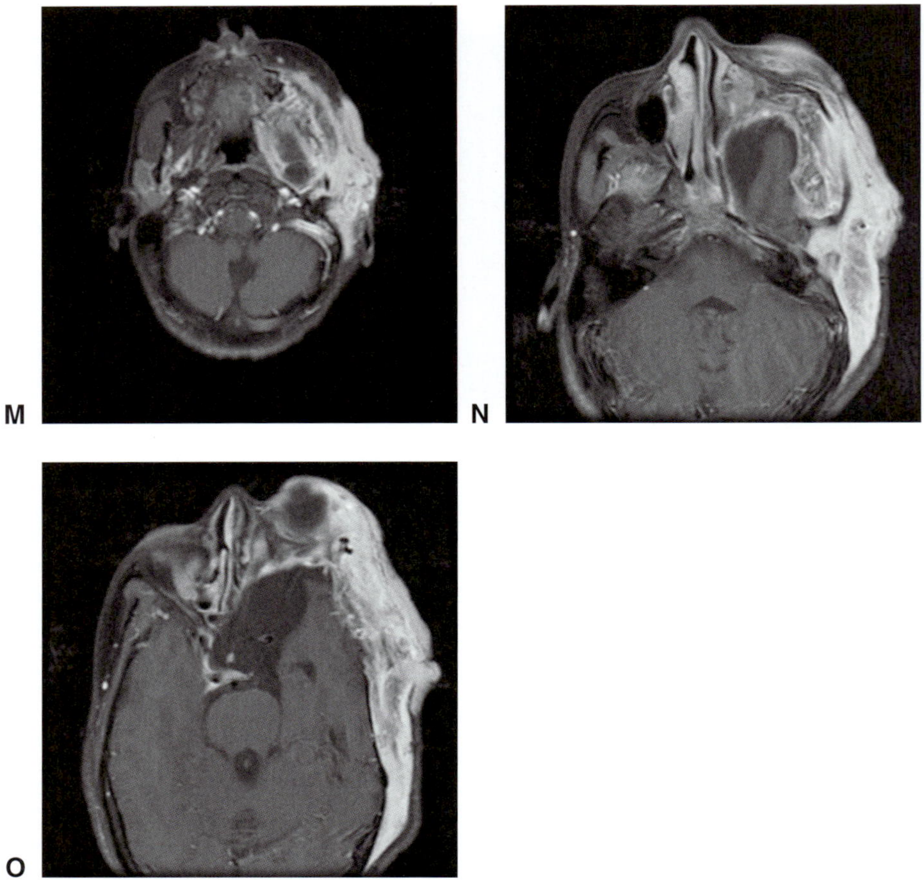

Figure 8.9. ***(continued)*** **M–O.** Axial T1 postcontrast: Heterogeneous but avid enhancement of the infiltrative scalp mass invading into the left orbit and masticator space.

Malignant Peripheral Nerve Sheath Tumor

Definition: Malignant peripheral nerve sheath tumor (MPNST) is a malignant tumor composed of Schwann cell or perineural cell differentiation, most commonly arising in a peripheral nerve or in extraneural soft tissue.

Epidemiology: Approximately half of all MPNST cases are associated with *NF1*, in which they often arise from a preexisting plexiform or intraneural neurofibroma and affect younger age groups. In contrast, most sporadic cases affect young to middle-aged adults and arise from large peripheral nerves without an associated benign precursor.

Molecular and genetic profile: MPNST associated with *NF1*, sporadic MPNST, and radiation-associated MPNST share highly recurrent genetic inactivation in *NF1*, cyclin-dependent kinase inhibitor 2A (*CDKN2A*), and the polycomb repressive complex 2 (*PRC2*) components *SUZ12* and erythema elevatum diutinum (*EED*).

Clinical features and standard therapy: Surgical resection is the primary treatment, and there is no effective chemotherapy or targeted agents. There is a higher recurrence rate for subtotally resected MPNST.

Imaging

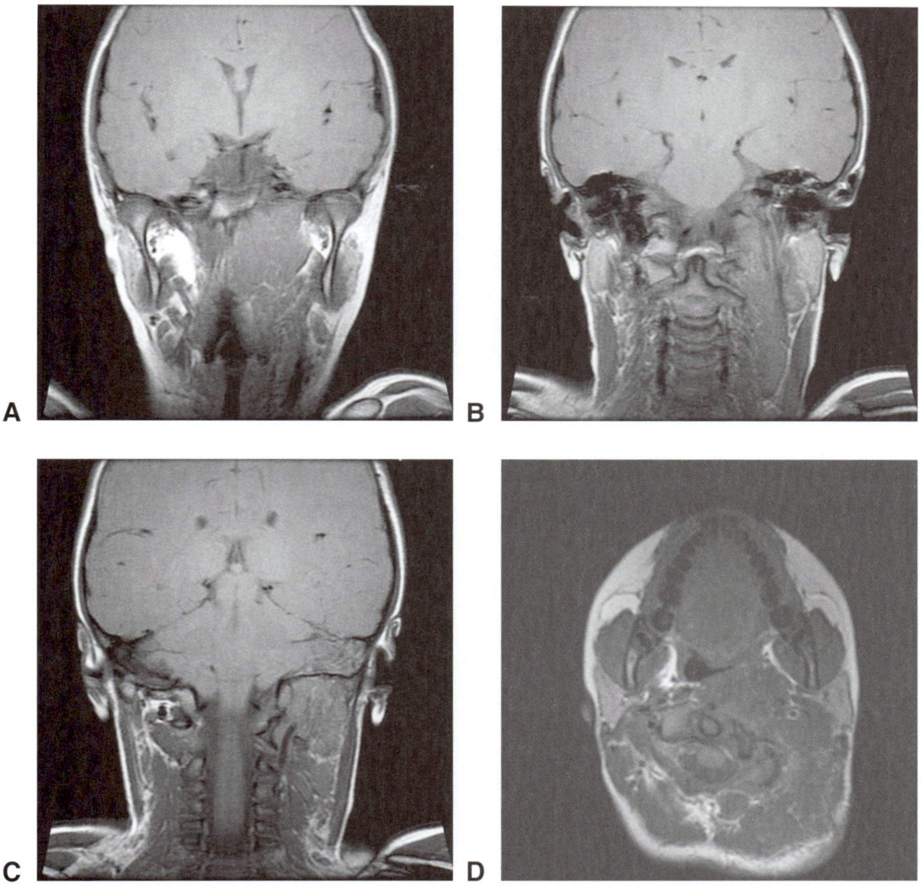

Figure 8.10. Imaging of malignant peripheral nerve sheath tumor. A–C. Coronal T1 precontrast: Homogeneously low-signal intensity ill-defined mass involving the left prevertebral space and posterior neck. **D–F.** Axial T1 precontrast: Homogeneously low-signal intensity ill-defined mass involving the left prevertebral space and posterior neck.

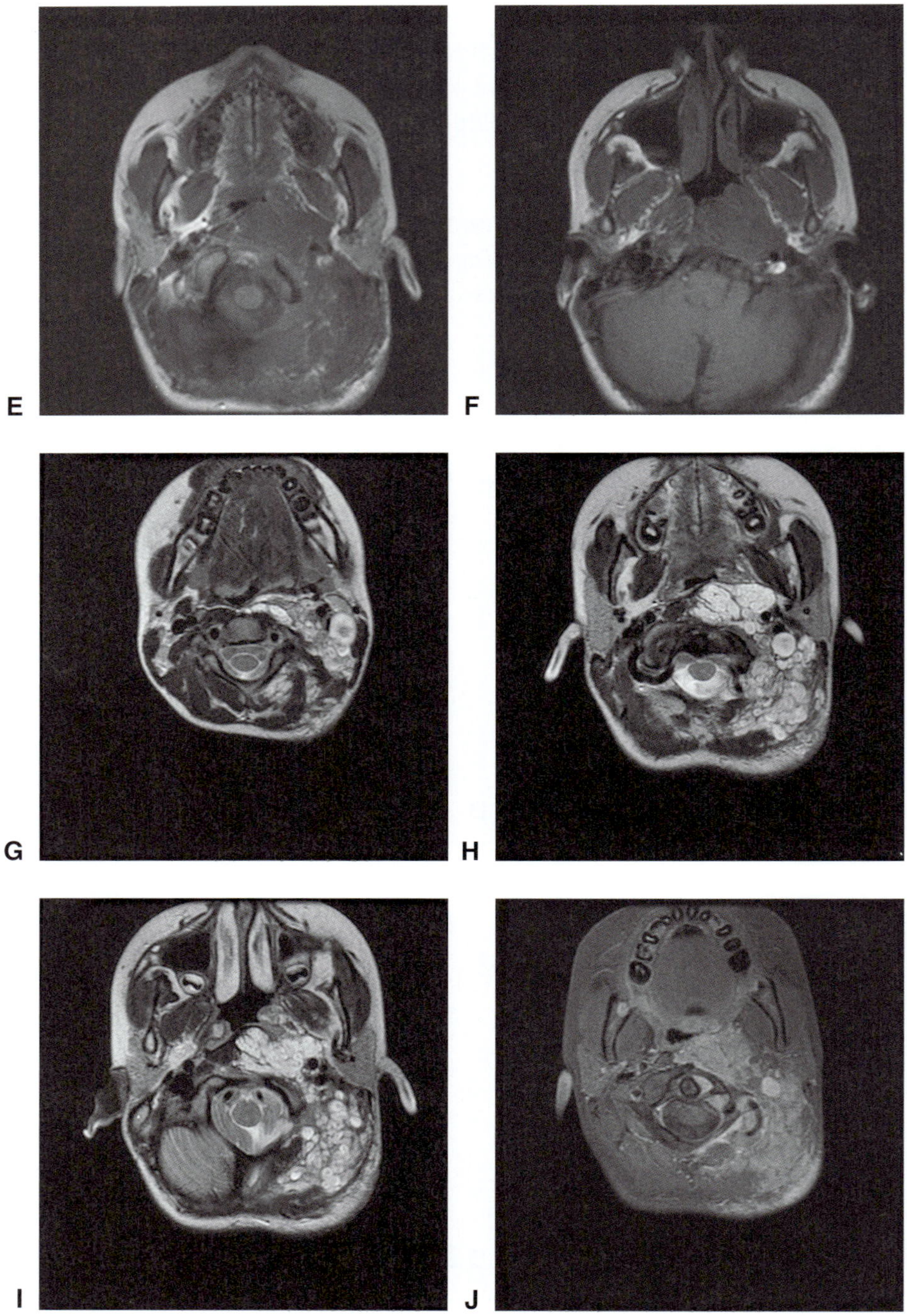

Figure 8.10. ***(continued)*** **G–I.** Axial T2: Heterogeneously high-signal intensity ill-defined mass with multiloculated cystic components involving the left prevertebral space and posterior neck. **J–L.** Axial T1 postcontrast: Heterogeneously enhancing mass involving the left prevertebral space and posterior neck.

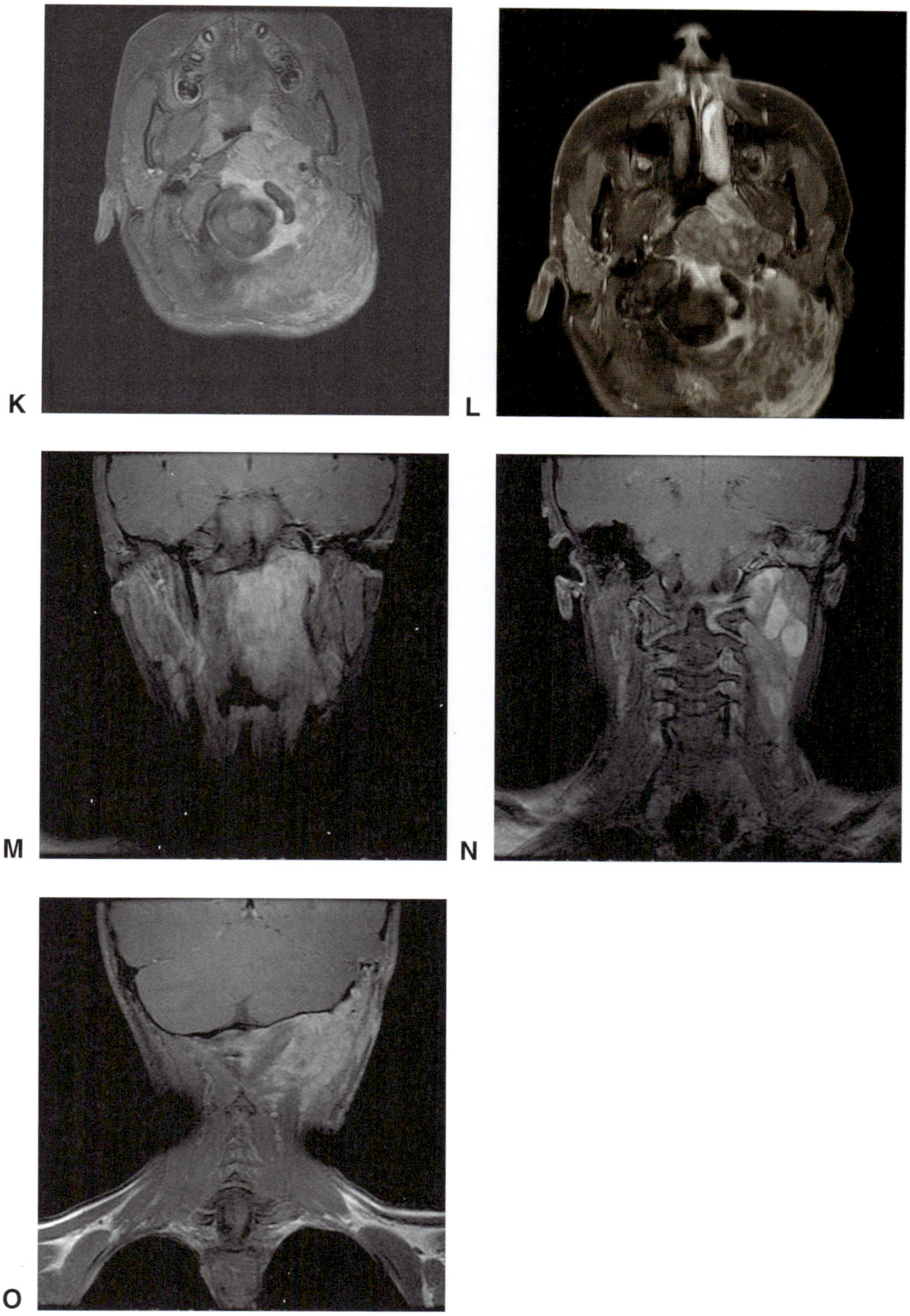

Figure 8.10. ***(continued)*** **M–O.** Coronal T1 postcontrast: Heterogeneously enhancing mass involving the left prevertebral space and posterior neck.

Bibliography

Ahlawat S, Blakeley JO, Langmead S, Berlzberg AJ, Faya LM. Current status and recommendations for imaging in neurofibromatosis type 1, neurofibromatosis type 2, and schwannomatosis. *Skeletal Radiol.* 2020;49:199–219.

Avery RA, Katowitz JA, Fisher MJ, et al. Orbital/periorbita plexiform neurofibromas in children with neurofibromatosis type 1: multidisciplinary recommendations for care. *Ophthalmology.* 2017;124:123–132.

Dombi E, Solomon J, Gillespie AJ, et al. NF1 plexiform neurofibroma growth rate by volumetric MRI: relationship to age and body weight. *Neurology.* 2007;68:643–647.

Hrehorovich PA, Franke HR, Maximin S, et al. Malignant peripheral nerve sheath tumor. *Radiographics.* 2003;23:790–794.

Lee JH, Lee HK, Choi CG, et al. Malignant peripheral nerve sheath tumor in the parapharyngeal space: tumor spread through the eustachian tube. *AJNR Am J Neuroradiol.* 2001;22:748–750.

Pilavaki M, Chourmouzi D, Kiziridou A, et al. Imaging of peripheral nerve sheath tumors with pathologic correlation: pictorial review. *Eur J Radiol.* 2004;52:229–239.

Skolnik AD, Loevner LA, Sampathu DM, et al. Cranial nerve schwannomas: diagnostic imaging approach. *Radiographics.* 2016;36:1463–1477.

Van Meerbeeck SFL, Verstraete KL, Janssens S, Mortier G. Whole body MR imaging in neurofibromatosis type 1. *Eur J Radiol.* 2009;69:236–242.

9

Tumors of the Pineal Region

Overview

Primary tumors of the pineal region are comprised largely of four different histologic subtypes—pineocytoma, pineal parenchymal tumor of intermediate differentiation (PPTID), pineoblastoma, and papillary tumor of the pineal region (PTPR). Each has unique cell of origin, gender and age predilection, imaging features, and prognosis.

	Age range (mean)	Female: male ratio	Cell of origin	WHO grade	Molecular/ genetic markers	Prognosis (median overall survival)
Pineocytoma	43	1:0.6	Pineolocyte	I		NA
PPTID	41		Pineolocyte	II or III	Chromosome 4q gain, 12Q gain, 22 loss	165 months
PTPR	35	1:106	Ependymocyte	II or III		70% 5-year survival
Pineoblastoma	18		Immature neuroepithelial cells	IV		77 months

PPTID, pineal parenchymal tumor of intermediate differentiation; PTPR, papillary tumor of the pineal region.

Tumor Types

Pineocytoma

Pineal parenchymal tumor of intermediate differentiation (PPTID)

Papillary tumor of the pineal region (PTPR)

Pineoblastoma

Pineocytoma

Definition: Pineocytoma is a well-differentiated pineal parenchymal tumor comprised of uniform cells forming large pineocytomatous rosettes and/or of pleomorphic cells showing gangliocytic differentiation. It is a WHO grade I tumor with no malignant potential or dissemination.

Epidemiology: This accounts for <1% of all intracranial neoplasms and 27% of pineal neoplasms.

Affected age group: The tumor can occur in any age but most frequently affects adults, with a mean age of 43 years; there is a female predominance, with a female-to-male ratio of 1:0.6.

Molecular and genetic profile: Cell of origin is likely the pinealocyte, a cell with photosensory and neuroendocrine functions. It is associated with immunoexpression of cone-rod homeobox (*CRX*) (a transcription factor involved in the development and differentiation of pineal cell lineage) and acetylserotonin methyltransferase (*ASMT*) (a critical enzyme for synthesis of melatonin, which is a hormone produced by the pineal gland). No syndromic associations or genetic susceptibilities are known.

CSF markers: None.

Clinical features and standard therapy: Surgical resection is the definitive treatment without adjuvant radiotherapy or chemotherapy.

Prognosis: The 5-year survival rate ranges from 86% to 91%, and the most important prognostic marker is the extent of surgical resection.

Imaging

The hallmark of pineocytoma is a lobulated solid mass with or without cystic or calcific component, usually <3 cm, which may cause obstructive hydrocephalus. The cystic component may be the dominant feature with minor solid tumor tissue.

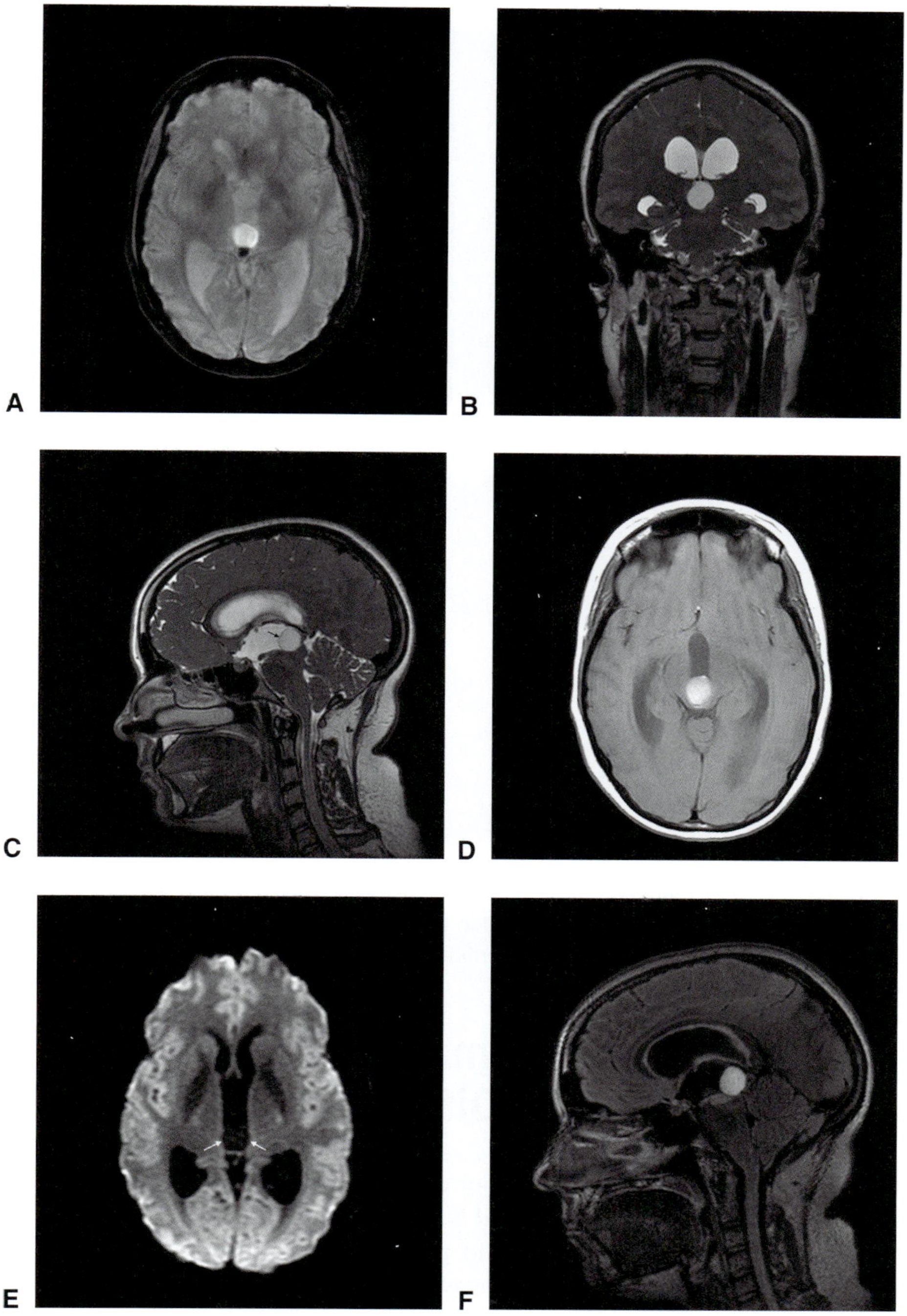

Figure 9.1. Imaging of pineocytoma. A. Axial Susceptibility-weighted imaging (SWI): Hyperintense cyctic mass. **B.** Coronal T2 fast spin echo (FSE): Hyperintense cyctic mass. **C.** Sagittal T2 FSE: Hyperintense cyctic mass. **D.** Axial T1 precontrast: Hyperintense cyctic mass. **E.** Axial diffusion-weighted imaging (DWI): No reduced diffusion within the cystic mass. **F.** Sagittal fluid-attenuated inversion recovery (FLAIR): Hyperintense cyctic mass.

G 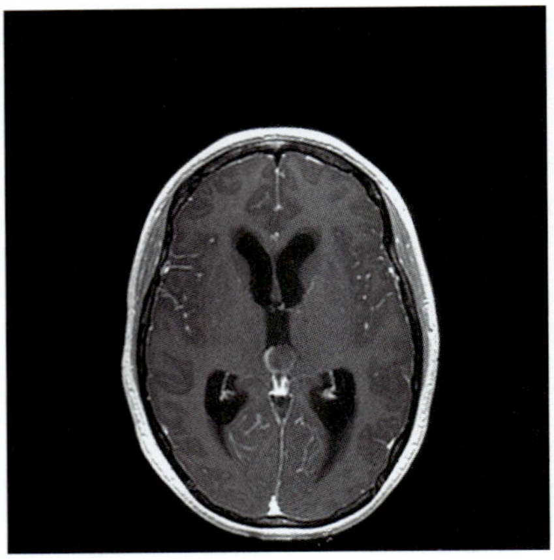

H 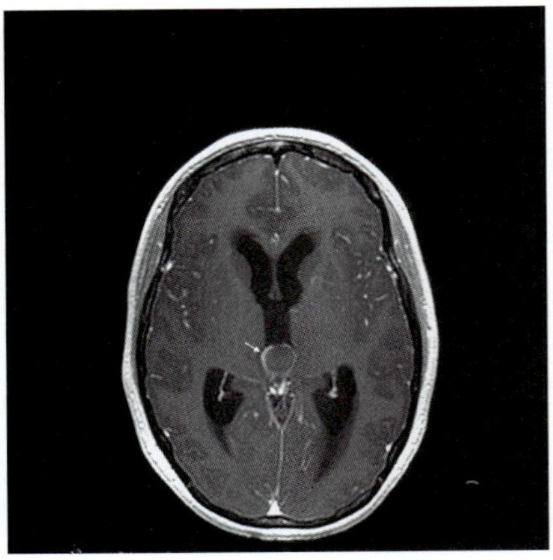

I 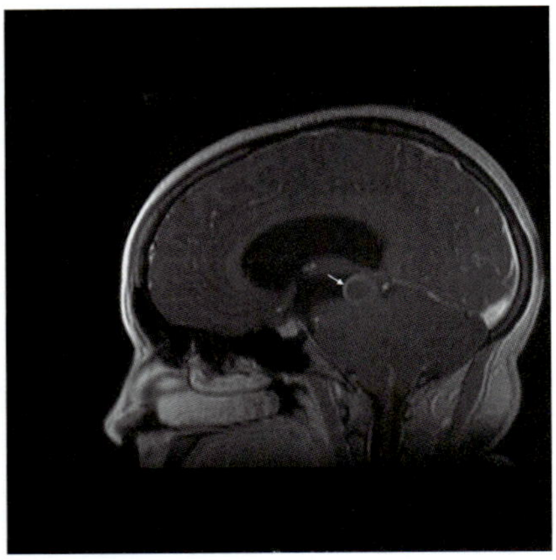

Figure 9.1. ***(continued)*** **G.** Axial T1 postcontrast: Thin rim of enhancement of the cystic mass. **H.** Axial T1 postcontrast: Thin rim of enhancement of the cystic mass. **I.** Sagittal T1 post contrast: Thin rim of enhancement of the cystic mass.

Pineal Parenchymal Tumor of Intermediate Differentiation

Definition: Pineal parenchymal tumor comprises diffuse sheets or large lobules of monomorphic round cells and is intermediate in malignancy between the malignancies of pineocytoma and pineoblastoma. Unlike pineocytoma, PPTID has a potential to recur and metastasize.

Epidemiology: This tumor accounts for approximately 45% of all pineal tumors, with a range of 21% to 54%.

Affected age group: PPTID can occur in patients of any age, but it most frequently affects adults, with a mean age of 41 years. There is slight female preponderance, with a female-to-male ratio of 1:0.

Molecular and genetic profile: ASMT-positive cells are much more prevalent in PPTID than pineocytoma. The most frequently observed chromosomal imbalances are 4q gain, 12q gain, and 22 loss.

Clinical features and standard therapy: Similar to other pineal region tumors, patients with PPTID present with signs and symptoms primarily related to increased intracranial pressure caused by obstructive hydrocephalus. Compression of the superior colliculus by PPTID can cause ocular movement abnormalities (i.e., Parinaud syndrome) such as paralysis of upward gaze, dilated pupils, and nystagmus. Surgical resection followed by radiation therapy is the standard of care.

Prognosis: PPTID, as its name suggests, is a malignant tumor of intermediate grade that has worse prognosis than pineocytoma but a better prognosis than pineoblastoma. Craniospinal dissemination at the time of diagnosis is rare but not uncommon in recurrent settings.

Imaging

PPTID is a relatively large solid mass centered in the pineal region and can be disseminated at the initial diagnosis.

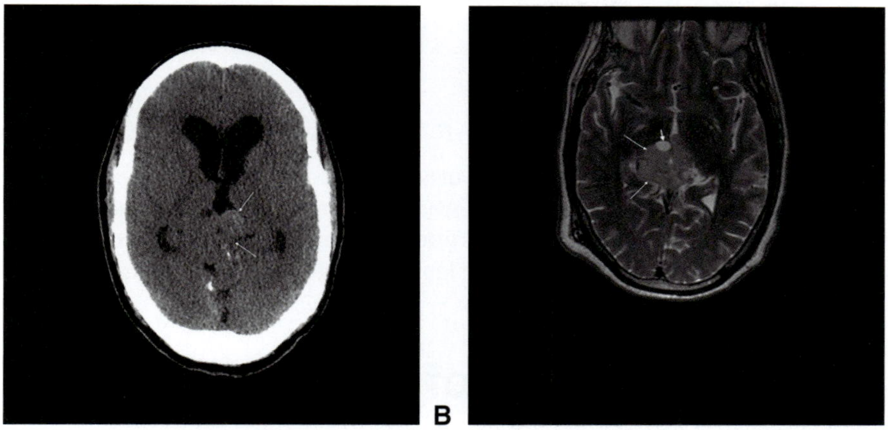

A B

Figure 9.2. Imaging of pineal parenchymal tumor of intermediate differentiation. A. CT, unenhanced: Lobulated iso-dense pineal mass (white arrows). **B.** Axial T2: Heterogeneously hypointense mass (long arrows) with prominent cystic component (short arrow).

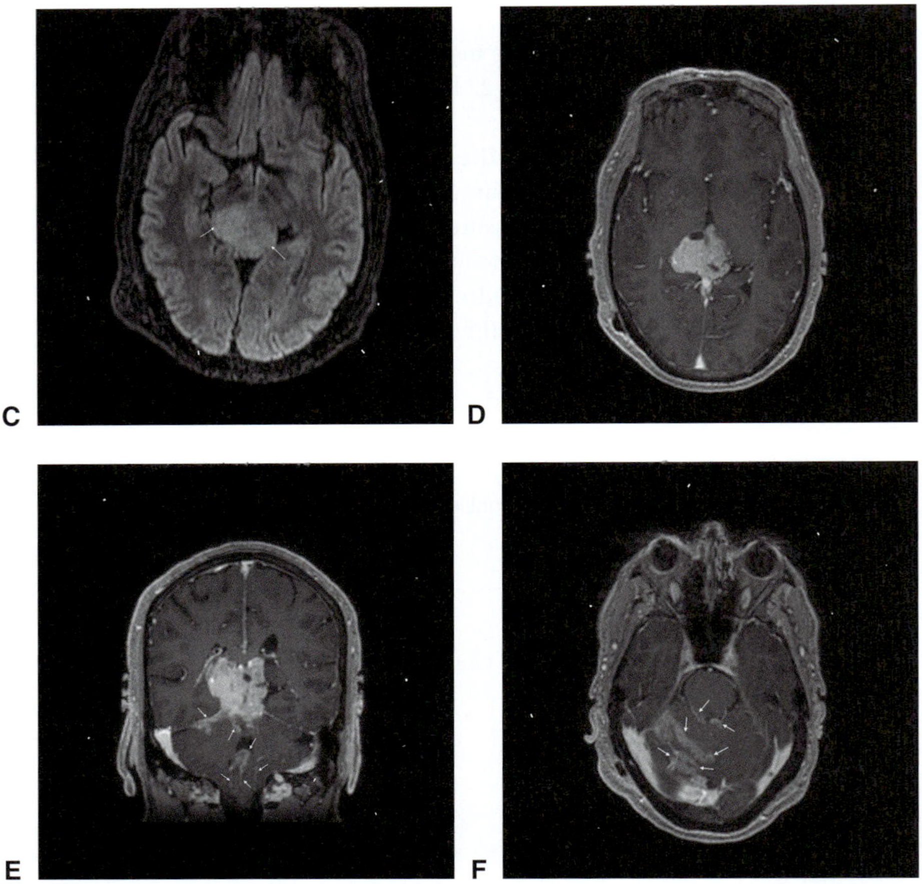

Figure 9.2. ***(continued)*** **C.** Axial FLAIR: Heterogeneously hyperintense mass (white arrows). **D.** Axial T1 postcontrast: Avid but heterogeneously enhancing mass. **E.** Coronal T1 postcontrast: Multiple sites of leptomeningeal spread of tumor (arrows). **F.** Axial T1 postcontrast: Multiple sites of leptomeningeal spread of tumor (arrows)

▶ Papillary Tumor of the Pineal Region

Definition: PTPR is a neuroepithelial tumor localized in the pineal region and comprised of a combination of papillary and solid tumor tissues. Biologic behavior and recurrence rate of PTPR fall between those of pineocytoma and PPTID, and its grade is considered WHO II to III, though the exact grading of PTPR remains unsettled.

Epidemiology: Due to its extreme rarity, incidence data are not available.

Affected age group: The published literature suggests that PTPR affects both children and adults, with reported age ranges from 1 to 71 years, with a median of 35 years. No gender predilection has been noted, with a female-to-male ratio of 1:1.06.

Molecular and genetic profile: Claudin expression profile similar to that of the subcommissural organ in human fetuses is seen in PTPR.

CSF markers: None.

Clinical features and standard therapy: Surgical resection is the mainstay, and no standard chemotherapy has been established to treat PTPR.

Prognosis: Local recurrence rate can be high and 5-year survival rate is around 70%. Lower extent of surgical resection is associated with decreased survival and increased recurrence rate.

Imaging

PTPR is a relatively large (2–5 cm), well-circumscribed, lobulated contour mass with cystic and solid components. The mass can be centered in the pineal region or the posterior commissure.

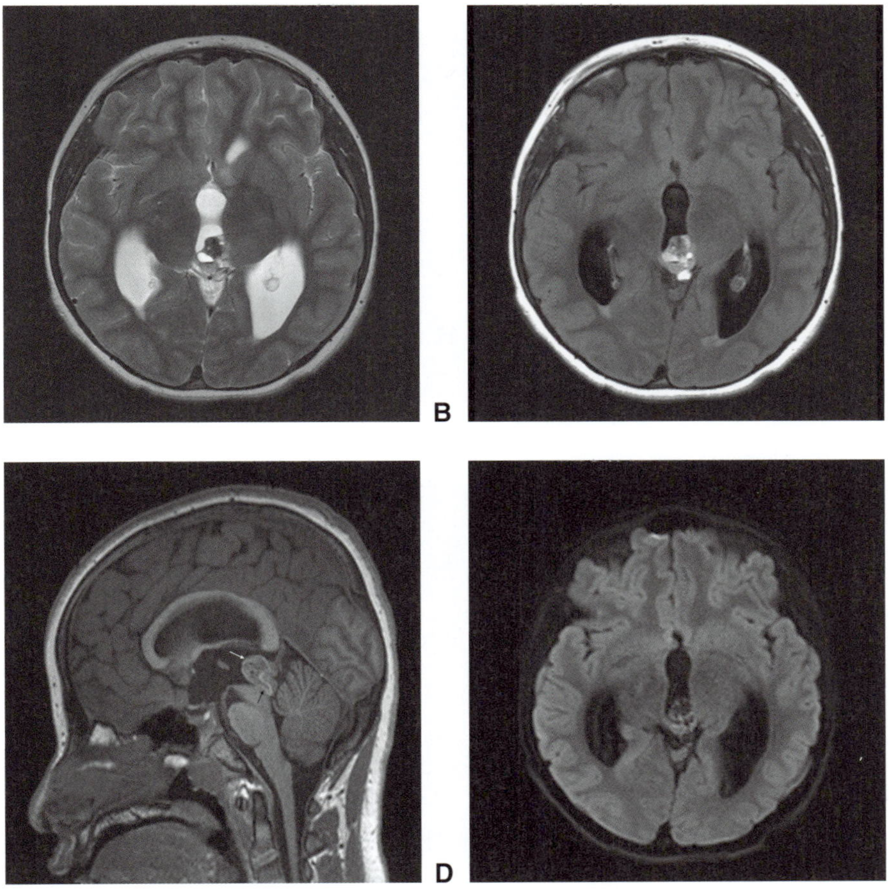

Figure 9.3. Imaging of papillary tumor of pineal region. A. Axial T2: Heterogeneous cystic and solid mass near the pineal region. **B.** Axial FLAIR: Heterogeneous cystic and solid mass near the pineal region. **C.** Sagittal T1 precontrast: Heterogeneous cystic and solid mass anterior to the pineal region near posterior commissure (white arrow) extending into the cerebral aqueduct (black arrow). **D.** Axial DWI: Rim of reduced diffusion.

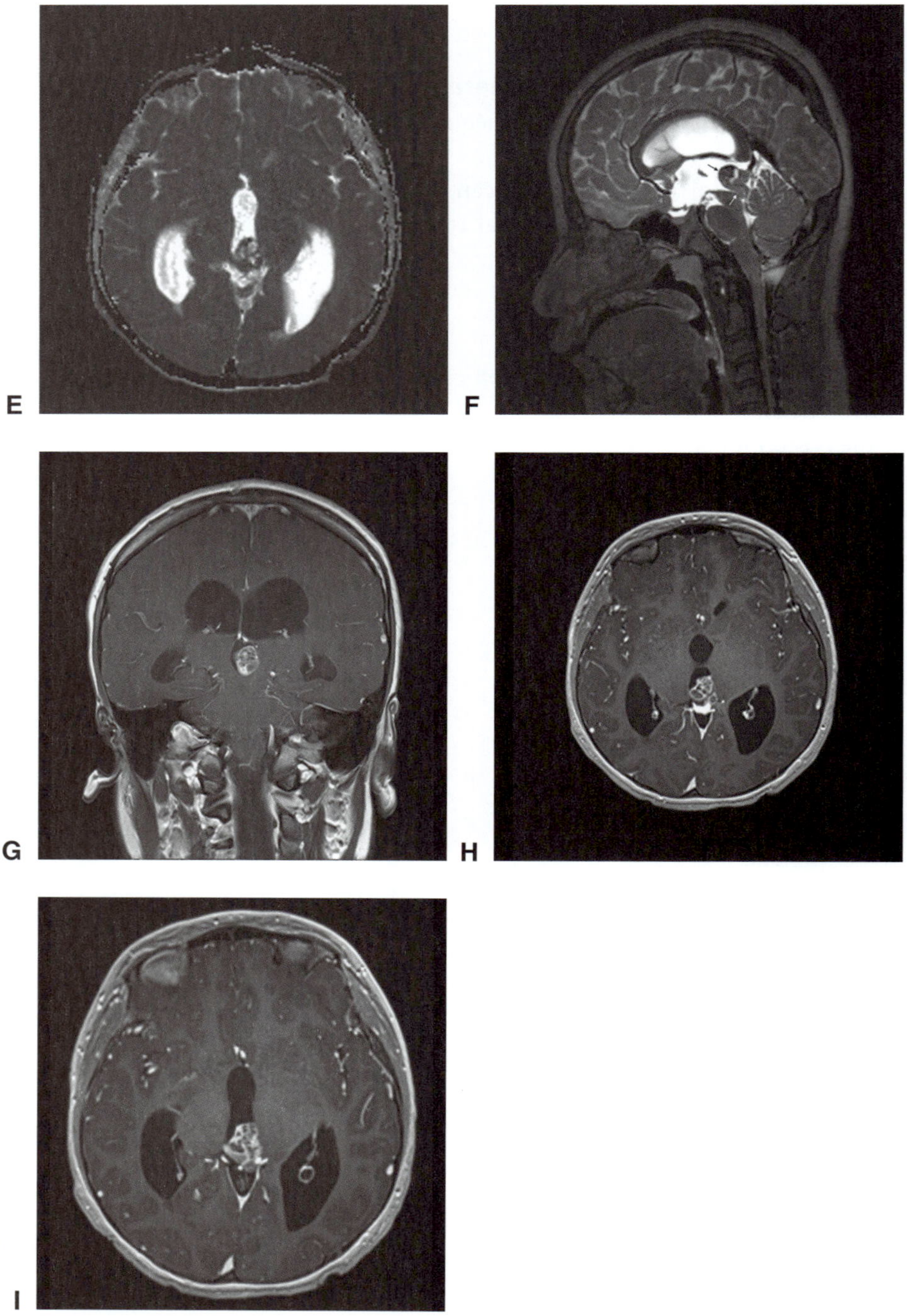

Figure 9.3. ***(continued)*** **E.** Axial apparent diffusion coefficient (ADC): Rim of reduced diffusion. **F.** Sagittal T2: Heterogeneous cystic and solid mass anterior to the pineal region near posterior commissure (black arrow) extending into the cerebral aqueduct (white arrow). **G.** Coronal T1 postcontrast: Avid but heterogeneous enhancement within the mass. **H–I.** Axial T1 postcontrast: Avid but heterogeneous enhancement within the mass.

Pineoblastoma

Definition: Pineoblastoma is a high-grade primary pineal parenchymal tumor comprised of poorly differentiated, highly cellular, malignant embryonal cells; small round blue cells.

Epidemiology: This rare malignant tumor accounts for 35% of all pineal parenchymal tumors.

Affected age group: Pineoblastoma most frequently affects children and young adults within the first two decades of life, with a mean patient age of 18 years at initial diagnosis. A alight female predominance is noticed, with a female-to-male ratio of 1:0.7.

Molecular and genetic profile: No distinct disease-defining markers have emerged, but pineoblastomas share similar molecular and cellular markers of PPTID, including the expression of *ASMT*, *CRX*, S-arrestin, and rhodopsin.

CSF markers: None.

Clinical features and standard therapy: Its presenting signs and symptoms are similar to those of PPTID or any other pineal region tumors that cause hydrocephalus or compression of superior colliculus. The standard of care is surgical resection, followed by radiotherapy and chemotherapy, including vincristine, cisplatin, nitrogen mustard, and procarbazine.

Prognosis: The 5-year survival rate is 60% to 65%, with worse prognosis in children <5 years of age. Extent of resection is an important predictor of long-term prognosis.

Imaging

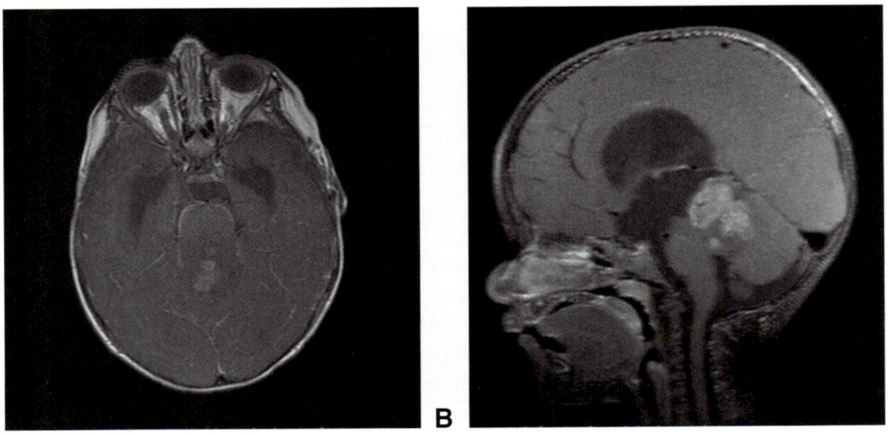

A B

Figure 9.4. Imaging of pineoblastoma. A. Axial T1-postcontrast: Heterogeneously enhancing pineal mass. **B.** Sagittal T1-postcontrast: Heterogeneously enhancing pineal mass.

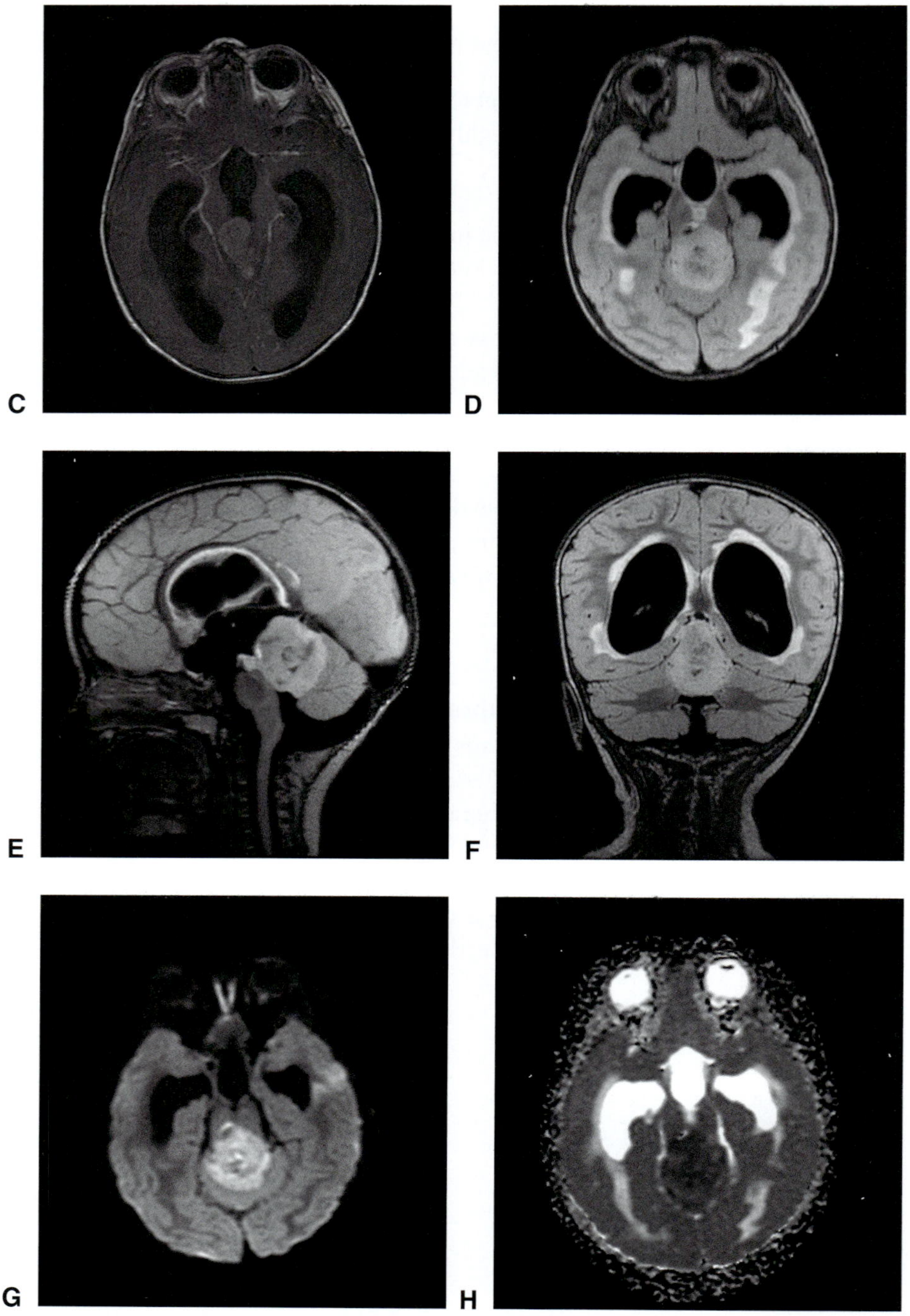

Figure 9.4. ***(continued)*** **C.** Axial T1-postcontrast: Heterogeneously enhancing pineal mass causing obstructive hydrocephalus. **D.** Axial FLAIR: Slightly hyperintense pineal mass causing obstructive hydrocephalus. **E.** Sagittal FLAIR: Slightly hyperintense pineal mass. **F.** Coronal FLAIR: Slightly hyperintense pineal mass. **G.** Axial DWI: Reduced diffusion within the mass due to high cellularity. **H.** Axial ADC: Reduced diffusion within the mass due to high cellularity.

I

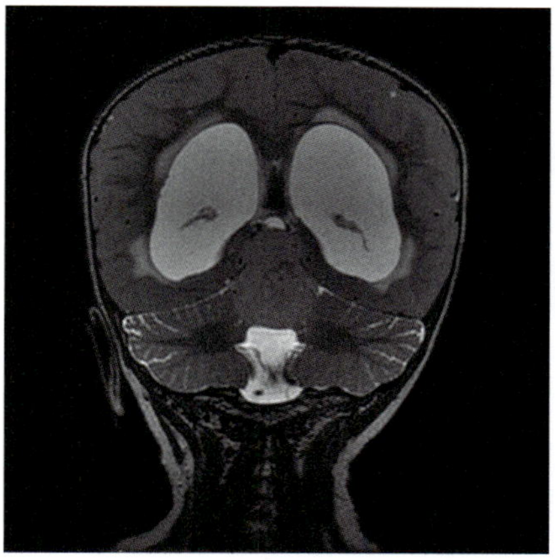

Figure 9.4. ***(continued)*** **I.** Coronal T2: Homogeneously low-signal intensity within the mass due to high cellularity.

Bibliography

Chang A, Fuller G, Debnam J, et al. MR imaging of papillary tumor of the pineal region. *AJNR Am J Neuroradiol.* 2008;29:187–189. doi:10.3174/ajnr.A0784

Drummond KJ, Rosenfeld JV. Pineal region tumours in childhood: a 30-year experience. *Childs Nerv Syst.* 1999;15(2–3):119–126.

Dumrongpisutikul N, Intrapiromkul J, Yousem DM. Distinguishing between germinomas and pineal cell tumors on MR imaging. *ASNR Am J Neuroradiol.* 2021;33:550–555.

Korogi Y, Takahashi M, Ushio Y. MRI of pineal region tumors. *J Neurooncol.* 2001;54: 251–261.

Smith AB, Rushing EJ, Smirniotopoulos JG. Lesions of the pineal region: radiologic-pathologic correlation. *Radiographics.* 2010;30:2001–2020. doi:10.1148/rg.307105131

10 Tumors of the Sellar Region

Overview

The genetic underpinnings of adamantinomatous and papillary craniopharyngiomas are very different, suggesting that they are each a distinct tumor entity although they share the same name. On the contrary, the three rare tumors of the sellar region—granular cell tumor, pituicytoma, and spindle cell oncocytoma—are thought to arise from multiple subtypes of pituicytes, hence sharing similar genetic expression.

	Age range (years)	Female: male ratio	Cell of origin	WHO grade	Molecular/ genetic markers	Prognosis
Adamantinomatous craniopharyngioma	Bi-modal (5–15, 45–60)	1:1	Rathke pouch epithelial cells	I	*CTNNB1* *WNT*	Guarded if unresectable
Papillary craniopharyngioma	40–60	1:1	Nonkeratinizing stratified squamous epithelial cells	I	*BRAF* V600E	Guarded if unresectable
Granular cell tumor	50–(female) 60–(male)	2:1	Epithelioid spindle cells of neurohypophysis or infundibulum	I	*TTF1* *CD68*, *S100*	Favorable
Pituicytoma	40–55	1:1.5	Pituicytes of neurohypophysis or infundibulum	I	*TTF1*	Favorable
Spindle cell oncocytoma	24–76	11	Pituicytes with mitochondrion-rich cytoplasm	I	*TTF1*	Favorable

Adamantinomatous Craniopharyngioma

Definition: Adamantinomatous craniopharyngioma is a benign, cystic and solid, epithelial tumor arising from embryonic remnants of the Rathke pouch epithelium.

Epidemiology: This tumor accounts for 1.2% to 4.6% of all intracranial tumors with bimodal age distribution.

Molecular and genetic profile: Catenin beta 1(*CTNNB1*) mutations and aberrant nuclear expression of beta-catenin in up to 95% of cases are seen.

Clinical features and standard therapy: Prominent cystic components of adamantinomatous craniopharyngioma are often multiloculated and multicompartmental, rendering complete surgical removal difficult, as is the infiltrative growth of the solid component. Recurrence is common when there is residual tumor after the initial surgery, and both chemotherapy and radiation therapies are largely ineffective.

Imaging

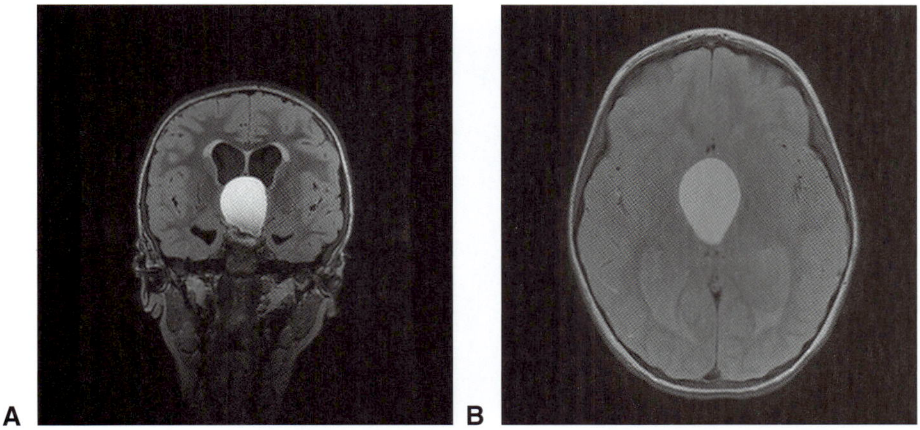

Figure 10.1. Imaging of adamantinomatous craniopharyngioma. A. Coronal FLAIR: Hyperintense cystic mass. **B.** Axial fluid-attenuated inversion recovery (FLAIR): Hyperintense cystic mass.

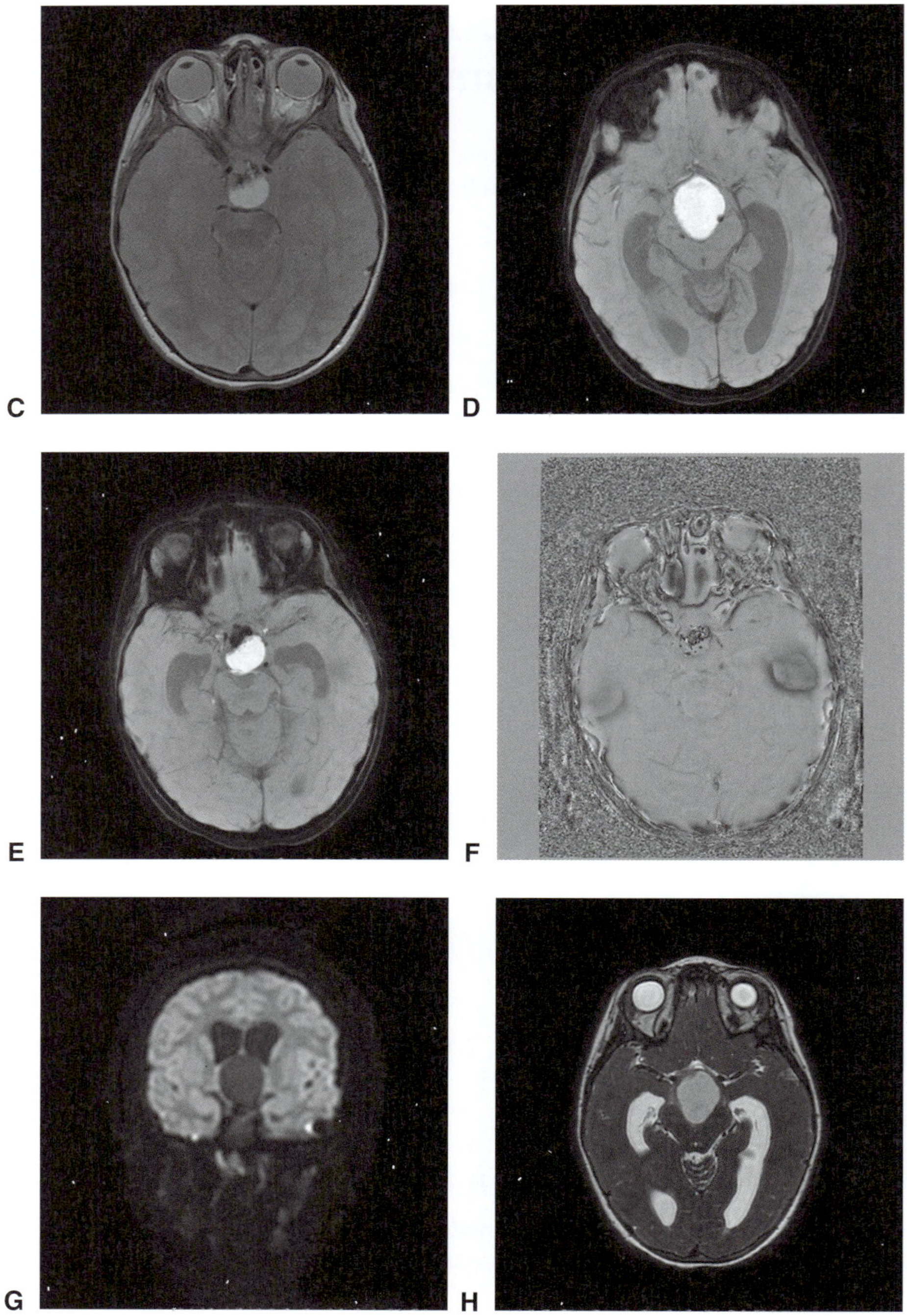

Figure 10.1. ***(continued)*** **C.** Axial FLAIR: Hyperintense cystic mass with anterior solid component. **D.** Axial susceptibility-weighted imaging (SWI): Hyperintense cystic mass. **E.** Axial SWI: Hyperintense cystic mass with anterior calcified solid component. **F.** Axial SWI (phase-filtered): Hypointense signal within the anterior calcified solid component. **G.** Coronal diffusion-weighted imaging (DWI): Increased diffusion within the cyst. **H.** Axial T2: Hyperintense cystic mass.

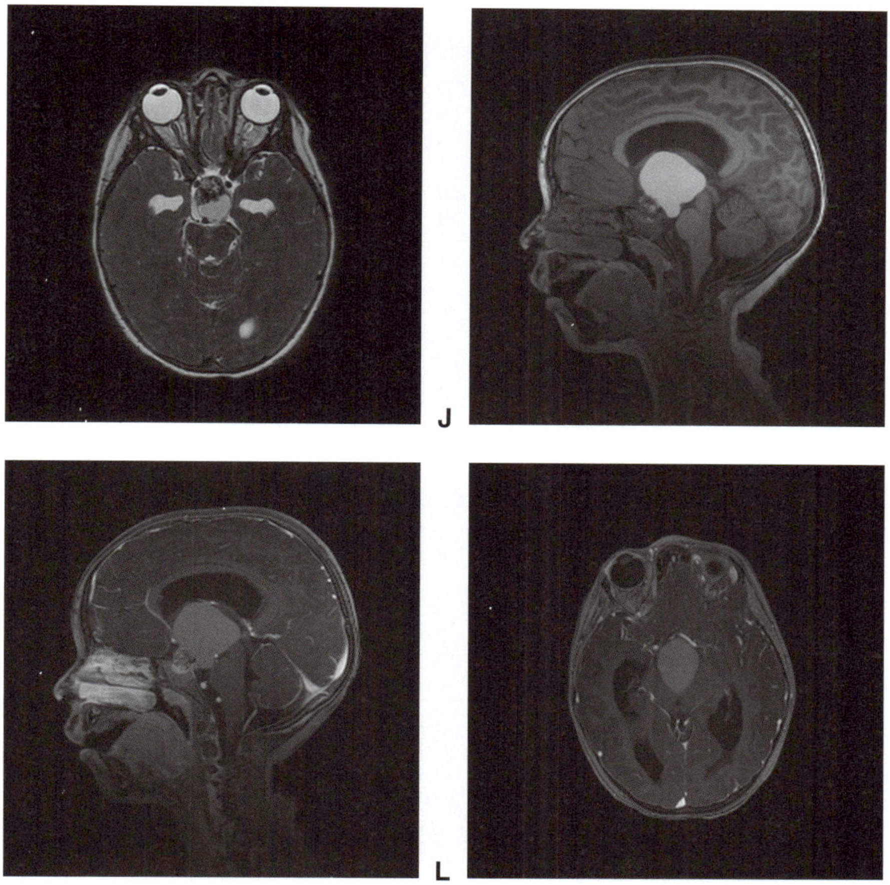

I J K L

Figure 10.1. ***(continued)*** **I.** Axial T2: Hyperintense cystic mass with anterior solid component. **J.** Sagittal T1 precontrast: Homogeneous hyperintense signal within the cyst. **K.** Sagittal T1 postcontrast: Heterogeneous enhancement within the anterior solid component. **L.** Axial T1 postcontrast: Heterogeneous enhancement within the anterior solid component.

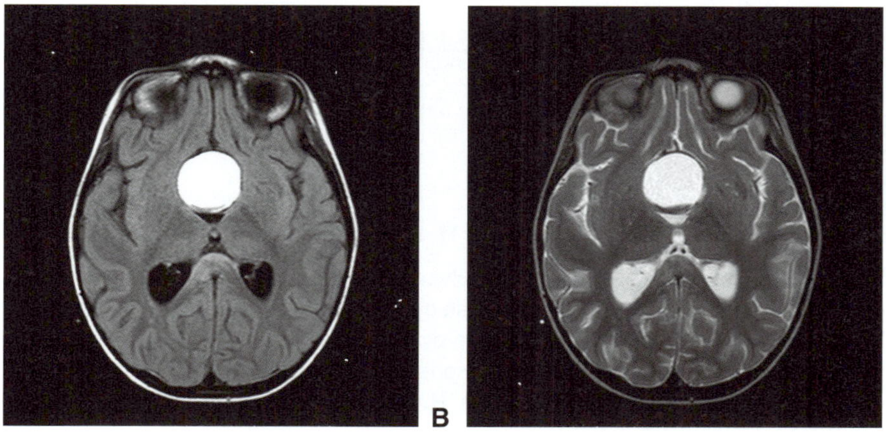

A B

Figure 10.2. **Imaging of adamantinomatous craniopharyngioma. A.** Axial FLAIR: Hyperintense cystic mass with layering blood products. **B.** Axial T2: Hyperintense cystic mass with layering blood products.

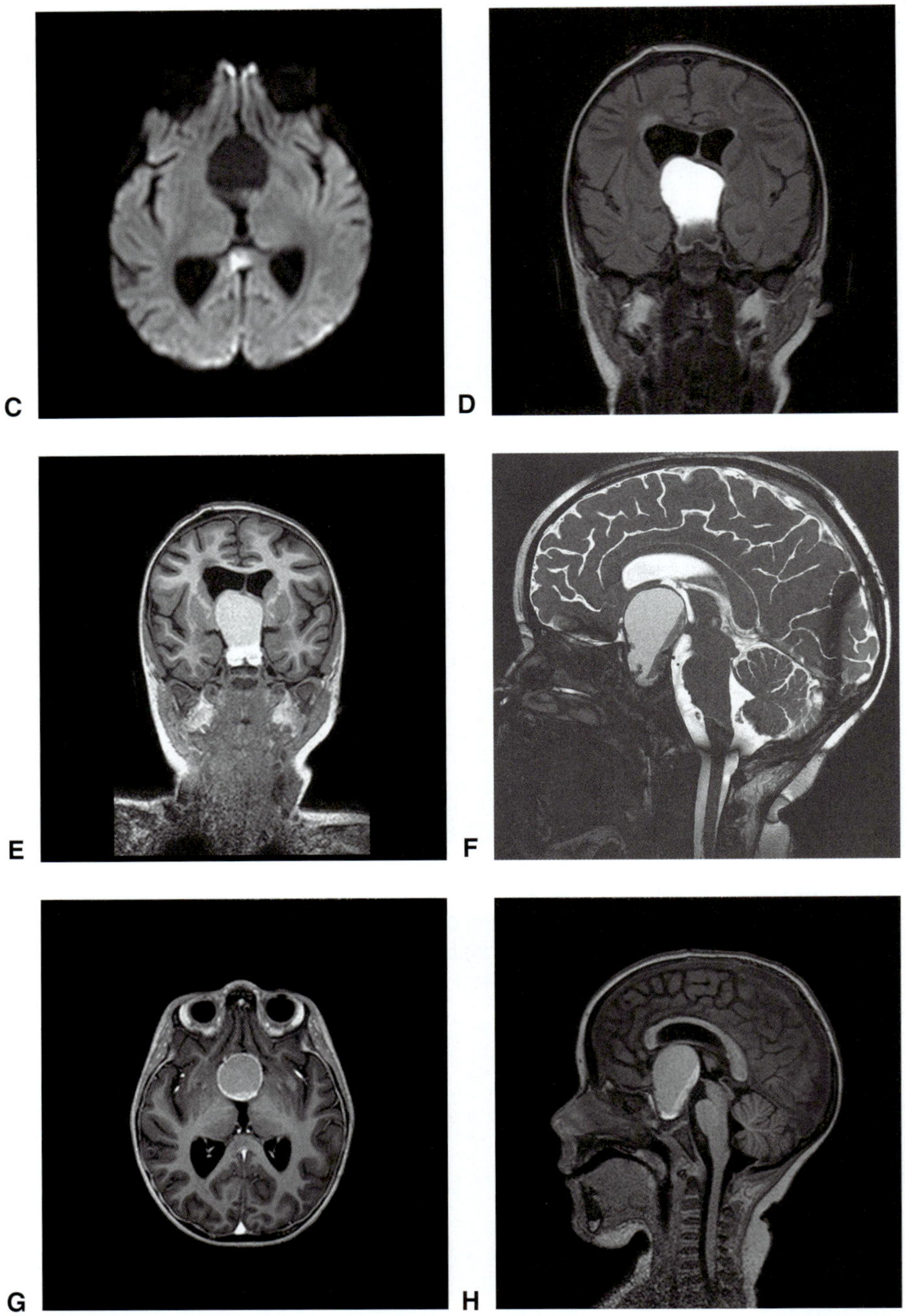

Figure 10.2. ***(continued)*** **C.** Axial DWI: Hypointense cystic mass with layering blood products. **D.** Coronal FLAIR: Hyperintense cystic mass with layering blood products. **E.** Coronal T1 precontrast: Hyperintense cystic mass. **F.** Sagittal FIESTA: Hyperintense cystic mass with layering blood products. **G.** Axial T1 postcontrast: Thin rind of enhancement around the cyst margin. **H.** Sagittal T1 precontrast: Homogeneous hyperintense signal within the cyst.

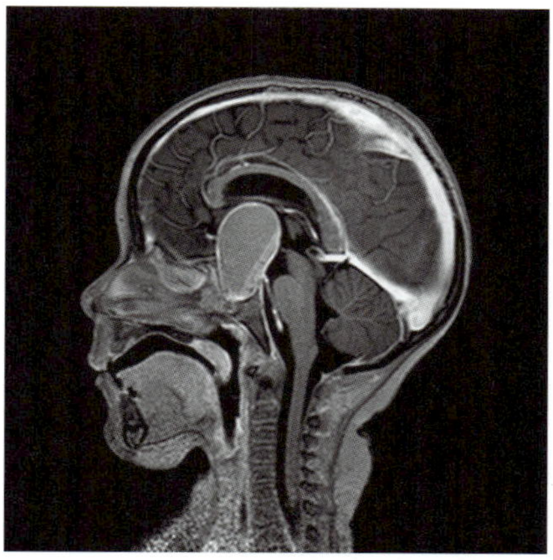

I

Figure 10.2. ***(continued)*** **I.** Sagittal T1 postcontrast: Thin rind of enhancement around the cyst margin.

Papillary Craniopharyngioma

Definition: Papillary craniopharyngioma is a benign, mostly solid, epithelial tumor arising from nonkeratinizing stratified squamous epithelium.

Epidemiology: The tumor accounts for 1.2% to 4.6% of all intracranial tumors and usually affects middle-aged individuals (40–60 years) and is extremely rare in the pediatric age group.

Molecular and genetic profile: *BRAF* V600E mutations are seen in up to 95% of cases.

Clinical features and standard therapy: In contrast to the adamantinomatous subtype, papillary craniopharyngiomas tend to be mostly solid. Surgical resection is the first-line treatment, but in the case of infiltrative growth, gross total resection may not be accomplished.

Imaging

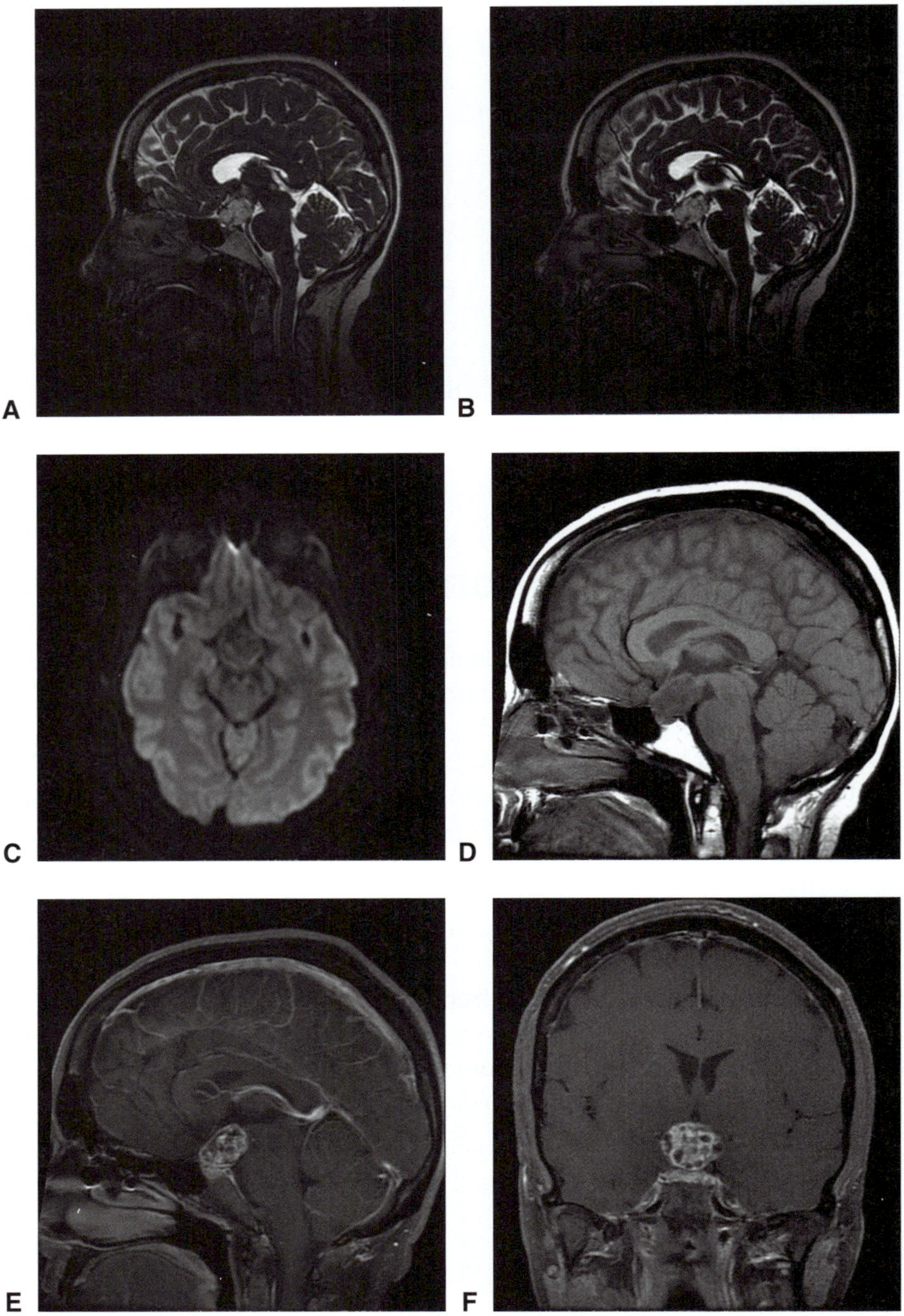

Figure 10.3. Imaging of papillary craniopharyngioma. A. Sagittal T2: Heterogeneously hyperintense suprasellar mass. **B.** Sagittal T2: Heterogeneously hyperintense suprasellar mass. **C.** Axial DWI: Increased diffusion within the mass. **D.** Sagittal T1 precontrast: Heterogeneously hypointense mass. **E.** Sagittal T1 postcontrast: Avid but heterogeneous enhancement of the mass. **F.** Coronal T1 postcontrast: Avid but heterogeneous enhancement of the mass.

Granular Cell Tumor of Neurohypophysis

Definition: Granular cell tumors of neurohypophysis are pituicytes expressing TTF-1 and containing lysosomal-rich cytoplasm.

Epidemiology: Adult female predominance with peak incidence in the fifth decade of life in women and the sixth decade of life in men has been noticed.

Molecular and Genetic Profile

Clinical features and standard therapy: Surgical removal is the primary treatment option, and the prognosis is excellent if gross total resection can be achieved. However, due to their firm and vascular nature with frequent lack of an obvious dissection plane render, complete surgical removal is a challenge, especially in large bulky tumors.

Imaging

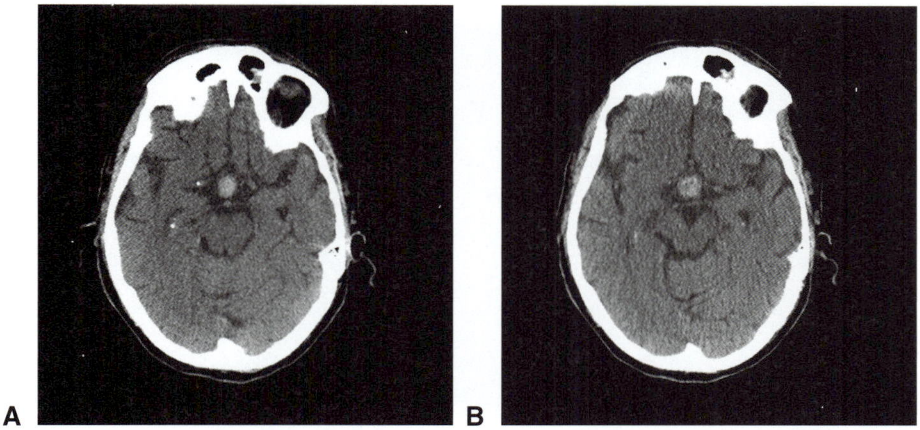

Figure 10.4. Imaging of granular cell tumor of neurohypophysis. A and B. Axial CT unenhanced: Hyperdense mass in the suprasellar region.

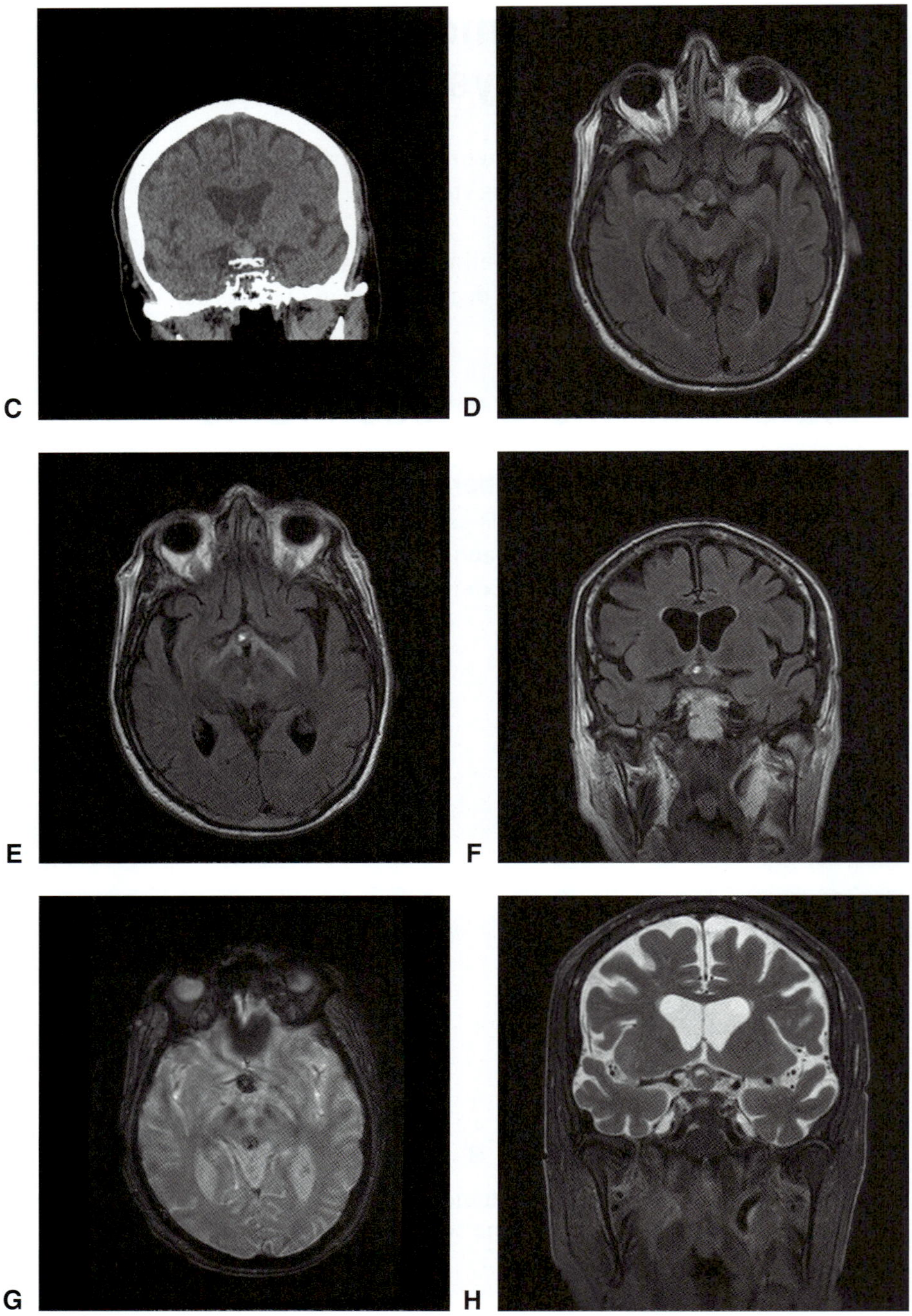

Figure 10.4. ***(continued)*** **C.** Coronal CT unenhanced: Hyperdense mass in the suprasellar region. **D and E.** Axial FLAIR: Heterogeneously isointense mass with edema tracking along bilateral optic track. **F.** Coronal FLAIR: Focal area of high-signal intensity in the superior aspect of the mass. **G.** Axial SWI: Prominent susceptibility signal within the mass. **H.** Coronal T2: Focal area of high-signal intensity in the superior aspect of the mass.

I 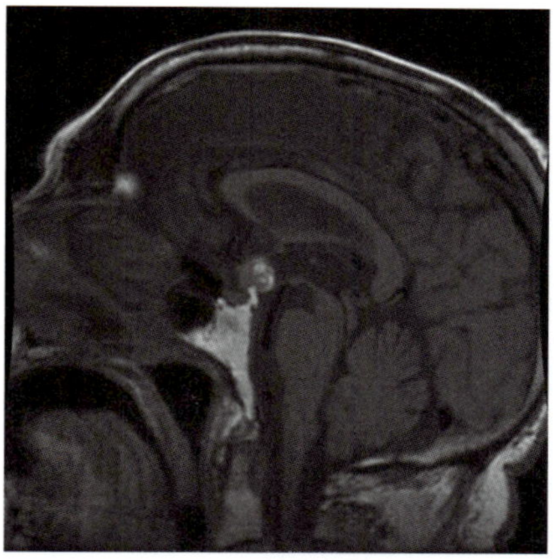

Figure 10.4. ***(continued)*** **I.** Sagittal T1: Focal area of high-signal intensity in the superior aspect of the mass.

Pituicytoma

Definition: Pituicytoma is a monomorphic spindle cell tumor composed of plump cells arranged in fascicles.

Epidemiology: This is a rare tumor with about 70 reported cases in the literature, mostly affecting adults of age 40 to 60 years (average 50 years) with a female-to-male ratio of 1:1.5.

Molecular and genetic profile: Nuclear expression of *TTF1* and strong immunoreactivity for S-100 protein are noticed.

Clinical features and standard therapy: Surgical resection is the first line of therapy, and there is no effective chemotherapy.

Imaging

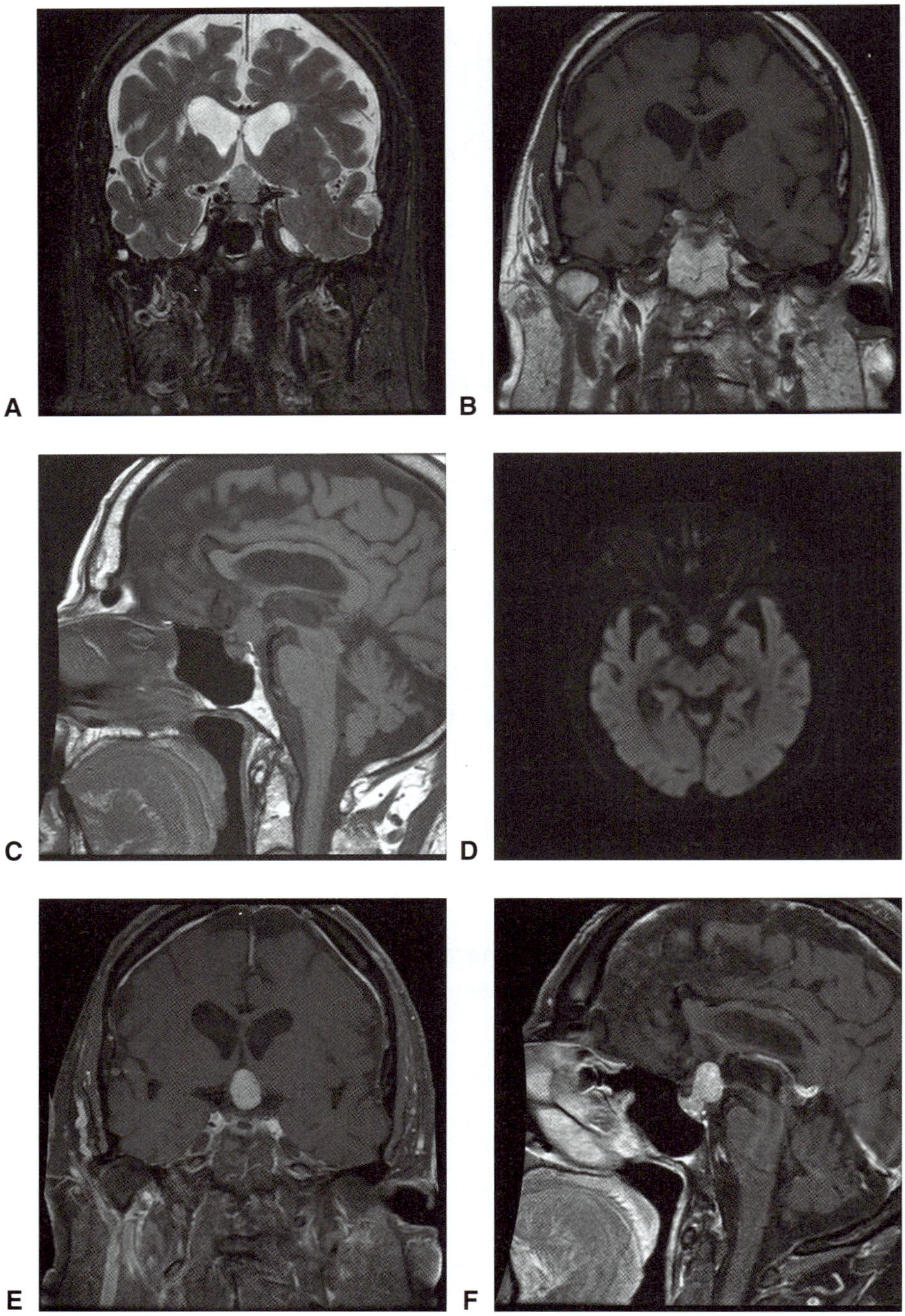

Figure 10.5. Imaging of pituicytoma. A. Coronal T2: Lobular suprasellar mass with isointense signal to brain parenchyma. **B.** Coronal T1 precontrast: Lobular suprasellar mass with isointense signal to brain parenchyma. **C.** Sagittal T1 precontrast: Lobular suprasellar mass with isointense signal to brain parenchyma. **D.** Axial DWI: Lobular suprasellar mass with isointense signal to brain parenchyma. **E.** Coronal T1 postcontrast: Avid and homogeneous enhancement within the mass. **F.** Sagittal T1 postcontrast: Avid and homogeneously enhancing suprasellar mass that abuts the posterior pituitary gland.

Spindle Cell Oncocytoma of the Adenohypophysis

Definition: Spindle cell oncocytoma of the adenohypophysis refers to epithelioid cells with numerous mitochondria.

Epidemiology: This is a rare tumor, with only 25 reported cases in the literature, in adults of age 24 to 76 years, with a mean age of 56 years and equal distribution between the sexes.

Molecular and genetic profile: Tumor cells stain for S100 protein, *BCL2*, *EMA*, and *MU213-UC* clone 131-1 and nuclear staining for *TTF1* are seen.

Clinical features and standard therapy: Surgical removal is the first-line therapy, and there is no effective chemotherapy; radiation therapy is not recommended after surgery regardless of the extent of resection and reserved for local recurrence. There are no reported cases of distant spread of tumor outside of the sellar region.

Imaging

A B

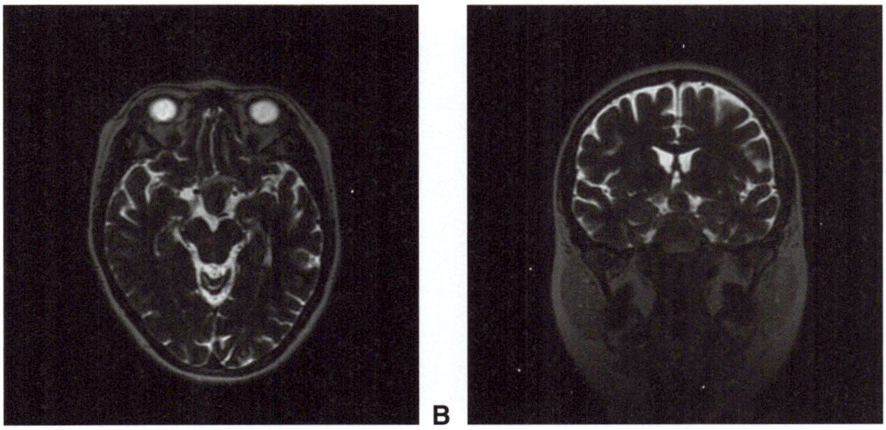

Figure 10.6. Imaging of spindle cell oncocytoma of the adenohypophysis. A. Axial T2: Homogeneously low-signal intensity suprasellar mass. **B.** Coronal T2: Homogeneously low-signal intensity suprasellar mass.

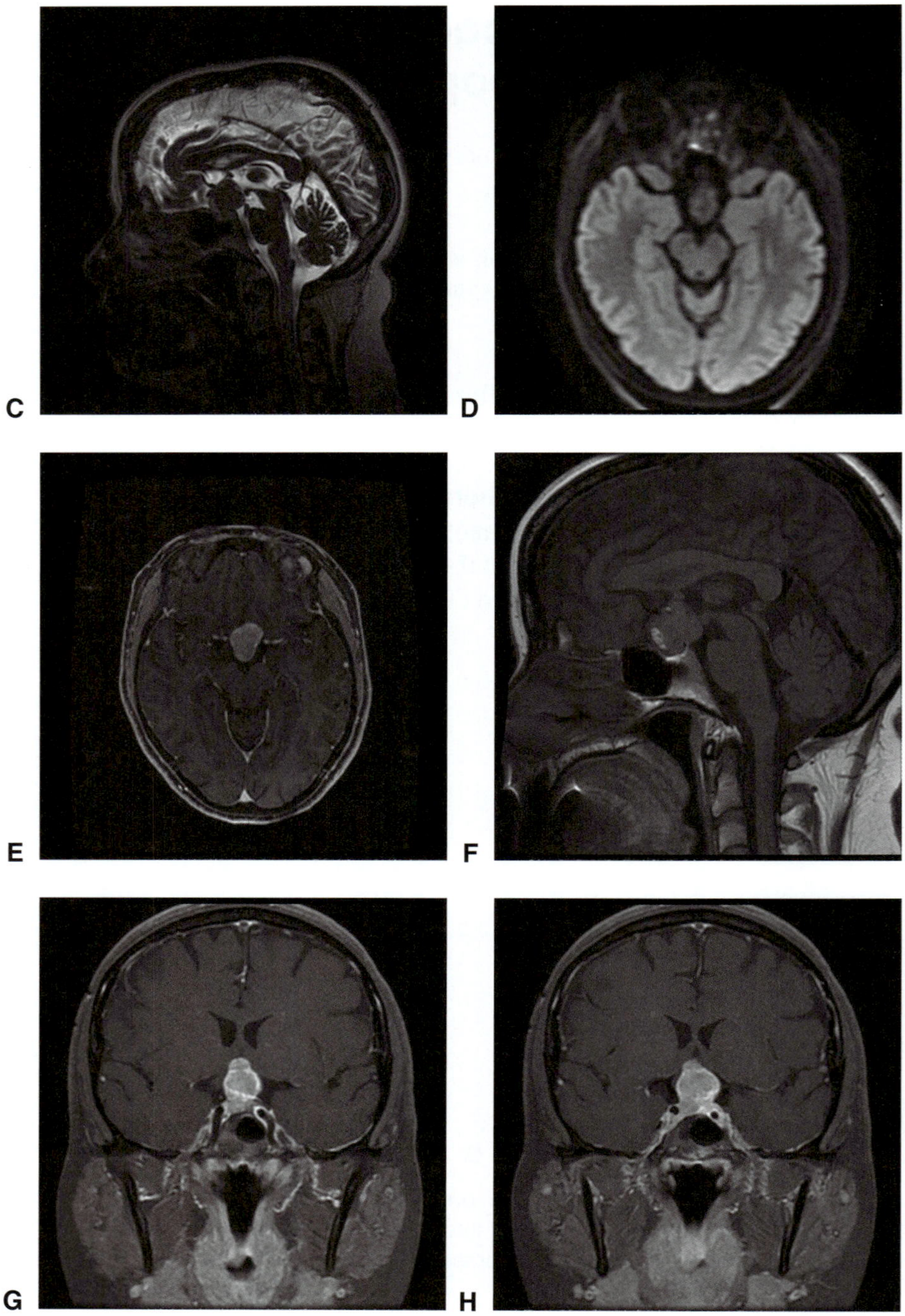

Figure 10.6. ***(continued)*** **C.** Sagittal T2: Homogeneously low-signal intensity suprasellar mass with sellar component. **D.** Axial DWI: No reduced diffusion within the mass. **E.** Axial T1 postcontrast: Avid enhancement within the mass. **F.** Sagittal T1 precontrast: Homogeneously low-signal intensity mass with discrete anterior region of high-signal intensity likely due to calcium. **G.** Coronal T1 postcontrast: Avid enhancement within the mass. **H.** Coronal T1 postcontrast: Avid enhancement within the mass.

I

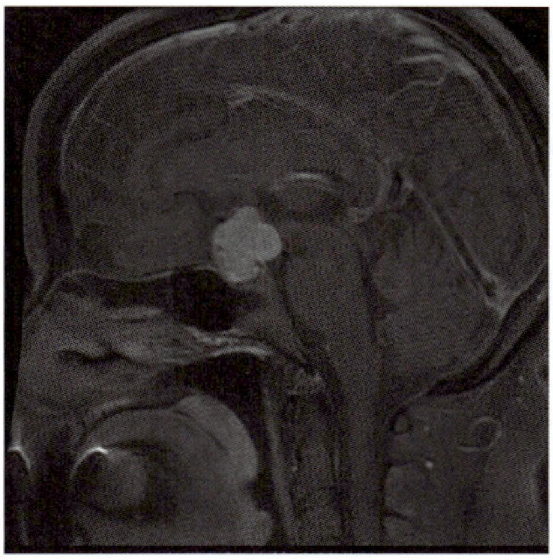

Figure 10.6. ***(continued)*** **I.** Sagittal T1 postcontrast: Avid enhancement within the mass.

Bibliography

Covington MF, Chin SS, Osborn AG. Pituicytoma, spindle cell oncocytoma, and granular cell tumor: clarification and meta-analysis of the world literature since 1893. *AJNR Am J Neuroradiol.* 2011;32:2067–2072.

Figarella-Branger D, Dufour H, Fernandez C, Bouvier-Labit C, Grisoli F, Pellissier JF. Pituicytomas, a mis-diagnosed benign tumor of the neurohypophysis: report of three cases. *Acta Neuropathol.* 2002;104:313–319.

Giantini Larsen AM, Cote DJ, Zaidi HA, et al. Spindle cell oncocytoma of the pituitary gland. *J Neurosurg.* 2018;131:517–525.

Holsken A, Sill M, Merkel J, et al. Adamantinomatous and papillary craniopharyngiomas are characterized by distinct epigenomic as well as mutational and transcriptomic profiles. *Acta Neuropathol Commun.* 2016;4:20.

Wilkinson MD, Fulham MJ, Besser M. Neuroimaging findings in a suprasellar granular cell tumor. *J Comput Assist Tomogr.* 2003;27:26–29.

Zada G, Lin N, Ojerholm E, Ramkissoon S, Laws ER. Craniopharyngioma and other cystic epithelial lesions of the sellar region: a review of clinical, imaging, and histopathological relationships. *Neurosurg Focus.* 2010; 28(4):E4.

11 Embryonal Tumors

Overview

Embryonal tumors of the central nervous system (CNS) are poorly differentiated, mitotically active, histologically and clinically aggressive, and highly cellular neoplasms and constitute the most common group of malignant brain tumors in children. Commonly referred to as small round blue cell tumors, the embryonal tumor group includes medulloblastoma, embryonal tumor with multilayered rosettes, atypical teratoid/rhabdoid tumor, CNS neuroblastoma, and high-grade neuroepithelial tumor with BCL-6 co-repressor (BCOR) internal tandem duplication as well as a spectrum of other CNS embryonal tumors that were previously called *CNS primitive neuroectodermal tumors*.

	Subtype	Age	Histology	Molecular/ genetic mutations	Prognosis
Medulloblastoma	WNT-activated	Children, teens	Classic Large cell/anaplastic	*CTNNB1*, *TP53*, *SMARCA4*, *DDX3X*	Favorable
	SHH-activated, TP53-mutant	Infants, adults	Large cell/anaplastic Desmoplastic/nodular	*ATOH1*, *PTCH1*, *TP53* germline	Very poor
	SHH-activated, TP53-wildtype	Infants, adults	Large cell/anaplastic Desmoplastic/nodular Extensive nodularity	*ATOH1*, *PTCH1*, *TP53*-wildtype	Intermediate to Poor
	Non-WNT/non-SHH group 3	Infants, children	Classic Large cell/anaplastic	*MYC*, *SMARCA4*, *OTX2*, *CTDNEP1*, *LRP1B*	Poor
	Non-WNT/non-SHH group 4	Infants, children, adults	Classic Large cell/anaplastic	*KDM6A* 17p deletion, 17q gain	Poor
Embryonal tumor with multilayered rosettes (ETMR)		0–4 yrs	Small cells forming multilayered rosettes, fibrillary zones; *LIN28*+	*C19MC*-altered at chromosome 19q; chromosome 2 gain	Poor

	Subtype	Age	Histology	Molecular/ genetic mutations	Prognosis
Atypical teratoid/ rhabdoid tumor (ATRT)		<3 yrs	Spindle-shaped cells clustered in papillary or trabecular pattern	*SMARCB1* locus at 22q11.2	Very poor
CNS neuroblastoma		4 wks-20 yrs	Zones of neurocytic differentiation & densely packed primitive embryonal cells	*FOXR2* *NKX2-1* 1p gain	Poor
High-grade neuroepithelial tumor with BCOR internal tandem duplication (HGNET-BCOR-ITD)		7 mos-22 yrs	Spindle to oval cells with fine chromatin, microcystic features, perivascular pseudo-rosettes, fibrillary cytoplasmic processes	Somatic internal tandem duplications in the 3rd end (exon 15) of *BCOR* gene	Poor

BCOR, BCL-6 co-repressor.

Medulloblastoma

Definition: Medulloblastoma is the most common embryonal neuroepithelial tumor arising in the cerebellum or posterior brain stem and most common malignant tumor of childhood consisting of densely packed small and round undifferentiated cells with high mitotic count.

Epidemiology: This is the most common CNS embryonal tumor of childhood and the second most common pediatric brain tumors after pilocytic astrocytoma; it accounts for up to 25% of all intracranial neoplasms in children. The median age at diagnosis of medulloblastoma is 9 years, with peaks incident at 3 and 7 years of age; it is more common in boys, with female-to-male ratio of 1:1.7. Among patients aged >3 years, the female-to-male ratio is 1:2. The various molecular groups and histopathological variants of medulloblastoma have different age distributions.

Molecular and genetic profile: Medulloblastomas are divided into four distinct molecular subtypes based on molecular profiles: WNT-activated, sonic hedgehog (SHH)-activated, non-WNT/non-SHH-activated group 3, and non-WNT/non-SHH-activated group 4.

Clinical features and standard therapy

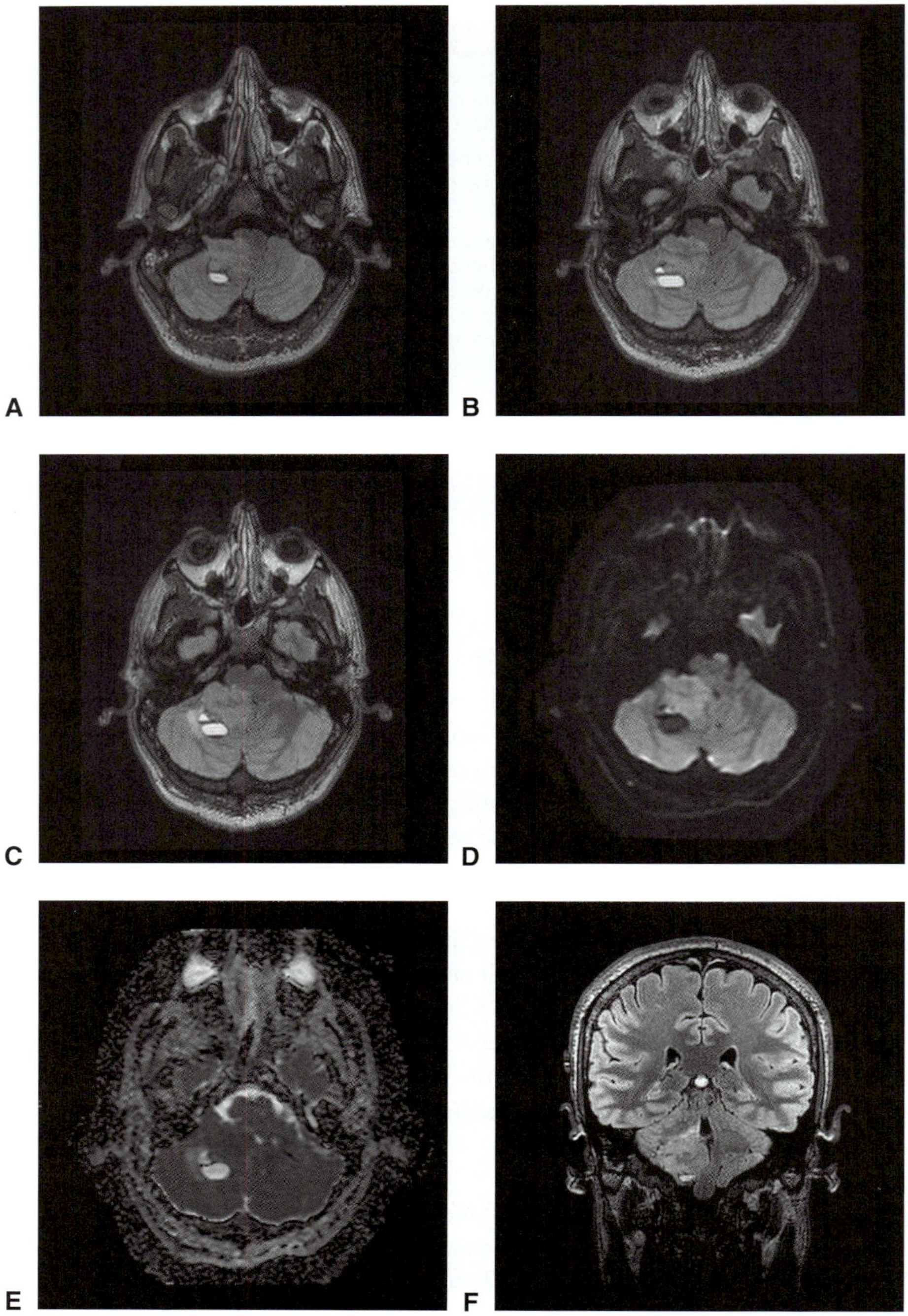

Figure 11.1. Imaging of medulloblastoma, WNT-activated. A–C. Axial T2: Heterogeneously isointense mass in the right cerebellopontine angle with posterior cystic components with fluid-fluid level. **D.** Axial diffusion-weighted imaging (DWI): Mildly hyperintense signal within the solid component. **E.** Axial apparent diffusion coefficient (ADC): Mildly reduced diffusion within the solid component. **F.** Coronal fluid-attenuated inversion recovery (FLAIR): Heterogeneously isointense mass.

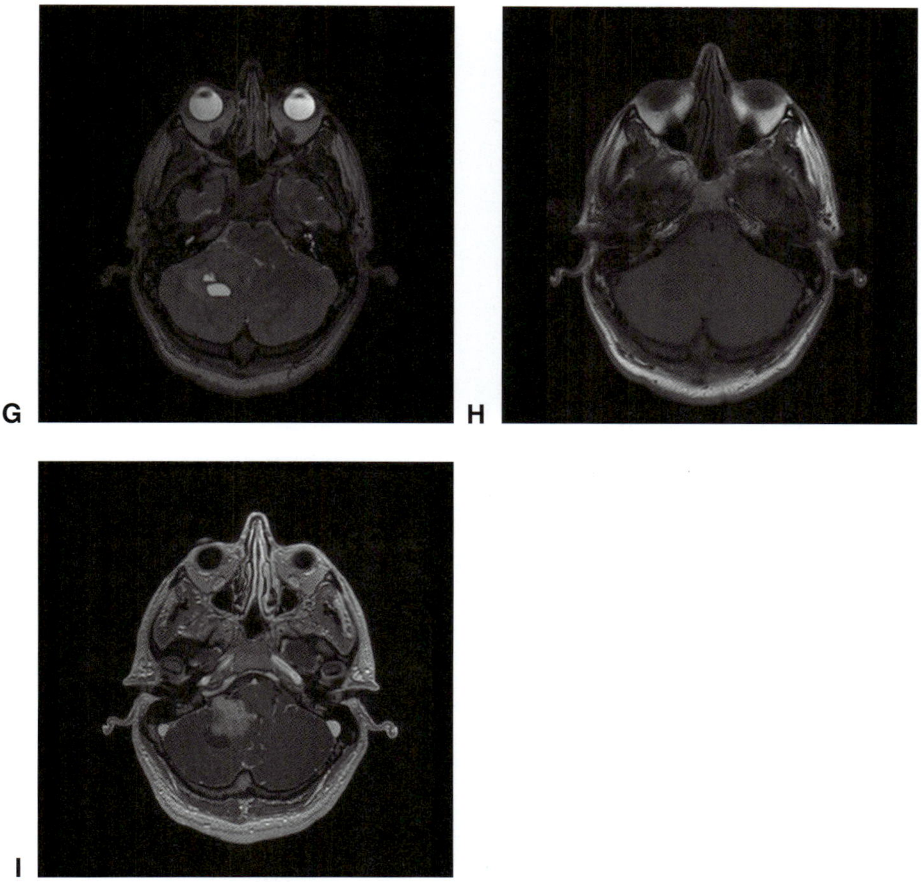

Figure 11.1. ***(continued)*** **G.** Axial FIESTA: Heterogeneously isointense mass in the right cerebellopontine angle with posterior cystic components with fluid-blood levels. **H.** Axial T1 precontrast: Homogeneously hypointense signal within the solid component. **I.** Axial T1 postcontrast: Avid enhancement within the solid component.

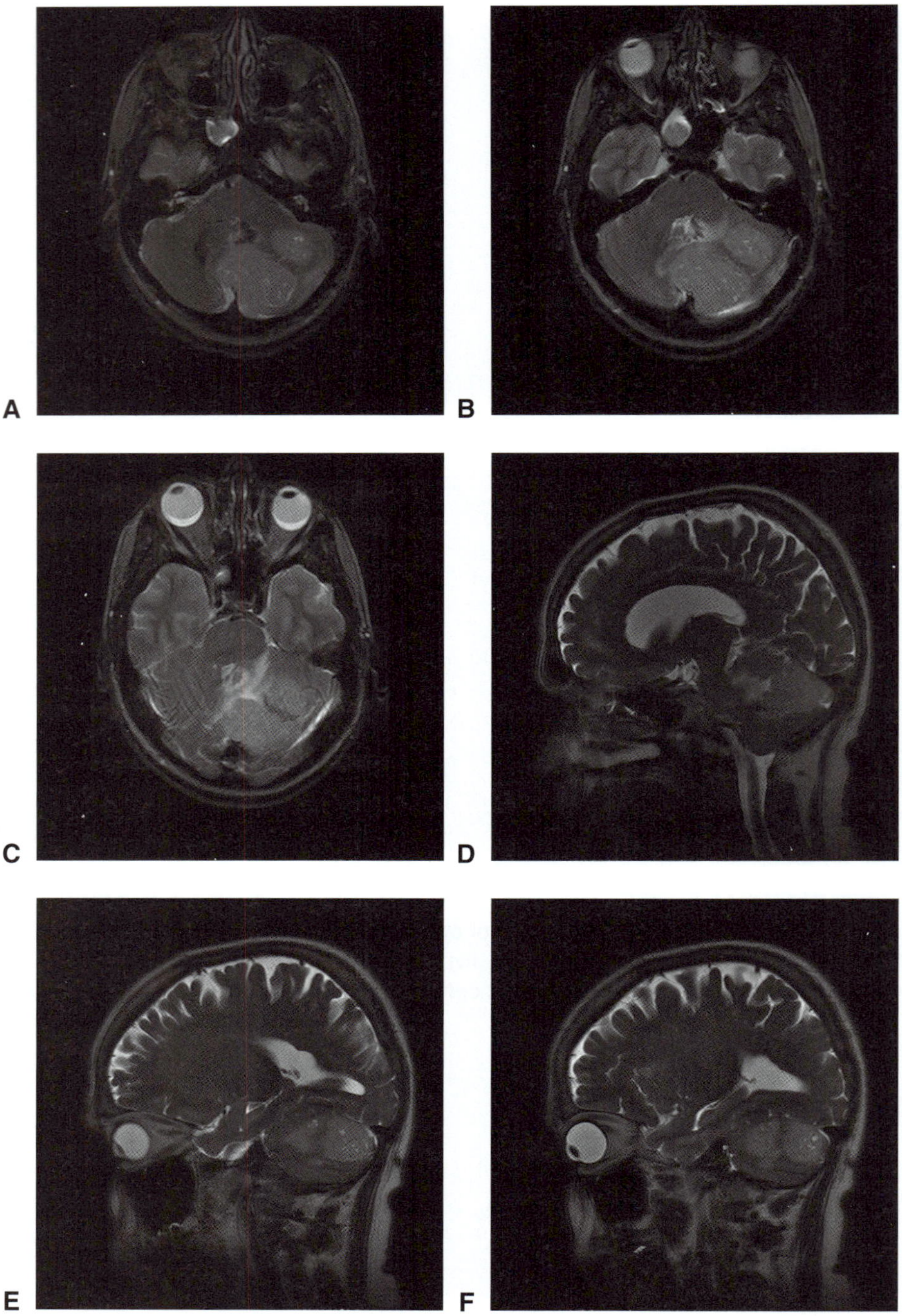

Figure 11.2. Imaging of medulloblastoma, SHH-activated. A–C. Axial T2: Heterogeneously slightly hyperintense solid mass in the left cerebellum. **D–F.** Sagittal T2: Slightly hyperintense solid mass with mild surrounding edema.

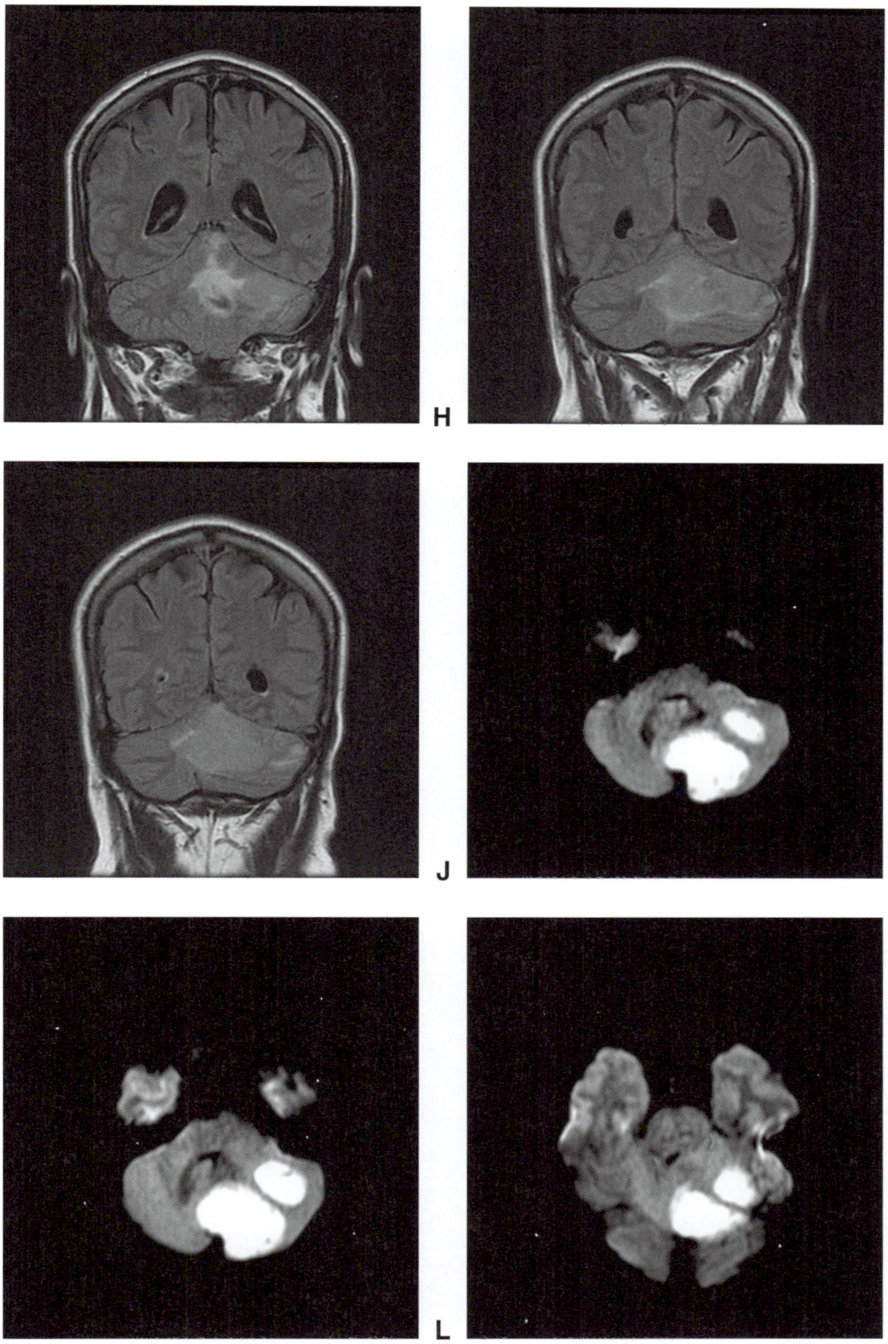

G H I J K L

Figure 11.2. ***(continued)*** **G–I.** Coronal FLAIR: Slightly hyperintense solid mass with mild surrounding edema. **J–L.** Axial DWI: Markedly reduced hypercellular mass.

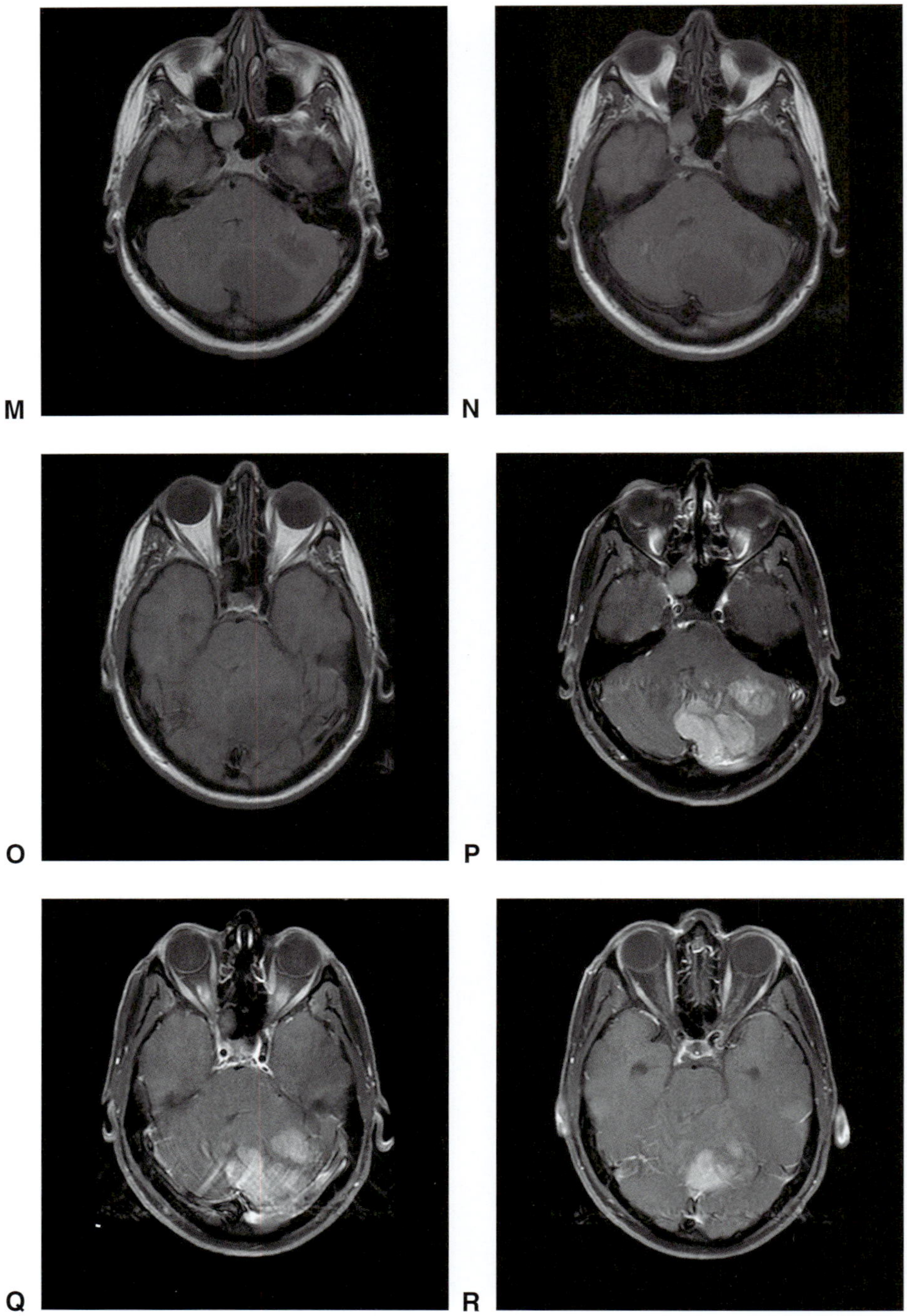

Figure 11.2. ***(continued)*** **M–O.** Axial T1 precontrast: Hypointense mass. **P–R.** Axial T1 postcontrast: Avid enhancement within the mass.

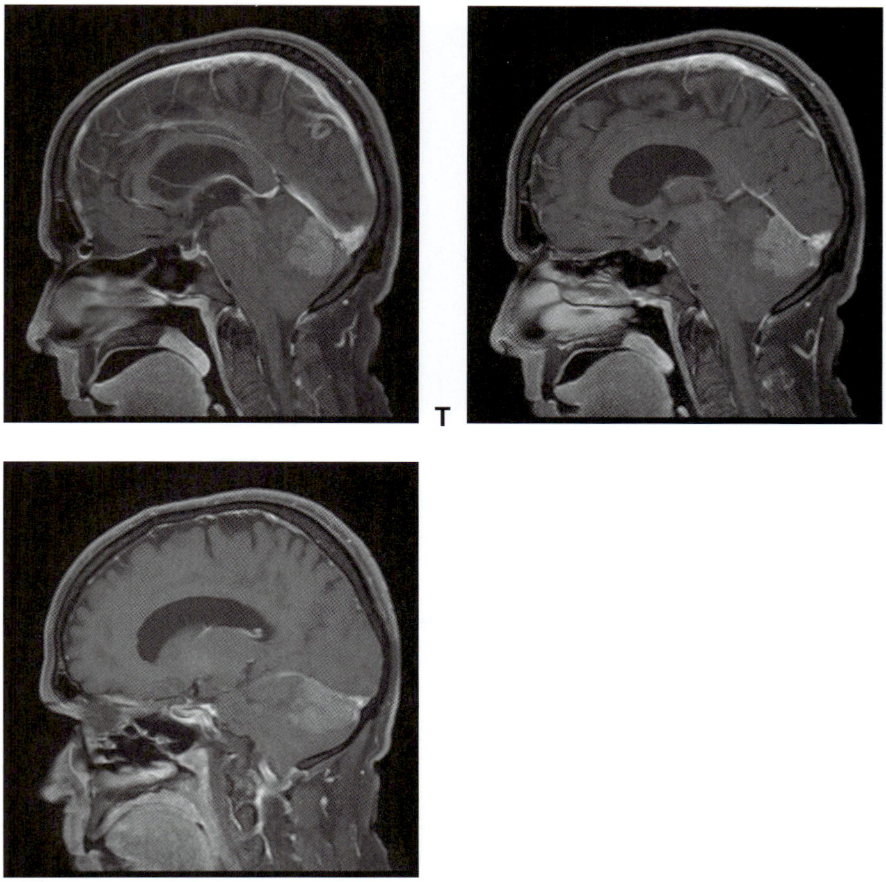

S T U

Figure 11.2. ***(continued)*** **S–U.** Sagittal T1 postcontrast: Avid enhancement within the mass and effacement of fourth ventricle due to mass effect.

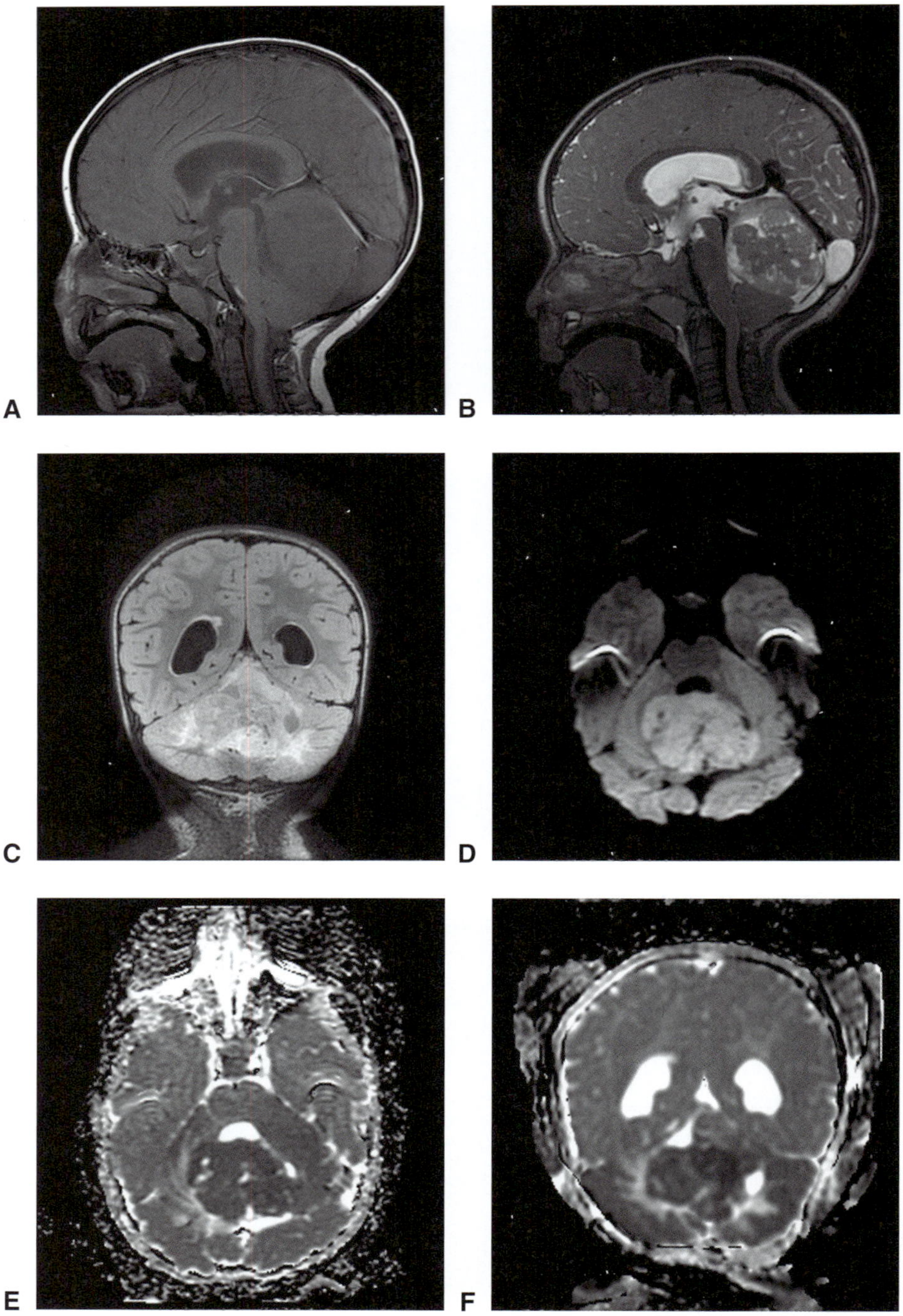

Figure 11.3. Imaging of medulloblastoma, non-WNT/non-SHH-activated, group 3. A. Sagittal T1 precontrast: Homogeneously hypointense midline mass. **B.** Sagittal T2: Heterogeneously hypointense mass. **C.** Coronal FLAIR: Mildly hyperintense mass with areas of cystic component and moderate surrounding edema. **D.** Axial DWI: Hyperintense mass. **E.** Axial ADC: Hypointense mass with reduced diffusion due to hypercellularity. **F.** Coronal ADC: Hypointense mass with reduced diffusion due to hypercellularity.

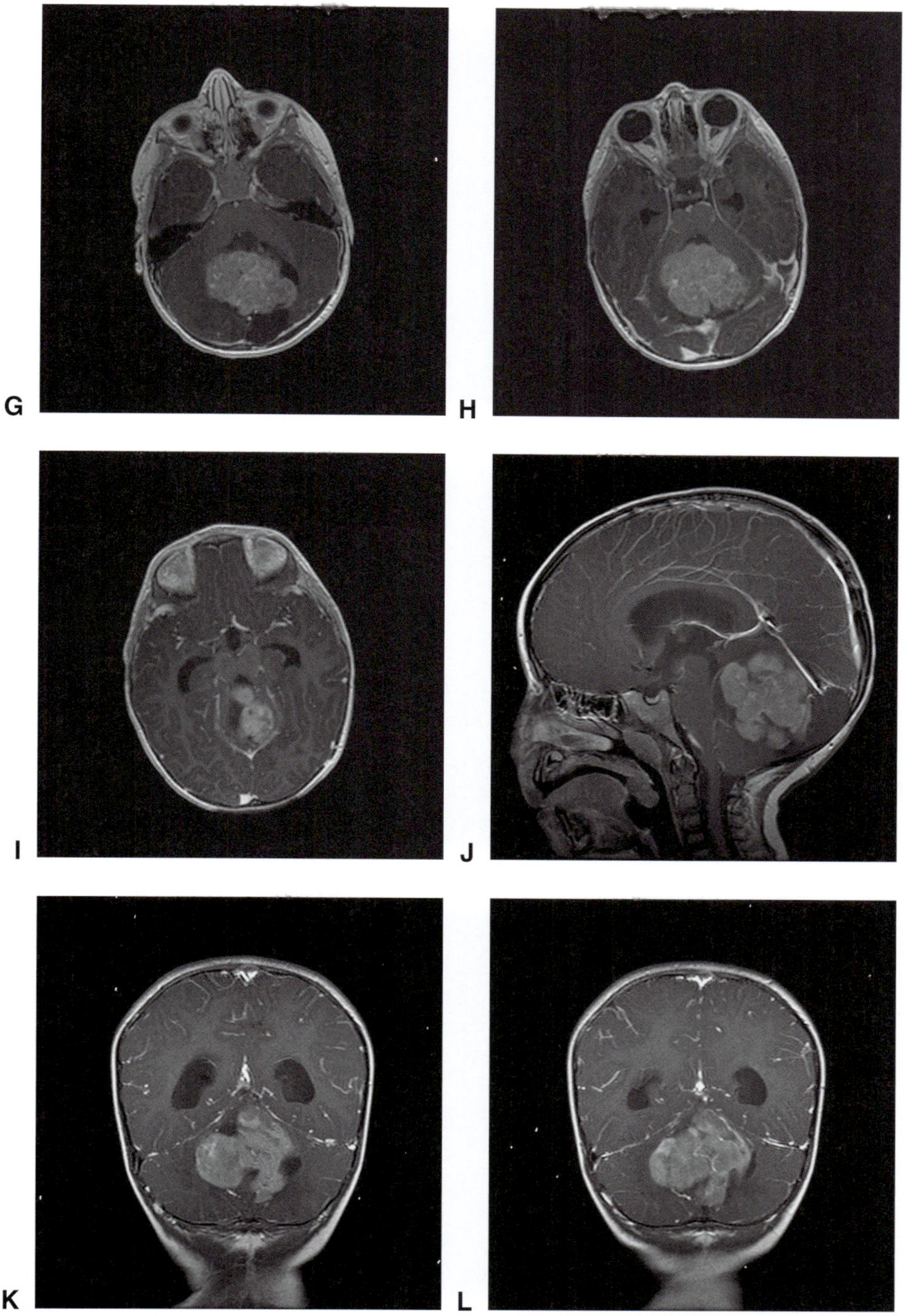

Figure 11.3. ***(continued)*** **G–I.** Axial T1 postcontrast: Avid enhancement of the dominant solid tumor with small peripheral cystic components. **J.** Sagittal T1 postcontrast: Multilobular contour of the mass with avid enhancement. **K–L.** Coronal T1 postcontrast: Multilobular contour of the mass with avid enhancement with small peripheral cystic components.

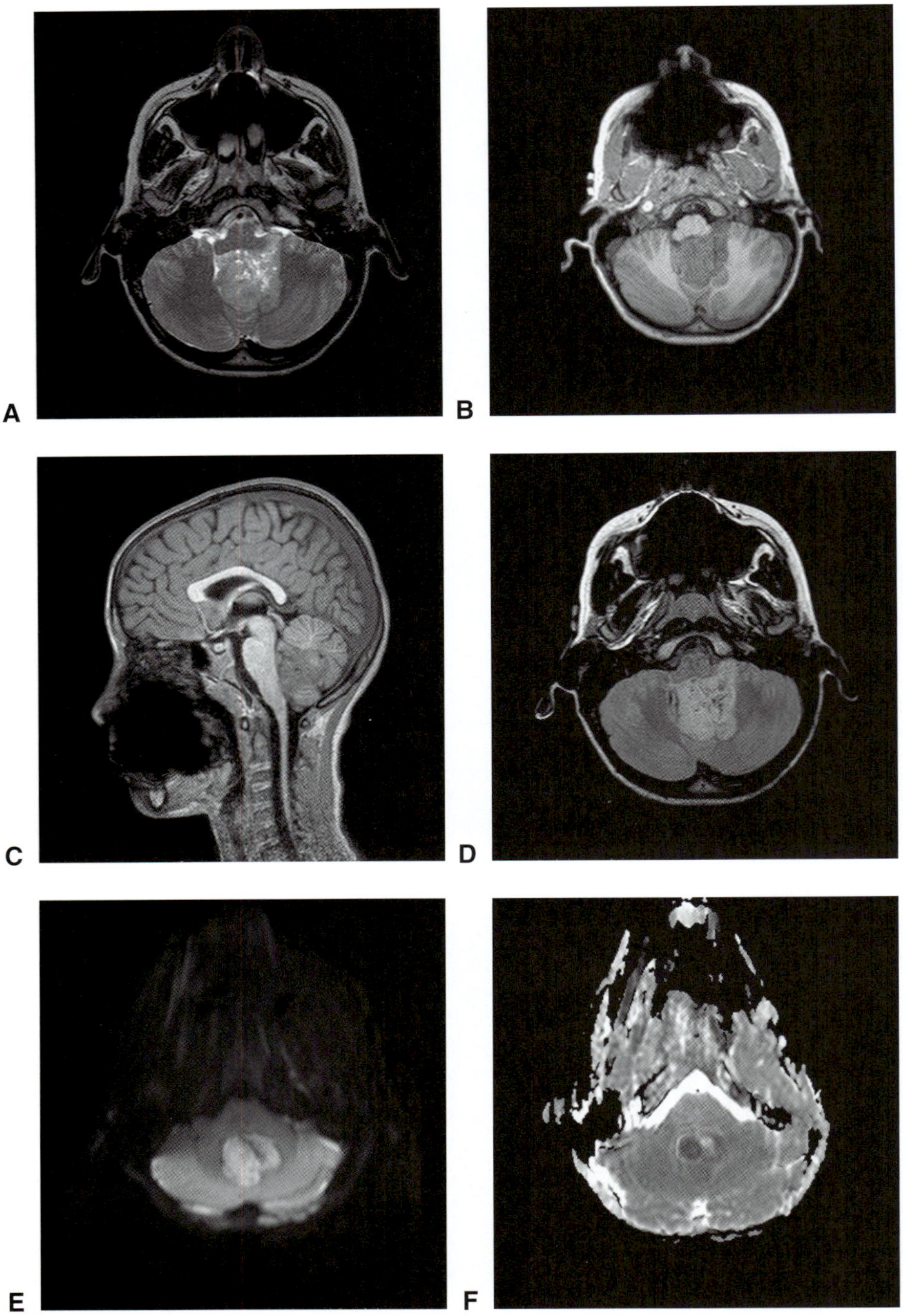

Figure 11.4. Imaging of medulloblastoma, non-WNT/non-SHH-activated, group 4. A. Axial T2: Heterogeneously and slightly hyperintense mass. **B.** Axial T1 precontrast: Hypointense midline mass extending to the foramen Luschka. **C.** Sagittal T1 precontrast: Hypointense midline mass filling the fourth ventricle. **D.** Axial FLAIR: Heterogeneously hyperintense mass extending to the foramen Luschka. **E.** Axial DWI: Hyperintense mass with central area of hypointensity within the cystic component. **F.** Axial ADC: Reduced diffusion within the solid component.

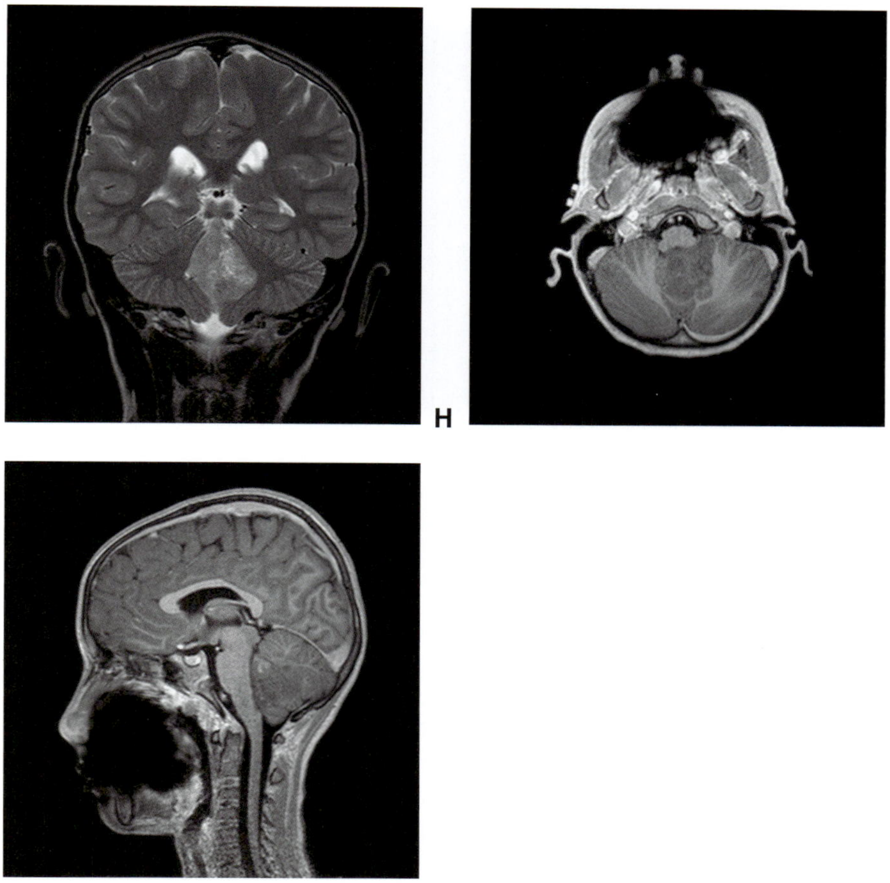

G H I

Figure 11.4. ***(continued)*** **G.** Coronal T2: Heterogeneously and slightly hyperintense mass. **H.** Axial T1 postcontrast: Minimal to absent enhancement within the mass. **I.** Sagittal T1 postcontrast: Small area of enhancement within the superior aspect of the mass.

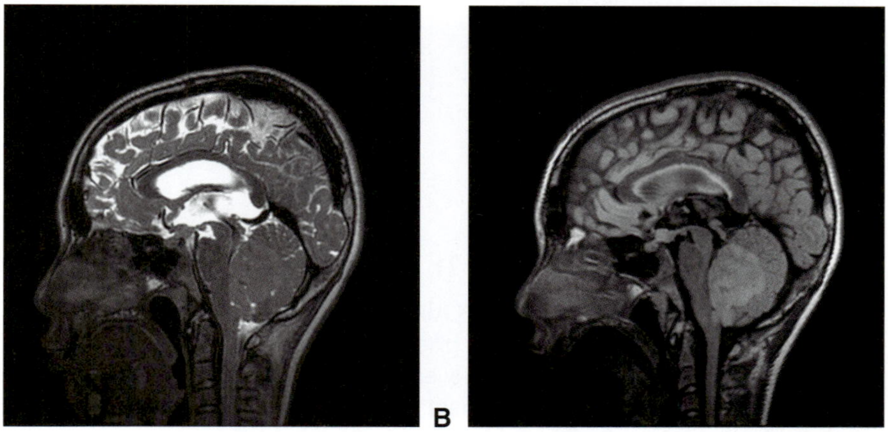

A B

Figure 11.5. **Imaging of disseminated medulloblastoma, group 4. A.** Sagittal T2: Heterogeneously hypointense mass. **B.** Sagittal FLAIR: Heterogeneously hyperintense mass.

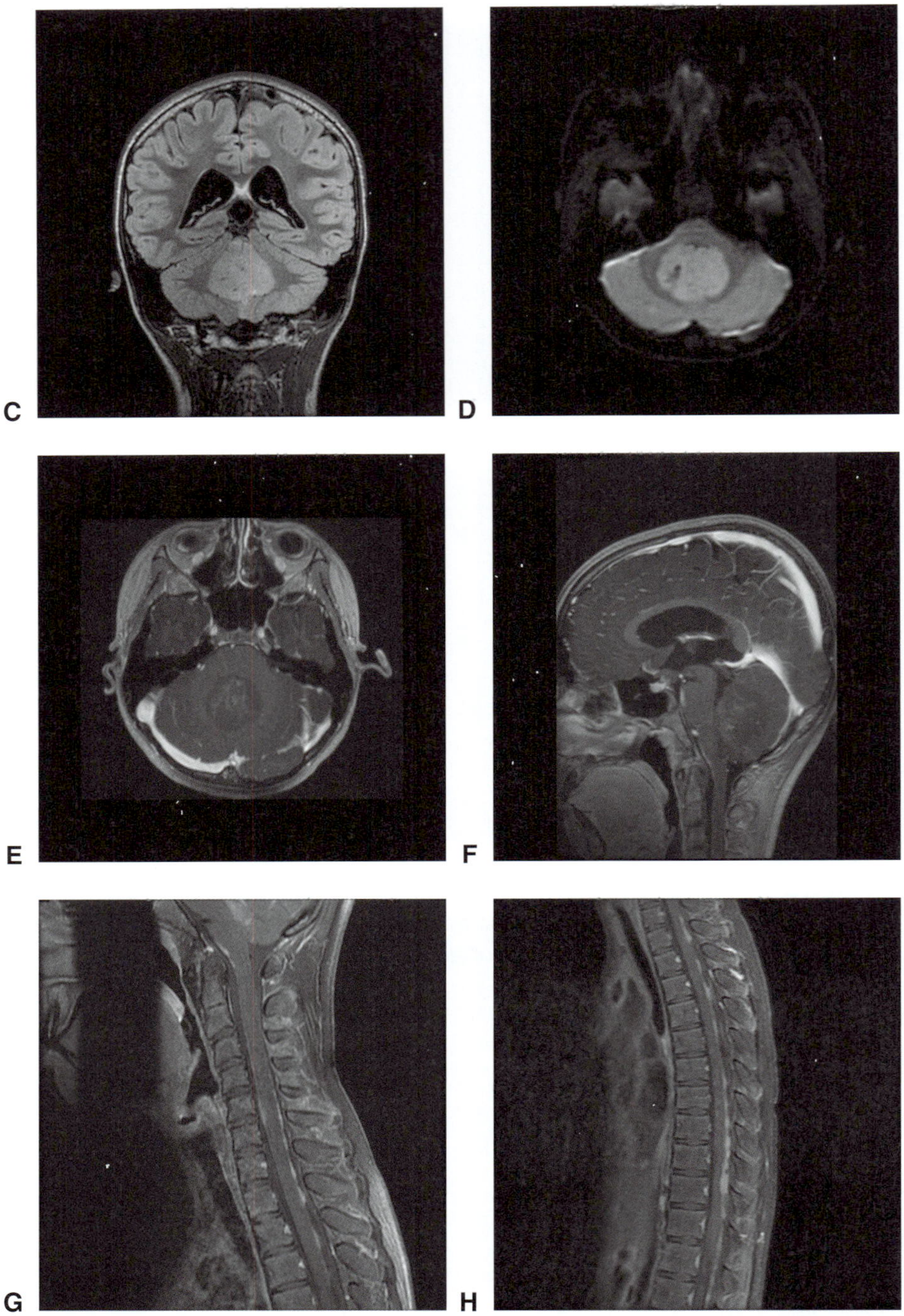

Figure 11.5. ***(continued)*** **C.** Coronal FLAIR: Heterogeneously hyperintense mass. **D.** Axial DWI: Homogeneously reduced diffusion except in small cystic area on the right. **E.** Axial T1 postcontrast: Mild patchy enhancement within the tumor. **F.** Sagittal T1 postcontrast: Mild patchy enhancement mostly within the anterior aspect of the tumor. **G.** Sagittal T1 postcontrast, cervical spine: Multifocal pial enhancement coating the ventral medulla and spinal cord, especially the dorsal surface. **H.** Sagittal T1 postcontrast, thoracic spine.

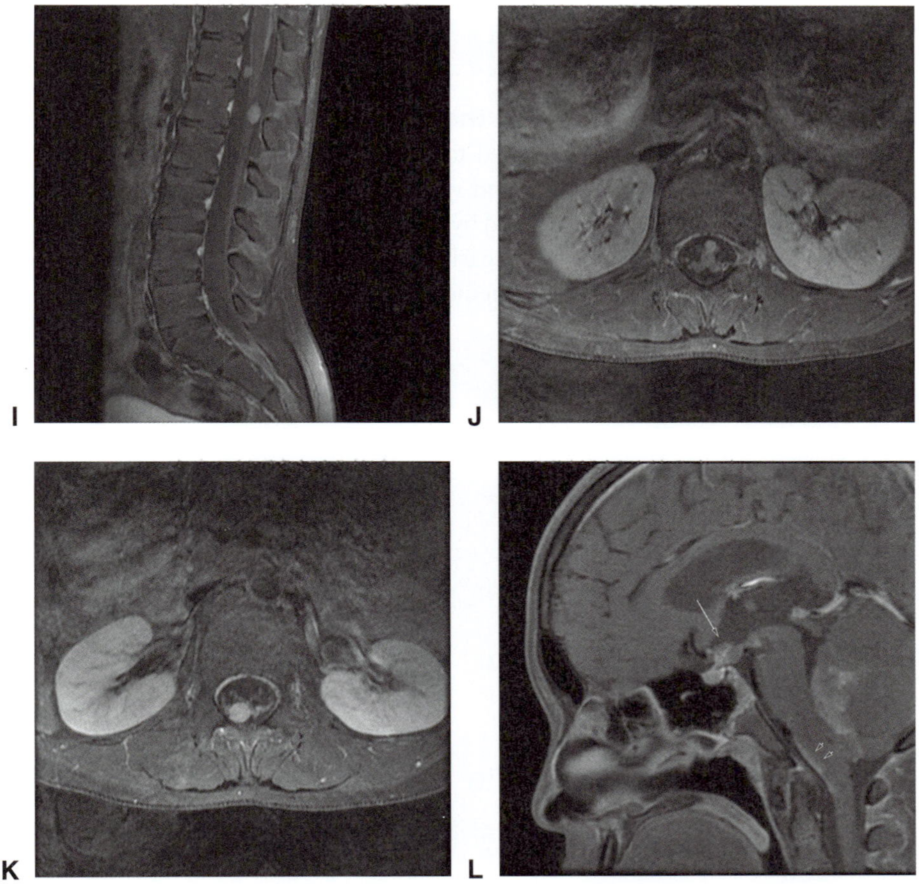

Figure 11.5. ***(continued)*** **I.** Sagittal T1 postcontrast, lumbar spine. **J.** Axial T1 post-contrast: Enhancing nodule on the ventral pial surface of distal conus medullaris. **K.** Axial T1 postcontrast: Enhancing nodule on the dorsal pial surface of the right nerve root of cauda equine. **L.** Sagittal T1 postcontrast, delayed imaging: Suprasellar mildly enhancing nodule (long arrow) and leptomeningeal enhancement along the ventral medullar (short arrows).

Embryonal Tumor with Multilayered Rosettes, C19MC-altered

Definition: Embryonal tumor with multilayered rosettes, C19MC-altered, is a malignant pediatric CNS embryonal tumor in young children with multilayered rosettes and amplification of the C19MC locus at chromosome 19q13.42.

Epidemiology: The exact incidence is unclear due to its rarity, but ETMR affects infants and young children, usually <4 years, with unknown gender predilection.

Molecular and genetic profile: C19MC-altered in chromosome 19q13.42 locus is seen.

Clinical features and standard therapy: Cerebral hemispheric lesions usually present with symptoms related to mass effect or seizure, whereas cerebellar lesions present with nausea and vomiting and symptoms of downward herniation. Surgical resection followed by radiation therapy is the current practice. Proton therapy has shown some early encouraging results but is not curative. Currently, there is no effective chemotherapy.

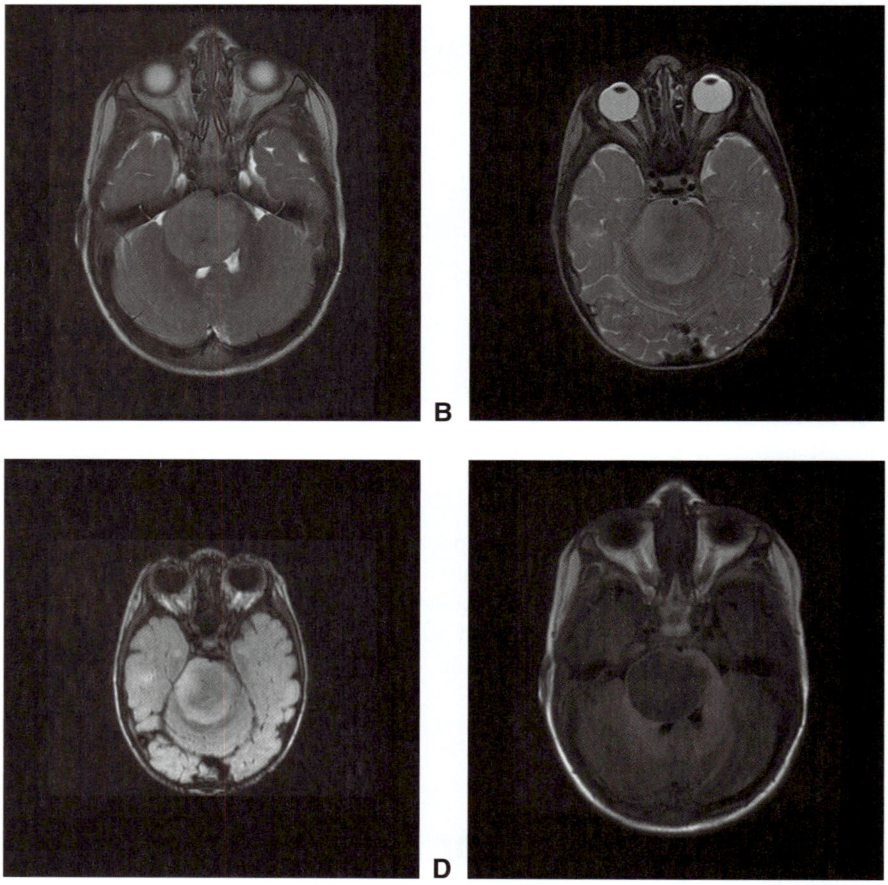

Figure 11.6. Imaging of embryonal tumor with multilayered rosettes. A. Axial T2: Homogeneously isointense pontine mass. **B.** Axial T2: Marked expansion of upper pons by the mass. **C.** Axial FLAIR: Heterogeneously hyperintense mass. **D.** Axial DWI: Mildly hyperintense mass.

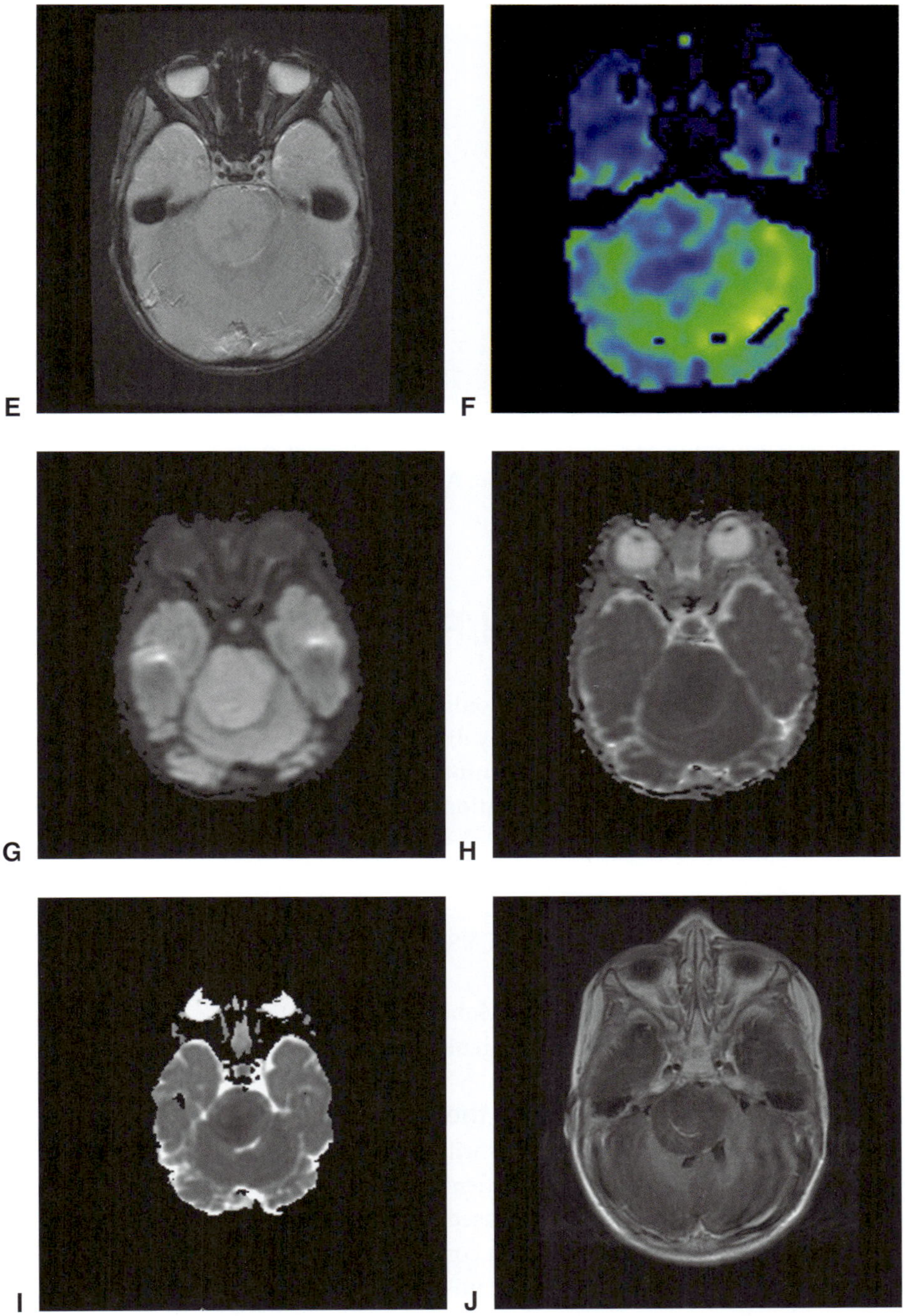

Figure 11.6. ***(continued)*** **E.** Axial ADC: Mildly hypointense mass. **F.** Axial ADC: Mildly hypointense mass. **G.** Axial T1 precontrast: Homogeneously hypointense mass. **H.** Axial T1 precontrast: Homogeneously hypointense mass. **I.** Axial SWI: Minimal susceptibility signal within the mass. **J.** Axial T1 postcontrast: Minimal central curvilinear enhancement within the mass.

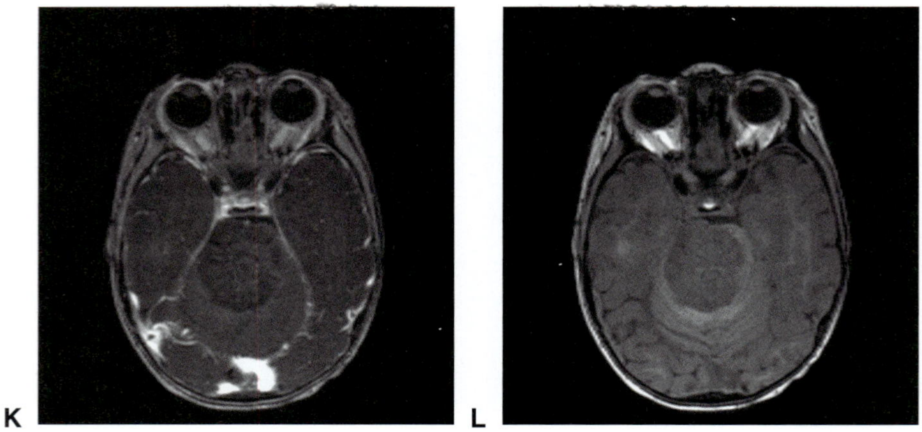

Figure 11.6. ***(continued)*** **K.** Axial T1 postcontrast: Minimal to absent enhancement within the superior aspect of the mass. **L.** Arterial spin labeling (ASL) perfusion: No hyperperfusion within the mass.

▶ Atypical Teratoid/Rhabdoid Tumor

Definition: Atypical teratoid/rhabdoid tumor (ATRT) is a malignant CNS embryonal tumor composed of poorly differentiated or primitive cells of polyphenotypic differentiation along neuroectodermal, epithelial, mesenchymal lines, and rhabdoid cells with inactivation of *SMARCB1* (*INI1*).

Epidemiology: ATRTs account for 1% to 2% of all pediatric brain tumors, but they are extremely rare in adult patients. In children <3 years, AT/RTs are estimated to account for >10% of all CNS tumors in infants.

Molecular and genetic profile: Mutation or loss of the *SMARCB1* locus at chromosome 22q11.2 is the defining genetic hallmark.

Clinical features and standard therapy: The presenting symptoms are variable and nonspecific, but patients with posterior fossa ATRT often present with nausea, vomiting, and ataxia. Patients with supratentorial ATRT can present with signs and symptoms of increased intracranial pressure, hydrocephalus, head tilt, and cranial nerve palsy, most commonly sixth and seventh nerve paresis. The use of radiation therapy remains controversial, especially for patients younger than 3 years of age due to CNS toxicity as a function of dose and younger age at the time of irradiation. Chemotherapy regimen includes doxorubicin, cyclophosphamide, vincristine, ifosfamide, cisplatin, etoposide, and methotrexate. Although not curative, trimodality therapy comprised of surgical resection, chemotherapy, and radiation therapy improves clinical outcomes, especially in younger patients with ATRT.

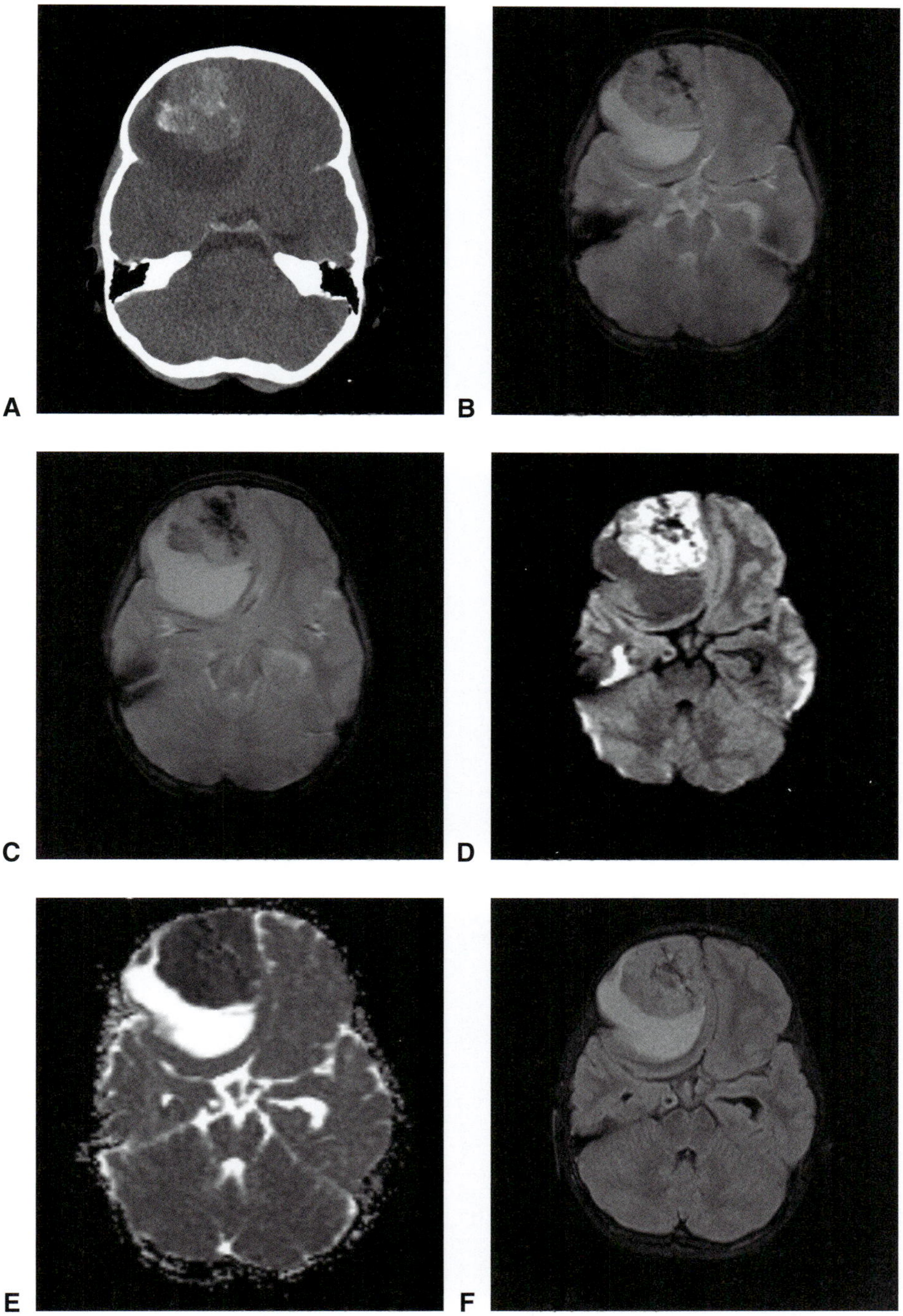

Figure 11.7. Imaging of atypical teratoid/rhabdoid tumor, supratentorial brain. **A.** Axial CT: Partially calcified right inferior frontal mass with prominent posterolateral cystic component. **B.** Axial SWI: Partially calcified right inferior frontal mass with prominent posterolateral cystic component. **C.** Axial SWI: Partially calcified right inferior frontal mass with prominent posterolateral cystic component. **D.** Axial DWI: Hyperintense signal within the solid component. **E.** Axial ADC: Reduced diffusion within the solid component. **F.** Axial FLAIR: Heterogeneously isointense solid tumor and hyperintense cystic component.

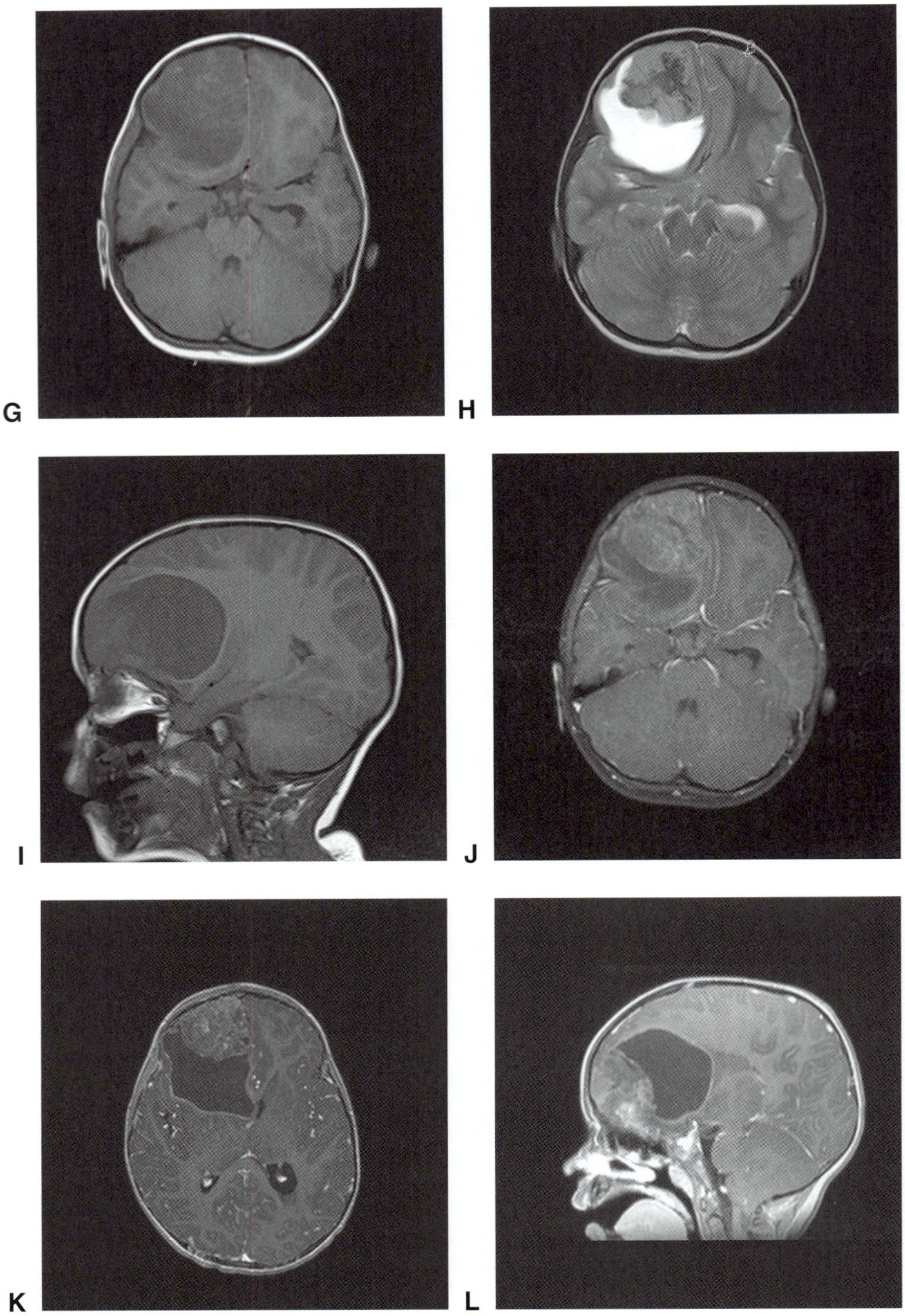

Figure 11.7. ***(continued)*** **G.** Axial T1 precontrast: Heterogeneously isointense solid tumor. **H.** Axial T2: Heterogeneously isointense solid tumor. **I.** Sagittal T1: Heterogeneously isointense solid tumor with prominent posterior cystic component. **J.** Axial T1 postcontrast: Heterogeneously enhancement within the solid tumor and thin rim enhancement of cystic component. **K.** Axial T1 postcontrast: Heterogeneously enhancement within the solid tumor and thin rim enhancement of cystic component. **L.** Sagittal T1 postcontrast: Heterogeneously enhancement within the solid tumor and thin rim enhancement of cystic component.

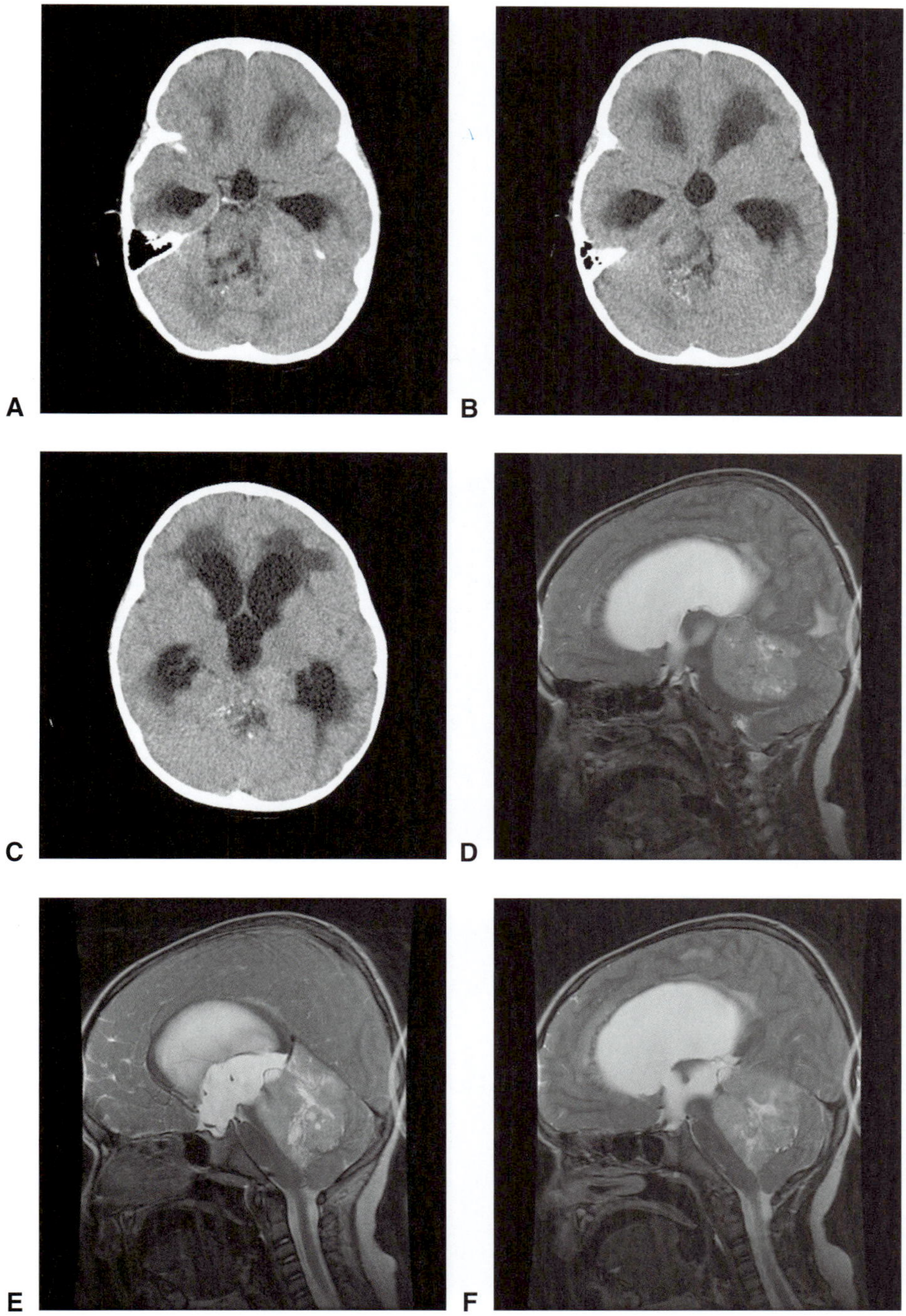

Figure 11.8. Imaging of atypical teratoid/rhabdoid tumor, posterior fossa. A–C. Axial CT: Heterogeneous mixed density midline posterior fossa mass. **D–F.** Sagittal T2: Heterogeneously isointense mass with internal areas of hyperintensity.

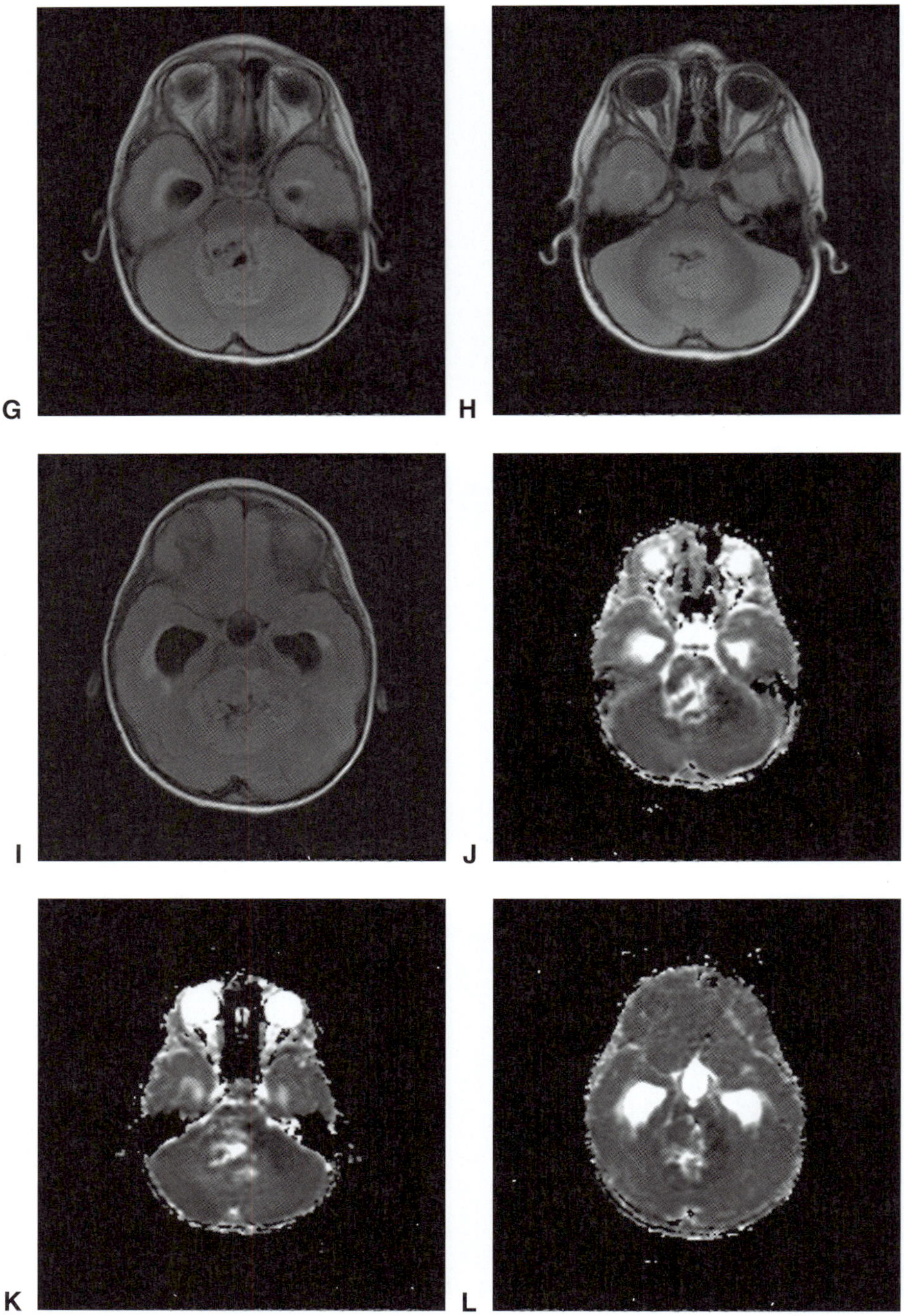

Figure 11.8. *(continued)* **G–I.** Axial FLAIR: Heterogeneously hyperintense mass with internal areas of hypointensity. **J–L.** Axial ADC: Peripheral areas of reduced diffusion.

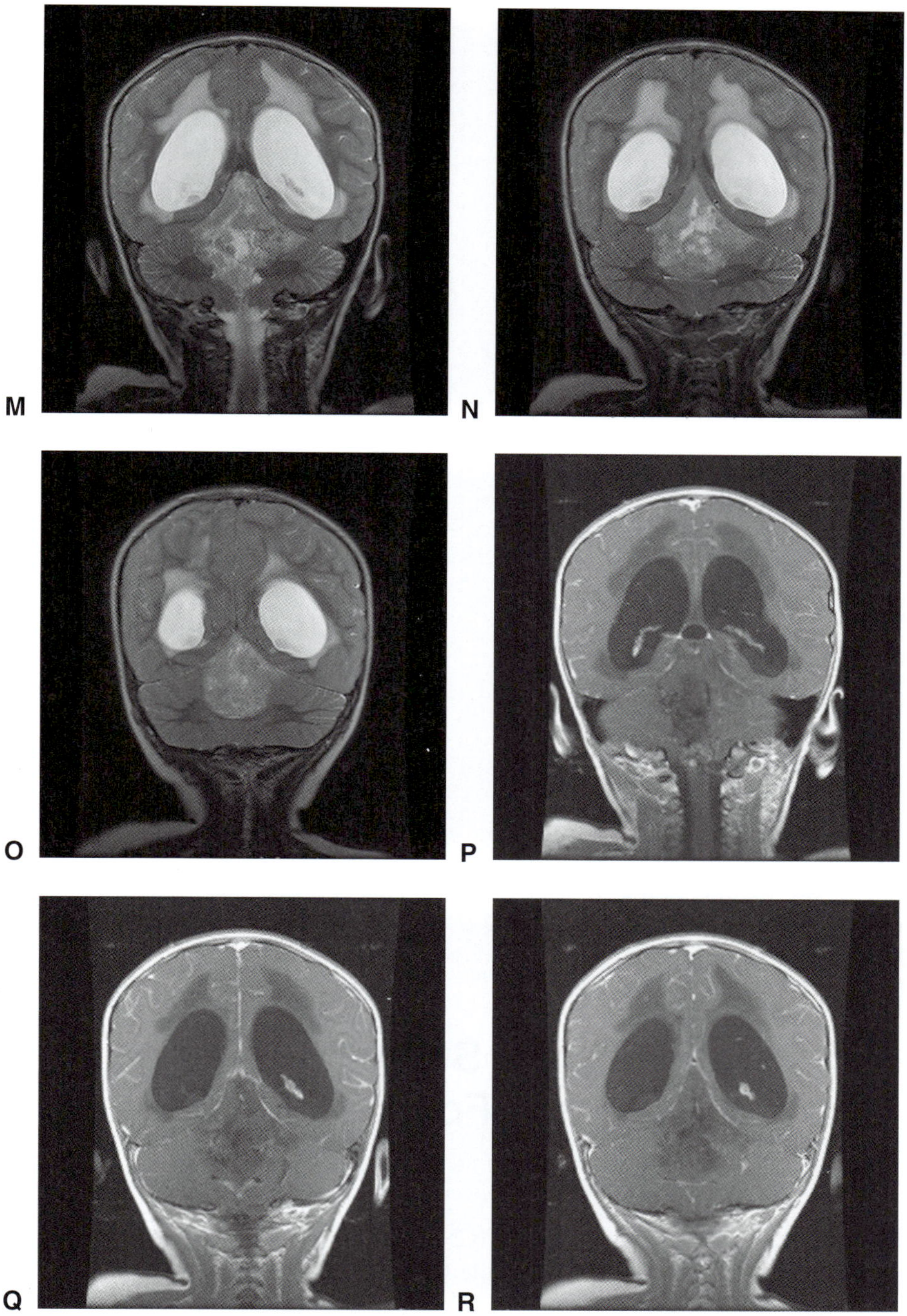

Figure 11.8. ***(continued)*** **M–O.** Coronal T2: Heterogeneously isointense mass with internal areas of hyperintensity. **P–R.** Coronal T1 postcontrast: Minimal enhancement within the mass and obstructive hydrocephalus.

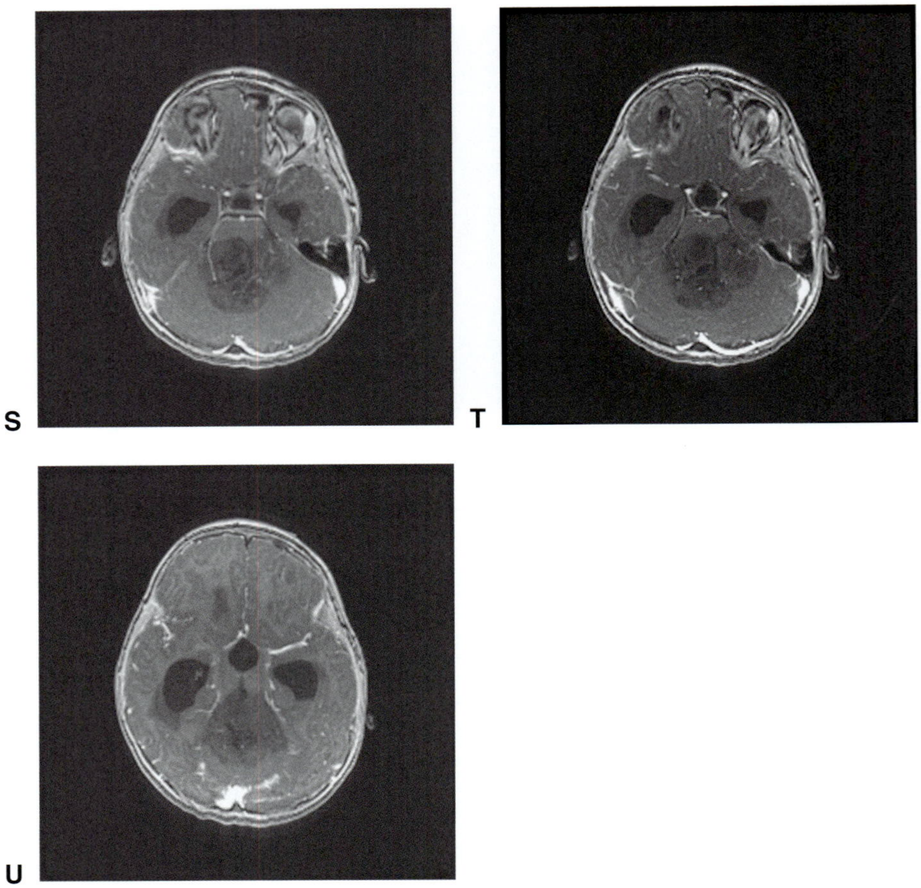

Figure 11.8. ***(continued)*** **S–U.** Axial T1 postcontrast: Minimal enhancement within the mass and obstructive hydrocephalus.

Central Nervous System Neuroblastoma, Forkhead Box R2 Activated

Definition: Central nervous system (CNS) neuroblastoma, forkhead box R2 (*FOXR2*) activated, is a rare high-grade CNS embryonal tumor composed of poorly differentiated neuroepithelial cells with high cellularity, groups of neurocytic cells, and variable occurrence of ganglion cells and without glial component.

Epidemiology: The exact incidence is unknown due to sparse literature on primary CNS neuroblastomas, but they primarily affect infants and young children, with unknown gender predilection; they can occur at both the intraventricular and the parenchymal locations.

Molecular and genetic profile: Activation of *FOXR2*, a transcription factor identified as a putative oncogene, is the genetic hallmark of CNS neuroblastoma.

Clinical features and standard therapy: Patients with CNS neuroblastoma present with signs and symptoms related to mass effect, midline shift, and increased intracranial pressure. Surgical debulking with an attempt at gross total resection followed by radiation therapy is the accepted practice. Currently, there is no effective chemotherapy. High rates of local recurrence have been reported.

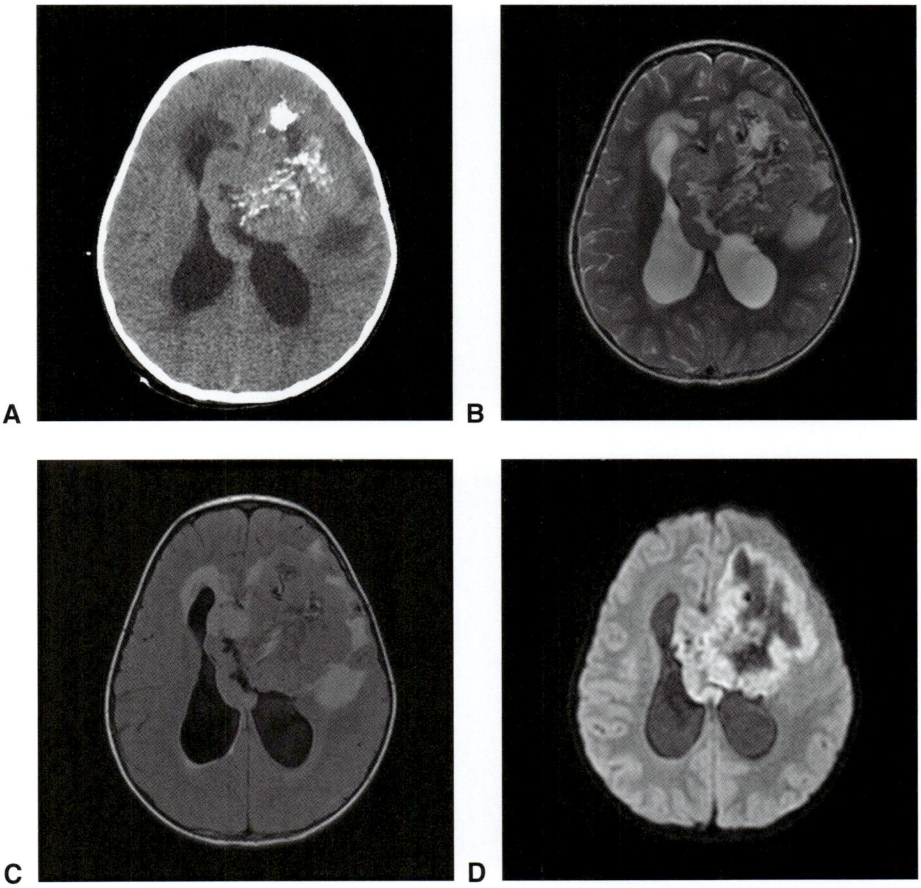

Figure 11.9. Imaging of CNS neuroblastoma, *FOXR2* activation. A. Axial CT: Large lobulated mass with prominent intratumoral areas of calcification. **B.** Axial T2: Heterogeneous isointense and hyperintense mass with areas of necrosis prominent intratumoral vessels. **C.** Axial FLAIR: Heterogeneous isointense and hyperintense mass with areas of necrosis prominent intratumoral vessels. **D.** Axial DWI: Hyperintense signal within the deep medial and peripheral parts of the tumor.

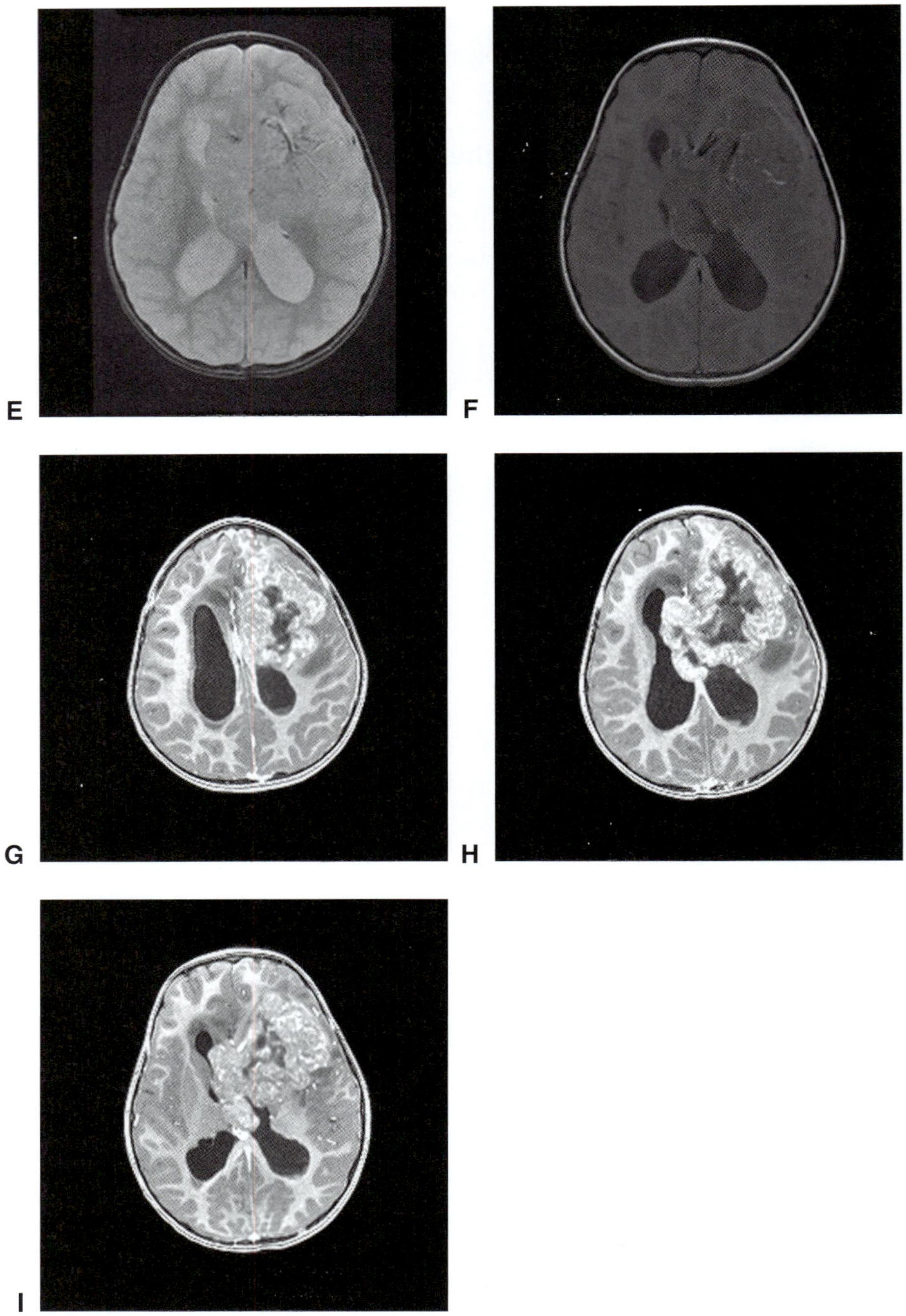

Figure 11.9. ***(continued)*** **E.** Axial gradient recalled echo (GRE): Mild susceptibility signal. **F.** Axial T1 precontrast: Heterogeneously hypointense mass. **G–I.** Axial T1 postcontrast: Avid enhancement within the deep medial and peripheral parts of the tumor and prominent central necrosis.

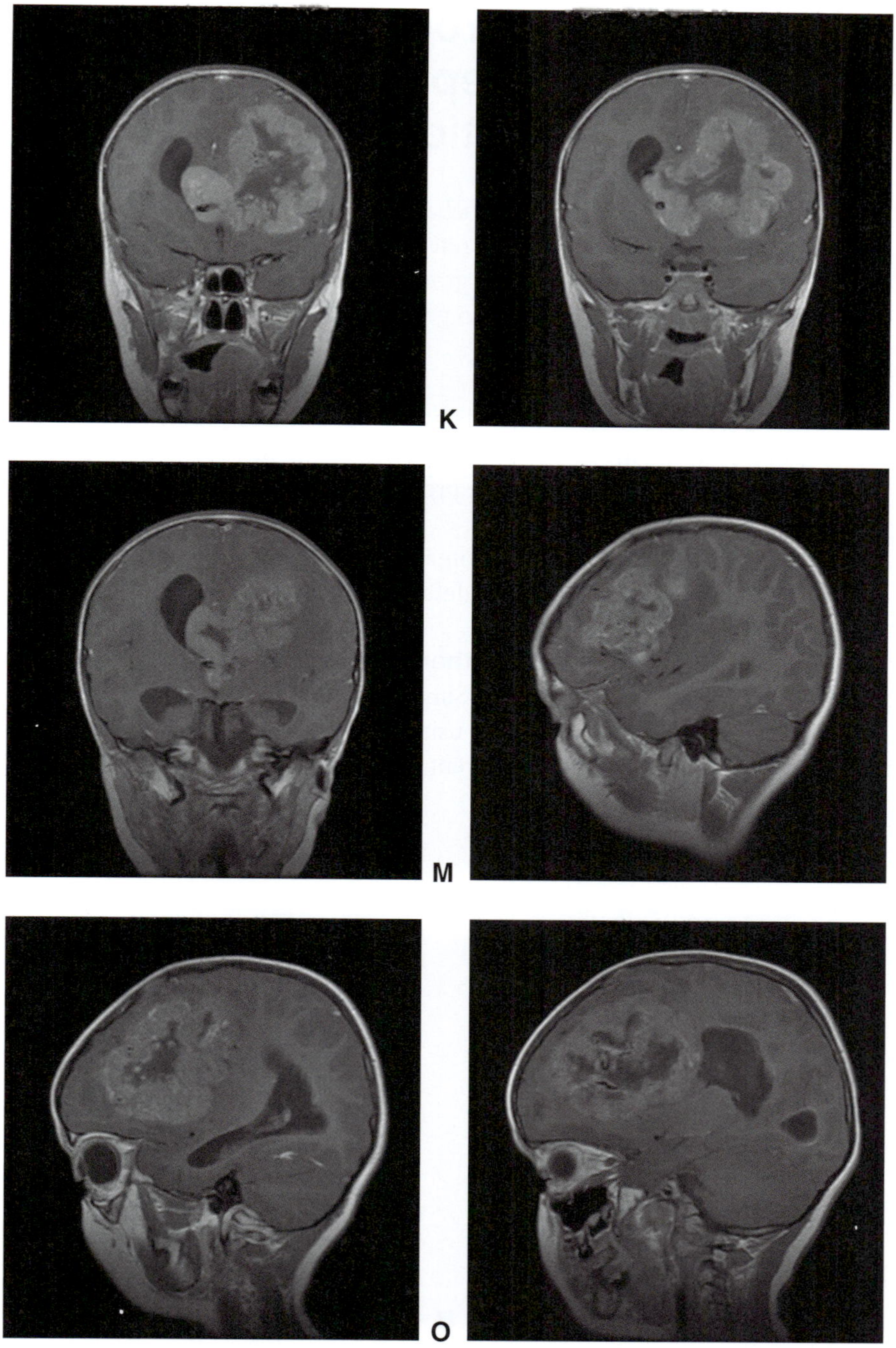

J K L M N O

Figure 11.9. ***(continued)*** **J–L.** Coronal T1 postcontrast: Avid enhancement within the deep medial and peripheral parts of the tumor and prominent central necrosis. **M–O.** Sagittal T1 postcontrast: Avid enhancement within the deep medial and peripheral parts of the tumor and prominent central necrosis.

High-Grade Neuroepithelial Tumor with BCL-6 Co-repressor Internal Tandem Duplication

Definition: High-grade neuroepithelial tumor with BCL-6 co-repressor (BCOR) internal tandem duplication refers to a highly malignant neuroepithelial tumor affecting the pediatric age group with distinct molecular mutations in *BCOR* gene, a co-repressor of *BCL6* gene, most commonly occurring in the posterior fossa.

Epidemiology: The tumor primarily affects infants and young children and rarely young adults, with an age range of 7 months to 22 years and a reported mean age of 5.5 years with slight male predominance.

Molecular and genetic profile: Somatic internal tandem duplication in the C-terminus, exon 15, of BCOR is the defining genetic marker.

Clinical features and standard therapy: Gait and balance disturbances, head tilt, cranial neuropathy are seen. Surgical debulking followed by radiotherapy and combination chemotherapies using methotrexate, vincristine, thiotepa, and stem cell transplantation are current practice, but overall clinical outcome remains poor.

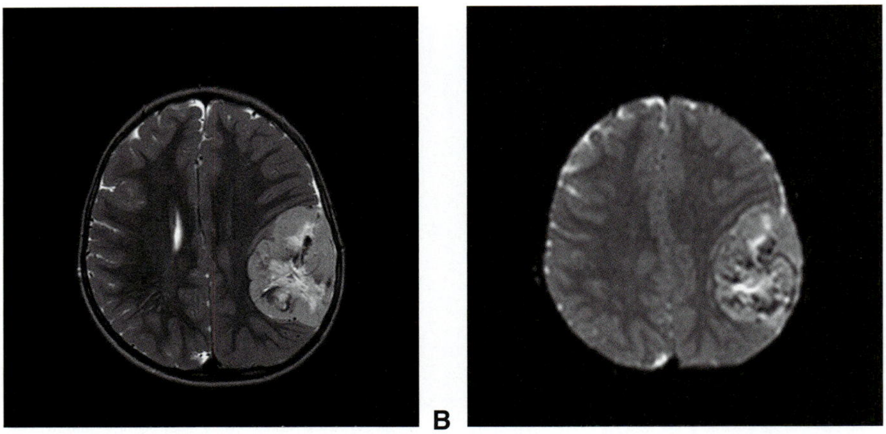

A B

Figure 11.10. Imaging of HGNET-BCOR-ITD, four different patients. A–C. Left frontal lobe. **A.** Axial T2: Heterogeneously hyperintense circumscribed mass. **B.** Axial ADC: Mildly reduced diffusion.

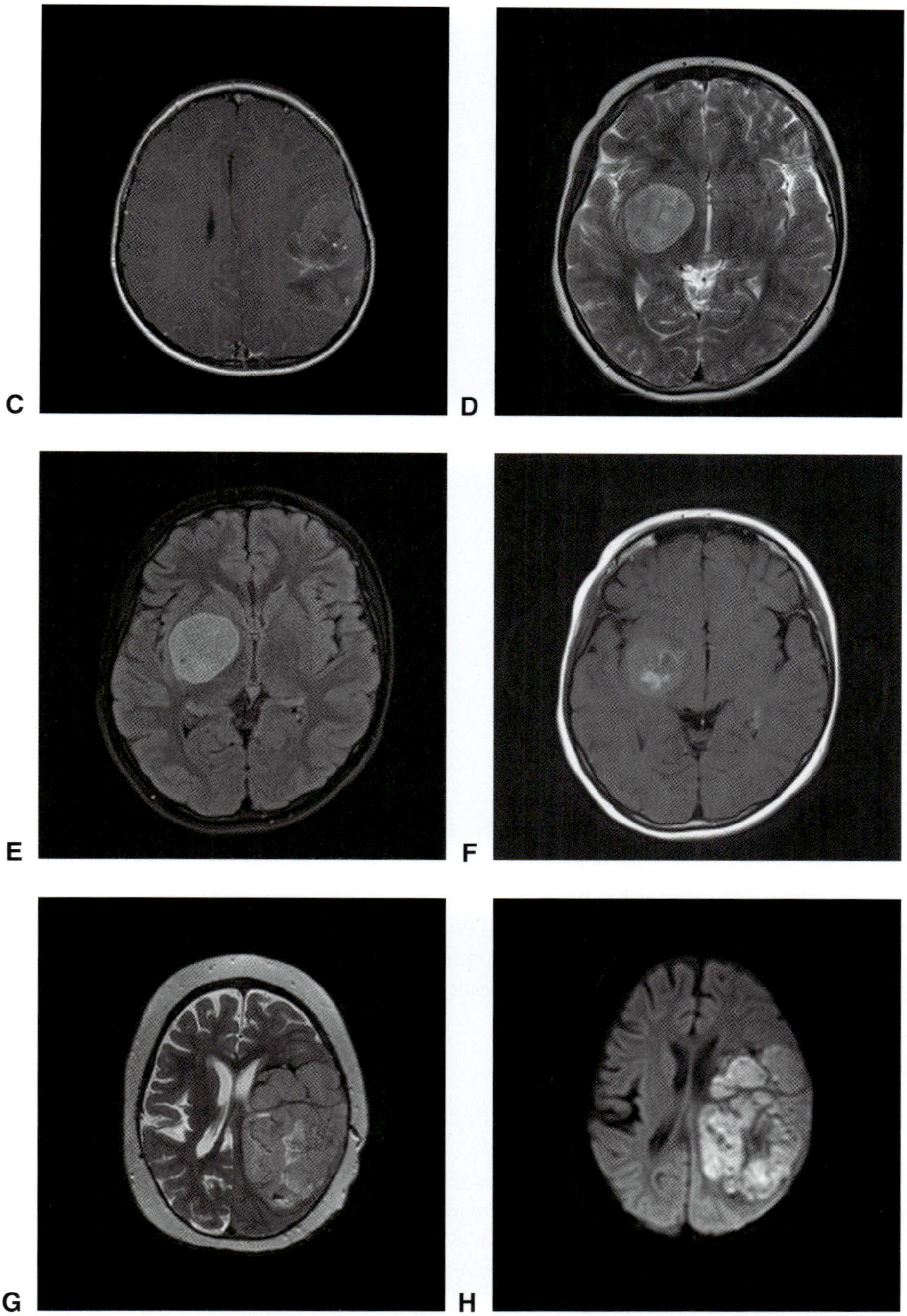

Figure 11.10. ***(continued)*** **C.** Axial T1 postcontrast: Mild heterogeneous enhancement. **D–F.** Right basal ganglia. **D.** Axial T2: Heterogeneously hyperintense circumscribed mass. **E.** Axial DWI: Mildly reduced diffusion. **F.** Axial T1 postcontrast: Mild heterogeneous enhancement. **G–I.** Left frontal lobe. **G.** Axial T2: Heterogeneously hyperintense circumscribed mass. **H.** Axial DWI: Reduced diffusion.

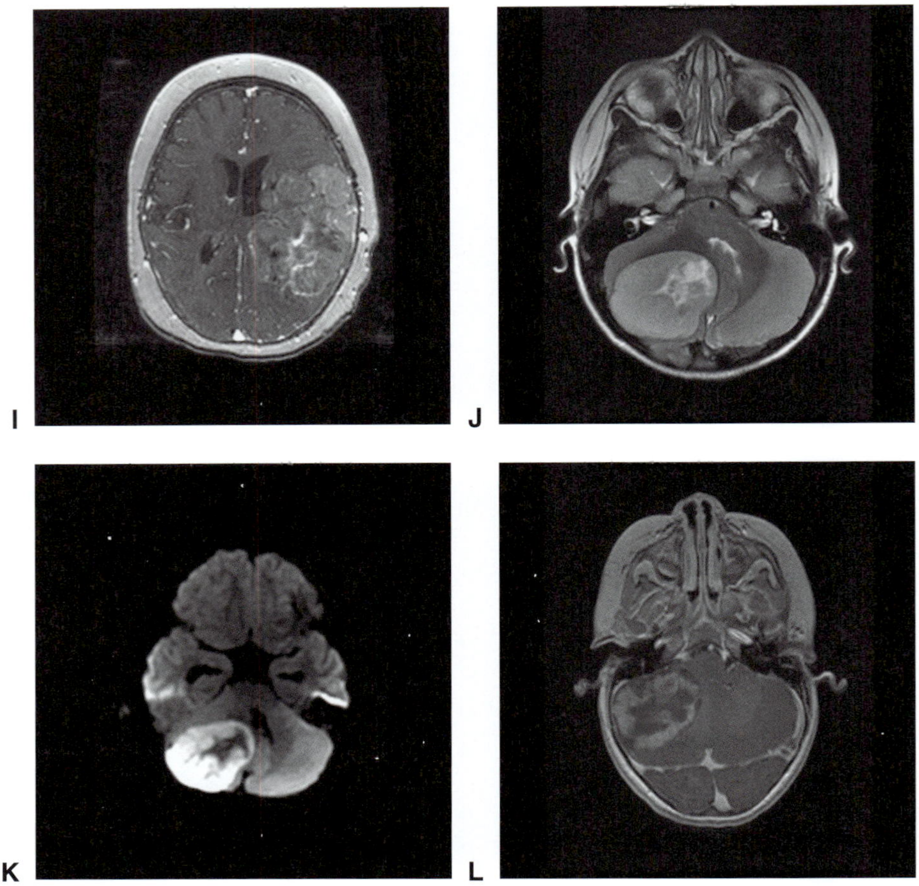

Figure 11.10. ***(continued)*** **I.** Axial T1 postcontrast: Mild heterogeneous enhancement. **J–L.** Right cerebellum. **J.** Axial T2: Heterogeneously hyperintense circumscribed mass with medial cystic component. **K.** Axial DWI: Prominent reduced diffusion in the solid tumor. **L.** Axial T1 postcontrast: Avid and nodular enhancement of the outer margin of tumor.

Bibliography

Ferris SP, Vega JV, Aboian M, et al. High-grade neuroepithelial tumor with BCOR exon 15 internal tandem duplication-a comprehensive clinical, radiographic, pathologic, and genomic analysis. *Brain Pathol.* 2020;30:46–62.

Juraschka K, Taylor MD. Medulloblastoma in the age of molecular subgroups: as review. *J Neurosurg Pediatr.* 2019;24:353–363.

Lambo S, von Hoff K, Korshunov A, et al. ETMR: a tumor entity in its infancy. *Acta Neuropathol.* 2020;140:249–266.

Lastowska M, Trubicka J, Sobocinska A, et al. Molecular identification of CNS NB-*FOXR2*, CNS EFT-CIC, CNS HGNET-MN1 and CNS HGNET-BCOR pediatric brain tumors using tumor-specific signature genes. *Acta Neuropathol Commun.* 2020;8:105.

Pei Y-C, Huang G-H, Yao X-H, et al. Embryonal tumor with multilayered rosettes, C19MC-altered: a newly defined pediatric brain tumor. *Int J Clin Exp Pathol.* 2019;12:3156–3163.

Perreault S, Ramaswamy V, Achrol AS, et al. MRI surrogates for molecular subgroups of medulloblastoma. *Am J Neuroradiol AJNR.* 2014;35:1263–1269.

Poh B, Koso H, Momota H, et al. Foxr2 promotes formation of CNS-embryonal tumors in a Trp53-deficient background. *Neuro Oncol.* 2019;21:993–1004.

Quinn TJ, Almahariq MF, Siddiqui AZ, et al. Trimodality therapy for atypical teratoid/rhabdoid tumor is associated with improved overall survival: A surveillance, epidemiology, and end results analysis. *Pediatr Blood Cancer.* 2019;66:e27969.

Shih R, Koeller KK. Embryonal tumors of the central nervous system: From the radiologic pathology archives. *Radiographics.* 2018;38:525–541

Sturm D, Orr BA, Toprak UH, et al. New brain tumor entities emerge from molecular classification of CNS-PNETs. *Cell.* 2016;164:1060–1072.

12 Diffuse Astrocytic and Oligodendroglial Tumors

Overview

Diffuse astrocytic and oligodendroglial tumors are diffuse gliomas comprising astrocytomas; oligodendrogliomas are the most common primary parenchymal neoplasms of the brain. The World Health Organization (WHO) classification is continuously being updated, and the latest version in 2016 included several molecular and genetic markers in the diagnosis and grading of diffuse gliomas. Krebs cycle enzymes isocitrate dehydrogenases (IDHs) 1 and 2 fundamentally changed the way diffuse gliomas are classified, studied, and treated. ATRX, a chromatin remodeling protein whose main function is the deposition of the histone variant H3.3, is a marker of diffuse astrocytoma, whereas chromosome 1p19q codeletion is a defining marker of diffuse oligodendroglioma. Diagnostic algorithms using a few genetic markers (*IDH*, *ATRX*, and chromosome 1p19q codeletion) brought robust and reproducible results that correlate with clinical outcomes in patients with diffuse glioma and how these tumors are understood and ushered in the era of new integrated molecular diagnostics. However, despite remarkable advances in multiple fronts, including neuropathological and neuroimaging diagnostics, neurosurgical technique, radiation therapy, and chemotherapy, diffuse gliomas remain one of the most challenging tumors to treat and cure effectively, mainly due to their widespread invasiveness, biologic progression, and resistance to therapy.

	Age range (mean)	Female: male ratio	Cell of origin	WHO grade	Molecular/ genetic markers	Prognosis
Diffuse astrocytoma	30–40 (38)	1:1.3	Astrocyte	II, III	*IDH*-mutant, *ATRX*	Guarded
Diffuse oligodendroglioma	35–44 (40)	1:1.5	Oligodendrocyte	II, III	*IDH*-mutant, 1p19q	Favorable to neutral
Glioblastoma	55–85 (64)	1:1.6	Astrocyte	IV	*TERT* mutation, *CDKN2A/N2B* *EGFR*, *PTEN*	Poor
Diffuse midline glioma	5–11 (7)	1:1	Astrocyte	IV	*H3 K27M*-mutant	Poor

Diffuse Astrocytoma

Definition: Diffuse astrocytoma is diffusely infiltrating astrocytoma with a mutation in either the *IDH1* or the *IDH2* gene and the presence of *ATRX* and *TP53* mutation. Gliomatosis cerebri, a type of diffuse astrocytoma but not a distinct WHO entity, is largely a clinicopathologic and an imaging-based diagnosis that implies extensive concurrent involvement of multiple cerebral lobes (at least three) by highly infiltrating diffuse astrocytoma.

Epidemiology: This tumor accounts for up to 15% of all astrocytic brain tumors and roughly 60% of primary parenchymal brain tumors. It affects all ages from childhood to older adults, with substantial increase in incidence with advancing age.

Affected age group: Diffuse astrocytoma affects adults in their mid-30s with the median age of 38 years; slight male predominance is seen.

Molecular and genetic profile: Over 80% of diffuse astrocytomas are either *IDH1* or *IDH2* mutant, >50% are *ATRX* or *TP53* mutant, and none have chromosome 1p19q codeletion.

Clinical features and standard therapy: Clinical symptoms at presentation depend on the location of tumor, but seizure is one of the most common ones followed by insidious or gradual onset of focal neurological deficits such as speech difficulties, motor or sensory or vision changes, and behavioral or personality changes. Some tumors are diagnosed incidentally such as when a head CT is done to assess for traumatic brain injury following a motor vehicle accident. Surgical resection is the first line of therapy to both diagnose and debulk the tumor. Giving adjuvant radiation therapy and chemotherapy depends on the extent of resection, location of tumor, age of the patient, and molecular characteristics of tumor.

Imaging

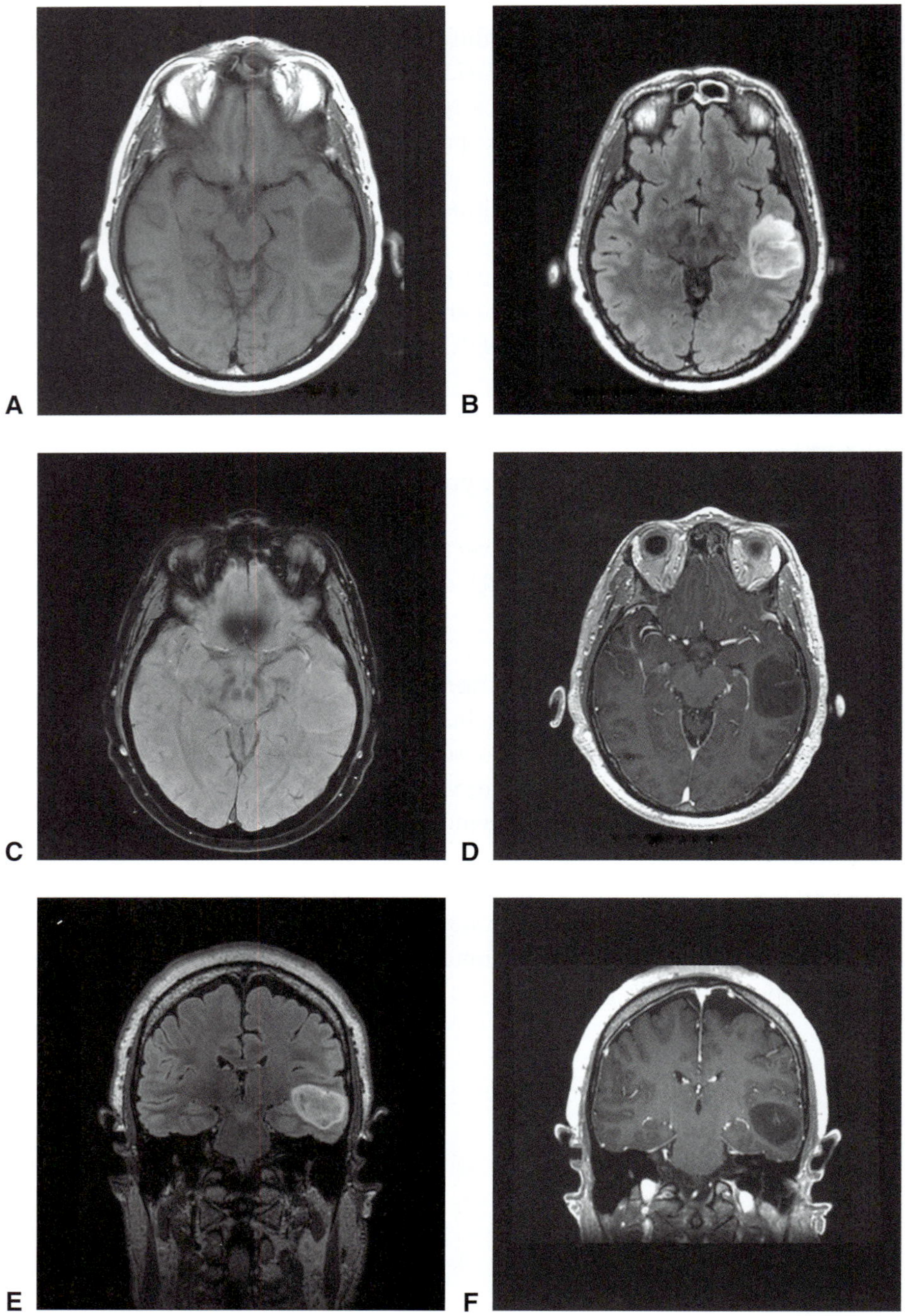

Figure 12.1. **Imaging of diffuse astrocytoma, *IDH-mutant*. A.** Axial T1 precontrast: Hypointense mass. **B.** Axial FLAIR: Heterogeneously hyperintense mass. **C.** Axial susceptibility-weighted imaging (SWI): No underlying blood products or calcium. **D.** Axial T1 postcontrast: No enhancement. **E.** Coronal FLAIR: Circumscribed margin. **F.** Coronal T1 postcontrast: Small vascular but no intratumoral enhancement.

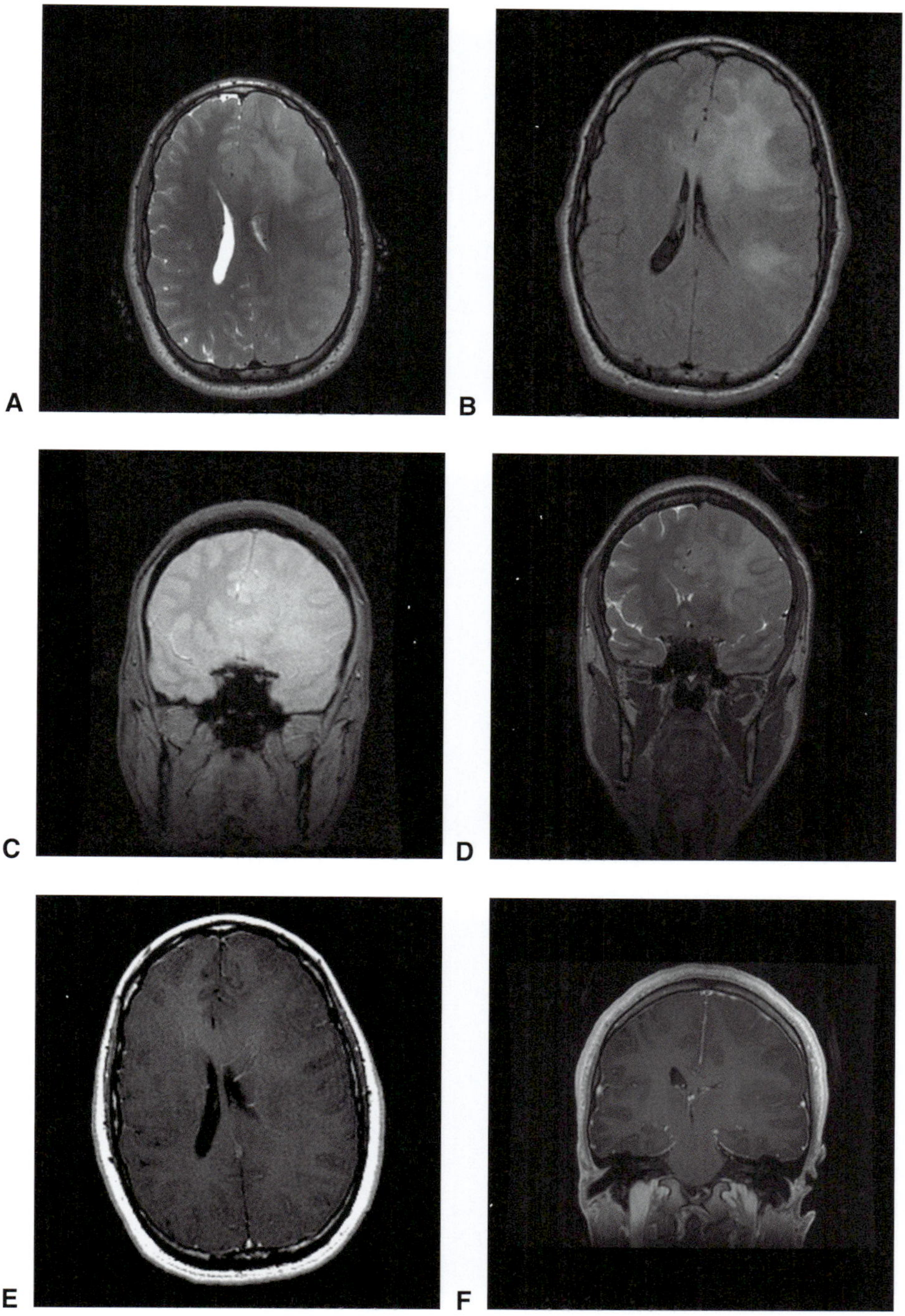

Figure 12.2. Imaging of diffuse astrocytoma, *IDH-mutant*. A. Axial T2: Hyperintense multifocal infiltrative mass. **B.** Axial FLAIR: Hyperintense multifocal infiltrative mass. **C.** Coronal gradient echo: No underlying blood products or calcium. **D.** Coronal T2: Extensive infiltrative pattern. **E.** Axial T1 postcontrast: No enhancement but mass effect on the adjacent ventricle. **F.** Coronal T1 postcontrast: No enhancement but mass effect on the adjacent ventricle.

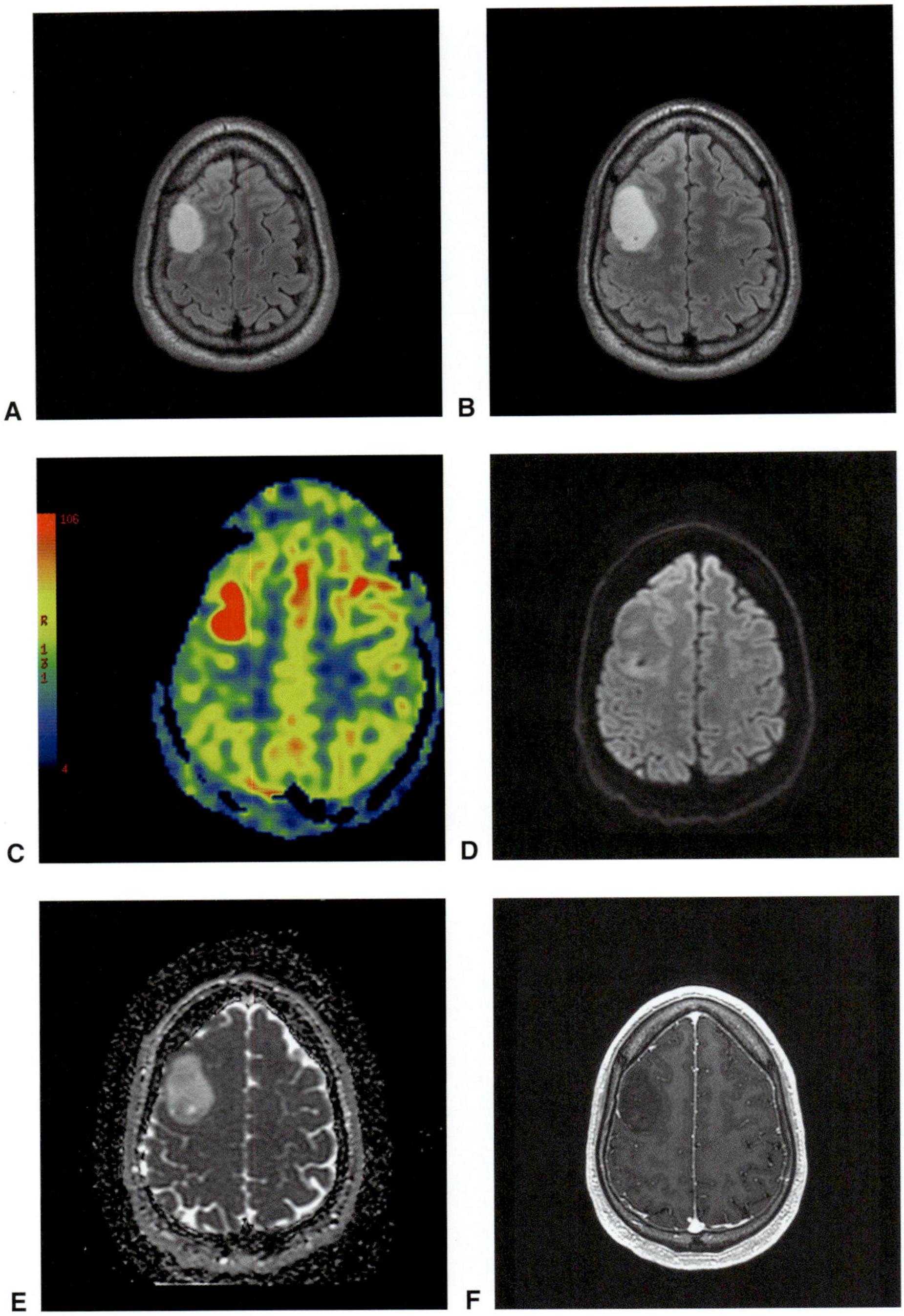

Figure 12.3. Imaging of diffuse anaplastic astrocytoma, *IDH-wildtype*. A. Axial FLAIR: Hyperintense mass with circumscribed margin. **B.** Axial FLAIR: Hyperintense mass with circumscribed margin. **C.** Axial arterial spin labeling (ASL): Hypervascular mass. **D.** Axial diffusion-weighted imaging (DWI): No reduced diffusion. **E.** Axial apparent diffusion coefficient (ADC): No reduced diffusion. **F.** Axial T1 postcontrast: No enhancement.

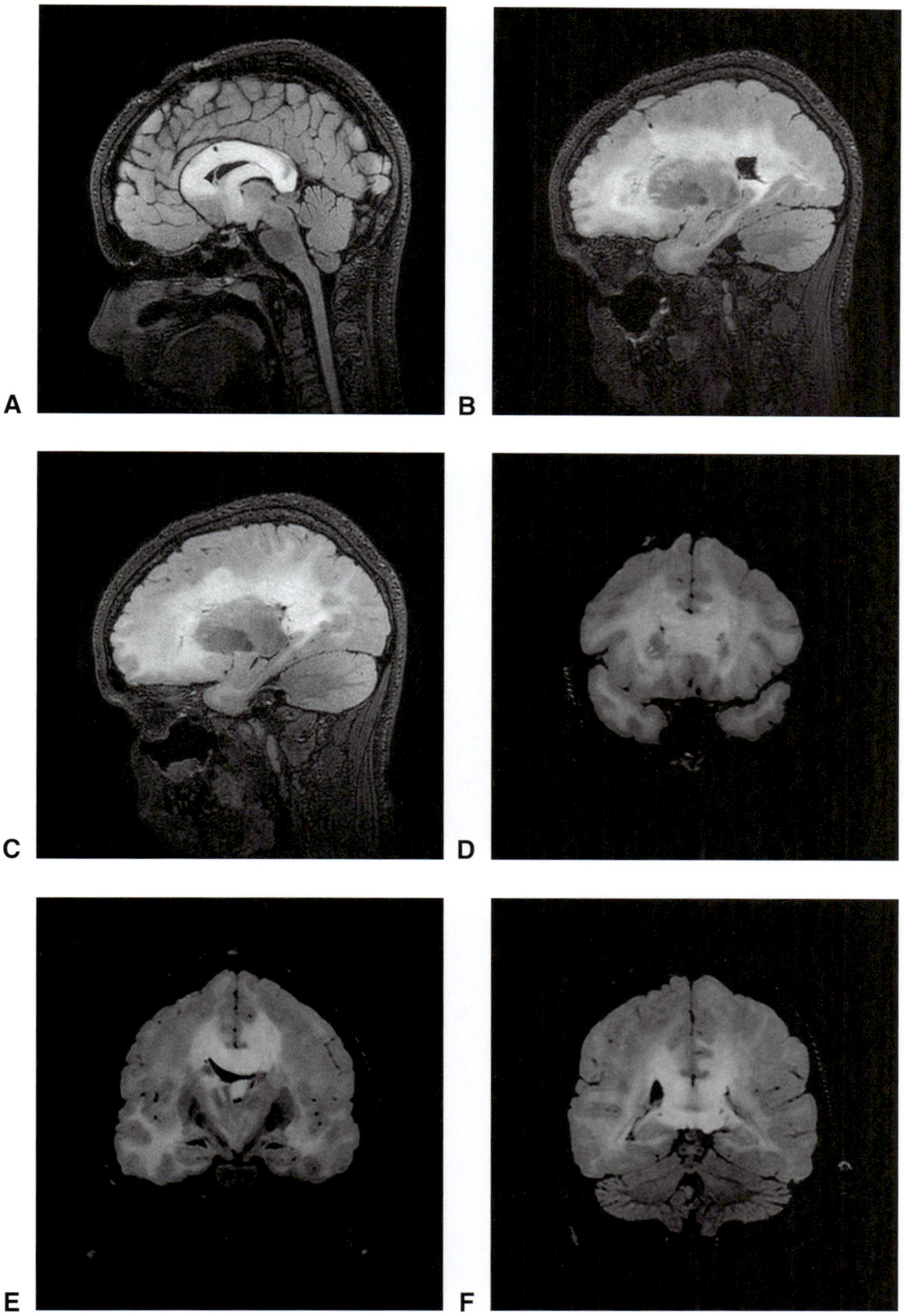

Figure 12.4. Imaging of gliomatosis cerebri, *IDH*-mutant. A–C. Sagittal FLAIR: Diffusely infiltrating hyperintense mass involving the entire corpus callosum and bilateral cerebral hemispheres. **D–F.** Coronal FLAIR: Diffusely infiltrating hyperintense mass involving the entire corpus callosum and bilateral cerebral hemispheres.

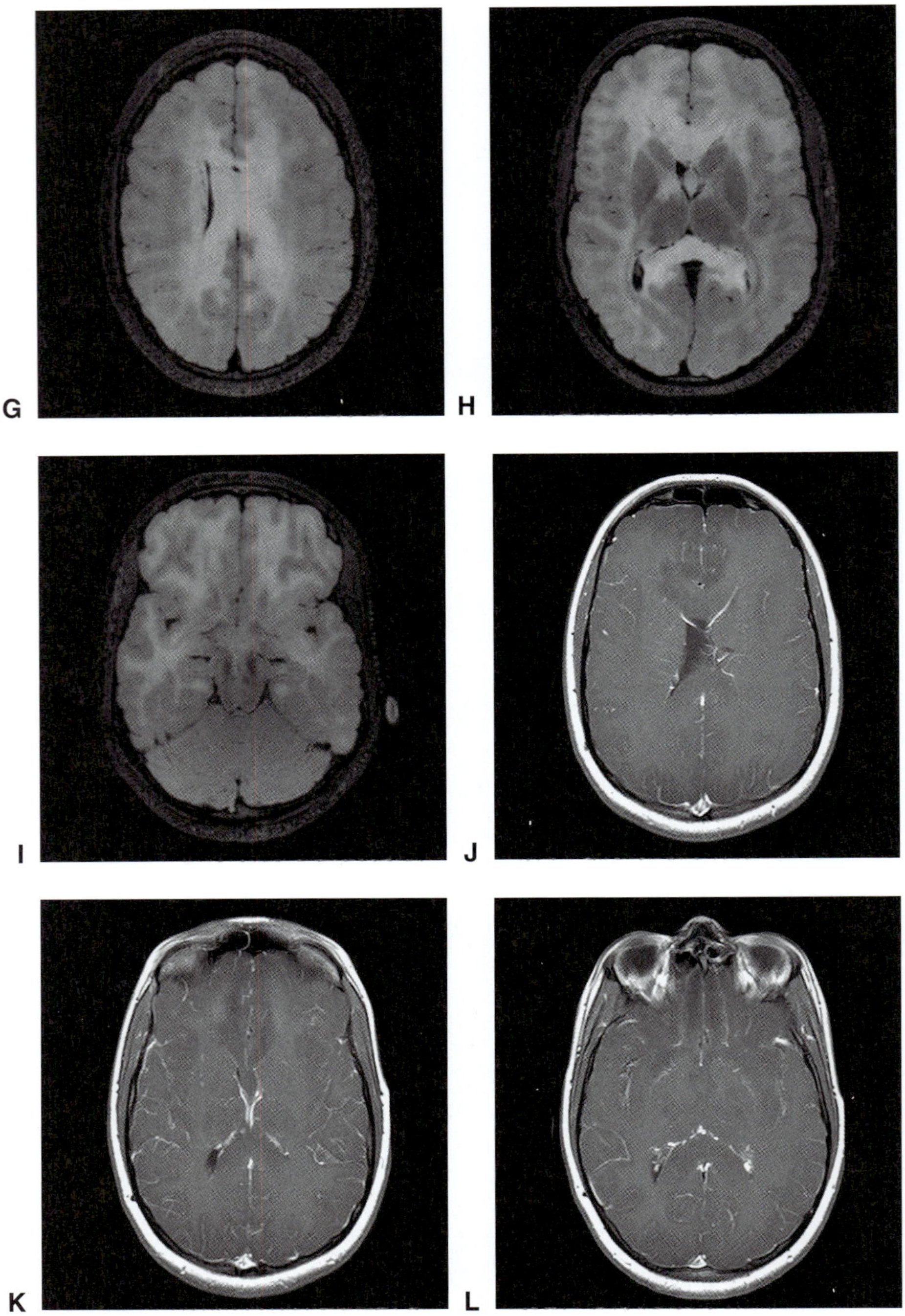

Figure 12.4. ***(continued)*** **G–I.** Axial FLAIR: Diffusely infiltrating hyperintense mass involving the entire corpus callosum and bilateral cerebral hemispheres. **J–L.** Axial T1 postcontrast: No enhancement associated with the diffusely infiltrating mass.

Diffuse Oligodendroglioma

Definition: Diffuse oligodendroglioma is a diffusely infiltrating, slow-growing glioma with *IDH1* or *IDH2* mutation and codeletion of chromosomal arms 1p and 19q comprising tumor cells resembling oligodendrocytes.

Epidemiology: The tumor accounts for ~3% of all primary parenchymal brain tumors and up to 15% of all diffuse gliomas, with a slight increase in incidence over the past 3 decades for yet undefined reasons.

Affected age group: Young to middle-aged adults with a peak incidence in the third and fourth decades is seen; it is distinctly uncommon in children. As with other gliomas, there is slight male predominance.

Molecular and genetic profile: Chromosome losses at 1p and 19q and *IDH* mutation are the defining molecular genetic hallmarks of oligodendroglioma.

Clinical features and standard therapy: Due to their frequent frontal lobe and cortical locations, oligodendrogliomas usually present with seizures in up to two thirds of the patients. Slow, protracted onset focal neurologic deficits can be seen as signs and symptoms of increased intracranial pressure, including headaches, nausea/vomiting, and papilledema.

Imaging

Oligodendrogliomas are a nonenhancing or minimally enhancing, cortically based, expansile mass with frontal lobe predominance and heterogeneously hyperintense on fluid-attenuated inversion recovery (FLAIR) and T2-weighted images with frequent intratumoral cystic components and curvilinear calcium deposits. Anaplastic oligodendrogliomas tend to enhance more with larger areas of cystic or necrotic component, mass effect, and prominent peritumoral edema.

Glioblastoma

Definition: Glioblastoma is the highest grade form (WHO grade IV) of diffuse astrocytoma with histologic hallmarks of microvascular proliferation, nuclear atypia, mitotic activity, and pseudo-pallisading necrosis.

Epidemiology: This tumor is the most common primary parenchymal brain tumor in adults, accounting for up to 20% of all intracranial neoplasms, 50% of all primary brain tumors, and 70% of all diffuse gliomas.

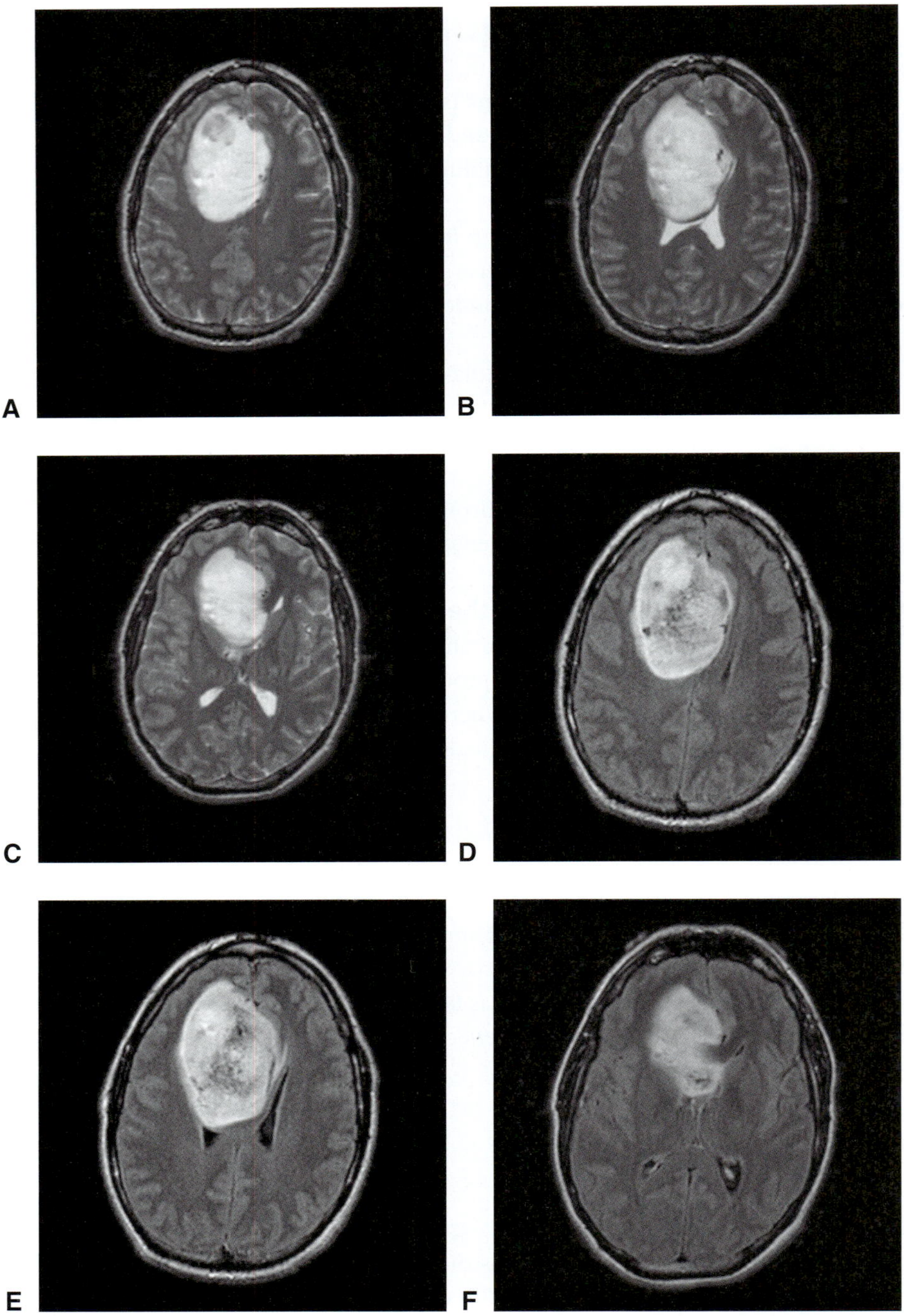

Figure 12.5. Imaging of oligodendroglioma, *IDH-mutant*, *1p19q co-deleted.* **A–C.** Axial T2: Heterogeneously hyperintense mass. **D–F.** Axial FLAIR: Heterogeneously hyperintense mass.

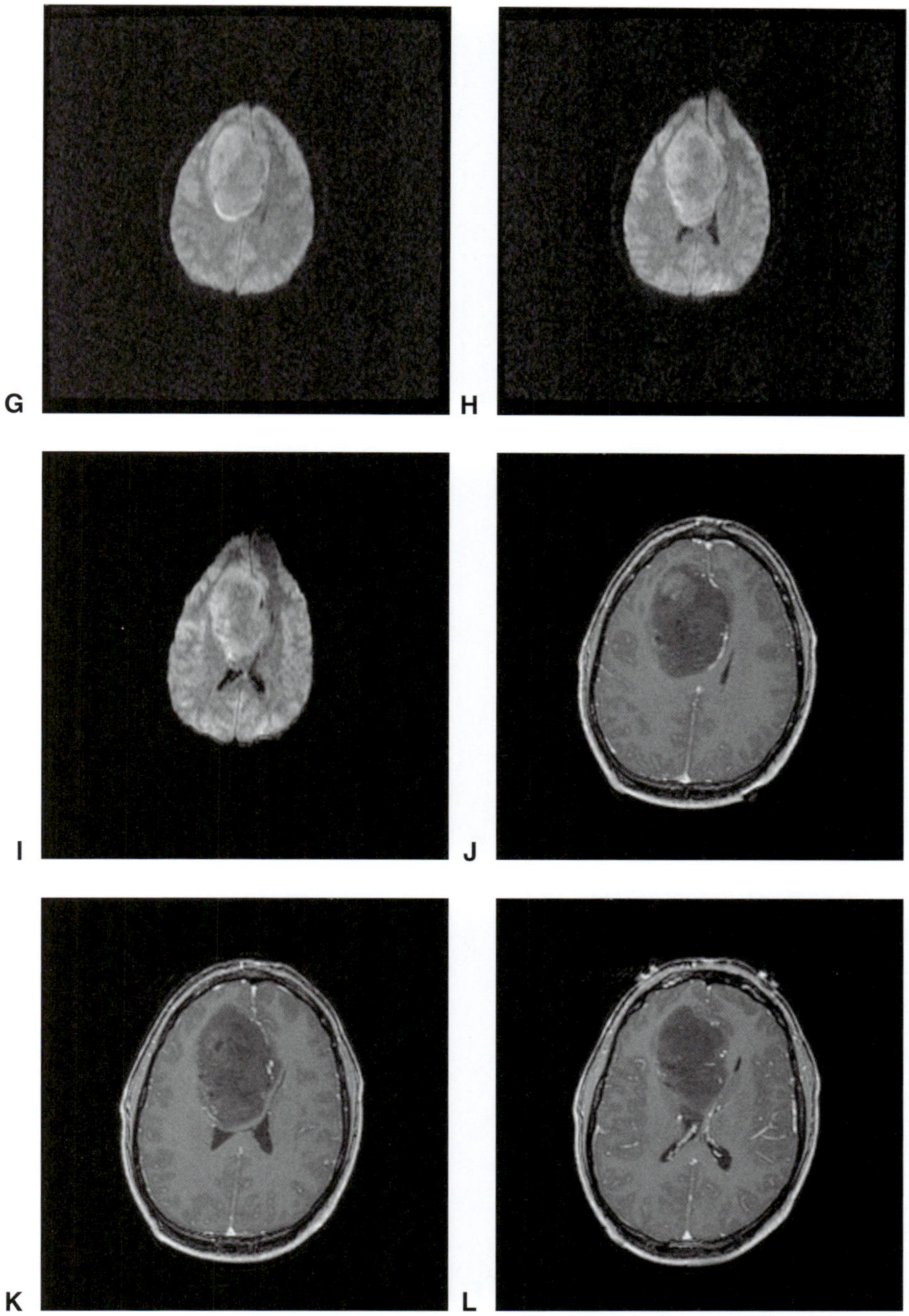

Figure 12.5. ***(continued)*** **G–I.** Axial DWI: Reduced diffusion around the peripheral margin of the mass. **J–L.** Axial T1 postcontrast: No enhancement.

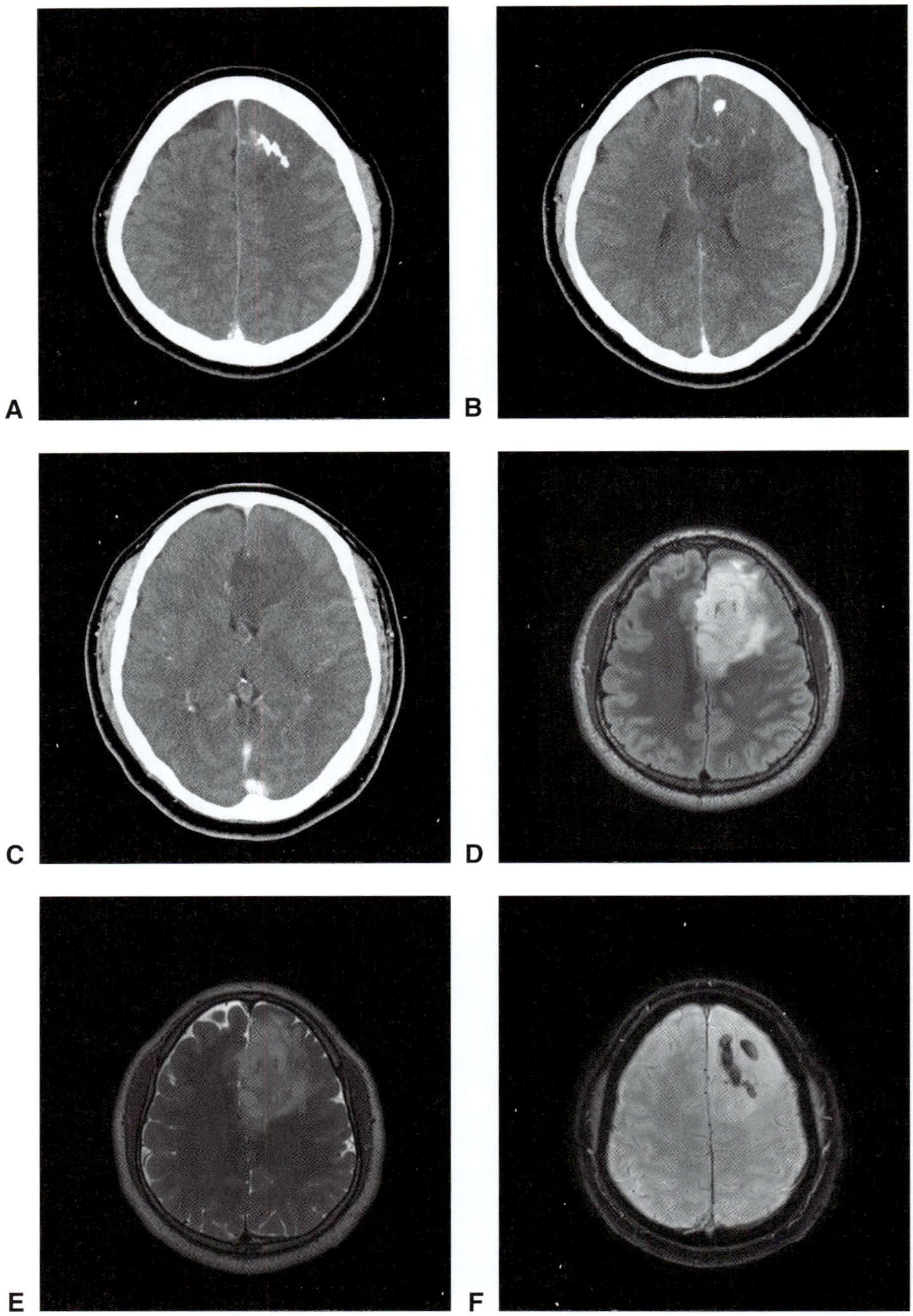

Figure 12.6. Imaging of anaplastic oligodendroglioma, *IDH*-mutant, *1p19q* codeleted. A–C. Axial CT with contrast: Heterogeneously low-density mass with curvilinear coarse calcium. **D.** Axial FLAIR: Heterogeneously hyperintense mass with infiltrative margin. **E.** Axial T2: Heterogeneously hyperintense mass with infiltrative margin. **F.** Axial SWI: Susceptibility corresponding to the calcium component of the mass.

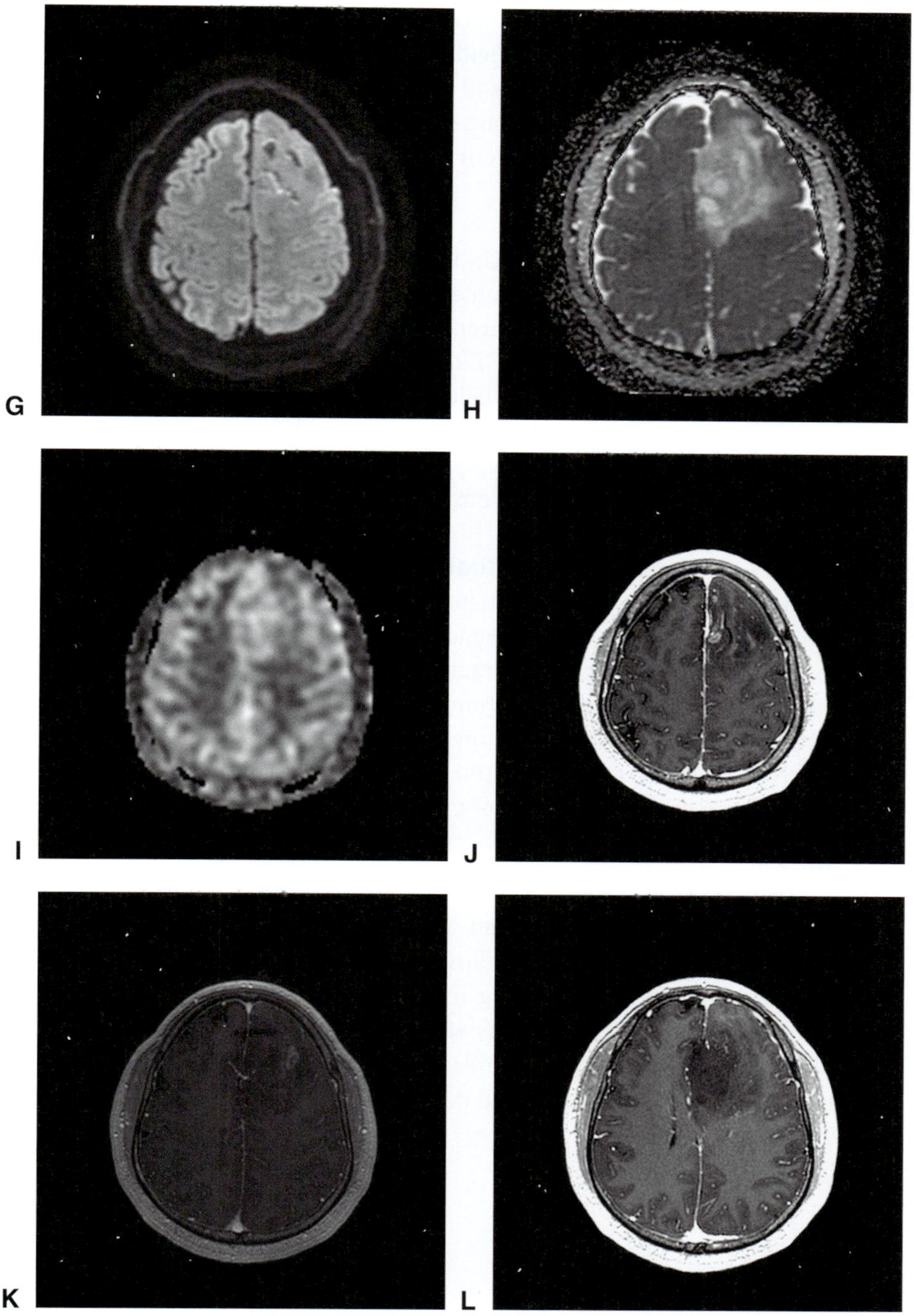

Figure 12.6. ***(continued)*** **G.** Axial DWI: Mildly reduced with calcium-related susceptibility artifact. **H.** Axial ADC: Heterogeneously and mildly reduced. **I.** Axial ASL: Mildly hypervascular. **J–L.** Axial T1 postcontrast: Mostly nonenhancing mass with scattered areas rim enhancement.

Affected age group: Glioblastoma occurs in all age groups but is particularly common in older adults, with peak incidence occurring in patients aged 55 to 85 years; it is rare in individuals aged <40 years. The median patient age at diagnosis of *IDH*-wildtype and *IDH*-mutant is 62 years and 48 years, respectively. Similar to other diffuse gliomas, there is male predominance, with female-to-male ratio of 1:1.6.

Molecular and genetic profile: Up to 90% of glioblastomas is *IDH*-wildtype with associated *TERT* promotor mutations (~80%), homozygous deletion of *CDKN2A*/*CDKN2B* (~60%), loss of chromosomes 10p (~50%) and 10q (~70%), epidermal growth factor receptor (*EGFR*) alterations (~55%), *TP53* mutations (~30%), and *PI3K* mutations (~25%). Glioblastoma, *IDH*-mutant, is considered a diffuse astrocytoma, with a continuum of lower to higher grade histopathologic features. Several histologic subtypes include giant cell, epithelioid, primitive neuronal component, and gliosarcoma—each with unique imaging features.

Clinical features and standard therapy: Unlike the lower-grade diffuse gliomas, the onset of symptoms in patients with glioblastoma is relatively rapid (usually <3 months), with seizure, headache, and focal neurologic deficit being the three most common. Longer protracted symptoms of glioblastoma suggest *IDH*-mutant subtype. Surgical resection followed by radiation therapy with concurrent temozolomide chemotherapy is the standard of care at initial diagnosis. There is a wide variety of treatment options at recurrence, but few are proven effective in controlling the tumor growth.

Imaging

Glioblastomas, *IDH*-wildtype, are an irregularly rim-enhancing, centrally necrotic mass involving the corpus callosum, deep or subcortical white matter and neighboring cortex with frequent intratumoral hemorrhage, mass effect, and peritumoral edema. Glioblastomas, *IDH*-mutant, show large nonenhancing cortically based mass with scattered areas of enhancement and subtle or frank intratumoral necrosis. Mass effect and peritumoral edema are less severe than the *IDH*-wild type variant.

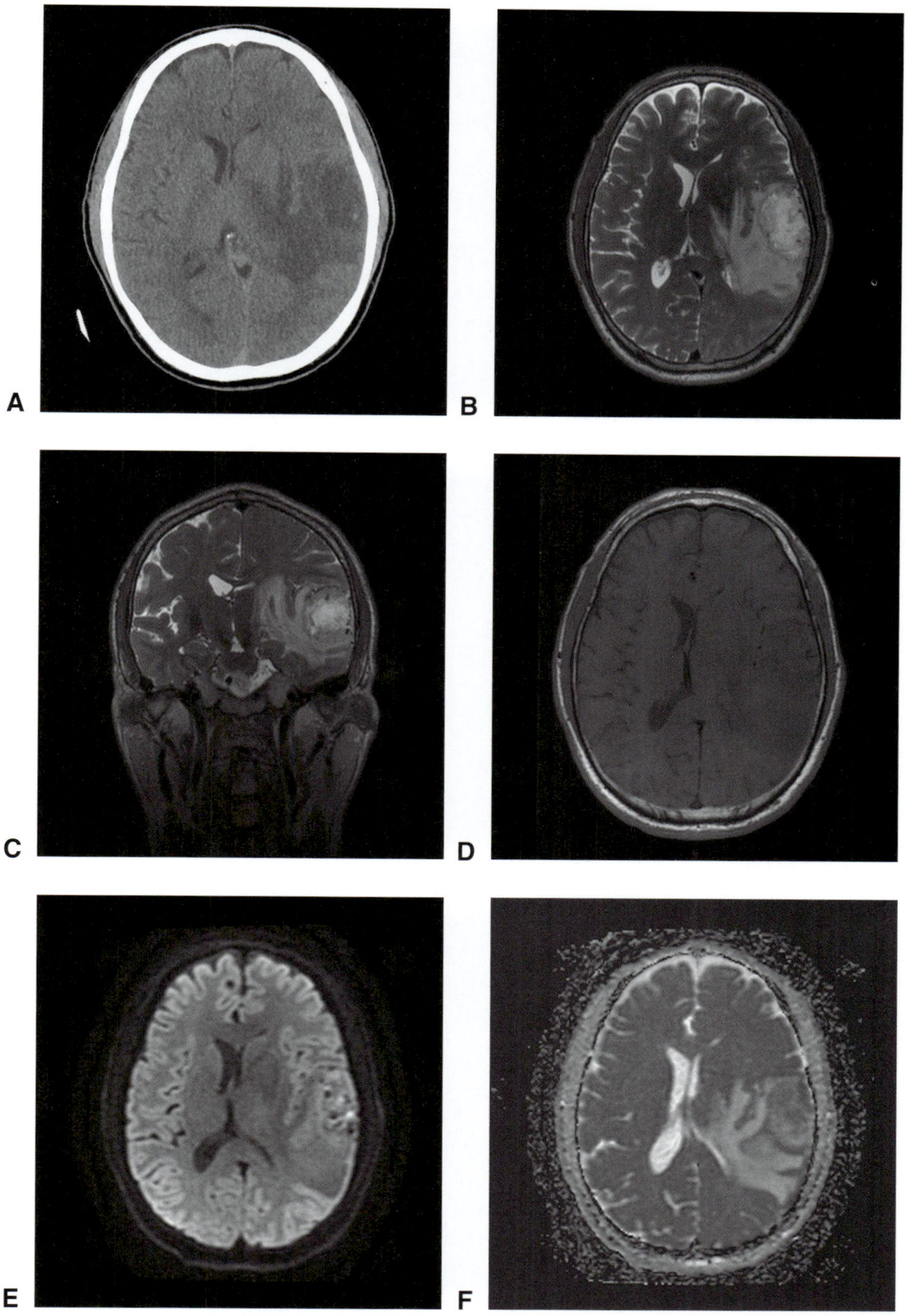

Figure 12.7. Imaging of glioblastoma, *IDH*-wildtype. A. Axial CT unenhanced: Low-density mass with surrounding edema. **B.** Axial T2: Heterogeneously hyperintense mass and hypointense rim with surrounding edema. **C.** Coronal T2: Heterogeneously hyperintense mass and hypointense rim with surrounding edema. **D.** Axial T1 precontrast: Hypointense mass with subtle areas of intrinsic T1 shortening. **E.** Axial DWI: Heterogeneously hyper- and hypointense regions within tumor and increased diffusion within the edema. **F.** Axial ADC: Heterogeneously hyper- and hypointense regions within tumor and increased diffusion within the edema.

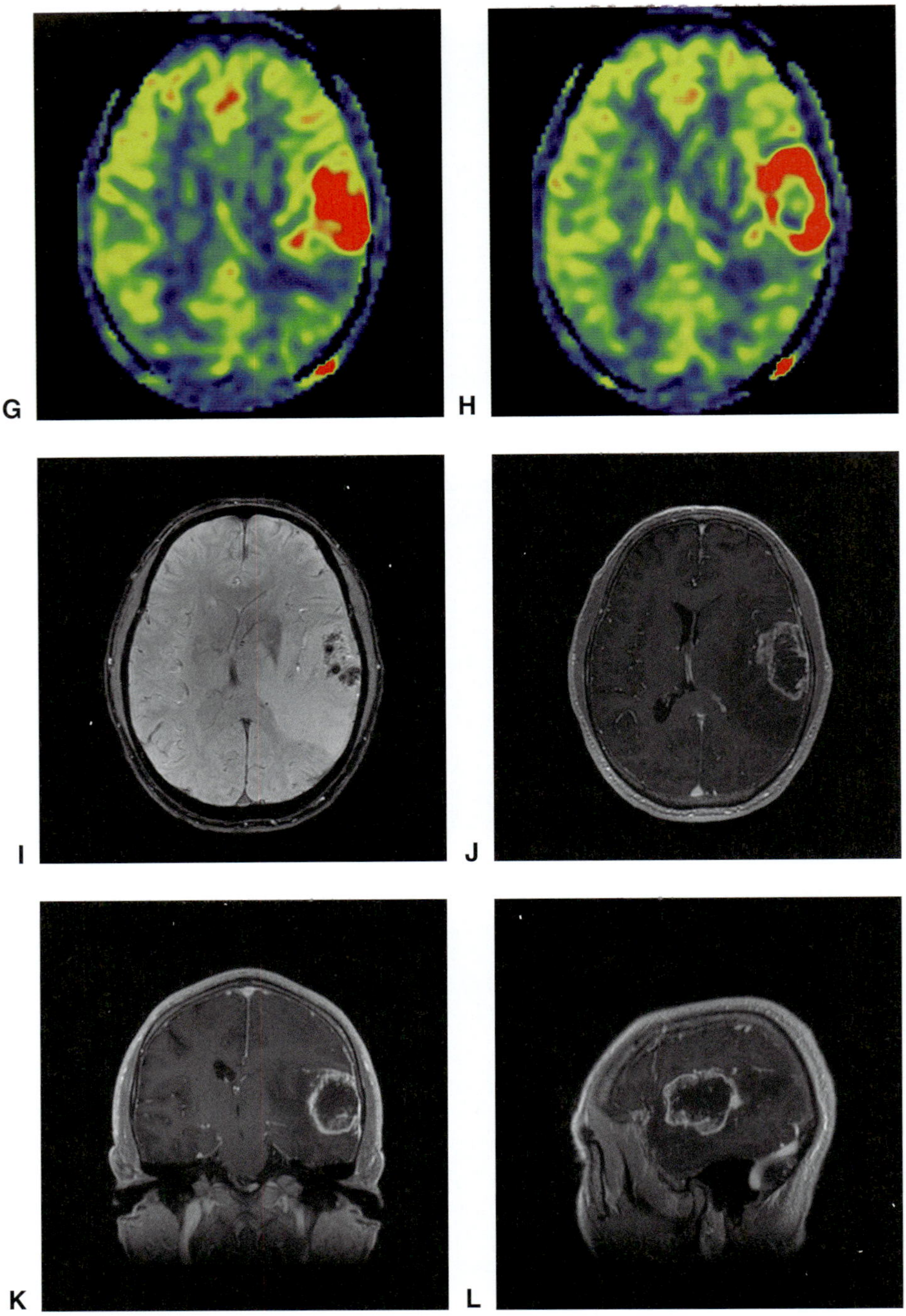

Figure 12.7. ***(continued)*** **G.** Axial ASL: Markedly hypervascular tumor. **H.** Axial ASL: Markedly hypervascular tumor. **I.** Axial SWI: Few nodular blood products within tumor. **J.** Axial T1 postcontrast: Irregularly rim-enhancing, centrally necrotic mass with peritumoral edema. **K.** Coronal T1 postcontrast: Irregularly rim-enhancing, centrally necrotic mass with peritumoral edema. **L.** Sagittal T1 postcontrast: Irregularly rim-enhancing, centrally necrotic mass with peritumoral edema.

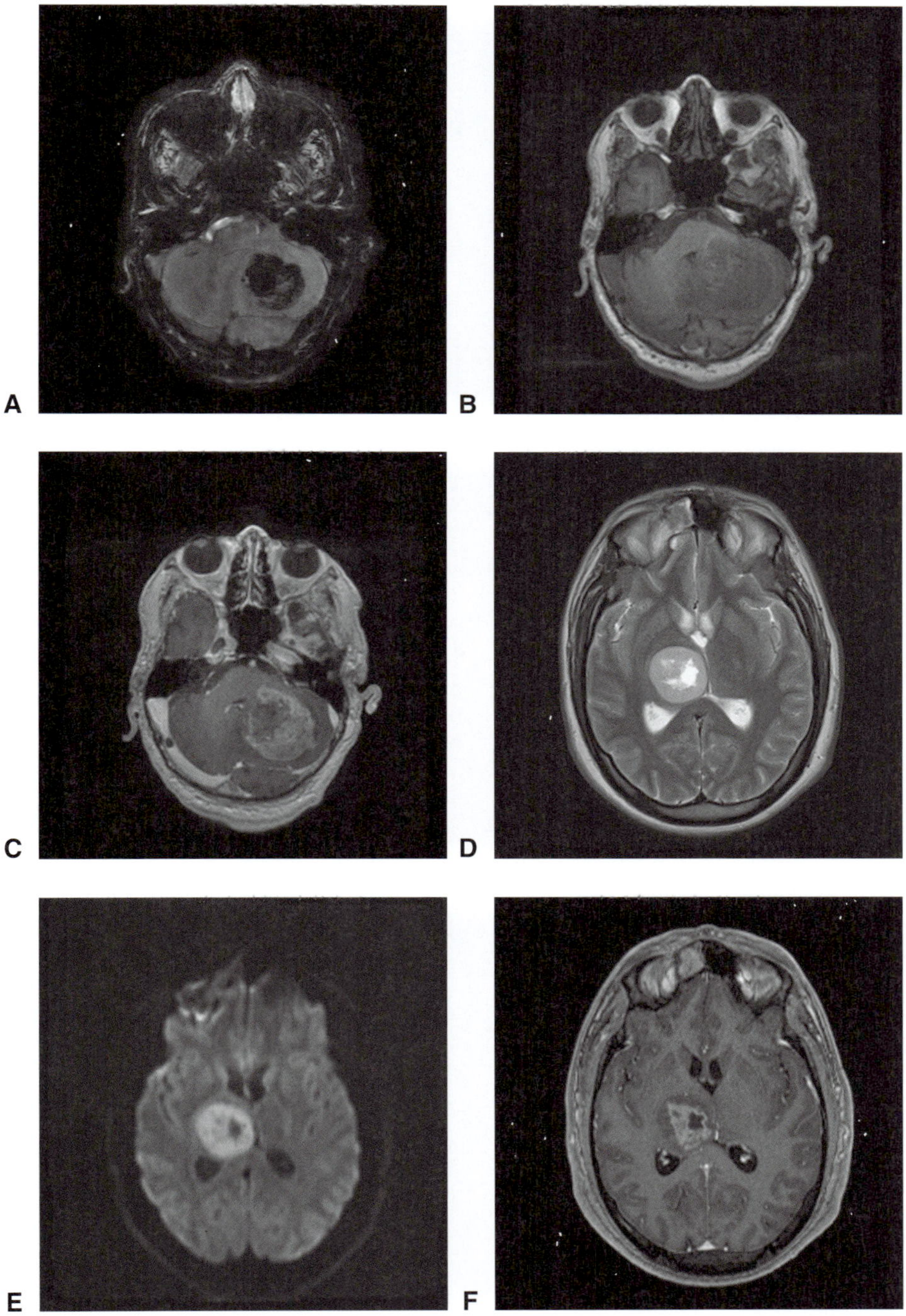

Figure 12.8. Imaging of glioblastomas, *IDH*-wildtype, four different locations. A–C. Cerebellar glioblastoma: Axial SWI (A), axial T1 precontrast (B), axial T1 postcontrast (C): Hemorrhagic irregularly enhancing and necrotic mass. **D–F.** Thalamic glioblastoma: Axial T2 (D), axial DWI (E), and axial T1 postcontrast (F): Circumscribed, heterogeneously mixed hyper- and iso-intense mass with irregularly enhancing and necrotic mass.

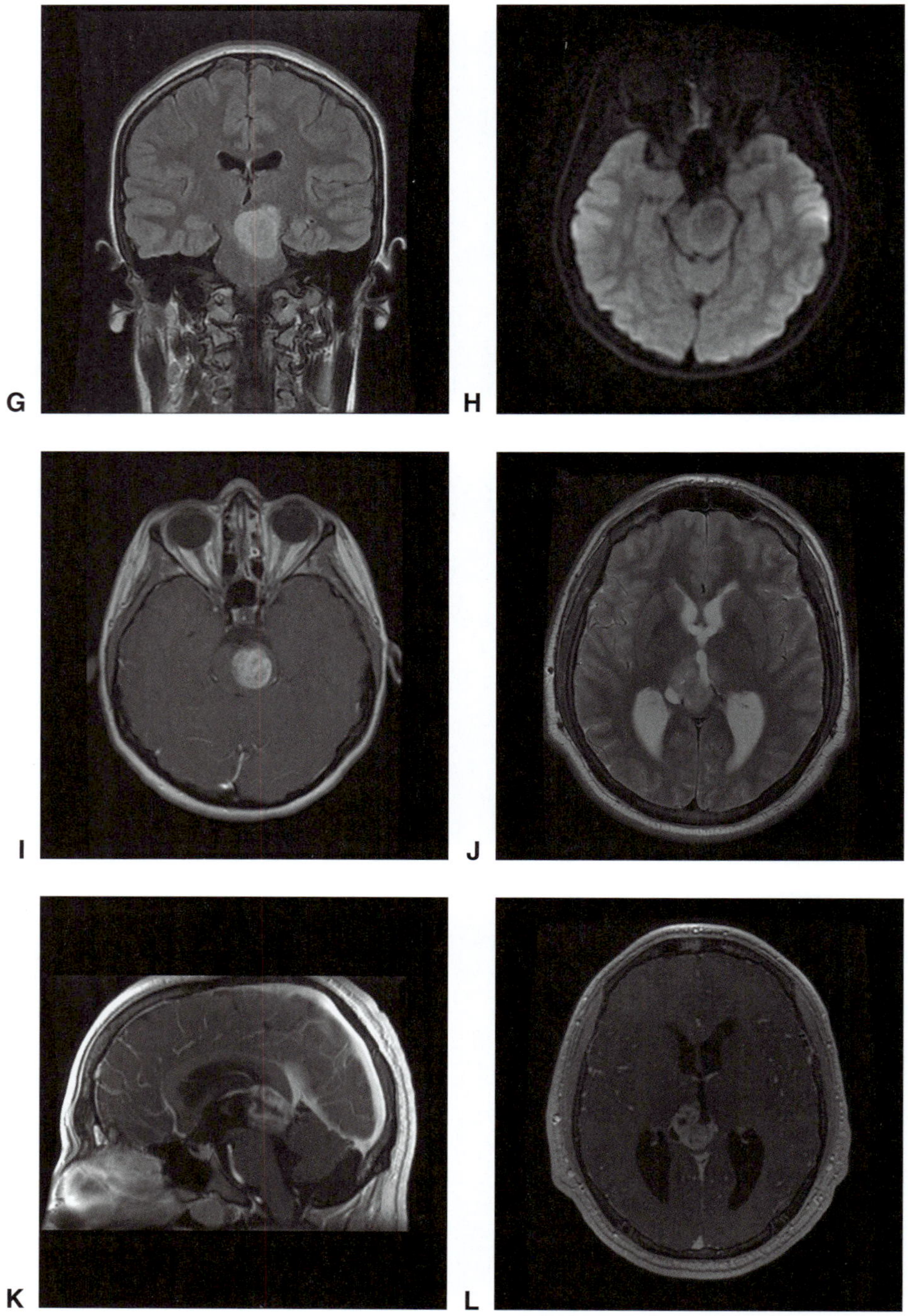

Figure 12.8. ***(continued)*** **G–H.** Pontine glioblastoma: Coronal FLAIR (G), axial DWI (H), axial T1 postcontrast (I): Circumscribed, heterogeneously hyperintense, avidly enhancing mass. **J–L.** Pineal glioblastoma: Axial T2 (J), sagittal T1 postcontrast (K), and axial T1 postcontrast (L).

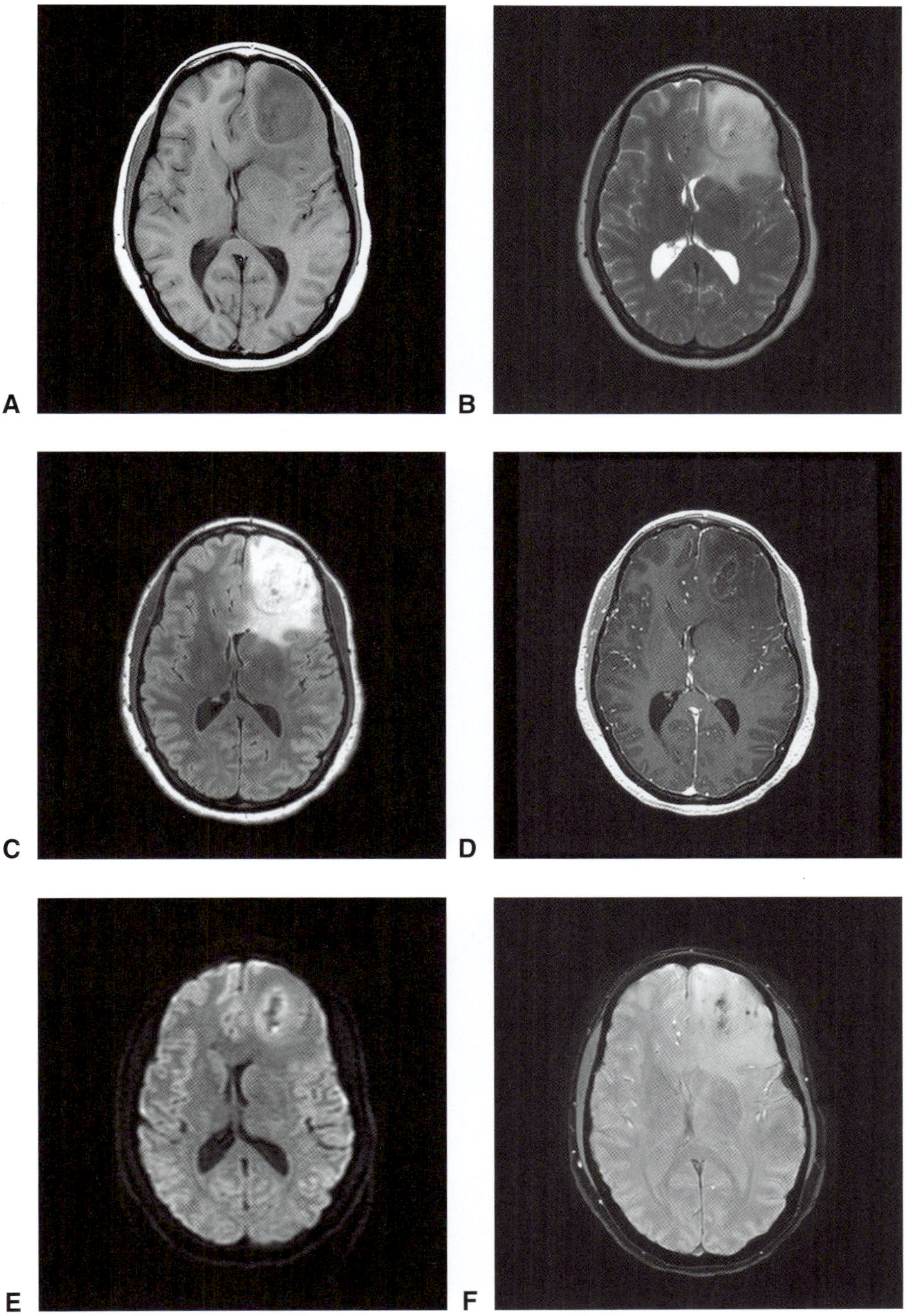

Figure 12.9. Imaging of glioblastoma, *IDH*-mutant. A. Axial T1 precontrast: Hypointense infiltrative mass with cortical expansion. **B.** Axial T2: Heterogeneously hyperintense mass. **C.** Axial FLAIR: Hyperintense mass. **D.** Axial T1 postcontrast: Nonenhancing cortical component and rim-enhancing, centrally necrotic white matter component. **E.** Axial DWI: Reduced diffusion corresponding to the enhancing rim. **F.** Axial SWI: Scattered areas of blood products.

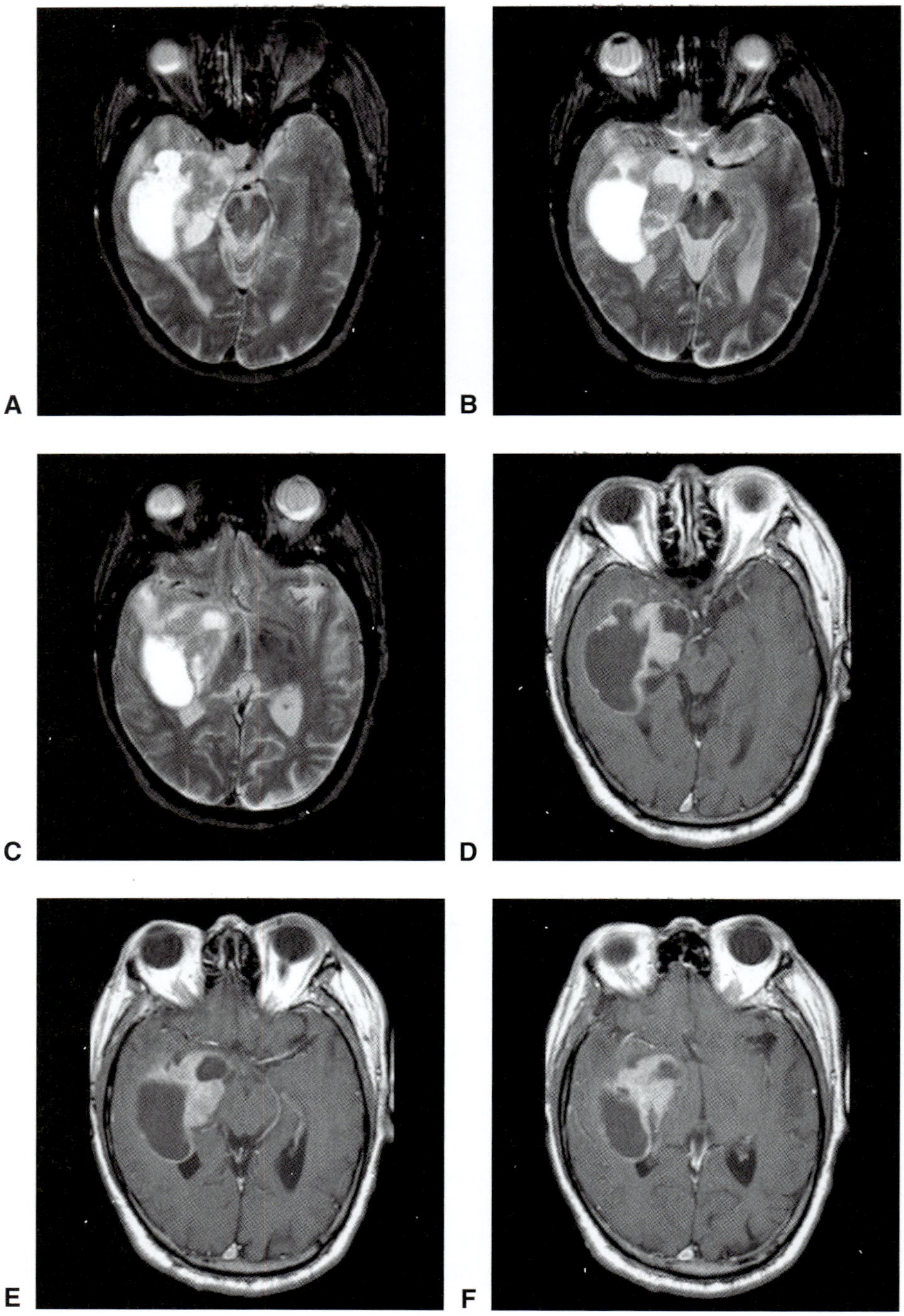

Figure 12.10. Imaging of giant cell glioblastoma. A–C. Axial T2: Circumscribed cystic and solid mass. **D–F.** Axial T1 postcontrast: Avidly enhancing solid component.

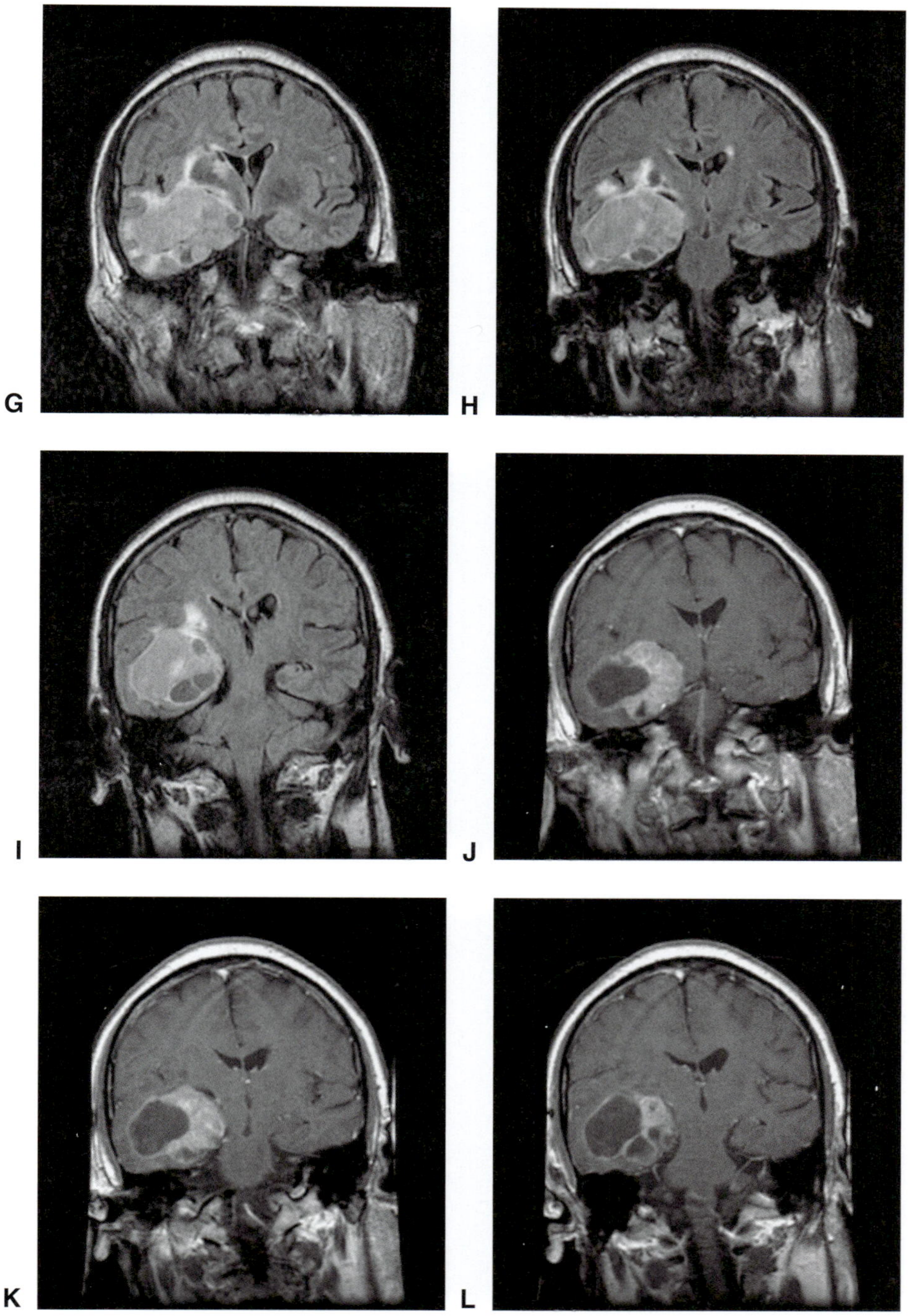

Figure 12.10. ***(continued)*** **G–I.** Coronal FLAIR: Mild peritumoral edema. **J–L.** Coronal T1 postcontrast: Medially located solid component.

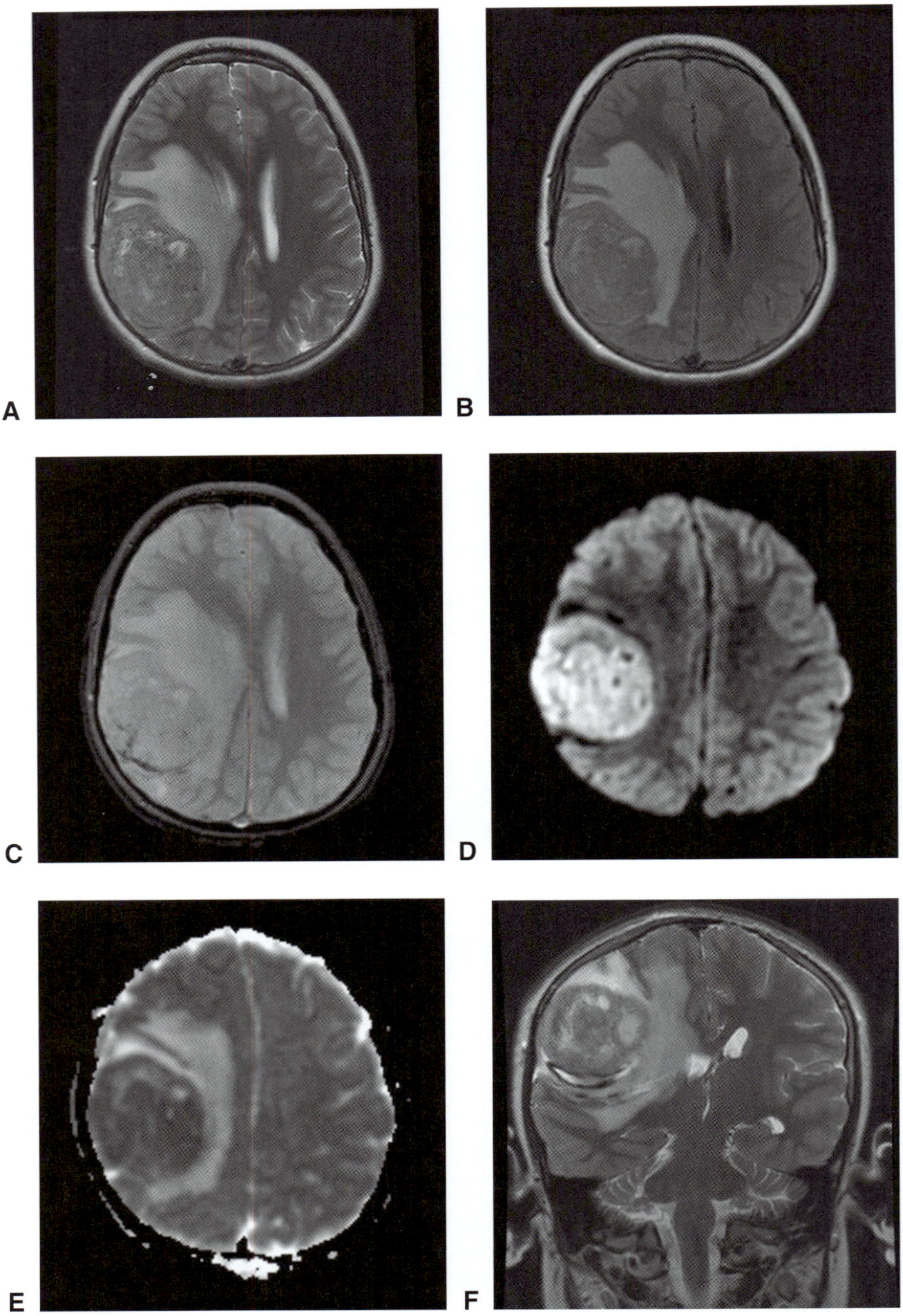

Figure 12.11. **Imaging of epithelioid glioblastoma. A.** Axial T2: Heterogeneously hypointense solid mass with small peripheral cystic components and marked peritumoral edema. **B.** Axial FLAIR: Heterogeneously hypointense solid mass with small peripheral cystic components and marked peritumoral edema. **C.** Axial SWI: Minimal blood products along the periphery of tumor. **D.** Axial DWI: Heterogeneously hyperintense cellular mass. **E.** Axial ADC: Heterogeneously hypointense cellular mass. **F.** Coronal T2: Hypointense solid mass with small peripheral cystic components and marked peritumoral edema.

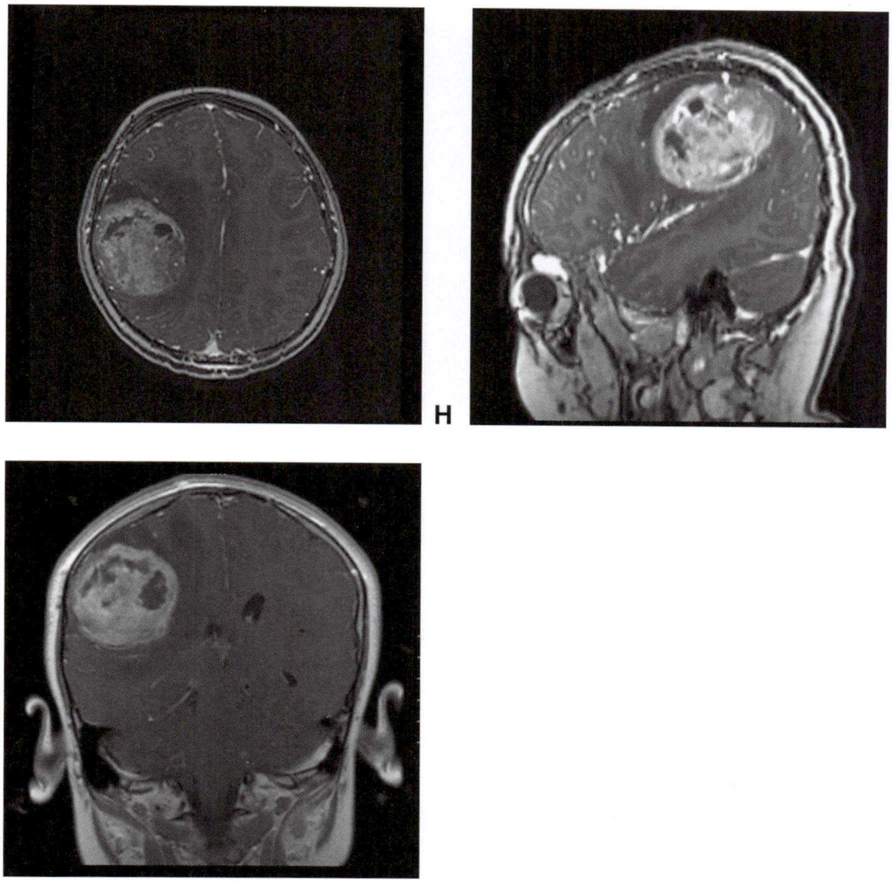

G H I

Figure 12.11. ***(continued)*** **G.** Axial T1 postcontrast: Heterogeneous but avid enhancement. **H.** Sagittal T1 postcontrast: Heterogeneous but avid enhancement. **I.** Coronal T1 postcontrast: Heterogeneous but avid enhancement

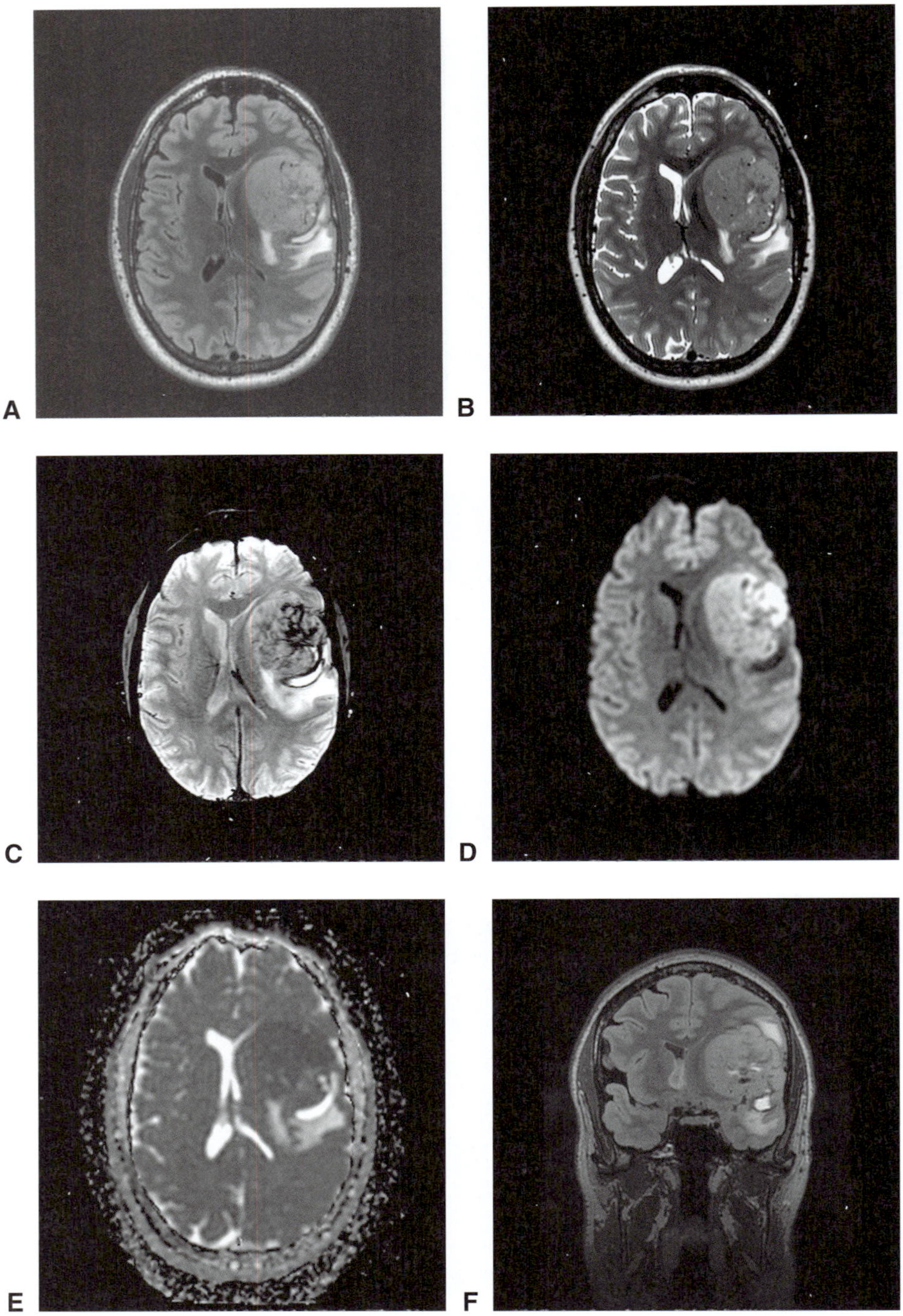

Figure 12.12. Imaging of glioblastoma with a primitive neuronal component. **A.** Axial FLAIR: Heterogeneously isointense solid mass with surrounding edema. **B.** Axial T2: Heterogeneously isointense solid mass with surrounding edema. **C.** Axial SWI: Heterogeneous and extensive blood products within the tumor. **D.** Axial DWI: Heterogeneously hyperintense mass. **E.** Axial ADC: Heterogeneously hypointense mass. **F.** Coronal FLAIR: Heterogeneously isointense solid mass with surrounding edema.

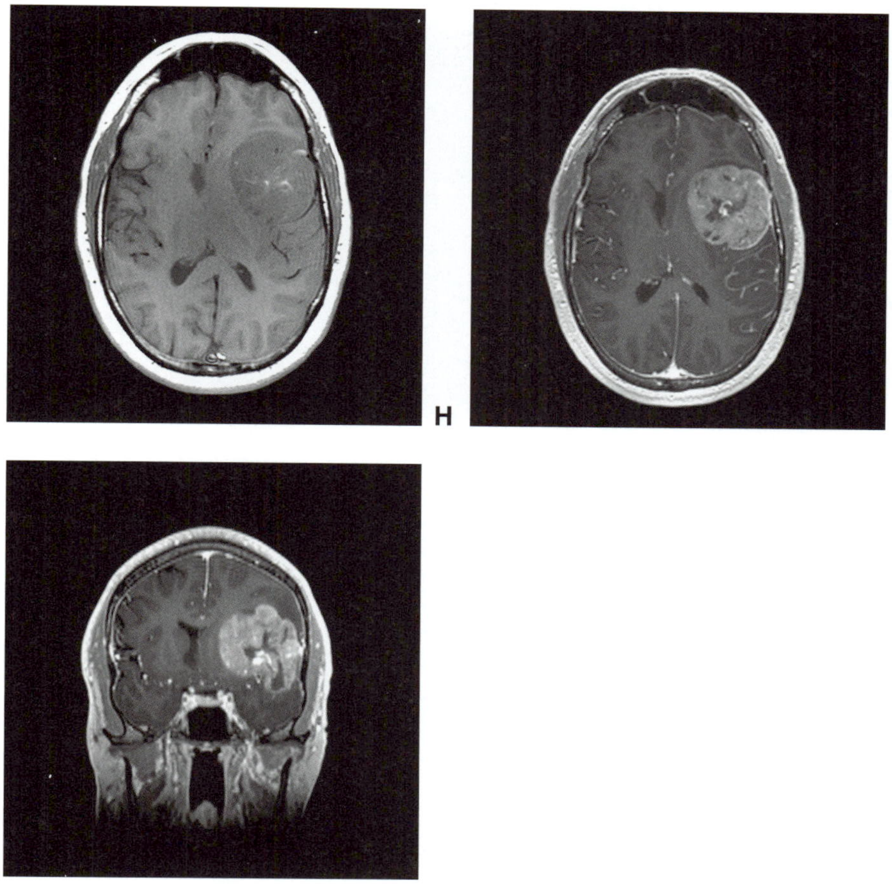
G H I

Figure 12.12. ***(continued)*** **G.** Axial T1 precontrast: Isointense mass with areas of T1 shortening due to blood products. **H.** Axial T1 postcontrast: Heterogeneous and avid enhancement with internal areas of necrosis. **I.** Coronal T1 postcontrast: Heterogeneous and avid enhancement with internal areas of necrosis.

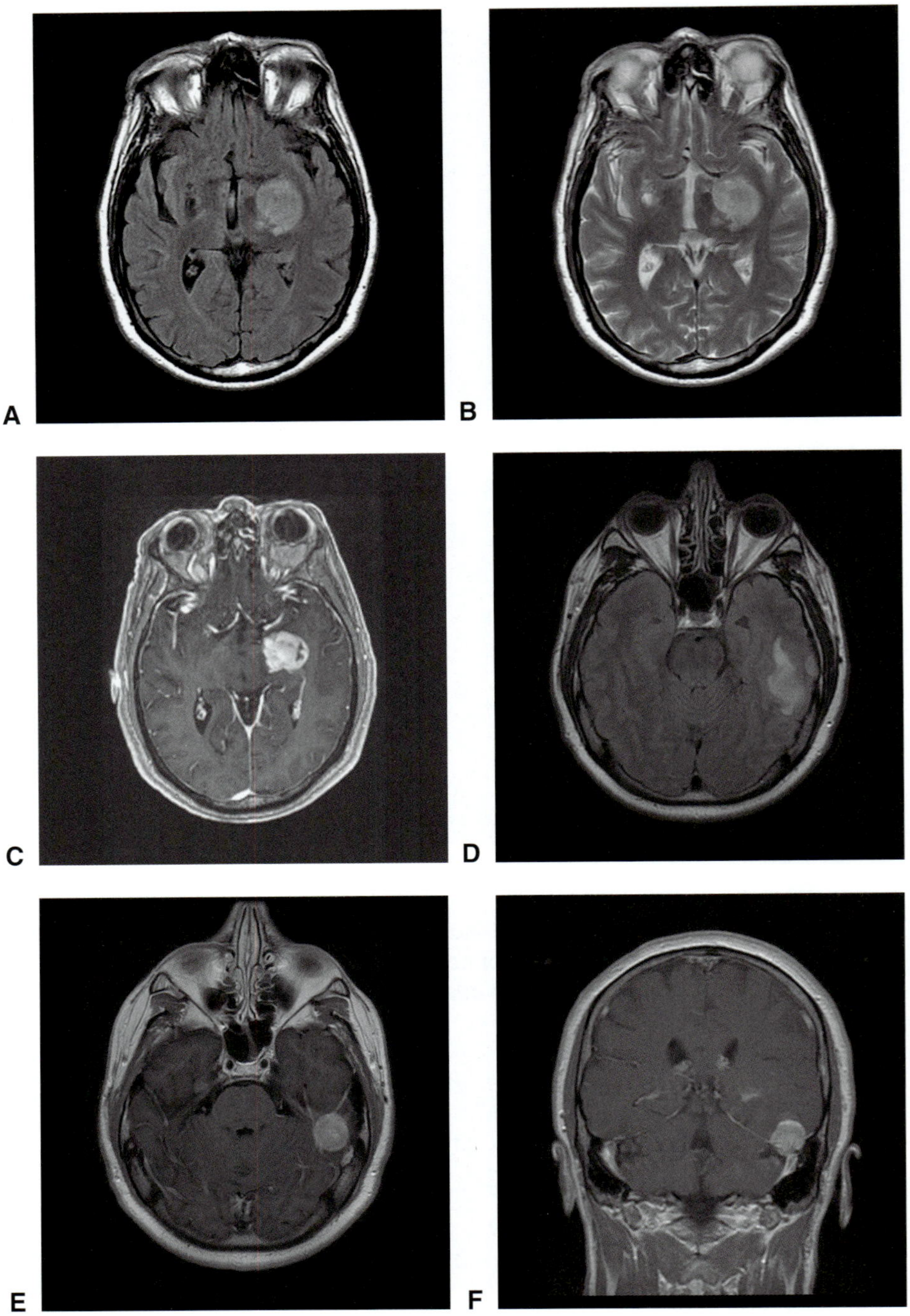

Figure 12.13. Imaging of gliosarcoma in four different patients. A–C. Left thalamic gliosarcoma. Axial FLAIR (A), Axial T2 (B), and Axial T1 postcontrast images: Circumscribed hyperintense mass with heterogeneous and avid enhancement but no surrounding edema. **D–F.** Left inferior temporal gliosarcoma. Axial FLAIR (D), Axial T1 postcontrast (E), and coronal T1 postcontrast (F) images: Superficially located avidly enhancing intraparenchymal mass with surrounding edema.

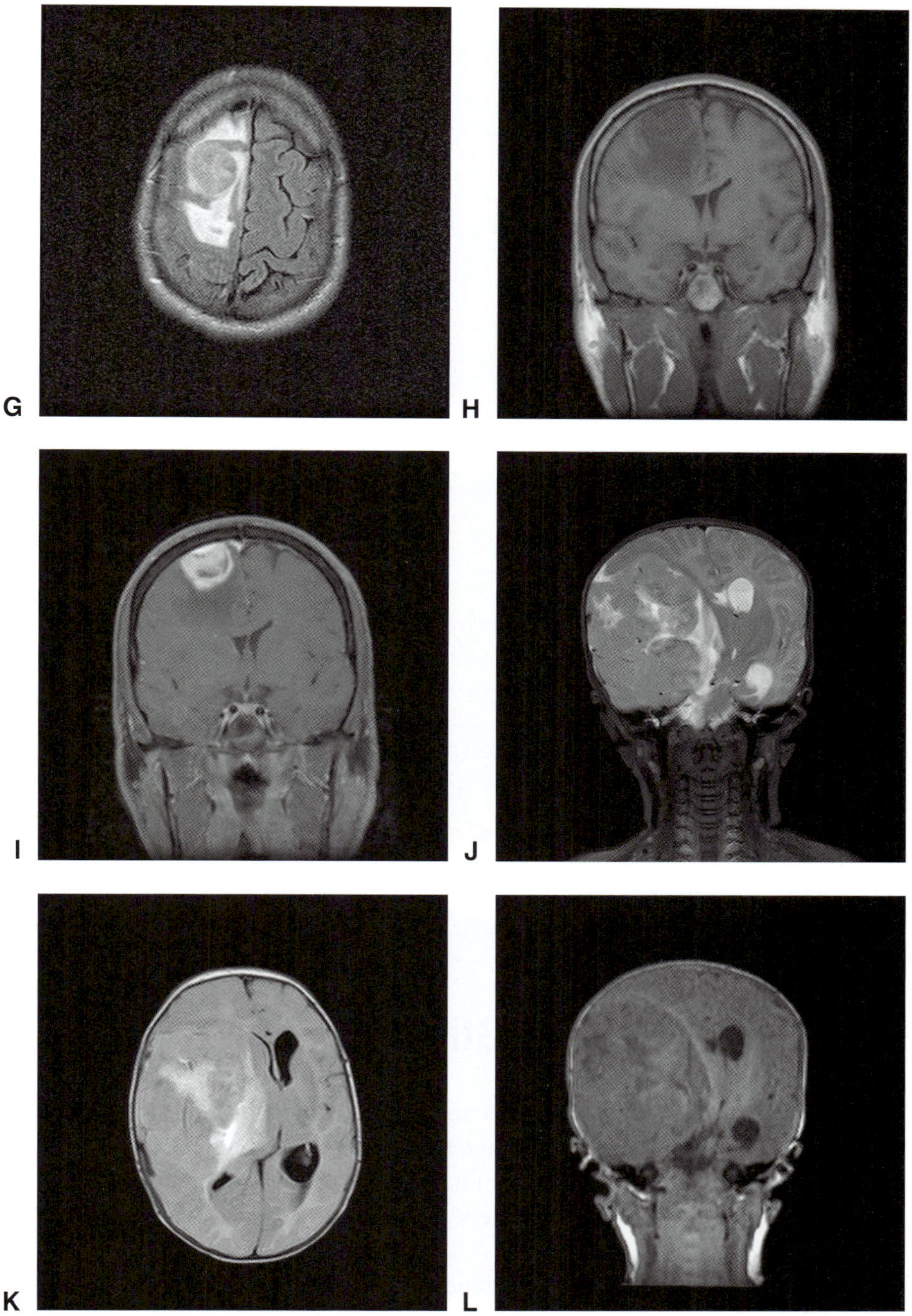

Figure 12.13. ***(continued)*** **G–I.** Right superior frontal gliosarcoma. Axial FLAIR (G), coronal T1 precontrast (H), and coronal T1 postcontrast images: Cortically based avidly enhancing mass with marked surrounding edema and mass effect. **J–O.** Right frontotemporal gliosarcoma in an infant. Coronal T2 (J), axial FLAIR (K), coronal T1 precontrast (L), axial ADC (M), axial T1 postcontrast (N), and coronal T1 postcontrast (O) images: Massive solid tumor with internal necrosis, avid enhancement, and high cellularity but mild degree of surrounding edema occupying large portion of the right cerebral hemisphere.

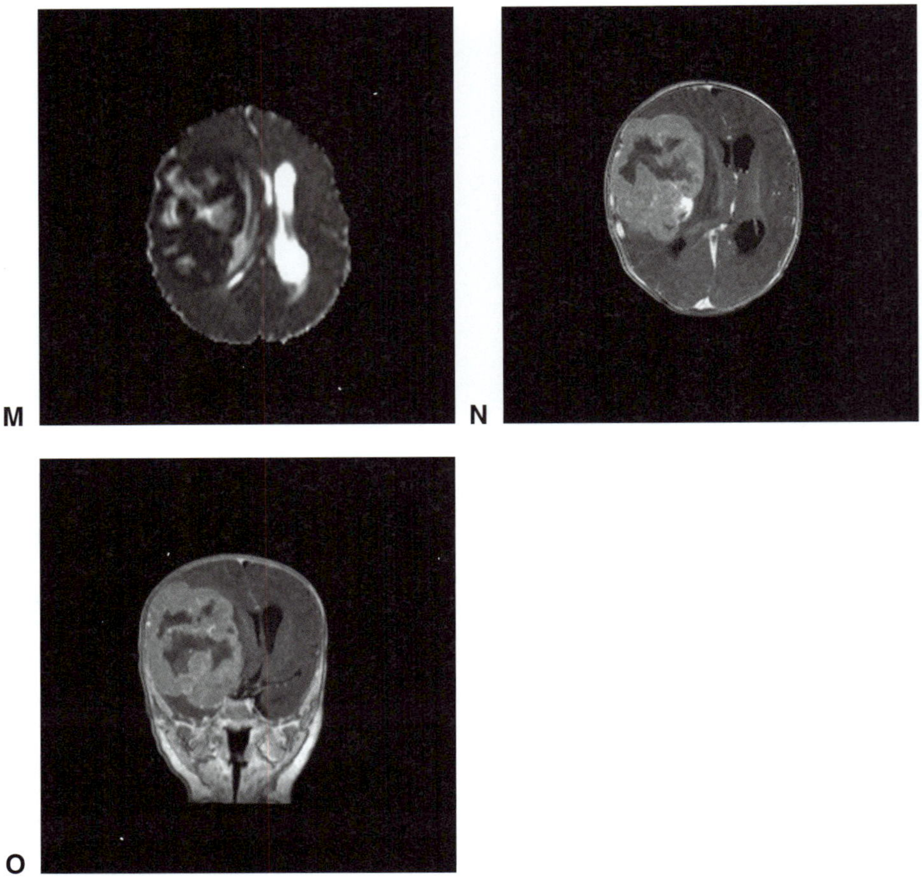

Figure 12.13. *(continued)*

Diffuse Midline Glioma

Definition: Diffuse midline glioma is an infiltrative malignant glioma located midline or paramidline of the central nervous system (CNS) with predominantly astrocytic differentiation and a *K27M* mutation in either *H3F3A* or *HIST1H3B/C* and occurring primarily in the brain stem, thalamus, and spinal cord.

Epidemiology: Because diffuse midline gliomas (DMGs) are not recognized as a distinct category in large brain tumor registries, their exact incidence is not available.

Affected age group: Young children are the most commonly affected age group, with the median age at diagnosis of 5 to 11 years, with pontine tumors arising earlier on average (~7 years) than their thalamic or spinal cord counterparts (~11 years). There is no gender predilection.

Molecular and genetic profile: Heterozygous mutations at position K27 in the histone coding genes *H3F3A*, *HIST1H3B*, and *HIST1H3C* in high-grade gliomas involving the pons, thalamus, and spinal cord are seen. Additional mutations in *H3 K27M*-mutant DMGs include *TP53* mutation (50%), *PDGFRA* amplification (30%), *CDK4/6* or *CCND1-3* amplification (20%), *ACVR1* mutation (20%), *PPM1D* mutation (15%), *MYC/PVT1* amplification (15%), *ATRX* mutation (15%), and *CDKN2A/B* homozygous deletion (<5%).

Clinical features and standard therapy: The clinical presentation of diffuse midline gliomas depends on location of the tumor. The pontine DMGs present with brain stem dysfunction, most notable cranial nerve IV to VII neuropathies, long tract signs, and ataxia. The thalamic DMGs present with signs of increased intracranial pressure, motor or sensory weakness or hemiparesis, and gait disturbance. The spinal DMGs present with myelopathy, gait disturbance, or long tract sensory or motor deficits. Due to their eloquent location, DMGs are usually not amenable to gross total resection without severely compromising function. Biopsy is commonly done to establish the diagnosis, and radiation therapy is the mainstay of treatment. Several chemotherapeutic agents targeting the molecular alterations of histone pathway are in clinical trials and await efficacy and survival benefit data.

Imaging

Diffuse midline glioma is an expansile mass with or without enhancement arising within the thalamus, pons, medulla, or spinal cord. It is hyperintense of FLAIR and T2-weighted imaging with increased diffusivity on diffusion-weighted imaging.

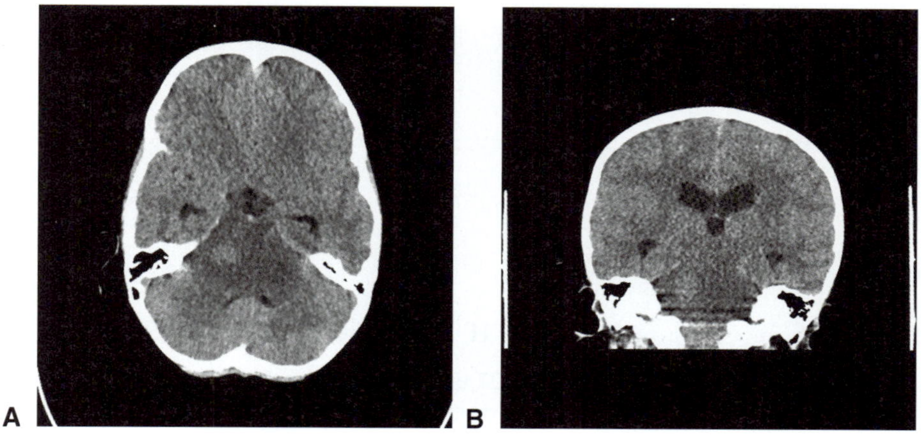

Figure 12.14. Imaging of diffuse midline glioma of the brain. A. Axial CT unenhanced: Expansile low-density pontine mass with focal high-density area on the right. **B.** Coronal CT unenhanced: Expansile low-density pontine mass with focal high-density area on the right.

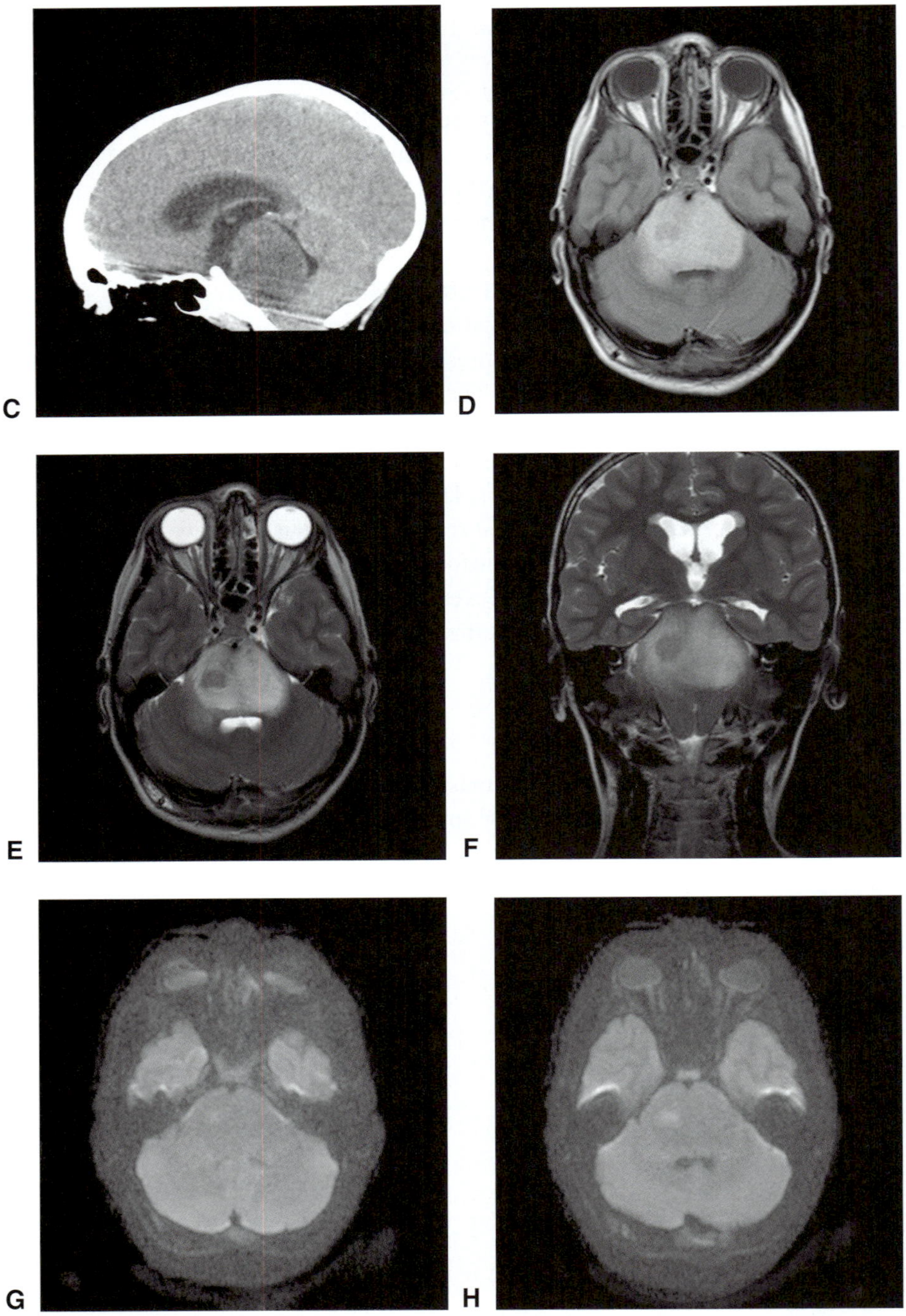

Figure 12.14. ***(continued)*** **C.** Sagittal CT unenhanced: Expansile low-density pontine mass with focal high-density area on the right. **D.** Axial FLAIR: Hyperintense except in the focal area on the right. **E.** Axial T2: Hyperintense except in the focal area on the right. **F.** Coronal T2: Hyperintense except in the focal area on the right. **G.** Axial DWI: Isointense to normal-appearing cerebellum. **H.** Axial DWI: Reduced diffusion in the focal area on the right.

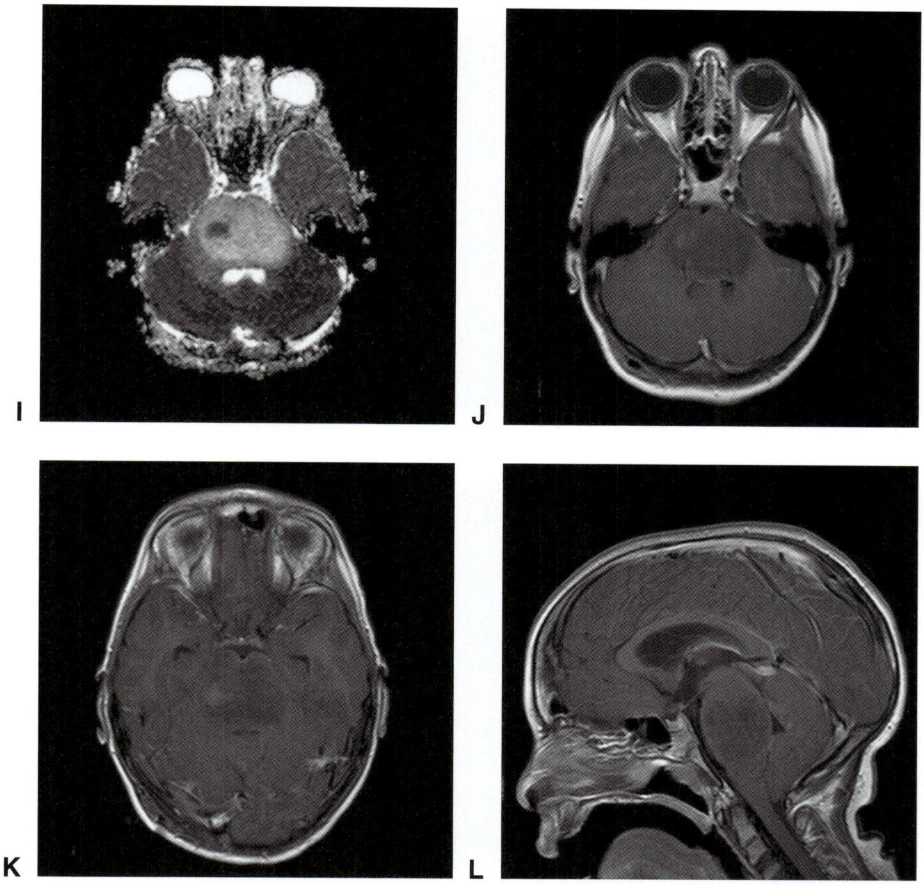

Figure 12.14. ***(continued)*** **I.** Axial ADC: Reduced diffusion in the focal area on the right. **J.** Axial T1 postcontrast: Mostly nonenhancing mass. **K.** Axial T1 postcontrast: Avid enhancement within the focal area on the right. **L.** Sagittal T1 postcontrast: Mostly nonenhancing mass.

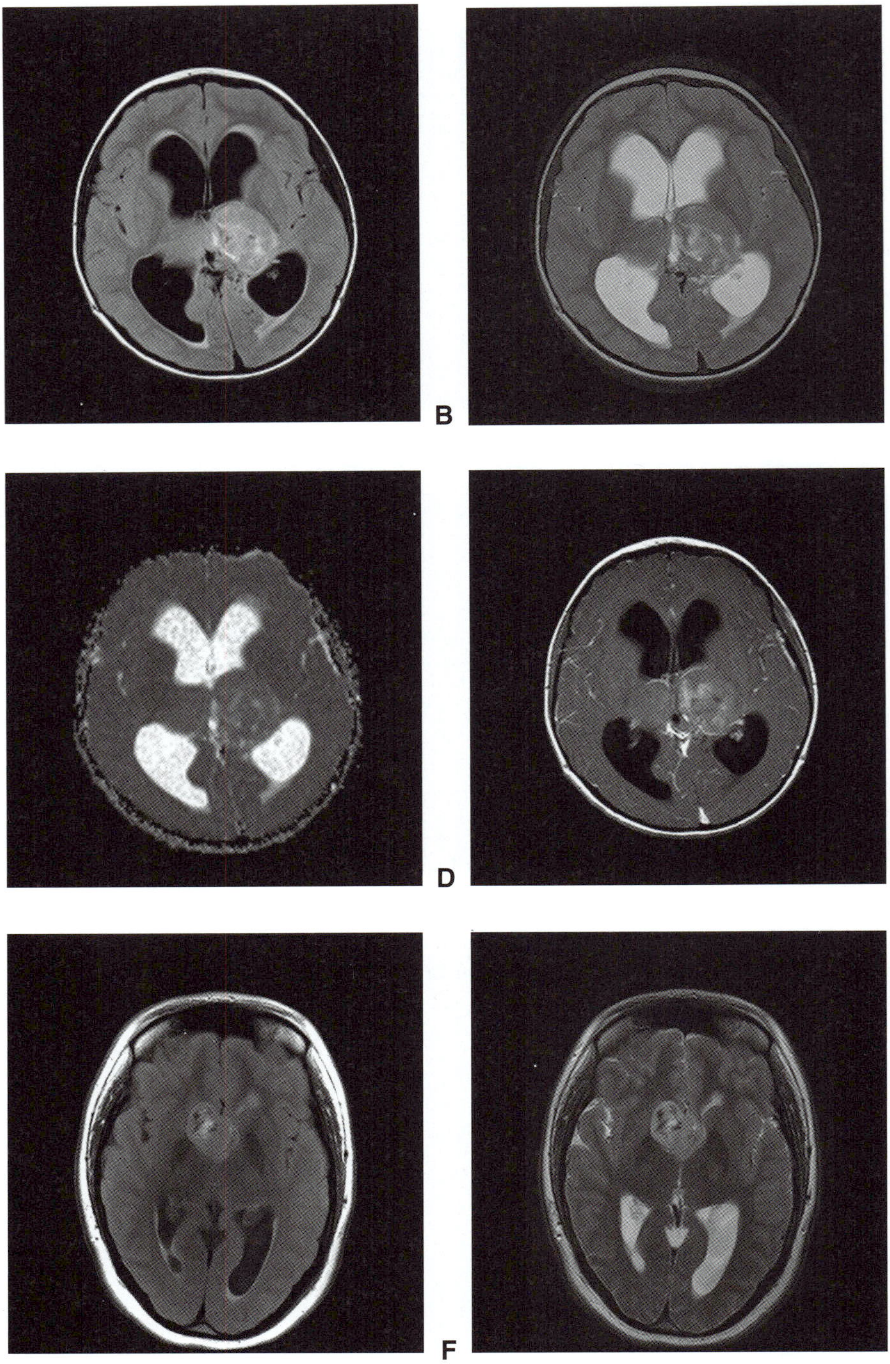

A B C D E F

Figure 12.15. Imaging of diffuse midline gliomas, four different patients. A–D. Thalamic DMG: Axial FLAIR (A), axial T2 (B), axial ADC (C), and axial T1 postcontrast (D): Heterogeneously hyperintense on FLAIR, hypointense on T2, mildly reduced on ADC, and enhancing mass. **E–H.** Hypothalamic DMG: Axial FLAIR (E), axial T2 (F), axial SWI (G), and axial T1 postcontrast (H): Heterogeneously hyperintense mass with blood products and irregular enhancement.

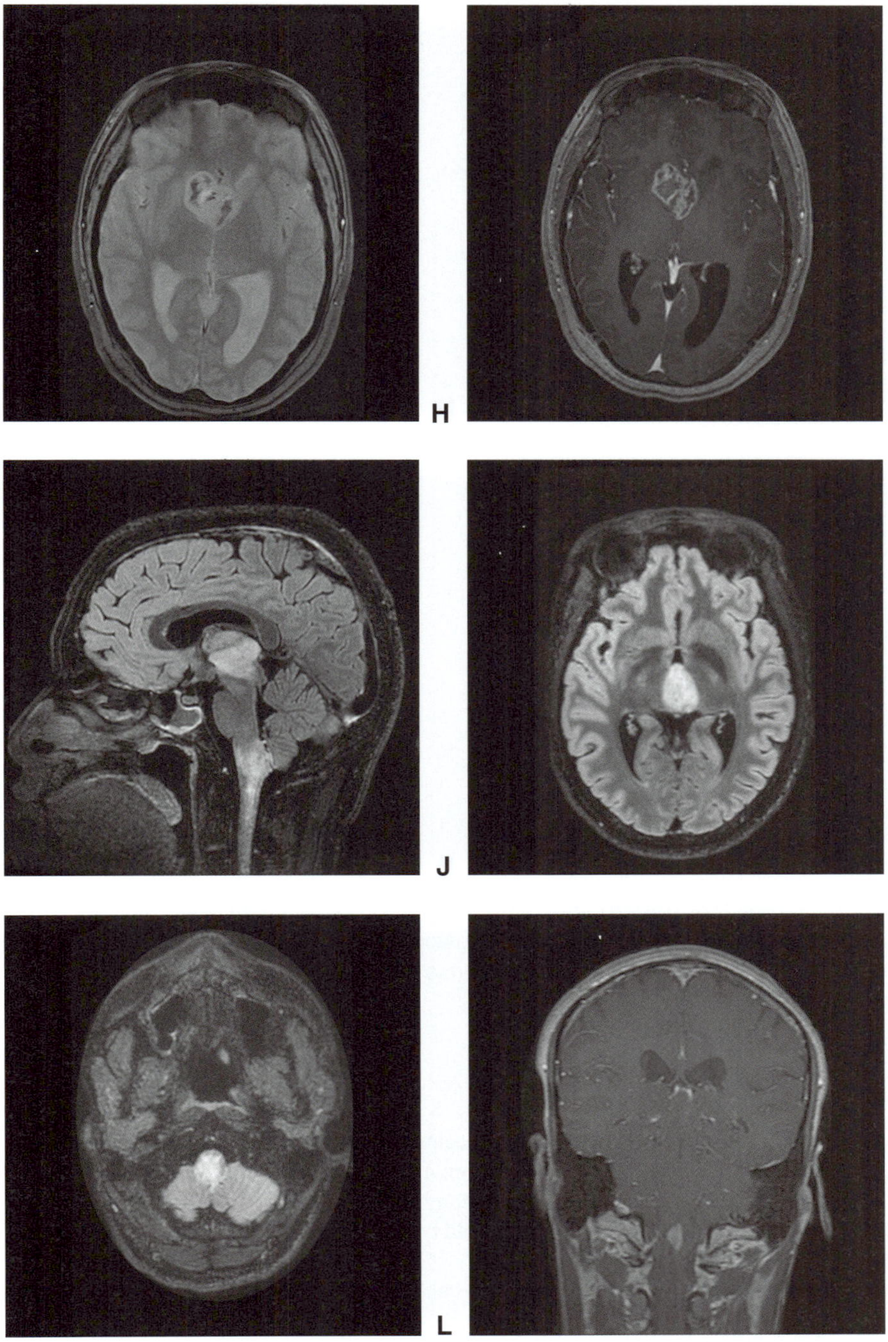

Figure 12.15. ***(continued)*** **I–L.** Intraventricular and medullary DMG: Sagittal FLAIR (I), axial FLAIR (J, K), and axial T1 postcontrast (L): Two discrete sites of tumor—third ventricular and medulla and cord—both are hyperintense on FLAIR but only the medullary lesion enhances.

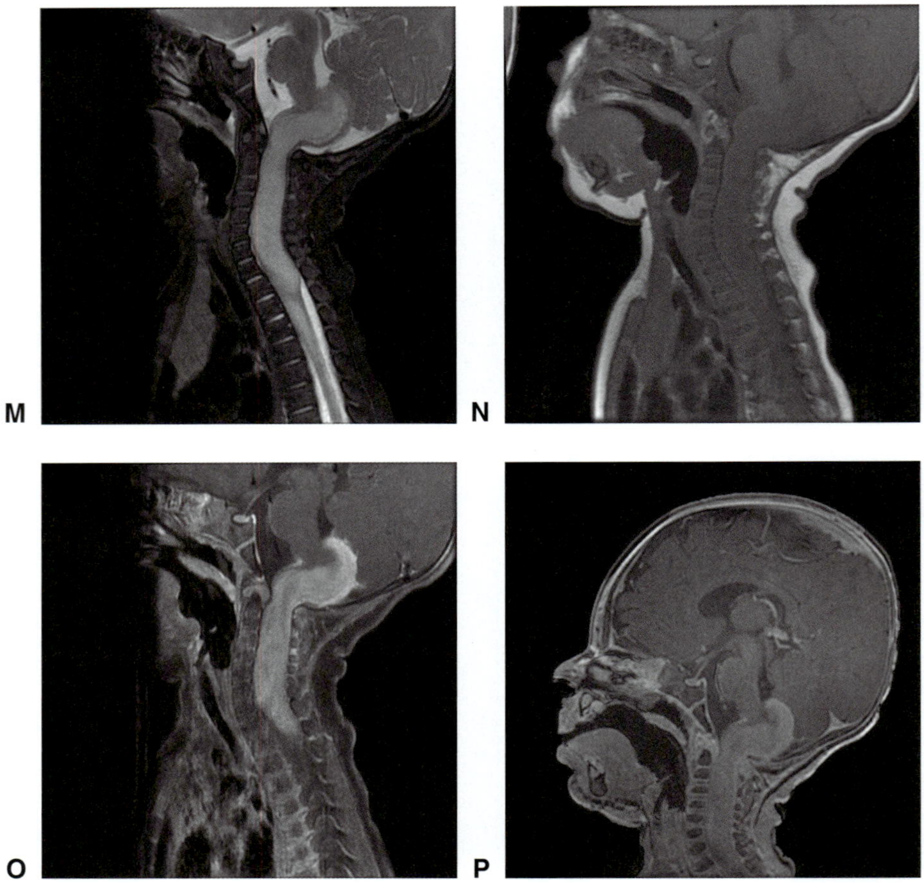

Figure 12.15. ***(continued)*** **M–P.** Medullary and cervical cord DMG: Sagittal T2 (M), sagittal T1 precontrast (N), sagittal T1 postcontrast (O, P): Expansile intramedullary mass, hyperintense on T2, and hypointense on T1, with avid enhancement.

Bibliography

Aboian MS, Solomon DA, Felton E, et al. Imaging characteristics of pediatric diffuse midline gliomas with histone H3 K27M mutation. *AJNR Am J Neuroradiol.* 2017;38:795–800.

Jung JS, Choi YS, Ahn SS et al. Differentiation between spinal cord diffuse midline glioma with histone H3 K27M mutation and wild type: Comparative magnetic resonance imaging. *Neuroradiology.* 2019;61:313–322.

Le Rhun E, Preusser M, Roth P, et al. Molecular targeted therapy of glioblastoma. *Cancer Treat Rev.* 2019;80:101896.

Nakajima N, Nobusawa S, Nakata S, et al. BRAF V600E, TERT promoter mutations and CDKN2A/B homozygous deletions are frequent in epithelioid glioblastomas: a histological and molecular analysis focusing on intratumoral heterogeneity. *Brain Pathol.* 2018;28:663–673.

Shirahata M, Ono T, Stichel D, et al. Novel, improved grading system(s) for IDH-mutant astrocytic gliomas. *Acta Neuropathol.* 2018;136:153–166.

Van den Bent MJ, Smits M, Kors JM, Chang SM. Diffuse infiltrating oligodendroglioma and astrocytoma. *J Clin Oncol.* 2017;35:2394–2401.

von Deimling A, Ono T, Shirahata M, Louis DB. Grading of diffuse astrocytic gliomas: a review of studies before and after the advent of IDH testing. *Semin Neurol.* 2018;38:19–23.

Wesseling P, van den Bent M, Perry A. Oligodendroglioma: pathology, molecular mechanisms and markers. *Acta Neuropathol.* 2015;129:809–827.

Xu G, Zheng H, Li JY. Next-generation whole exome sequencing of glioblastoma with a primitive neuronal component. *Brain Tumor Pathol.* 2019;36:129–134.

Yi X, Cao H, Tang H, et al. Gliosarcoma: a clinical and radiological analysis of 48 cases. *Eur Radiol.* 2019;29:429–438.

13 Circumscribed Astrocytic Tumors

Overview

Circumscribed astrocytic tumors of the central nervous system are characterized by well-delineated margin on pathology and imaging and usually lack infiltrative changes in the neighboring brain.

	Age range (mean)	Female: male ratio	Cell of origin	WHO grade	Molecular/genetic markers	Prognosis
Pilocytic astrocytoma	0–14	1:1	Bipolar cells with Rosenthal fibers	I	*BRAF V600E*	100% 5-year survival
Pilomyxoid astrocytoma	0–14	Unknown	Bipolar cells with myxoid background	I or II ?	*BRAF V600E*	Unknown but less favorable than pilocytic
Pleomorphic xanthoastrocytoma	10–30 (26)	1:1	Pleomorphic multinucleated cells	II	*BRAF V600E*	90% 5-year survival
Subependymal giant cell astrocytoma	0–20	Unknown	Ganglionic astrocyte	I	Inactivation of *TSC1* or *TSC2* genes; activation of mTOR pathway	100% 5-year survival

▶ Pilocytic Astrocytoma

Definition: Pilocytic astrocytoma is a well-circumscribed astrocytic neoplasm composed of variable proportions of compacted bipolar cells with Rosenthal fibers and loose, textured multipolar cells with microcysts and eosinophilic granular bodies. The supratentorial pilocytic astrocytomas are genetically characterized tandem duplications of chromosome 7q34 involving the *BRAF* gene resulting in oncogenic *BRAF* fusion proteins.

Epidemiology: Pilocytic astrocytomas account for up to 6% of all gliomas, and they are the most common primary brain tumors during the first two decades of life, especially in children. They account for almost 33% of all brain tumors in the 0- to 14-year age group.

Affected age group: This tumor primarily affects children ages 0 to 14 years, with a mean age of 7 years, and young adults, with a mean age of 22 years, but can occasionally occur in older patients in the fifth to seventh decades.

Molecular and genetic profile: Molecular and genetic alterations in pilocytic astrocytomas depend on the location of tumor. The most common genetic abnormality is in duplication of 7q34, encompassing the *BRAF* gene. Mutation hotspots result in valine to glutamate substitution at position 600, often referred to as *BRAF* V600E mutation. It remains unclear if this mutation has any prognostic significance.

Pilocytic astrocytoma is strongly associated with neurofibromatosis 1 (NF1), where up to 15% of individuals develop pilocytic astrocytomas, particularly of the optic nerve pathway but also in other sites; the tumor can be multiple.

CSF markers: None.

Clinical features and standard therapy: Surgical resection is the mainstay of therapy to either resect or obtain tissue for definitive diagnosis. Currently, there is no standard chemotherapy regimen, and radiotherapy is considered to control symptoms or slow down the tumor growth.

Imaging

Pilocytic astrocytomas are circumscribed tumors with variable imaging features depending on the location, with more homogeneous enhancement of the hypothalamic and optic pathway tumor and an enhancing nodule and a cyst pattern in the posterior fossa tumor.

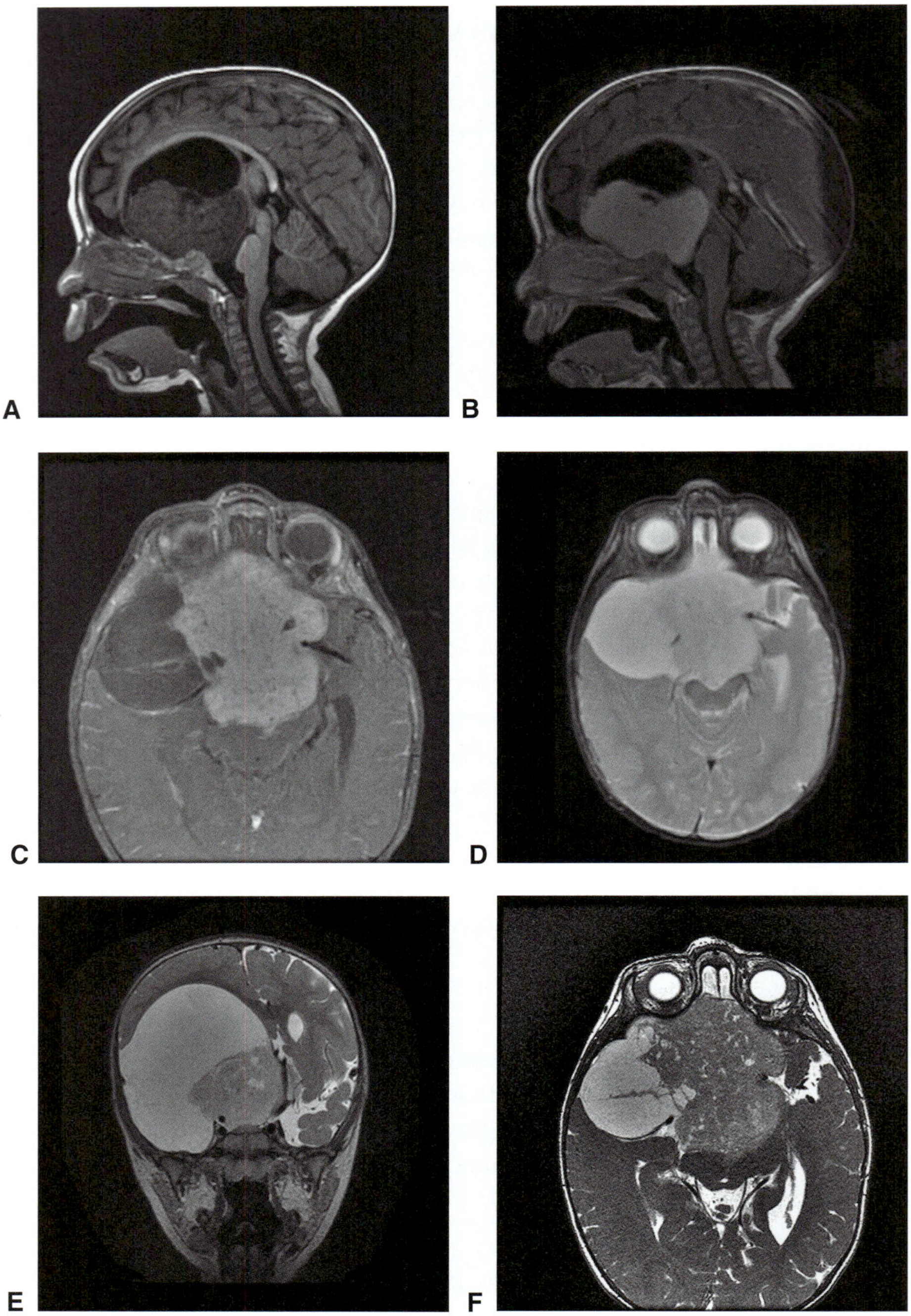

Figure 13.1. Five-year-old child with large optic pathway pilocytic astrocytoma. **A.** Sagittal T1-precontrast: Hypointense to surrounding brain. **B.** Sagittal T1-postcontrast: Avid enhancement of tumor. **C.** Axial T1-postcontrast: Avid enhancement of tumor. **D.** Axial T2 FSE: Hyperintense to surrounding brain and a large right-sided cystic component on the right. **E.** Coronal T2 FSE: Hyperintense to surrounding brain and a large cystic component enveloping the solid tumor. **F.** FIESTA: Slightly hyperintense to surrounding brain.

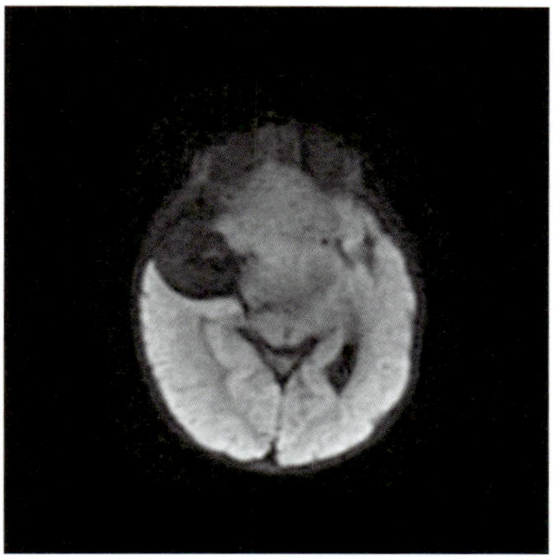

G

Figure 13.1. ***(continued)*** **G.** diffusion-weighted imaging (DWI): Slightly increased diffusion within the solid tumor.

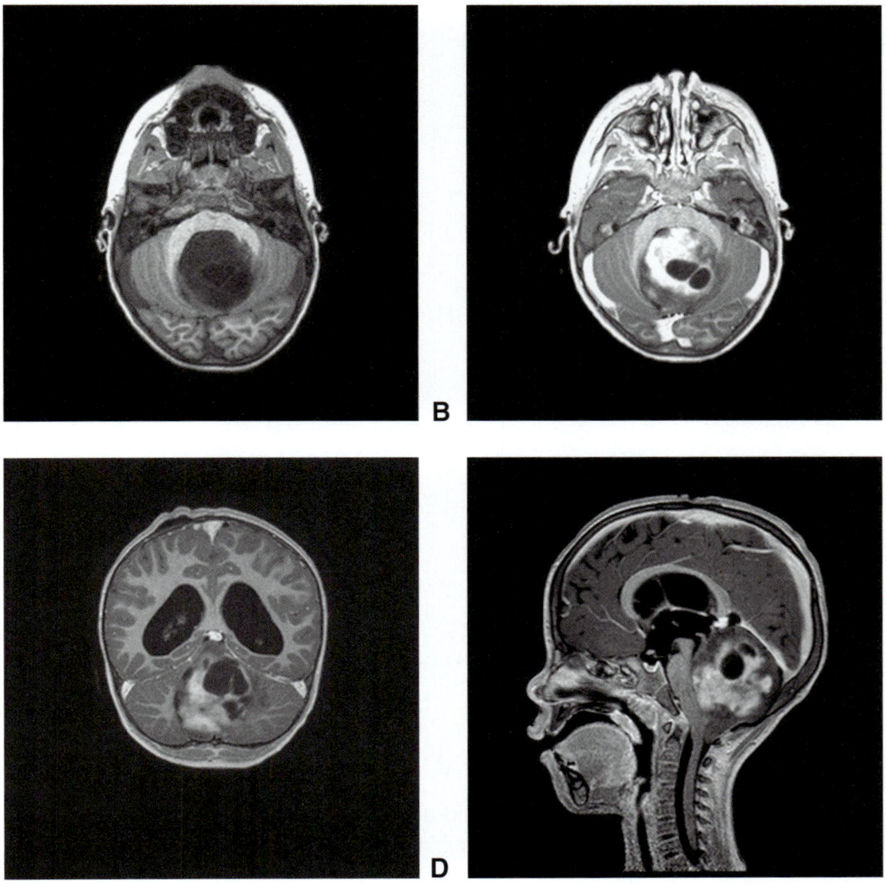

A B C D

Figure 13.2. Six-year-old child with posterior fossa pilocytic astrocytoma. A. Axial T1-precontrast: Hypointense to surrounding brain. **B.** Axial T1-postcontrast: Avidly enhancing mass with internal septated cystic component. **C.** Coronal T1-postcontrast: Increased diffusion. **D.** Sagittal T1-postcontrast: Avidly enhancing mass with internal septated cystic component.

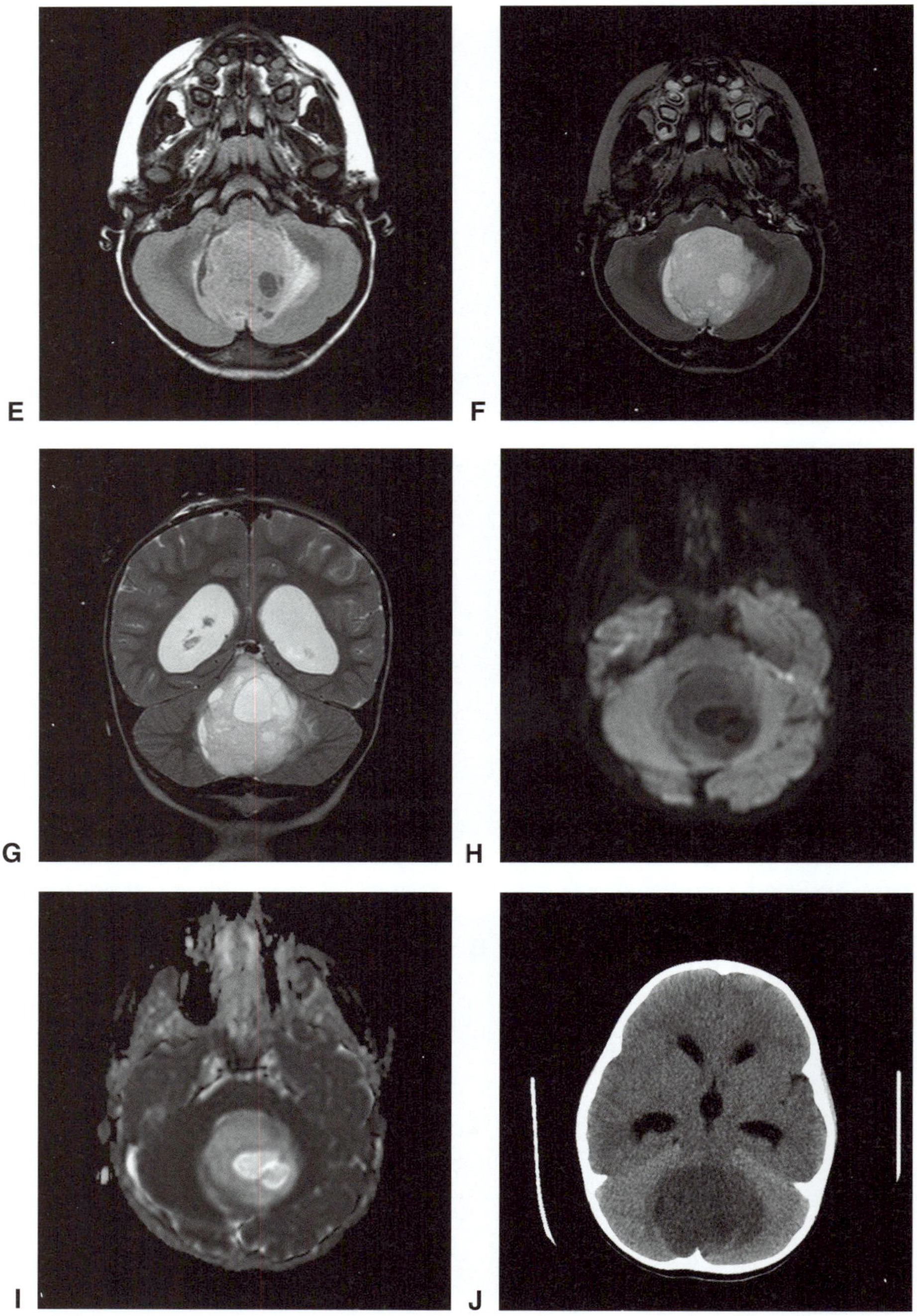

Figure 13.2. ***(continued)*** **E.** Axial fluid-attenuated inversion recovery (FLAIR): Hyperintense to surrounding brain with minimal surrounding edema. **F.** Axial T2 FSE: Hyperintense to surrounding brain with minimal surrounding edema. **G.** Coronal T2 FSE: Hyperintense to surrounding brain. **H.** Axial DWI: Increased diffusion. **I.** Axial apparent diffusion coefficient (ADC): Increased diffusion. **J.** Axial CT unenhanced: Low-density mass without calcium.

Pilomyxoid Astrocytoma

Definition: Pilomyxoid astrocytoma is a variant of pilocytic astrocytoma histologically but with distinct myxoid features and angiocentric arrangement of monomorphous, bipolar tumor cells.

Epidemiology: True incidence is unknown because pilomyxoid astrocytoma is very rare and often considered as a part of the much more common pilocytic astrocytoma. Pilomyxoid astrocytoma is more frequently seen in the pediatric age group.

Molecular and genetic profile: Although scant molecular genetic data are available due to its rarity, pilomyxoid astrocytoma can share the common genetic abnormality of pilocytic astrocytoma, namely *KIAA1549-BRAF* fusion.

CSF markers: None.

Clinical features and standard therapy: Similar to pilocytic astrocytoma, surgery is the mainstay of therapy, and no standard chemotherapy or radiotherapy guideline is available.

Imaging

Pilomyxoid astrocytomas are circumscribed tumors with avid enhancement and relatively larger size and more solid when compared to pilocytic astrocytomas.

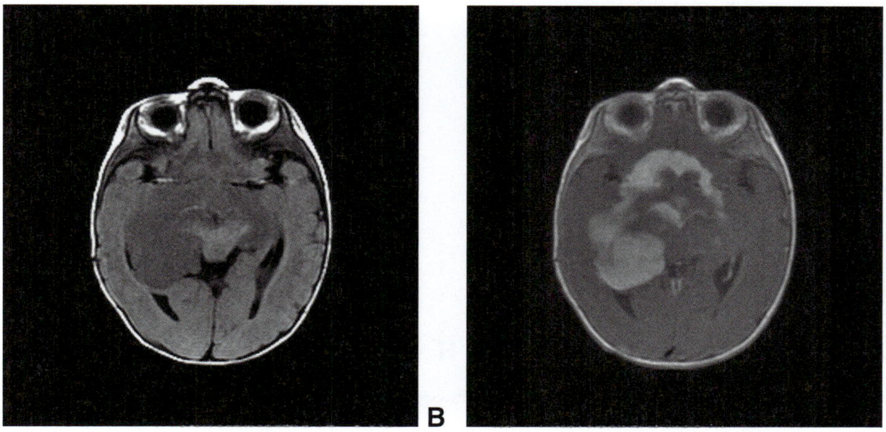

A B

Figure 13.3. A. Axial T1-precontrast: Hypointense to surrounding brain. **B.** Axial T1-postcontrast: Avid, fairly homogeneous enhancement.

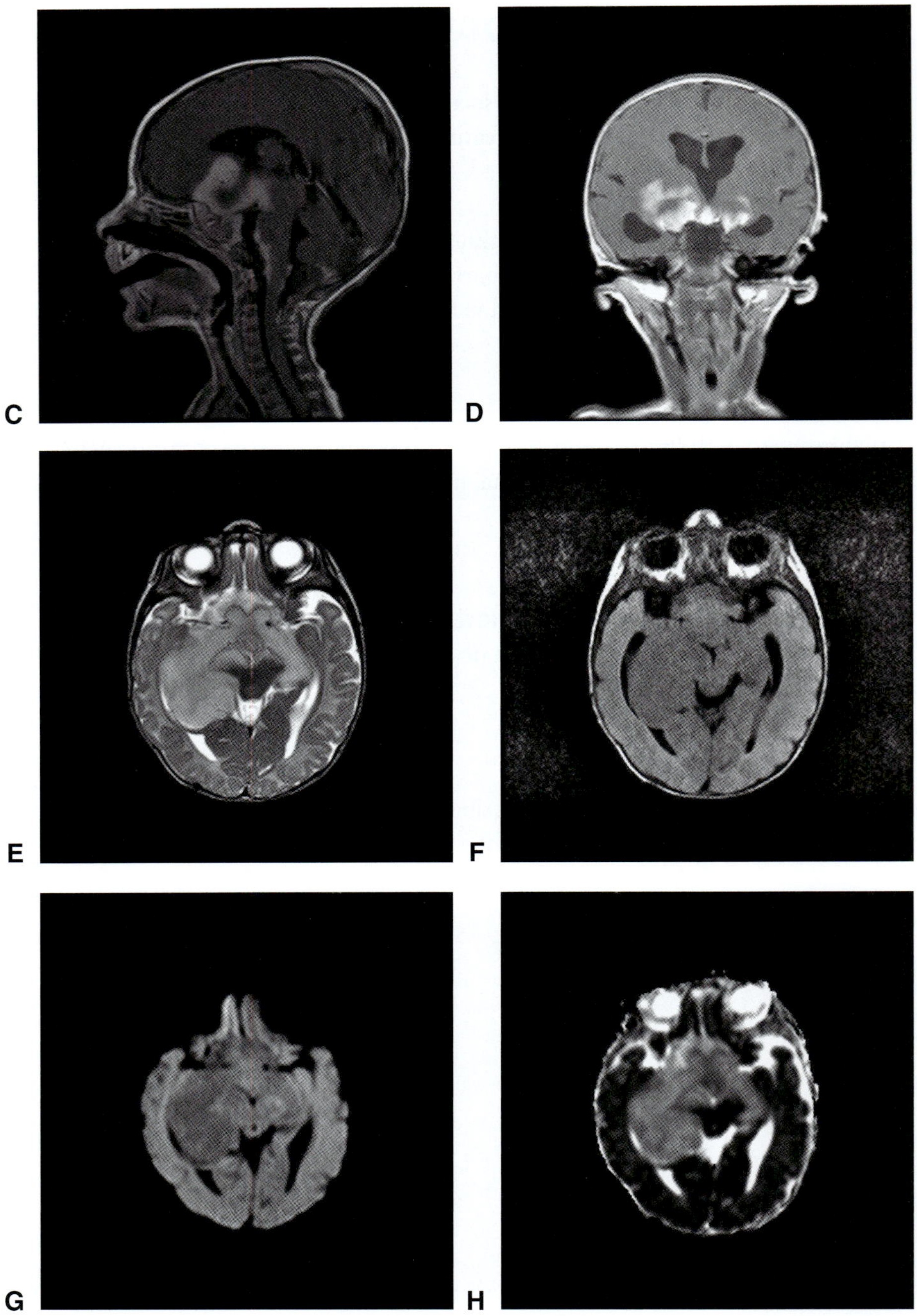

Figure 13.3. ***(continued)*** **C.** Sagittal T1-postcontrast. **D.** Coronal T1-postcontrast. **E.** T2 FSE: Hypo- or isointense to surrounding brain. **F.** FLAIR: Iso- to slightly hyperintense to surrounding brain. **G.** DWI: Increased diffusion. **H.** ADC: Increased diffusion.

Pleomorphic Xanthoastrocytoma

Definition: Pleomorphic xanthoastrocytoma is a WHO grade II astrocytic neoplasm involving the cerebral cortex with prominent large pleomorphic and multinucleated cells and comprised of spindle and lipidized cells in a background of dense pericellular reticulin network and eosinophilic granular bodies. Up to 30% can have histologic features of higher grade and more aggressive clinical and biological course and have been designated as anaplastic pleomorphic xanthoastrocytoma (PXA), WHO grade III. Anaplastic PXA is more likely to disseminate widely within the cerebrospinal fluid and can involve the spine.

Epidemiology: This is a rare tumor, <1% of all brain tumors, affecting children and young adults but can be seen in older adult patients. No gender predilection is seen.

Affected age group: Pleomorphic xanthoastrocytoma mostly affects children and young adults with a mean age of 26 years old but rarely can be seen in older adult patients in the seventh or eighth decade.

Molecular and genetic profile: *BRAF V600E* mutations can be seen in up to 60%, especially in grade II PXA.

CSF markers: None.

Clinical features and standard therapy: Surgical resection is the mainstay of therapy for PXA. Although there is no standard chemotherapy, a clinical trial using *BRAF* V600E inhibitor has been proposed in those PXAs with the *BRAF* V600E mutation.

Imaging

PXA can occur anywhere in the brain, with predilection for temporal lobe, and can involve the spinal cord. Usually, there is a solid enhancing component with or without cyst. PXA can be disseminated within the brain and spine at initial presentation. Anaplastic PXA tends to show intratumoral necrosis, higher cellularity, and dissemination along CSF spaces including the spine.

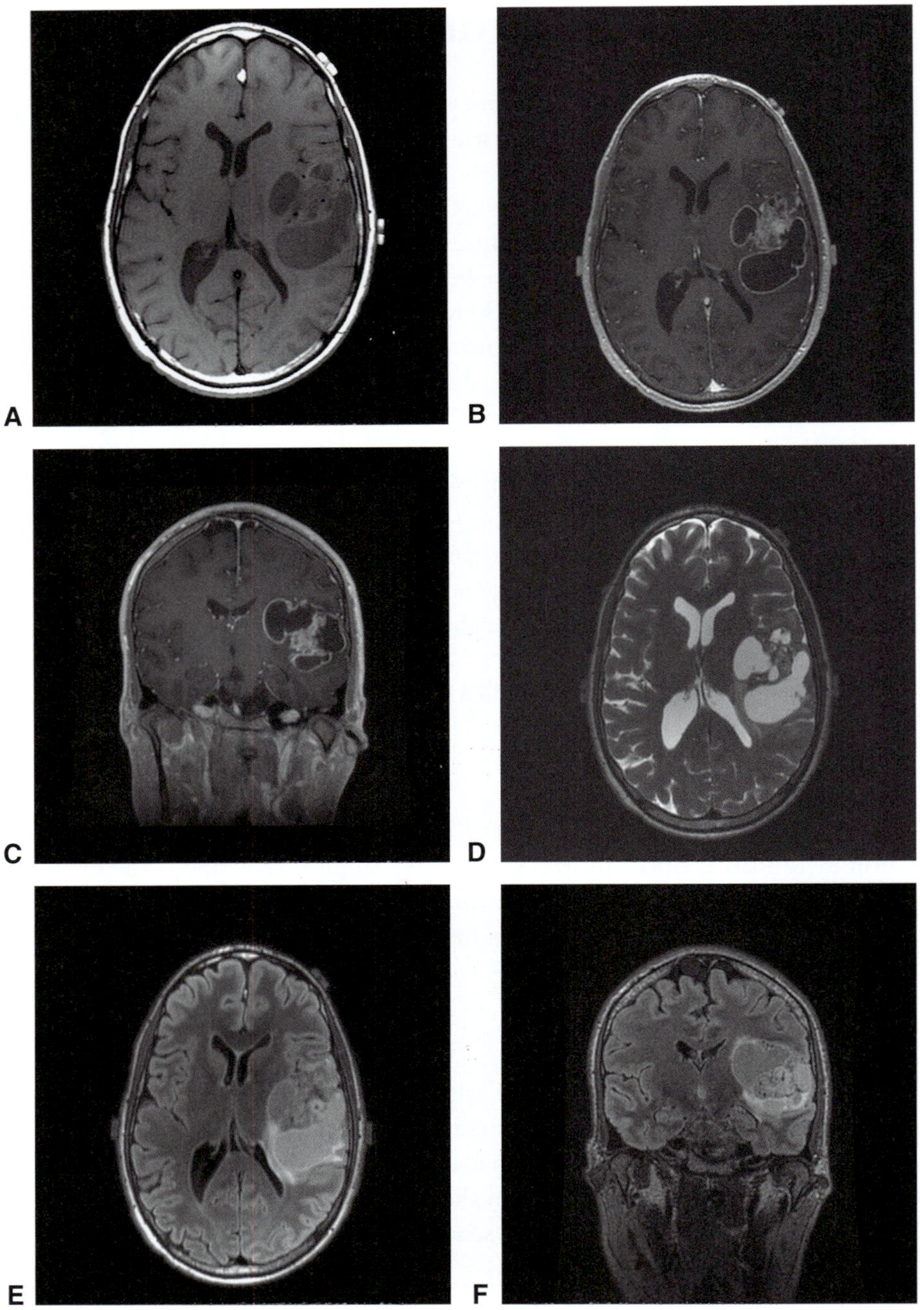

Figure 13.4. Imaging of pleomorphic xanthoastrocytoma. A. Axial T1-precontrast: Hypo- or isointense to surrounding brain with solid and cystic component. **B.** Axial T1-postcontrast: Avid but heterogeneous enhancement of the solid component, which is often superficially located; variable size and rim enhancement of cystic component. **C.** Coronal T1-postcontrast: Avid but heterogeneous enhancement of the solid component, which is often superficially located; variable size and rim enhancement of cystic component. **D.** T2 FSE: Hypo- or isointense to surrounding brain. **E.** Axial FLAIR: Iso- to slightly hyperintense to surrounding brain. **F.** Coronal FLAIR.

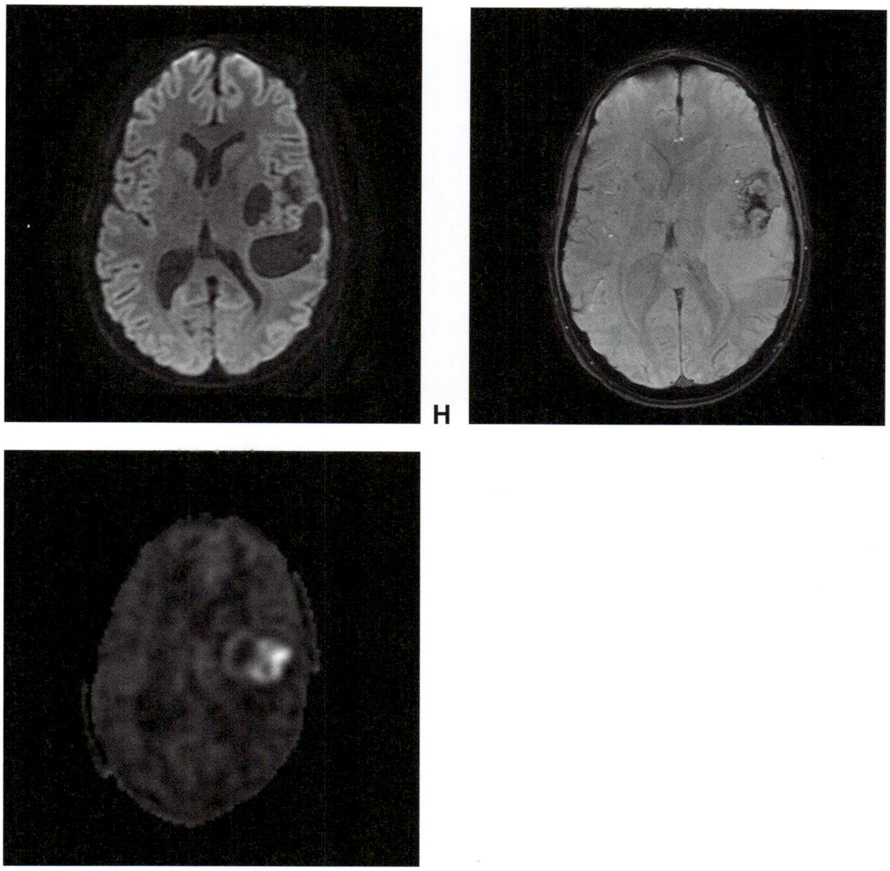

Figure 13.4. ***(continued)*** **G.** DWI: Increased diffusion. **H.** Susceptibility-weighted imaging (SWI): Heterogeneous blood products. **I.** Arterial spin labeling (ASL) Perfusion: Hypervascular solid component.

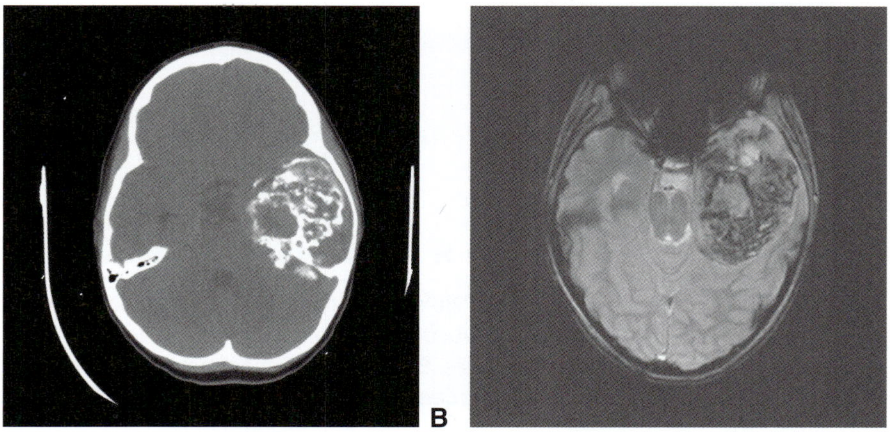

Figure 13.5. **Imaging of anaplastic pleomorphic xanthoastrocytoma. A.** Axial CT bone window: Calcified mass filling the left middle cranial fossa. **B.** Axial SWI: Calcified mass filling the left middle cranial fossa.

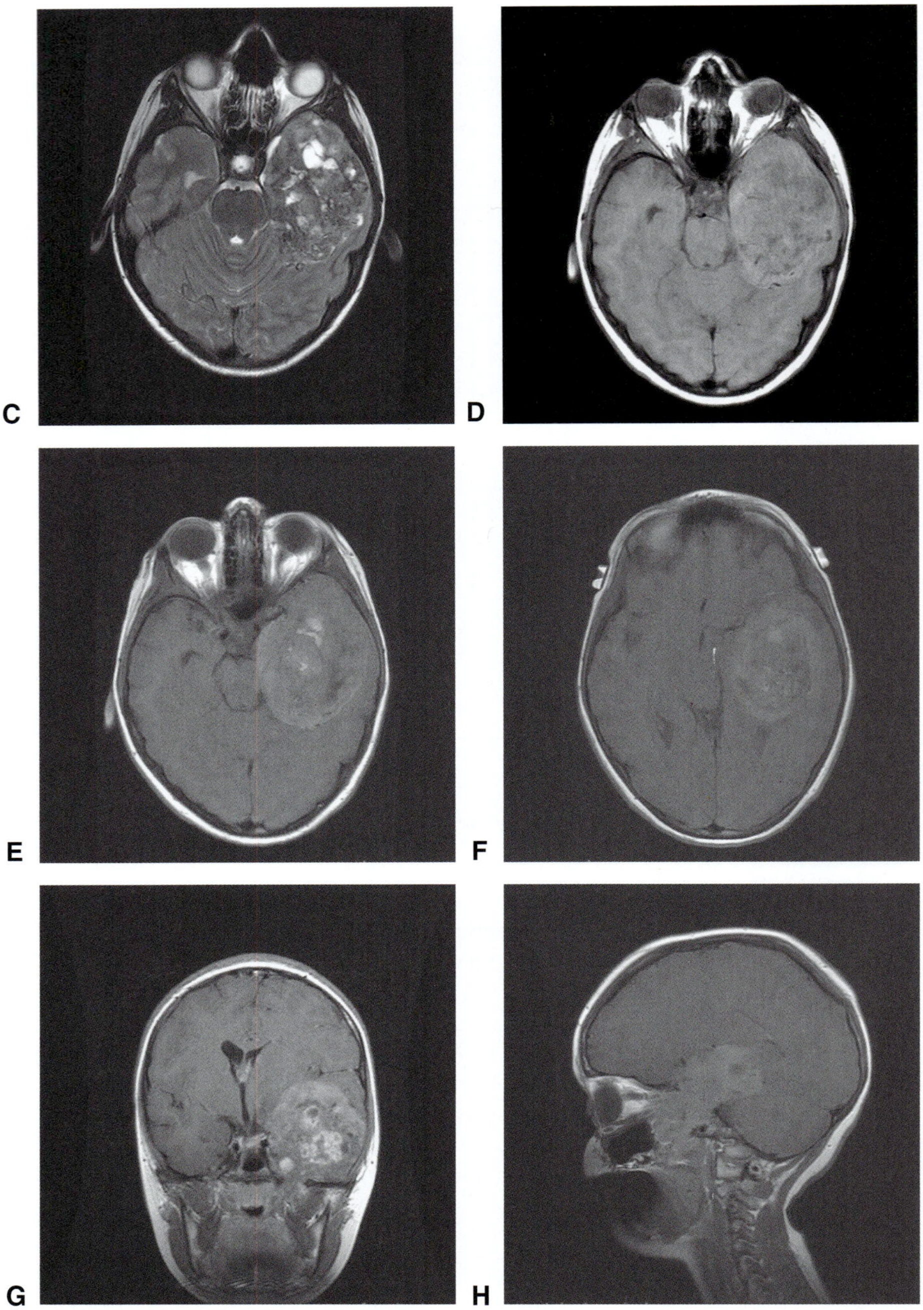

Figure 13.5. ***(continued)*** **C.** Axial T2: Heterogeneously low-signal intensity mass with areas of cystic components. **D.** Axial T1-precontrast: Heterogeneous mass with subtle areas of intratumoral necrosis. **E.** Axial T1-postcontrast: Heterogeneous enhancement with more avidly enhancing central components. **F.** Axial T1-postcontrast: Heterogeneous enhancement with more avid enhancing central components. **G.** Coronal T1-postcontrast: Heterogeneous enhancement with more avidly enhancing central components. **H.** Sagittal T1-postcontrast: Mass destroys the middle fossa and extends extracranially into the skull base.

I

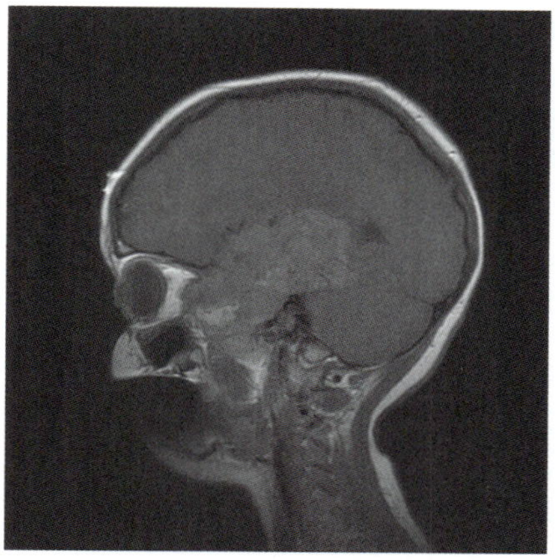

Figure 13.5. *(continued)* **I.** Sagittal T1-postcontrast: Mass destroys the middle fossa and extends extracranially into the skull base.

Subependymal Giant Cell Astrocytoma

Definition: Subependymal giant cell astrocytoma is a WHO grade I, slow-growing, circumscribed, benign astrocytic neoplasm composed of large ganglionic astrocytes arising in the walls of the lateral ventricle near the foramen of Monro in children or young adults and tightly linked with the tuberous sclerosis complex.

Epidemiology: Subependymal giant cell astrocytoma (SEGA) is a disease-defining tumor of tuberous sclerosis, occurring in up to 15% of patients with this disorder. However, SEGA has been reported in patients without tuberous sclerosis.

Affected age group: This tumor most commonly affects children or young adults (2–30 years) in the first two decades of life, usually less than 20 years of age but can occur in infants.

Molecular and genetic profile: SEGA is the principal central nervous system (CNS) neoplasm associated with tuberous sclerosis. The two-hit mechanism of genetic abnormality in SEGA involves inactivation of the *TSC1* gene at 9q or *TSC2* gene at 16p and activation of mTOR pathway.

CSF markers: None.

Clinical features and standard therapy: Although surgical resection is the mainstay, gross total resection of SEGA may not be possible due to its location near the foramen of Monro and caudate. The overall prognosis of patients with SEGA is very good provided that gross total resection is achieved and no complication has occurred. Although there is no standard chemotherapy for SEGA, inhibition of mTOR1 pathway using everolimus is showing some promise for those patients with residual or recurrent SEGA.

Imaging

SEGA is a lobulated or polypoid mass with avid enhancement located in and around foramen of Monro, or rarely entirely within the lateral ventricle.

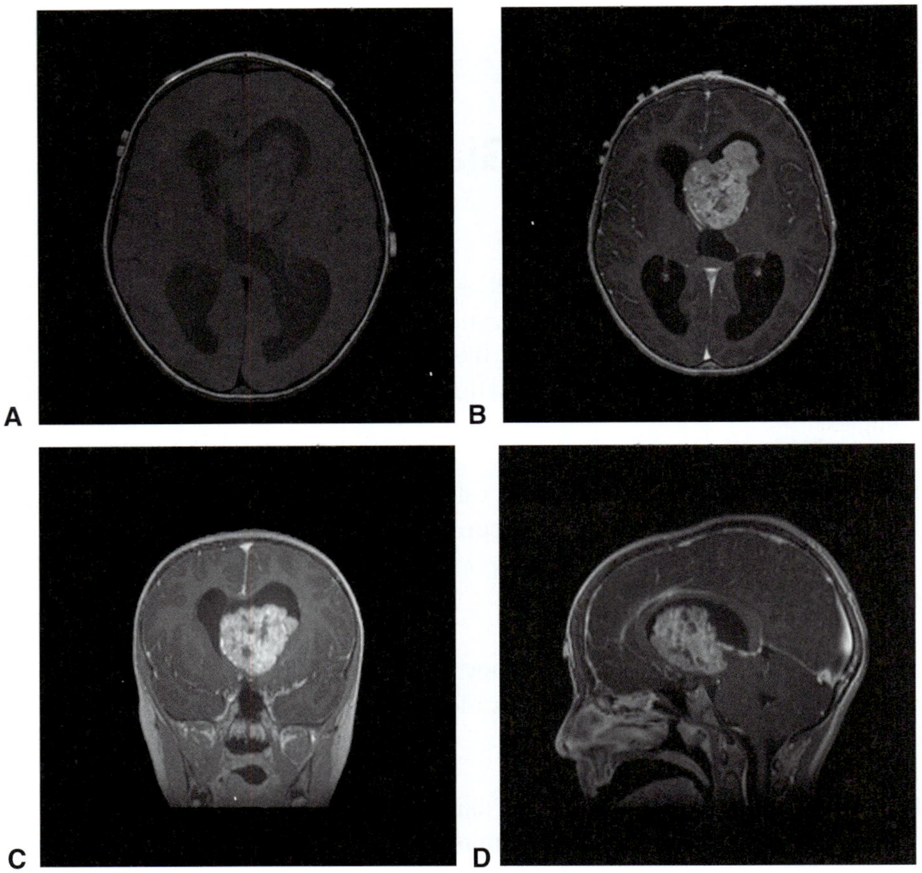

Figure 13.6. Imaging of SEGA. A. T1-precontrast: Hypo- or isointense to surrounding brain. **B.** Axial T1-postcontrast: Avid but heterogeneous enhancement except in areas of calcium. **C.** Coronal T1-postcontrast: Avid but heterogeneous enhancement except in areas of calcium. **D.** Sagittal T1-postcontrast: Avid but heterogeneous enhancement except in areas of calcium.

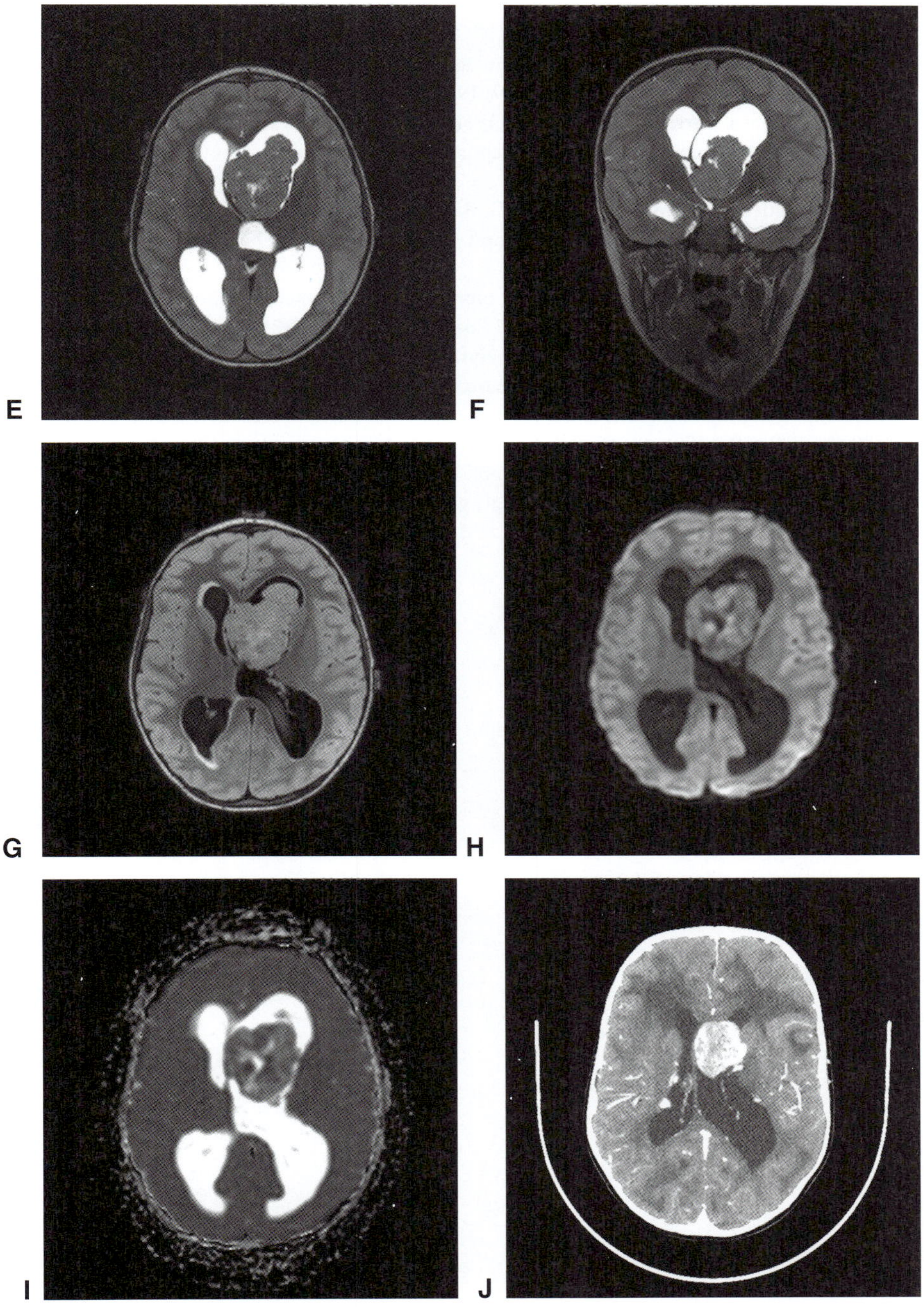

Figure 13.6. ***(continued)*** **E.** Axial T2 FSE: Hyper- or isointense to surrounding brain. **F.** Coronal T2 FSE: Hyper- or isointense to surrounding brain. **G.** FLAIR: Iso- to slightly hyperintense to surrounding brain. **H.** DWI: Isointense to brain. **I.** ADC: Isointense to brain. **J.** CT: Hyperdense, calcified mass associated with numerous subependymal tubers.

Bibliography

Arslanoglu A, Cirak B, Horska A, et al. MR imaging characteristics of pilomyxoid astrocytomas. *AJNR Am J Neuroradiol.* 2003;24(9):1906–1908.

Ceppa EP, Bouffet E, Griebel R, Robinson C, Tihan T. The pilomyxoid astrocytoma and its relationship to pilocytic astrocytoma: report of a case and a critical review of the entity. *J Neurooncol.* 2007;81(2):191–196.

Crespo-Rodriguez AM, Smirniotopoulos JG, Rushing EJ. MR and CT imaging of 24 pleomorphic xanthoastrocytomas (PXA) and a review of the literature. *Neuroradiology.* 2007;49:307–315.

Kalantari BN, Salamon N. Neuroimaging of tuberous sclerosis: spectrum of pathologic findings and frontiers in imaging. *AJR Am J Roentgenol.* 2008;190(5):W304–W309.

Schindler G, Capper D, Meyer J, et al. Analysis of *BRAF* V600E mutation in 1,320 nervous system tumors reveals high mutation frequencies in pleomorphic xanthoastrocytoma, ganglioglioma and extra-cerebellar pilocytic astrocytoma. *Acta Neuropathol.* 2011;121(3):397–405.

She D, Liu J, Xing Z, Zhang D, Cao D, Zhang Z. MR imaging features of anaplastic pleomorphic xanthoastrocytoma mimicking high-grade astrocytoma. *AJNR Am J Neuroradiol.* 2018;39:1446–1452.

14

Ependymal Tumors

Overview

Ependymal tumors of the CNS arise from the ependymal cells that line the ventricles of the brain or the central canal of the spinal cord and can affect any age group, although they are more common in children. Approximately 60% of ependymal tumors occur in the cerebral hemispheres, 30% in the posterior fossa, and 10% in the spinal canal. The two slow-growing grade I tumors are subependymoma and myxopapillary ependymoma, whereas more aggressive-grade tumors are ependymoma (grade II) and anaplastic ependymoma (grade III). Anaplastic ependymomas are more common in posterior fossa in children and supratentorial brain in adults. There are three rare distinct histological variants—papillary, clear cell, and tanycytic ependymomas. A recently defined distinct molecular subtype of ependymoma, the *RELA* fusion-positive, is an aggressive variant (grade II or III) of ependymoma occurring in the supratentorial brain in children and carries a worse prognosis. Although historically considered a single entity, ependymomas from each of the three anatomic compartments (supratentorial, posterior fossa, spinal canal) are considered biologically and genetically distinct entities.

	Age range (mean year)	Female: male ratio	Cell of origin	WHO grade	Molecular/ genetic markers	Prognosis
Subependymoma	55–64 (60)	1:2.3	Subependymal glia	I	Rare familial occurrence	Favorable
Myxopapillary ependymoma	20–34 (27)	1: 2.2	Radial glial cell (lumbosacral roots)	I	Polyploidy	Favorable
Supratentorial ependymoma	18–24 (21)	1:1	Radial glial cell	II or III	*RELA* fusion gene *YAP1* fusion gene	Guarded
Posterior fossa ependymoma	Bimodal (5 and 35)	1:1	Radial glial cell	II	Polyploidy *NF2* mutation	Variable
Spinal ependymoma	30–40 (35)	1:1	Radial glial cell	I or II	Polyploidy 6q deletion	Variable

Subependymoma

Definition: Subependymoma is a benign, slow-growing, often incidentally detected, intraventricular glial neoplasm arising from the subependymal glia and represents a lower-grade counterpart to ependymoma.

Epidemiology: Due to its rarity and asymptomatic clinical course, the true incidence of subependymoma is difficult to determine. It affects patients of all ages but is more common in middle-aged and older individuals.

Affected age group: The tumor usually affects middle-aged to older adults, with a mean age group of 55 to 64 years old, and without gender predilection.

Molecular and genetic profile: Chromosome 6 copy number alterations are only seen in lateral ventricule, posterior fossa, and spinal subependymomas and never in supratentorial subependymomas. Familial occurrence is well documented, but the underlying specific genetic susceptibility remains unknown.

Clinical features and standard therapy: Gross total resection of tumor leads to cure, although recurrence can be seen in rare cases.

Imaging

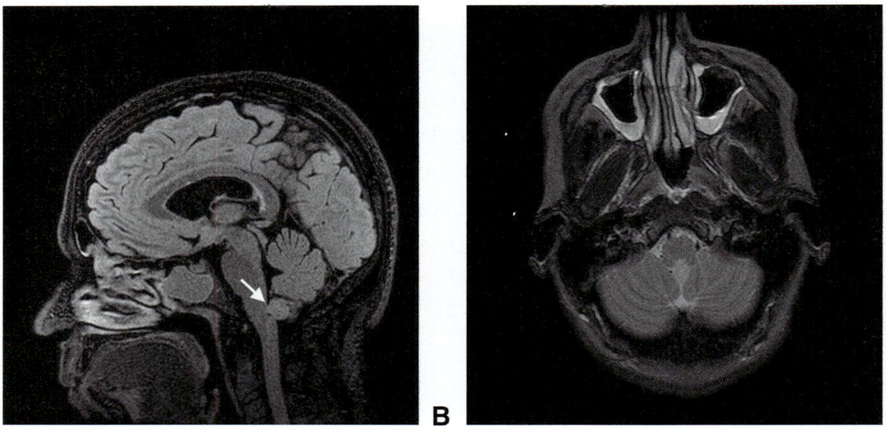

A B

Figure 14.1. Imaging of subependymoma at the obex. A. Sagittal fluid-attenuated inversion recovery (FLAIR): Slightly hyperintense ovoid mass at the obex (arrow). **B.** Axial T2: Slightly hyperintense ovoid mass at the obex.

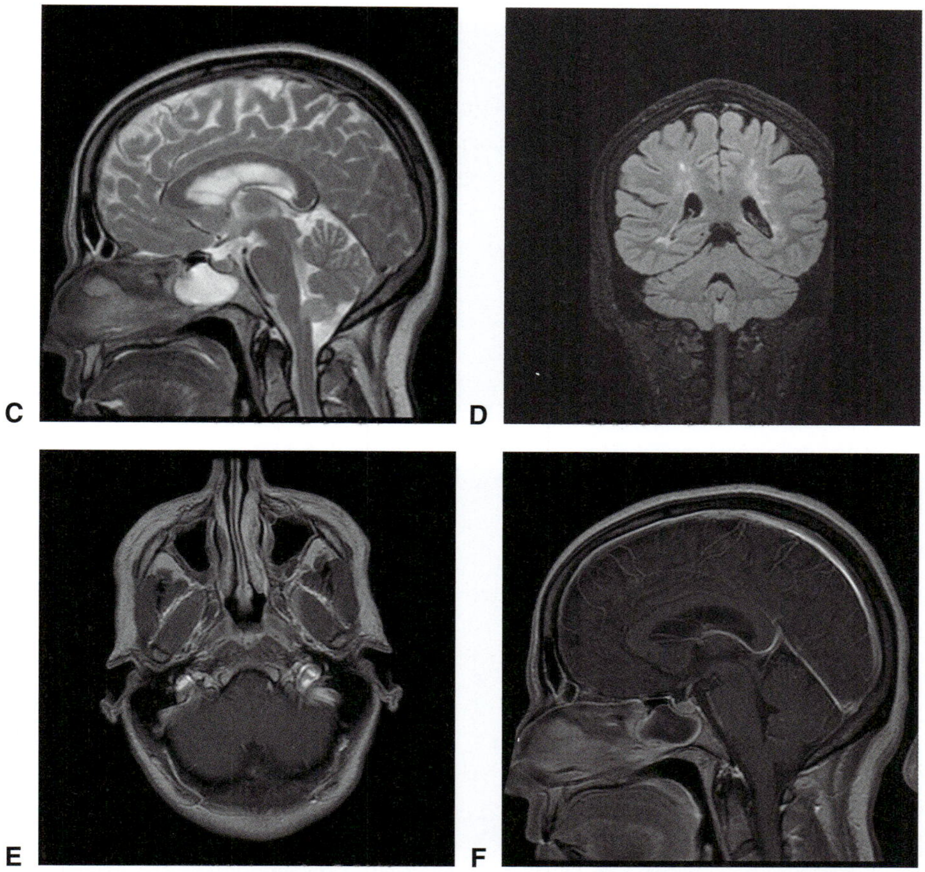

Figure 14.1. ***(continued)*** **C.** Sagittal T2: Slightly hyperintense ovoid mass at the obex. **D.** Coronal FLAIR: Slightly hyperintense ovoid mass at the obex. **E.** Axial T1-postcontrast: No enhancement within the mass. **F.** Sagittal T1-postcontrast: No enhancement within the mass.

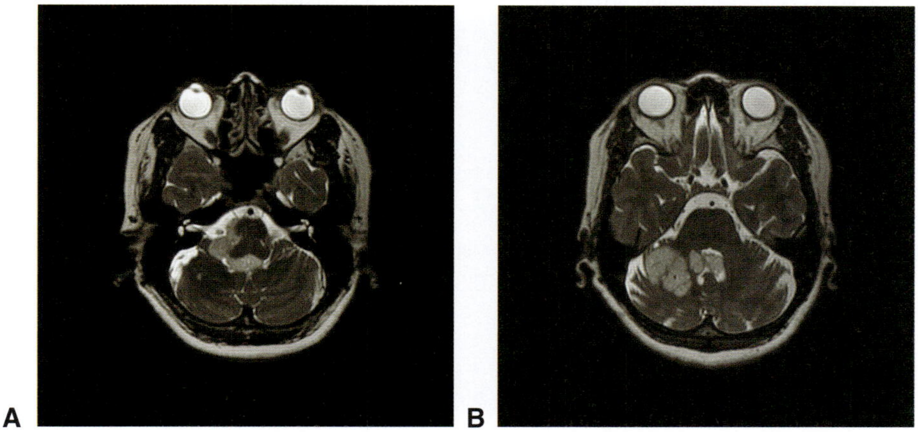

Figure 14.2. **Imaging of subependymoma of the posterior fossa. A.** Axial T2: Multilobulated slightly hyperintense mass within the fourth ventricle and right foramen of Luschka. **B.** Axial T2: Multilobulated slightly hyperintense mass within the fourth ventricle and right foramen of Luschka.

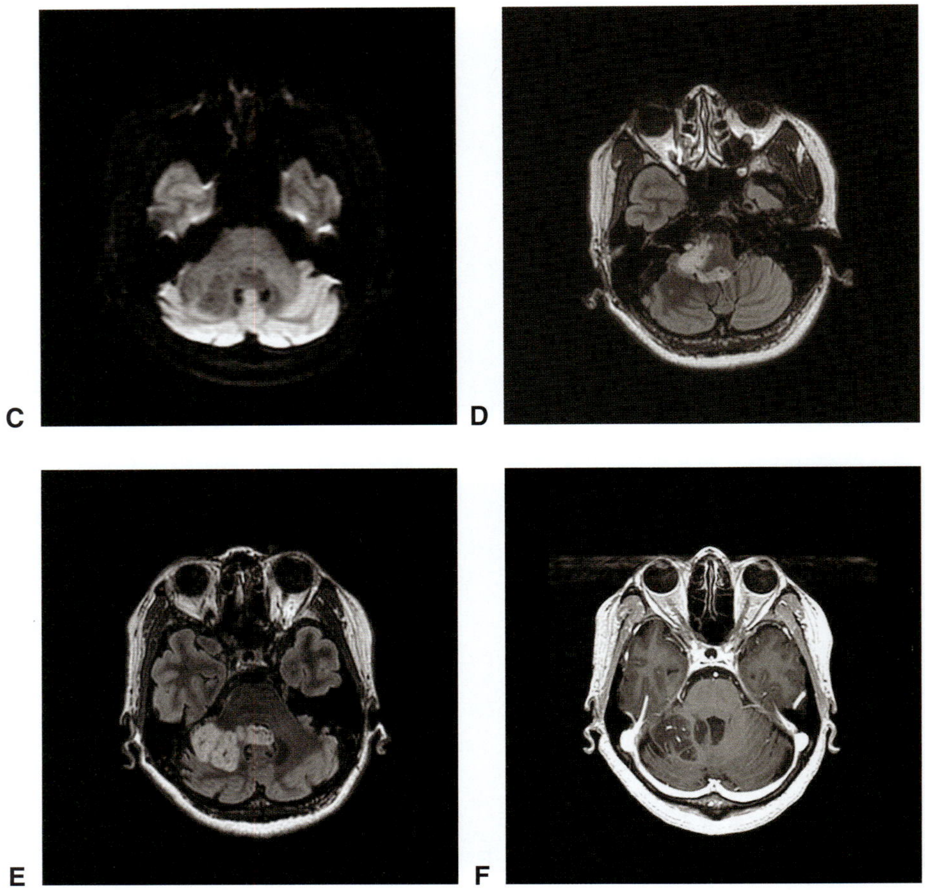

Figure 14.2. ***(continued)*** **C.** Axial diffusion-weighted imaging (DWI): No reduced diffusion within the mass. **D.** Axial FLAIR: Multilobulated slightly hyperintense mass within the fourth ventricle and right foramen of Luschka. **E.** Axial FLAIR: Multilobulated slightly hyperintense mass within the fourth ventricle and right foramen of Luschka. **F.** Axial T1-postcontrast: No enhancement within the mass; few vessels are seen within the mass.

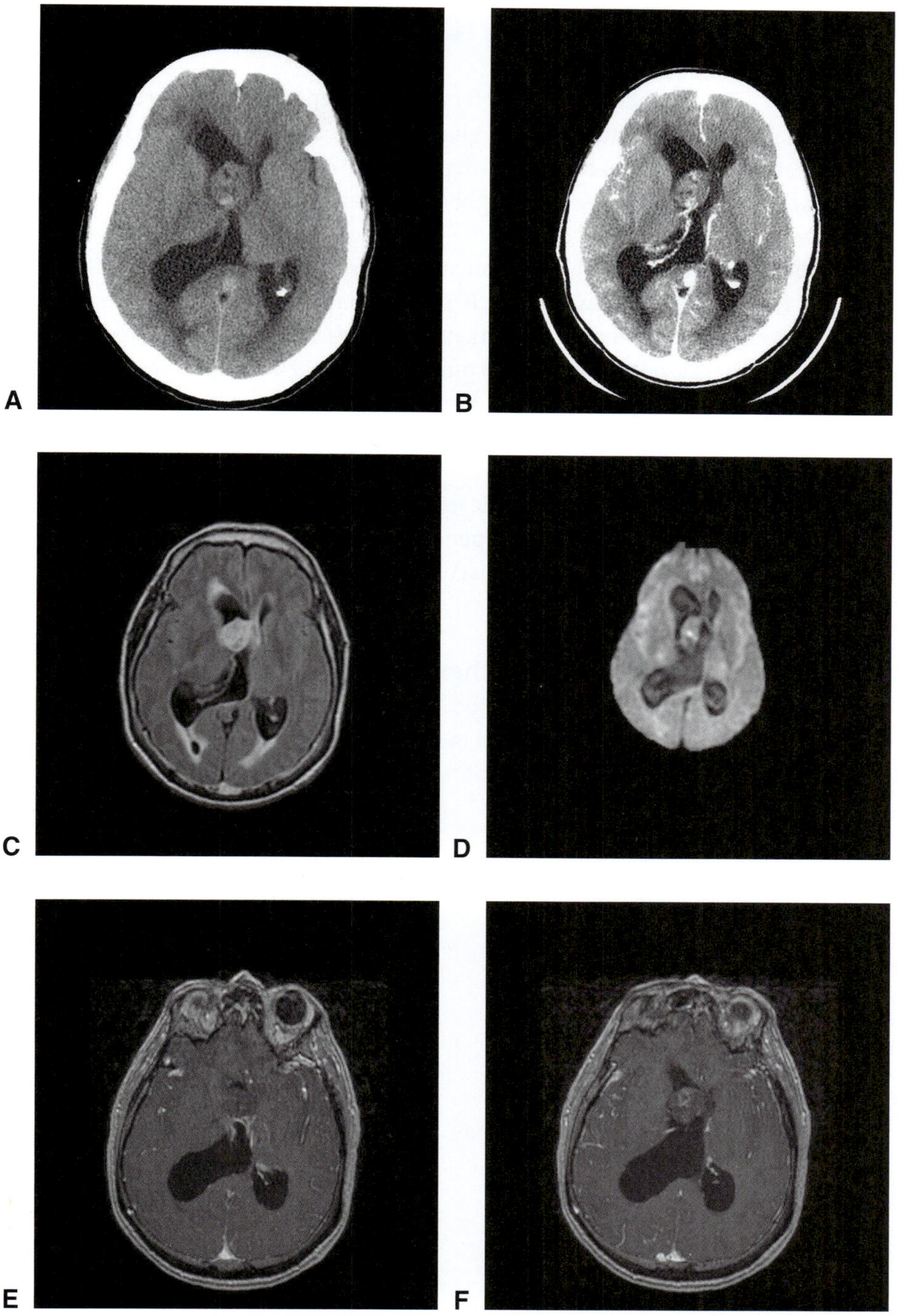

Figure 14.3. Imaging of subependymoma of the lateral ventricle. A. Unenhanced axial CT: Right intraventricular mass with focal calcification causing obstructive hydrocephalus. **B.** Enhanced axial CT: Mild enhancement within the mass. **C.** Axial FLAIR: Hyperintense mass. **D.** Axial DWI: Mildly reduced diffusion. **E.** Axial T1-postcontrast: No enhancement within the mass. **F.** Axial T1-postcontrast: Irregular rim enhancement within the mass.

▶ Classic Ependymoma

Definition: Classic ependymoma refers to intraventricular posterior fossa, spinal canal, or cerebral hemispheric glial tumor composed of uniform small ependymal cells growing in an expansive pattern. It has low cell density and low mitotic activity and rarely invades neighboring structures.

Epidemiology: The tumor affects patients of any age, but the intraventricular posterior fossa ependymomas are much more common in children, where the incidence decreases with increasing patient age; in children aged <3 years, up to 30% of all central nervous system (CNS) tumors are intraventricular posterior fossa ependymomas. On the contrary, spinal ependymomas are much more common in adults and account for up to 60% of all primary spinal neoplasm in adults.

Molecular and genetic profile: Based on DNA methylation profiles, nine molecular subgroups (Table 14.1) of ependymoma were found across three anatomical sites: the supratentorial compartment, posterior fossa, and spinal compartment.

Clinical features and standard therapy: Gross total resection of tumor leads to cure although recurrence can be seen, especially in anaplastic variants. To minimize local recurrence, adjuvant radiation therapy is often used, especially when there is any residual tumor, but it does not prevent distant recurrence.

TABLE 14.1 Nine Molecular Subgroups of Ependymoma

Anatomical location	Group	Genetic features	Dominant pathology	Age at diagnosis	Clinical prognosis
Supratentorial	ST-EPN-RELA	RELA fusion gene	Classic/anaplastic	Infancy to adulthood	Poor
	ST-EPN-YAP1	YAP1 fusion gene	Classic/anaplastic	Infancy to adulthood	Good
	ST-SE	Balanced genome	Subependymoma	Adulthood	Good
Posterior fossa	PF-EPN-A	Balanced genome	Classic/anaplastic	Infancy	Poor
	PF-EPN-B	Genome-wide polyploidy	Classic/anaplastic	Childhood to adulthood	Good
	PF-SE	Balanced genome	Subependymoma	Adulthood	Good
Spinal	SP-EPN	*NF2* mutation	Classic/anaplastic	Childhood to adulthood	Good
	SP-MPE	Genome-wide polyploidy	Myxopapillary	Adulthood	Good
	SP-SE	6q deletion	Subependymoma	Adulthood	Good

Imaging

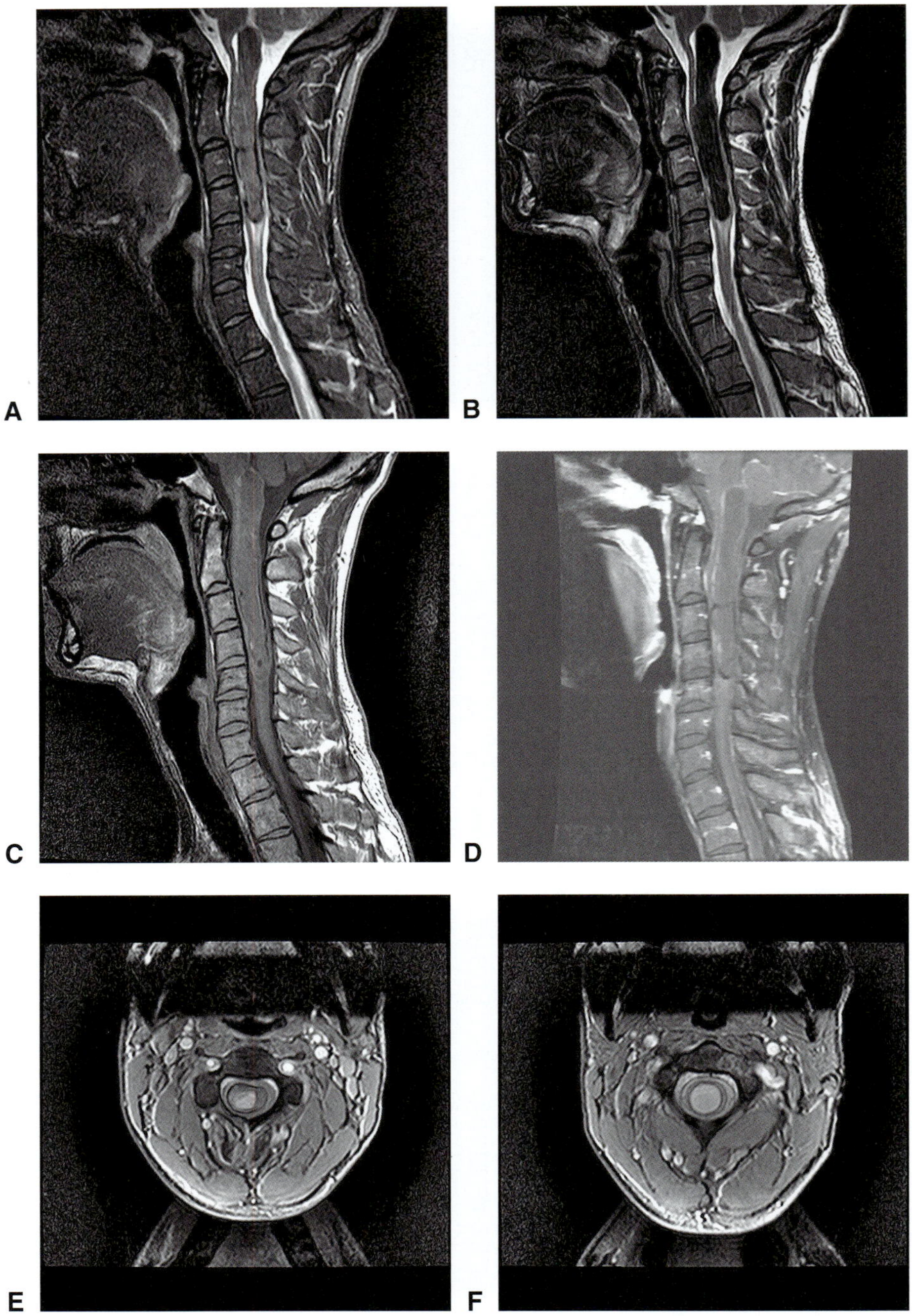

Figure 14.4. Imaging of spinal ependymoma. A. Sagittal Short tau inversion recovery (STIR*): Large hypointense intramedullary mass spanning from medullar to spinal cord at C4 level. **B.** Sagittal T2: Marked hypointense signal within the mass represents blood products. **C.** Sagittal T1-precontrast: Mass is near isointense with a rim of bright and dark signal due to blood products of varying age. **D.** Sagittal T1-postcontrast: No enhancement within the mass. **E.** Axial gradient echo: Hyperintense intramedullary cystic mass. **F.** Axial gradient echo: Hyperintense intramedullary cystic mass.

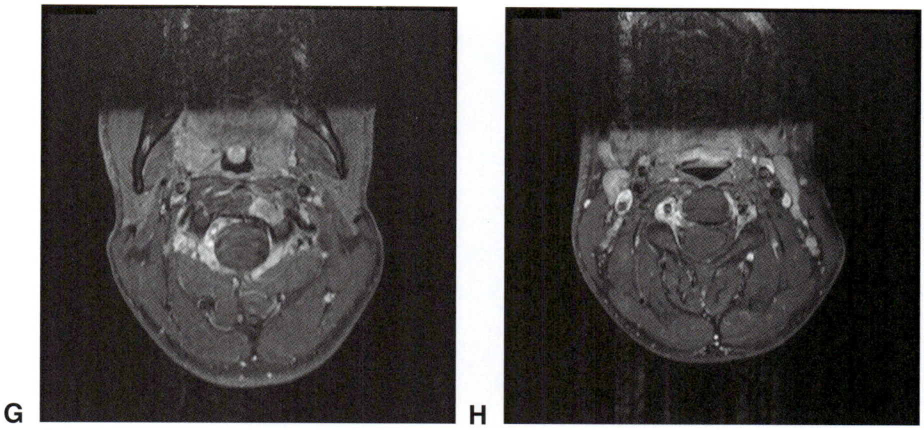

Figure 14.4. ***(continued)*** **G.** Axial T1 postcontrast: Hypointense intramedullary cystic mass without robust enhancement. **H.** Axial T1 postcontrast: Hypointense intramedullary cystic mass without robust enhancement.

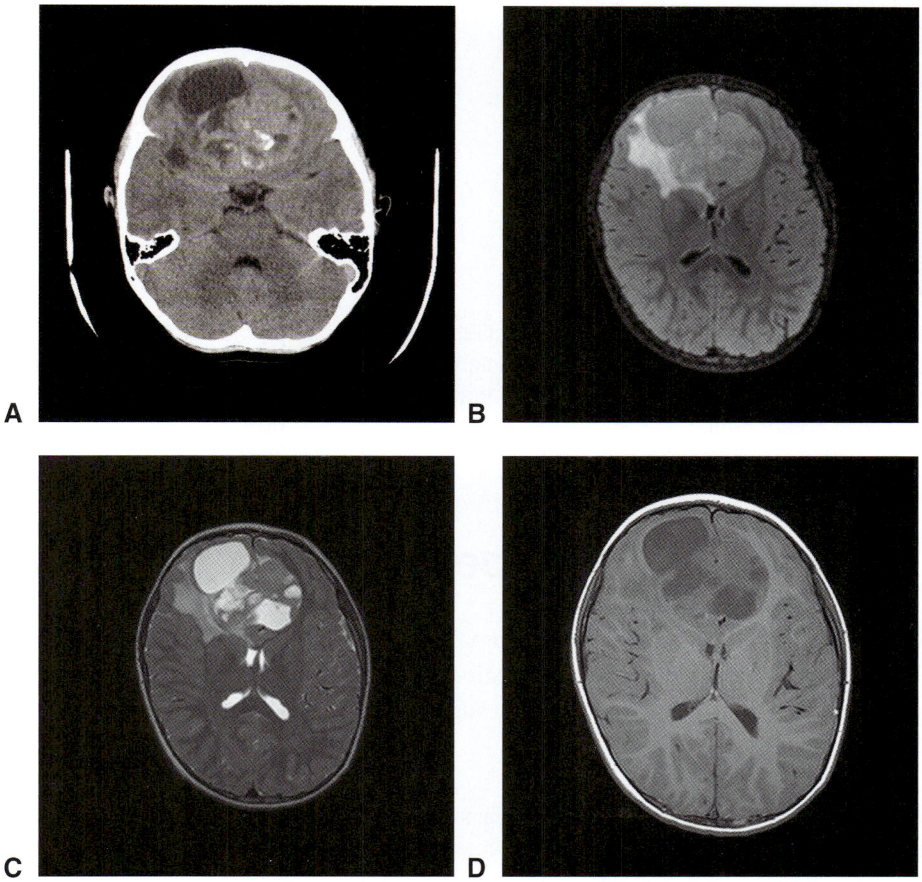

Figure 14.5. Imaging of supratentorial ependymoma. A. Axial unenhanced CT: Mixed solid and cystic midline intraparenchymal mass with scattered calcium. **B.** Axial FLAIR: Hypointense solid mass with cystic components and mild right frontal edema. **C.** Axial T2: Hypointense solid mass with cystic components and mild right frontal edema. **D.** Axial T1-precontrast: Hypointense solid mass with cystic components.

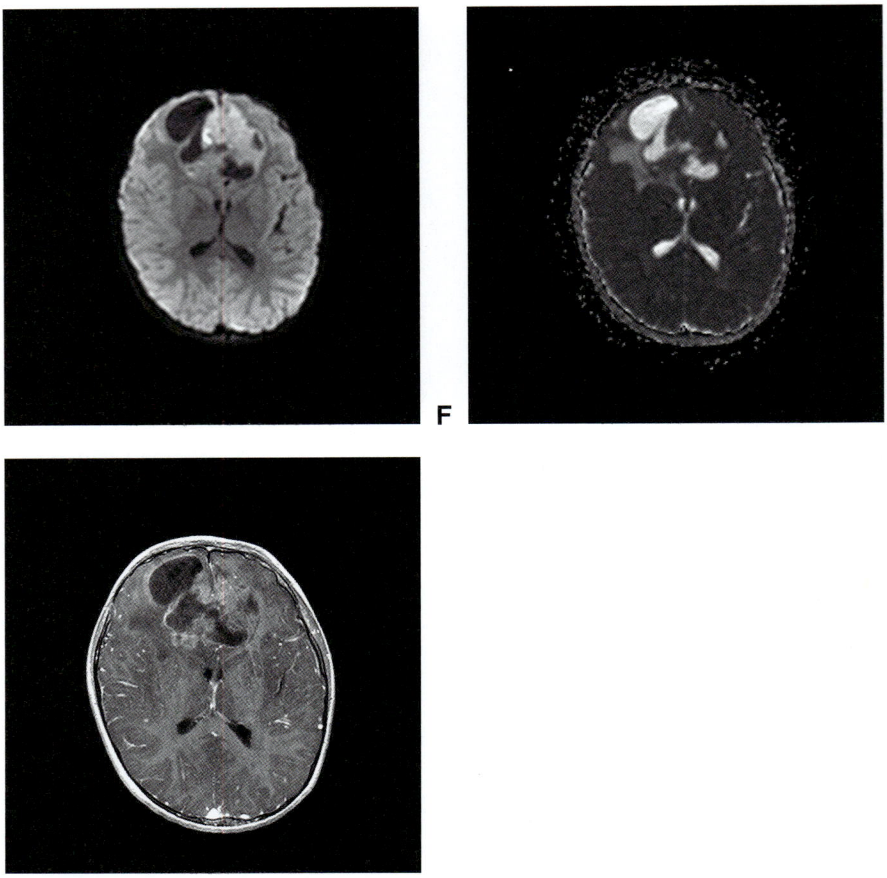

E F G

Figure 14.5. ***(continued)*** **E.** Axial DWI: Mildly reduced diffusion within the solid component. **F.** Axial apparent diffusion coefficient (ADC): Mildly reduced diffusion within the solid component. **G.** Axial T1-postcontrast: Heterogeneous enhancement within the solid component.

Myxopapillary Ependymoma

Definition: Myxopapillary ependymoma is a benign, slow-growing ependymal tumor arising exclusively from the region of the conus medullaris and cauda equina and can disseminate widely throughout the spinal canal and rarely into the brain.

Epidemiology: The myxopapillary variant accounts for approximately 10% of all ependymomas.

Affected age group: This usually affects young adults, with a mean age group of 20 to 35 years and male predilection.

Molecular and genetic profile: Genome-wide polyploidy is seen (see Table 14.1).

CSF markers: None.

Clinical features and standard therapy: Gross total resection of tumor leads to cure although recurrence can be seen in rare cases. To minimize local recurrence, adjuvant radiation therapy is often used, especially when there is any residual tumor, but it does not prevent distant recurrence.

Imaging

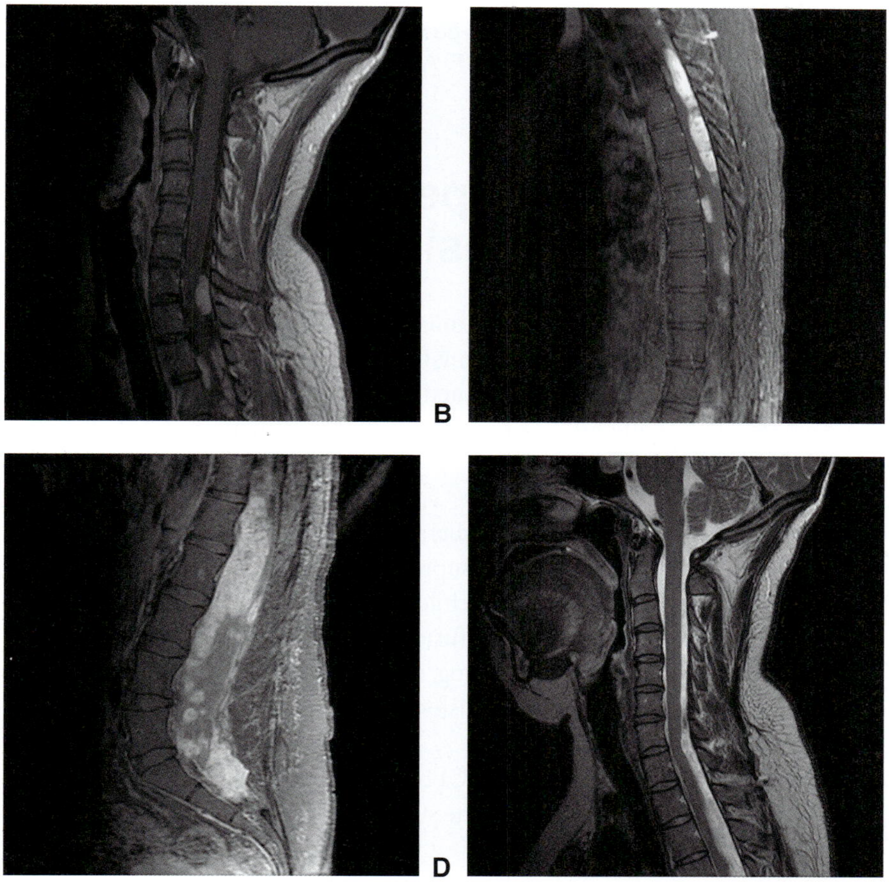

Figure 14.6. Imaging of disseminated myxopapillary ependymoma. A. Sagittal T1-postcontrast: Avidly enhancing intradural extramedullary nodules in the cervical spine. **B.** Sagittal T1-postcontrast: Avidly enhancing intradural extramedullary bulky masses in the thoracic spine. **C.** Sagittal T1-postcontrast: Avidly enhancing intradural extramedullary massive tumor filling the thecal sac in the lumbar spine. **D.** Sagittal T2-postcontrast: Hyperintense dorsal mass deforming the cervical cord.

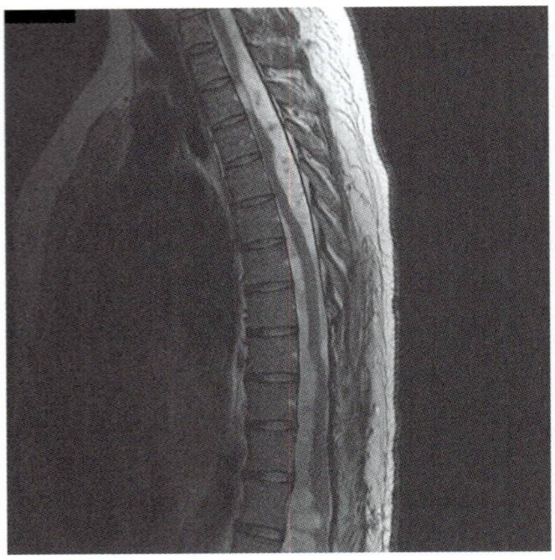
E

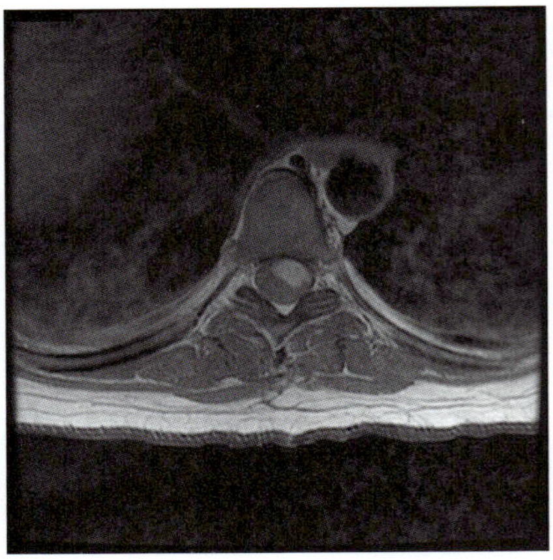
F

Figure 14.6. *(continued)* **E.** Sagittal T2-postcontrast: Hyperintense ventral and dorsal bulky masses deforming the cord. **F.** Axial T1-postcontrast: Ventral enhancing mass deforming the cord.

Supratentorial Ependymoma, RELA-Fusion Positive

Definition: Supratentorial ependymoma, RELA-fusion positive, is a circumscribed intraparenchymal tumor arising from ependymal cells of the supratentorial compartment. Genetically defined RELA fusion-positive ependymoma accounts for 70% of all childhood supratentorial ependymomas, which is rare in adults.

Epidemiology: Almost 90% of pediatric ependymomas are intracranial, of which around one-third arise in the supratentorial compartment, with a mean age of around 8 years at diagnosis. In children, up to two thirds of supratentorial ependymoma involves the oncogenic fusions of genes RELA (v-rel avian reticuloendotheliosis viral oncogene homolog A). There is no gender predilection in supratentorial ependymoma, RELA-fusion positive.

Molecular and genetic profile: C11orf95-RELA fusion is the most common molecular abnormality seen in the supratentorial ependymoma, especially in the pediatric age group.

Clinical features and standard therapy: Surgical resection is the primary therapy followed by radiation therapy. No effective chemotherapy is currently available.

Imaging

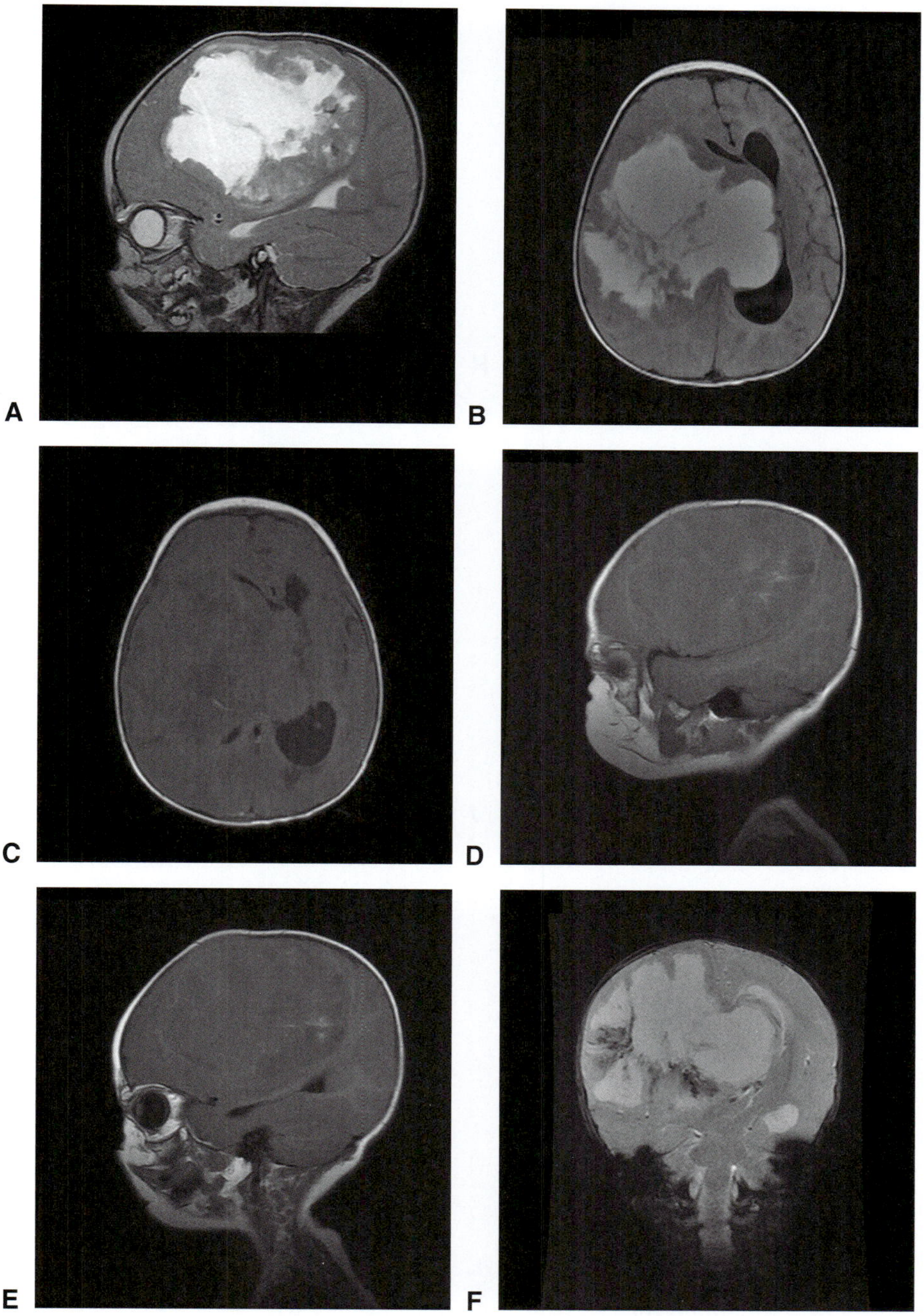

Figure 14.7. Imaging of supratentorial ependymoma, RELA fusion-positive. **A.** Sagittal T2: Hyperintense large lobulated mass. **B.** Axial FLAIR: Hyperintense large lobulated mass invading into the lateral ventricle. **C.** Axial T1-precontrast: Isointense large lobulated mass invading into the lateral ventricle. **D.** Sagittal T1-precontrast: Isointense large lobulated mass with subtle hyperintense internal septations. **E.** Sagittal T1-precontrast: Isointense large lobulated mass with subtle hyperintense internal septations. **F.** Coronal gradient echo: Peripheral rim of blood products.

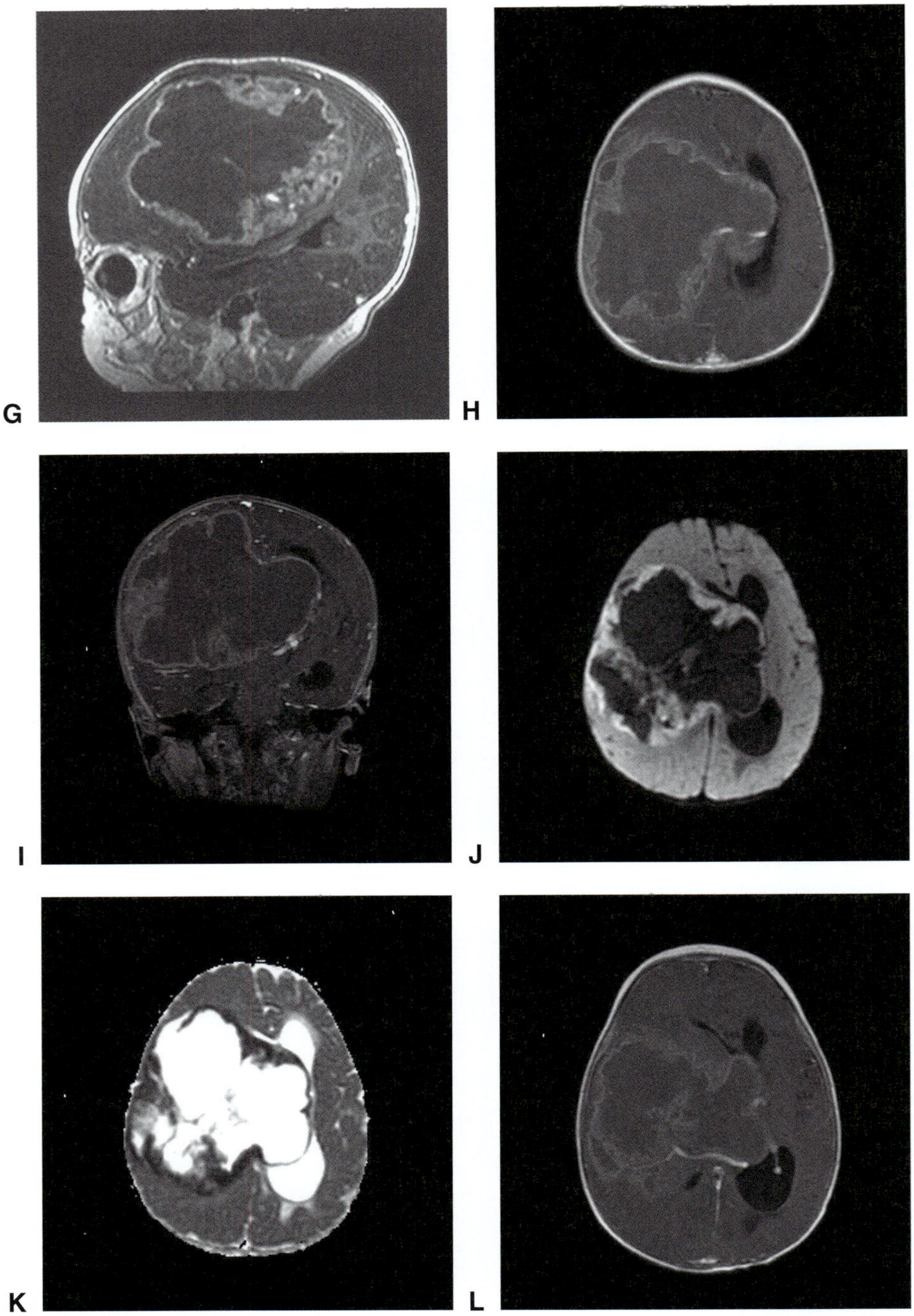

Figure 14.7. ***(continued)*** **G.** Sagittal T1-postcontrast: Irregular rim enhancement of the mass. **H.** Axial T1-postcontrast: Irregular rim enhancement of the mass. **I.** Coronal T1-postcontrast: Irregular rim enhancement of the mass. **J.** Axial DWI: Reduced diffusion corresponds to the irregular rim enhancement. **K.** Axial ADC: Reduced diffusion corresponds to the irregular rim enhancement. **L.** Axial T1-postcontrast: Irregular rim enhancement corresponds to the cellular component of tumor.

Bibliography

Hanna MH, Bansal A, Belani P. A review of radiographic imaging findings of ependymal tumors. *Neurosurg Cases Rev.* 2019;2:28.

Onish S, Yamasaki F, Nakano Y, et al. RELA fusion-positive anaplastic ependymoma: molecular characterization and advanced MR imaging. *Brain Tumor Pathol.* 2018;35:41–45.

Ragel BT, Osborn AG, Whang K, et al. Subependymomas: an analysis of clinical and imaging features. *Neurosurgery.* 2006;58(5):881–890.

Weber DC, Wang Y, Miller R, et al. Long-term outcome of patients with spinal myxopapillary ependymoma: treatment results from the MD Anderson Cancer Center and institutions from the Rare Cancer Network. *Neuro-oncology.* 2015;17(4):588–595.

Yuh EL, Barkovich AJ, Gupta N. Imaging of ependymomas: MRI and CT. *Childs Nerv Syst.* 2009;25(10):1203–1213.

15 Other Gliomas

Overview

There are three rare gliomas—chordoid glioma, angiocentric glioma, and astroblastoma—that do not fall into a specific glioma category or classification. Each has unique molecular and genetic profiles, predilection for certain locations and ages, and imaging features.

	Age range (yr) (mean)	Female: male ratio	Cell of origin	WHO grade	Molecular/genetic markers	Prognosis
Chordoid glioma	5–71(46)	2:1	Ependymal cell	II	11q13 and 9p21 losses	Favorable
Angiocentric glioma	<18	1:1	Radial glia	I	*MYB* focus 6q23	Favorable
Astroblastoma	<30	1:1	Astroblast	I or II	19 and 20q gains	Depends on histology

▶ Chordoid Glioma of the Third Ventricle

Definition: Chordoid glioma of the third ventricle is a low-grade, solid intraventricular glial neoplasm located in the third ventricle with indolent and noninvasive growth pattern and histologically composed of epithelioid cells expressing Glial fibrillary acidic protein (GFAP) in a background of mucinous stroma and lymphoplasmacytic infiltrate.

Epidemiology: This rare tumor occurs primarily in adults, with a female-to-male ratio of 2:1.

Affected age group: There is wide variation in age, with reported cases ranging from 5 to 71 years of age. Most patients are adults aged 35 to 60, with a mean age of 46 years.

Molecular and genetic profile: The most distinct immunohistologic feature is strong, diffuse positivity for glial fibrillary acidic protein as well as vimentin and CD34. Neuronal and neuroendocrine markers are absent. Chromosomal heterozygosity losses at 11q13 and 9p21 are noted.

CSF markers: None.

Clinical features and standard therapy: Surgical resection is the definitive therapy, and gross total resection usually results in cure. However, local recurrence can be seen in the setting subtotal resection.

Imaging

Chordoid glioma of the third ventricle is a solid, well-circumscribed tumor attached to the anterior wall or the roof of the third ventricle or inseparable from the hypothalamus.

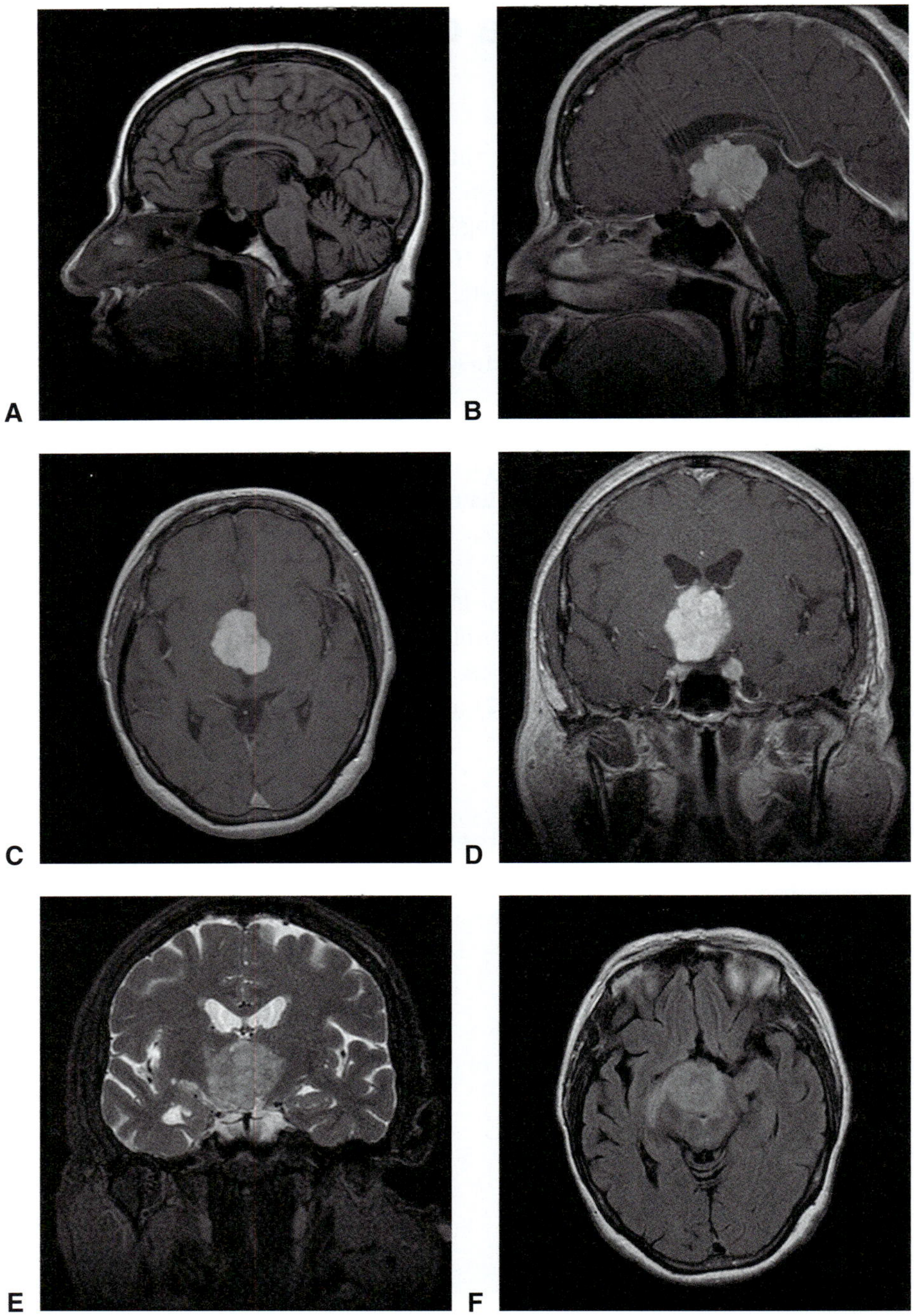

Figure 15.1. **Chordoid glioma. A.** Sagittal T1-precontrast: Hypointense to surrounding brain. **B.** Sagittal T1-postcontrast: Solid, homogeneous enhancement. **C.** Axial T1-postcontrast: Solid, homogeneous enhancement. **D.** Coronal T1-postcontrast: Solid, homogeneous enhancement. **E.** Coronal T2: Heterogeneous, mild hyperintense to brain. **F.** Fluid-attenuated inversion recovery (FLAIR): Mildly hyperintense to surrounding brain.

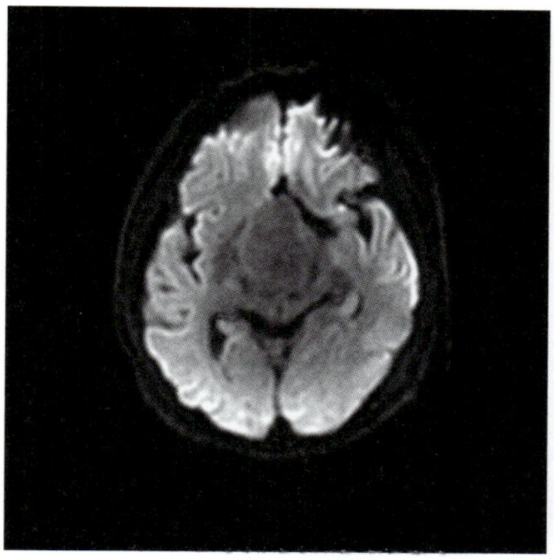

G

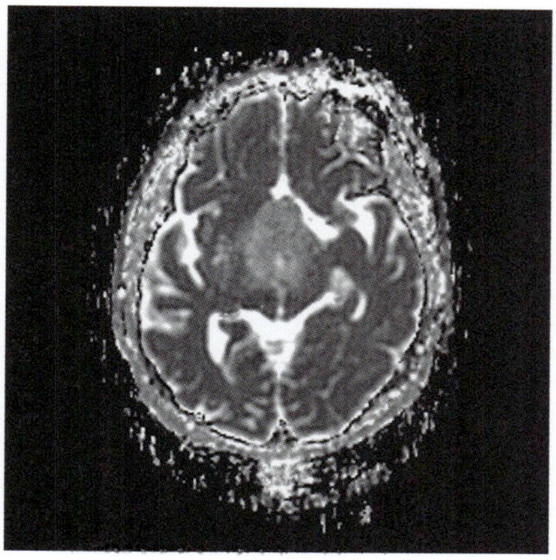

H

Figure 15.1. ***(continued)*** **G.** Diffusion-weighted imaging (DWI): Low signal on diffusion. **H.** Apparent diffusion coefficient (ADC): High signal on ADC.

Angiocentric Glioma

Definition: Angiocentric glioma is a circumscribed, superficially located, cortically based, benign cerebral tumor with angiocentric growth pattern and ependymal differentiation

Epidemiology: Due to the rarity of angiocentric glioma, the true incidence of this tumor is not known.

Affected age group: This tumor primarily occurs in children and young adults without gender predilection.

Molecular and genetic profile: Rearrangement of *MYB* locus on chromosome 6q23 is seen.

Clinical features and standard therapy: Chronic and intractable seizure is the most common clinical presentation, and gross total surgical resection achieves cure.

Imaging

Cortically based tumor with subcortical extension in the supratentorial brain and variable degree of enhancement, minimal mass effect, and a stalk-like extension toward neighboring ventricle.

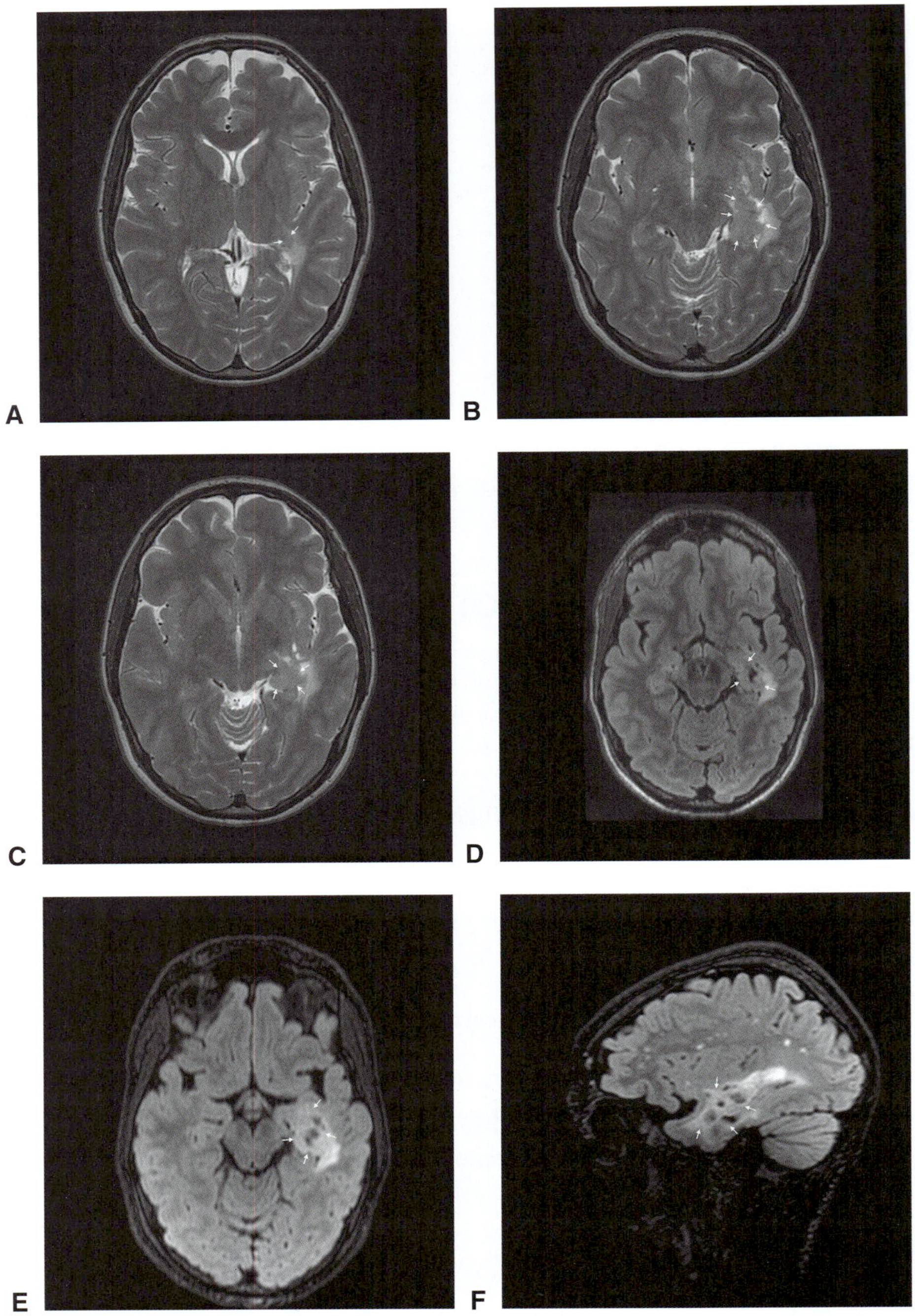

Figure 15.2. Angiocentric glioma. A–C. Axial T2: Lobular contour, hypointense mass (white arrows). **D–E.** Axial FLAIR: Heterogeneously hyperintense mass (white arrows). **F.** Sagittal FLAIR: Heterogeneously hyperintense mass (white arrows) with internal cystic changes.

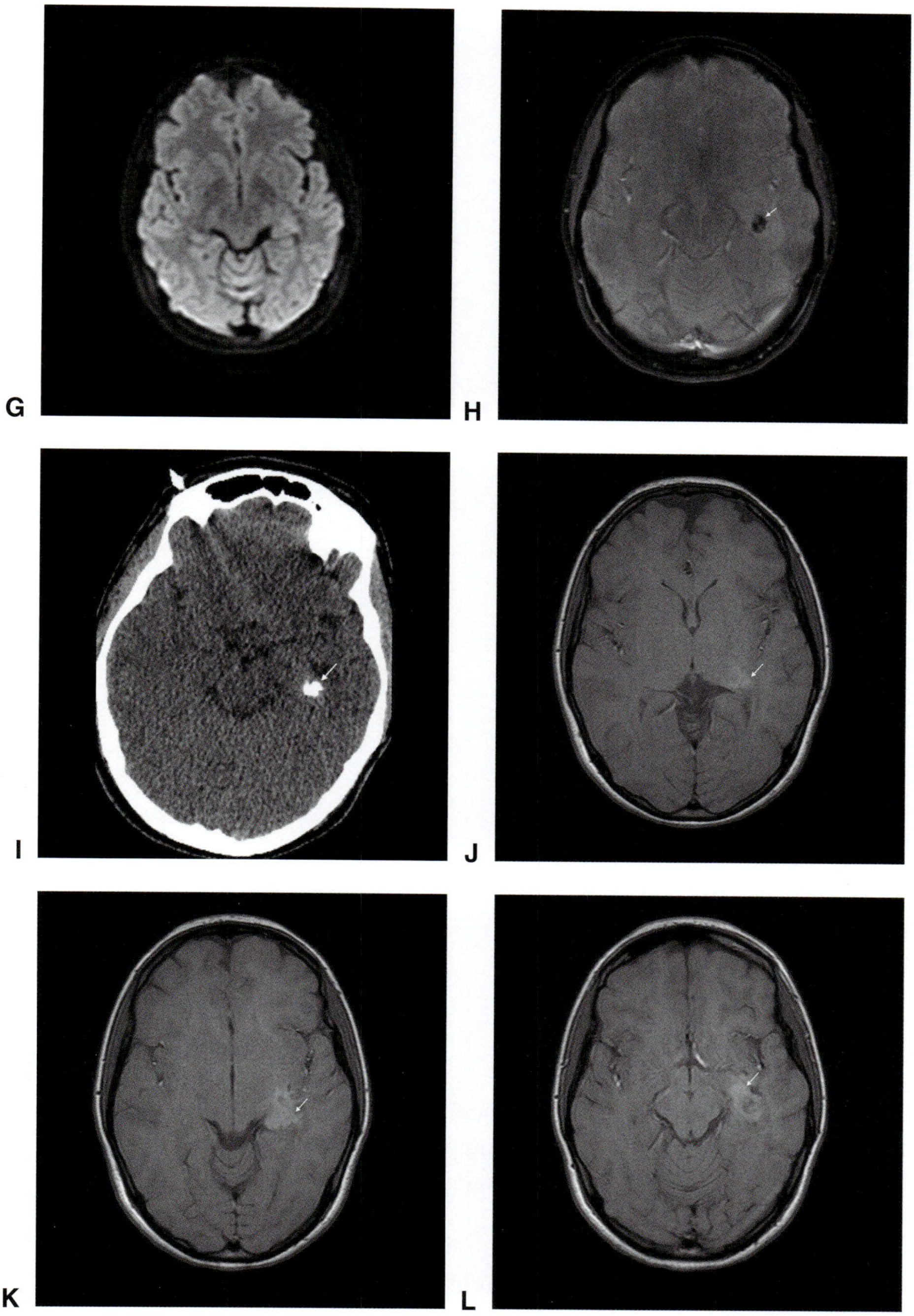

Figure 15.2. ***(continued)*** **G.** Axial DWI: No reduced diffusion within the mass. **H.** Axial Susceptibility-weighted imaging (SWI): Focal susceptibility within the mass (white arrow). **I.** Axial CT, bone window: Chunky intratumoral calcium confirmed on CT (white arrow). **J–L.** Axial T1-precontrast: Mild intrinsic T1 shortening within the mass (arrows).

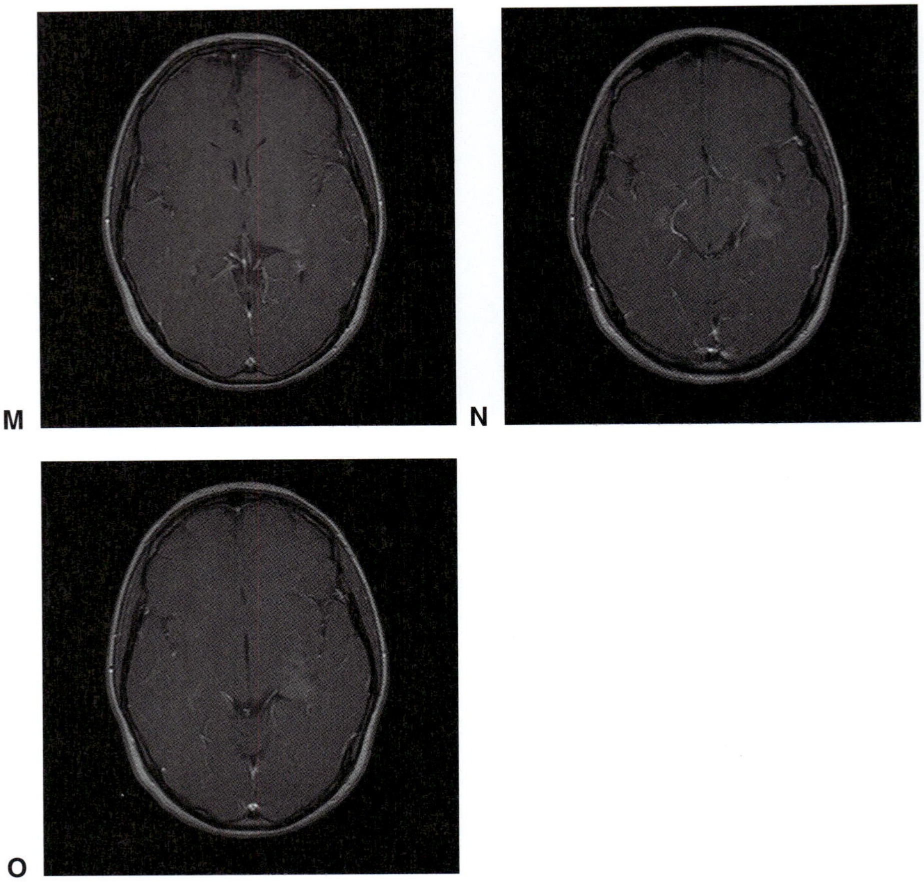

Figure 15.2. ***(continued)*** **M–O.** Axial T1-postcontrast: Minimal to absent enhancement within the mass.

Astroblastoma

Definition: Astroblastoma is an unusual cerebral hemispheric tumor, distinct from conventional glial neoplasms, composed of cells that resemble spongioblastoma and astrocytes; it can be benign (well-differentiated) or malignant (anaplastic).

Epidemiology: Rare neoplasm without standard histopathologic diagnostic criteria results in incomplete epidemiologic information on astroblastoma.

Affected age group: This rare tumor is most commonly seen in children, adolescents, and young adults.

Molecular and genetic profile: Deoxyribonucleic Acid (DNA) copy number alterations—gains of chromosomes 19 and 20q can be seen.

CSF markers: None.

Clinical features and standard therapy: Surgical resection is the mainstay for potential chance of cure. Incomplete resection can result in recurrence and growth of residual tumor, at which time repeat resection and/or radiation therapy are the recommended therapy.

Imaging

Large and circumscribed, lobulated, solid, and cystic masses located in the superficial or peripheral location of supratentorial brain have been noted. The solid component can contain calcium. The size of peritumoral edema is variable but usually much less than expected for the size of tumor.

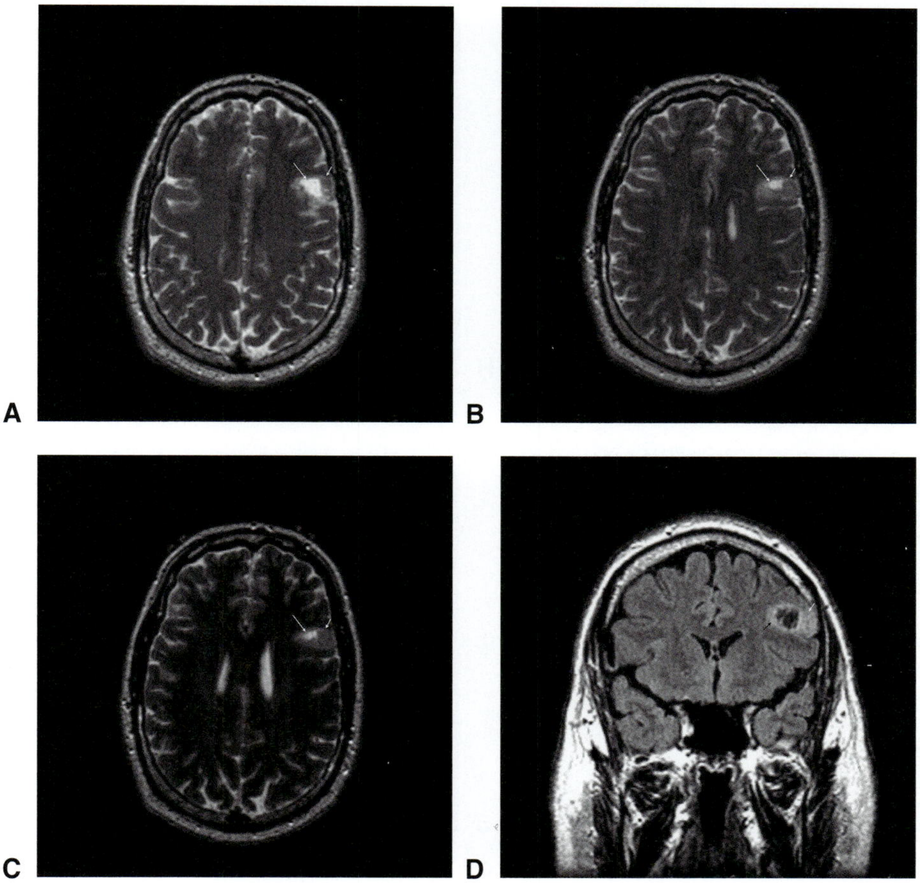

Figure 15.3. **Benign Astroblastoma at initial diagnosis (A–I) and at recurrence 11 years later (J–R). A–C.** Axial T2: Cortical, isointense solid nodule (short arrows) associated with a deeper cystic component (long arrows). **D–F.** Coronal FLAIR: Cortical nodule (white arrows) and medial nodule (black arrows) encase the cystic component.

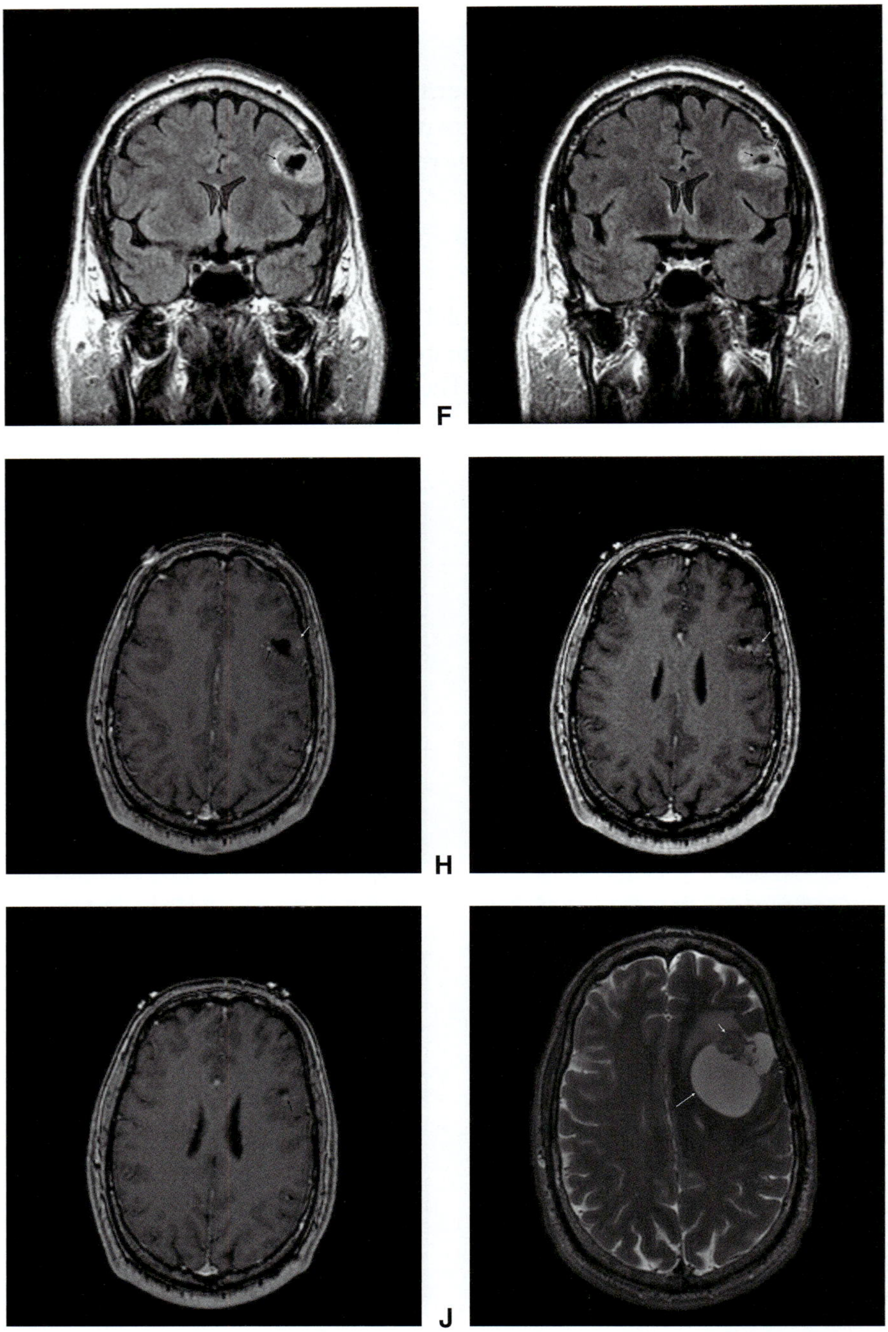

Figure 15.3. ***(continued)*** **G–I.** Axial T1-postcontrast: Mild enhancement of the cortical nodule (white arrows) and moderate enhancement of the deeper nodules (black arrows). **J–L.** Axial T2: Dominant cystic component (long arrows) and peripheral solid nodule (short arrows).

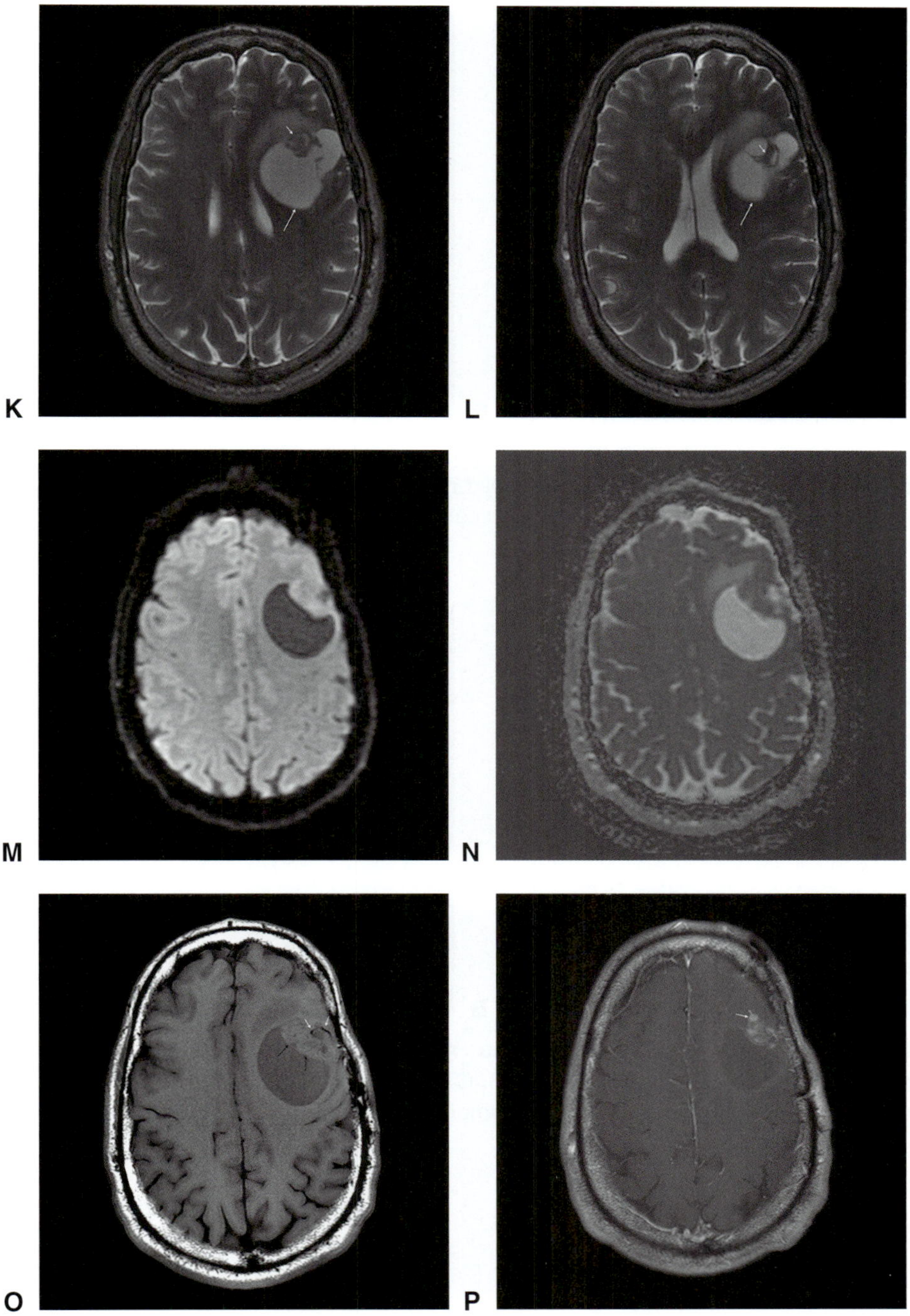

Figure 15.3. ***(continued)*** **M.** Axial DWI: Cerebrospinal fluid (CSF)-like fluid within the cyst. **N.** Axial ADC: Mildly reduced diffusion within the solid nodule. **O.** Axial T1-precontrast: Prominent vessels (white arrows) associated with the solid nodule (black arrows).

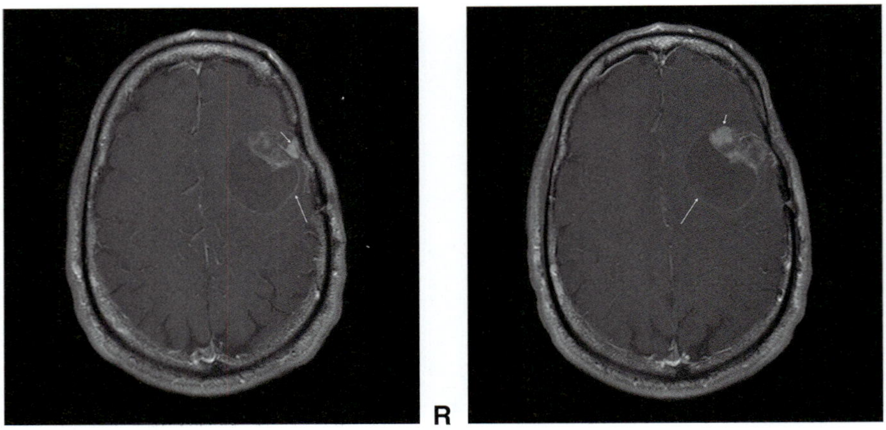

Q R

Figure 15.3. ***(continued)*** **P–R.** Axial T1-postcontrast: Avid but heterogeneous enhancement (short arrows) within the solid nodule and a thin rim of enhancement (long arrows) around the dominant cystic component.

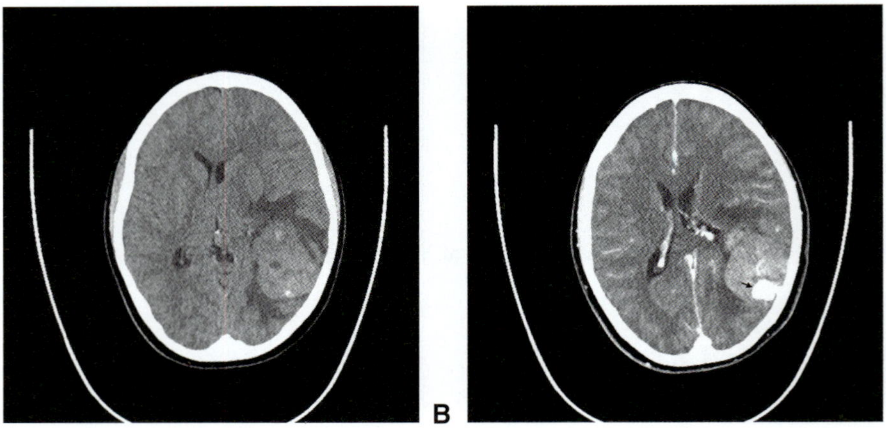

A B

Figure 15.4. **Malignant Astroblastoma. A. CT**, unenhanced: Lobulated hyperdense mass with surrounding edema. **B.** CT, enhanced: Heterogeneous enhancement within the mass and chunky intratumoral calcium (black arrow).

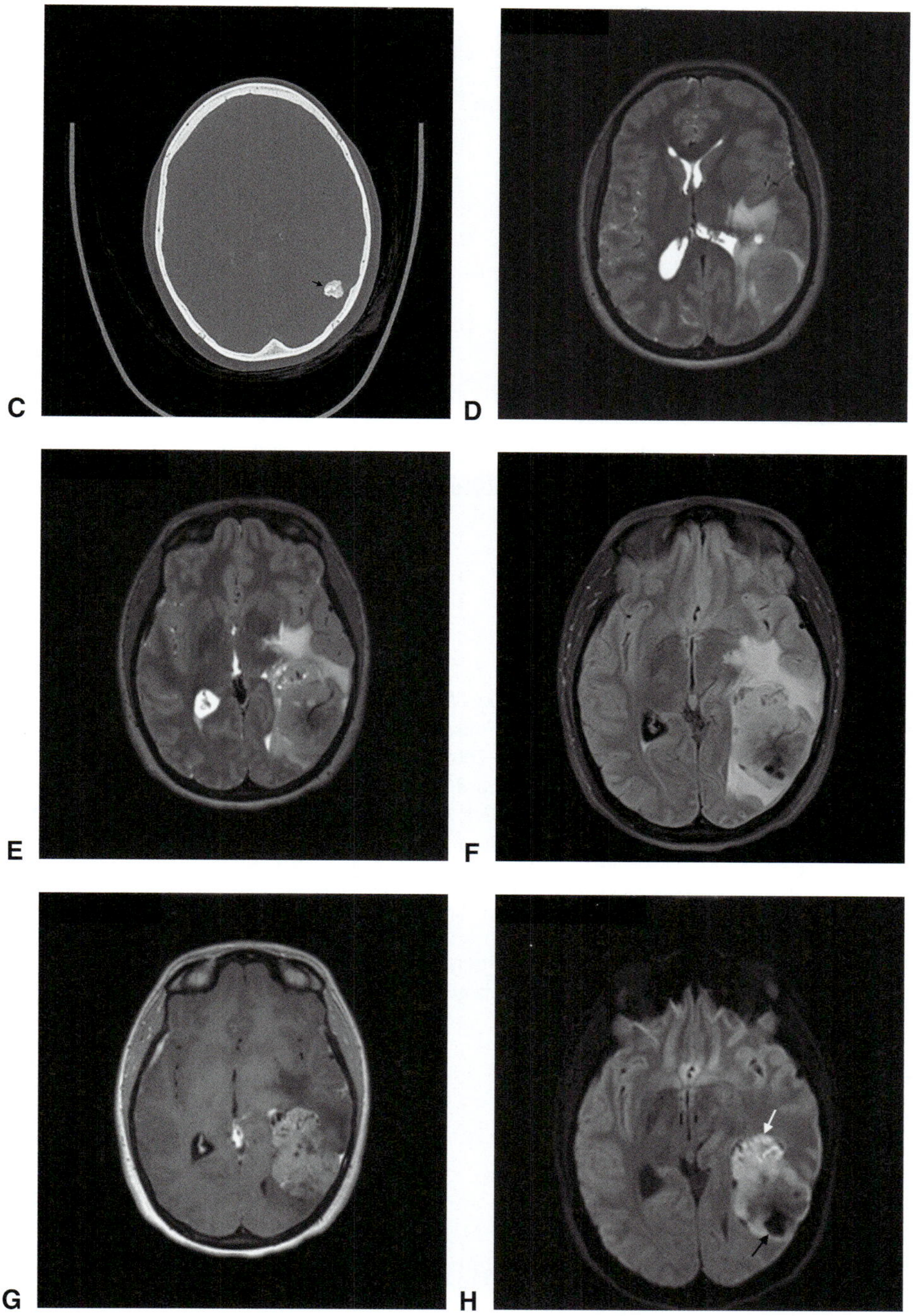

Figure 15.4. ***(continued)*** **C.** CT, bone window: Chunky intratumoral calcium is better delineated (black arrow). **D.** Axial T2: Heterogeneously isointense mass with moderate surrounding edema. **E.** Axial T2: Heterogeneously isointense mass with moderate surrounding edema. **F.** Axial FLAIR: Heterogeneously isointense mass with moderate surrounding edema. **G.** Axial T1-postcontrast: Avid but heterogeneous enhancement within the mass. **H.** Axial DWI: Reduced diffusion within the anterior aspect of the mass (white arrow) and posterior signal drop out (black arrow) within the chunky intratumoral calcium.

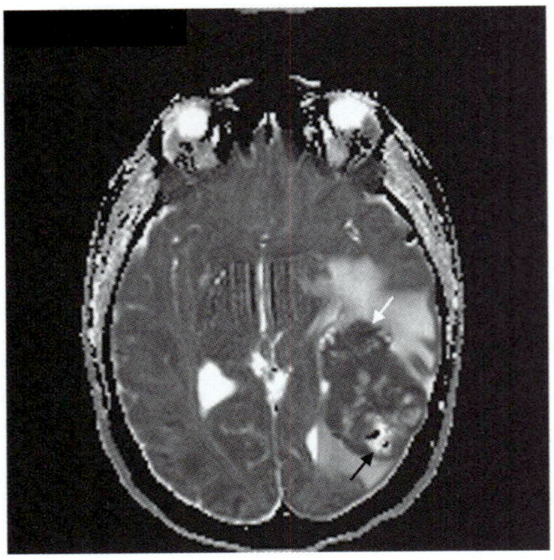

I

Figure 15.4. ***(continued)*** **I.** Axial ADC: Reduced diffusion within the anterior aspect of the mass (white arrow) and posterior signal drop out (black arrow) within the chunky intratumoral calcium.

Bibliography

Brat DJ, Scheithauer BW, Staugaitis SM, et al. Third ventricular chordoid glioma: a distinct clinicopathologic entity. *J Neuropathol Exp Neurol.* 1998;57(3):283–290.

Ganapathy S, Kleiner LI, Mirkin DL, et al. Unusual manifestations of astroblastoma: a radiologic-pathologic analysis. *Pediatr Radiol.* 2009;39(2):168–171.

Pomper MG, Passe TJ, Burger PC, et al. Chordoid glioma: a neoplasm unique to the hypothalamus and anterior third ventricle. *AJNR Am J Neuroradiol.* 2001;22(3):464–469.

Port JD, Brat DJ, Burger PC, et al. Astroblastoma: radiologic-pathologic correlation and distinction from ependymoma. *AJNR Am J Neuroradiol.* 2002;23(2):243–247.

Shakur SF, McGirt MJ, Johnson MW, et al. Angiocentric glioma: a case series. *J Neurosurg Pediatr.* 2009;3(3):197–202.

Wang M, Tihan T, Rojiani AM, et al. Monomorphous angiocentric glioma: a distinctive epileptogenic neoplasm with features of infiltrating astrocytoma and ependymoma. *J Neuropathol Exp Neurol.* 2005;64(10):875–881.

16

Choroid Plexus Tumors

Overview

Two types of choroid plexus tumors are presented—choroid plexus papilloma and choroid plexus carcinoma—both of which are strongly associated with familial cancer syndromes and primarily affect the pediatric age group.

	Age range (yr) (mean)	Female: male ratio	Cell of origin	WHO Grade	Molecular/genetic markers	Prognosis
Choroid plexus papilloma (CPP)	<15 (2.3)	1:1.2	Neuro-epithelial cells of choroid	I	*MGMT* promoter methylation Aicardi syndrome	Favorable
Choroid plexus carcinoma	<10	1:1	Neuro-epithelial cells of choroid	III	Germline *TP53* mutation (Li–Fraumeni syndrome) *SMARCB1* gene mutation	Guarded

▶ Choroid Plexus Papilloma

Definition: Choroid plexus papilloma is a benign solid neoplasm arising from the neuroepithelial cells of the choroid plexus epithelium, growing within the ventricles and producing Cerebrospinal fluid (CSF).

Epidemiology: This tumor primarily affects children, with about 80% of all choroid plexus tumors occurring in the first decade of life. Most choroid plexus tumors occur sporadically, except in two hereditary syndromes—Aicardi syndrome (defect in X chromosome leading to malformations) and Li–Fraumeni syndrome (autosomal dominant syndrome linked to germline mutations of *p53* tumor suppressor gene).

Affected age group: Pediatric CPPs tend to occur in the lateral, or less frequently in the third, ventricle whereas the fourth ventricle is more commonly involved in adult CPPs. A meta-analysis of CPP location found that the median patient age was 1.5 years for lateral/third ventricles, 22.5 years for fourth ventricle, and 35.5 years for cerebellopontine angle.

Molecular and genetic profile: This tumor is often associated with MGMT promoter methylation and less commonly with Aicardi syndrome (X-linked syndrome with triad of corpus callosal dysgenesis, chorioretinal lacunae, and infantile spasms).

CSF markers: None.

Clinical features and standard therapy: Gross total resection usually achieves cure of choroid plexus papilloma, with a 5-year survival of near 100% or 100%. However, recurrence locally or at a distant site, especially when the tumor is incompletely resected, is not unusual and contributes to shorter survival.

Imaging

CPP is a polypoid or lobular solid intraventricular mass with avid enhancement, hypercellularity, hypervascularity, and microcystic and calcium components. Hydrocephalus often accompanies the mass.

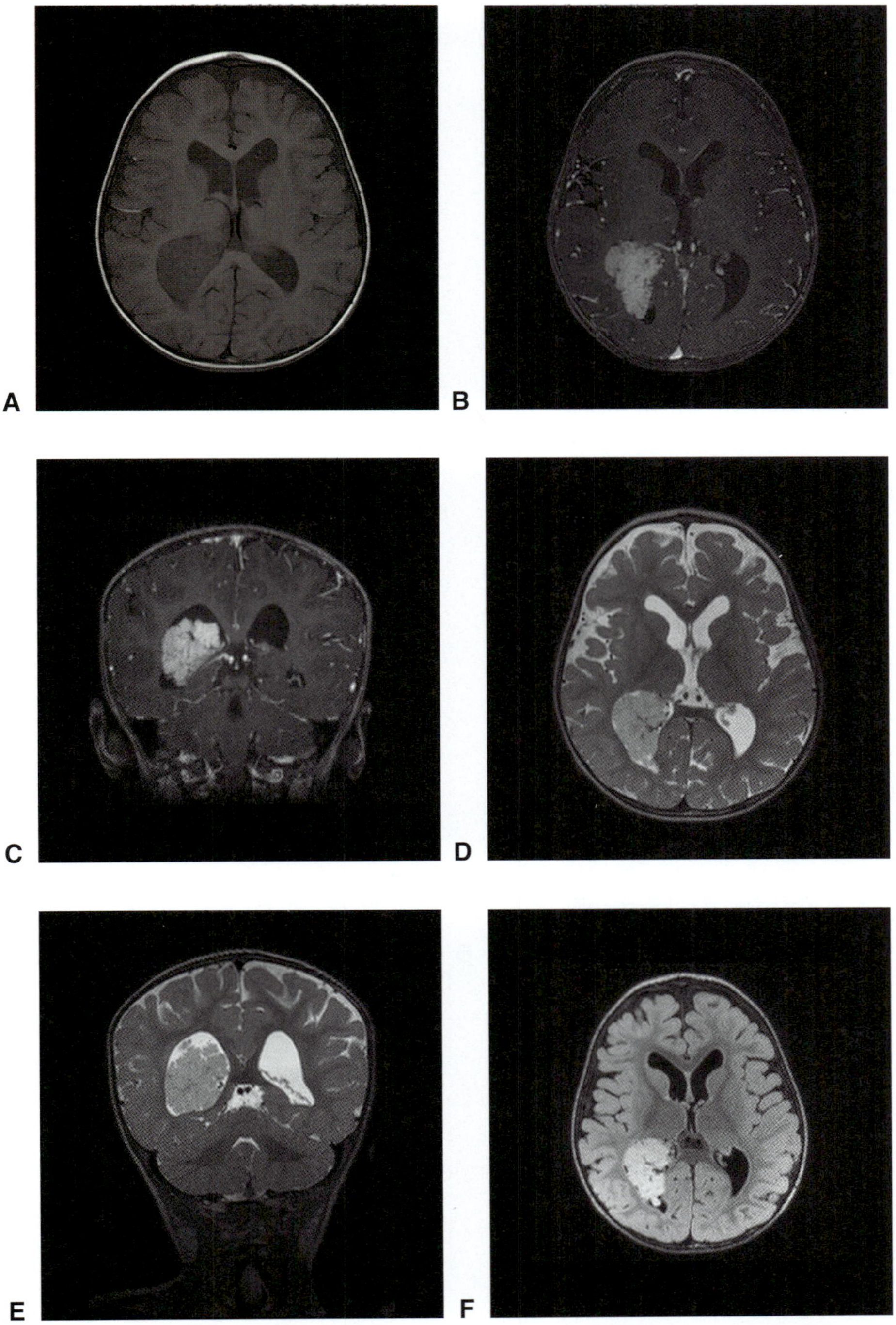

Figure 16.1. Imaging of Choroid Plexus Papilloma in a child. A. T1-precontrast: Hypo- or isointense to surrounding brain. **B**. Axial T1-postcontrast: Avid enhancement. **C**. Coronal T1-postcontrast: Avid enhancement. **D**. Axial T2 Fast spin echo (FSE): Hypointense to surrounding brain. **E**. Coronal T2 FSE: Hypointense to surrounding brain. **F**. Coronal Fluid-attenuated inversion recovery (FLAIR): Iso- to slightly hyperintense to surrounding brain.

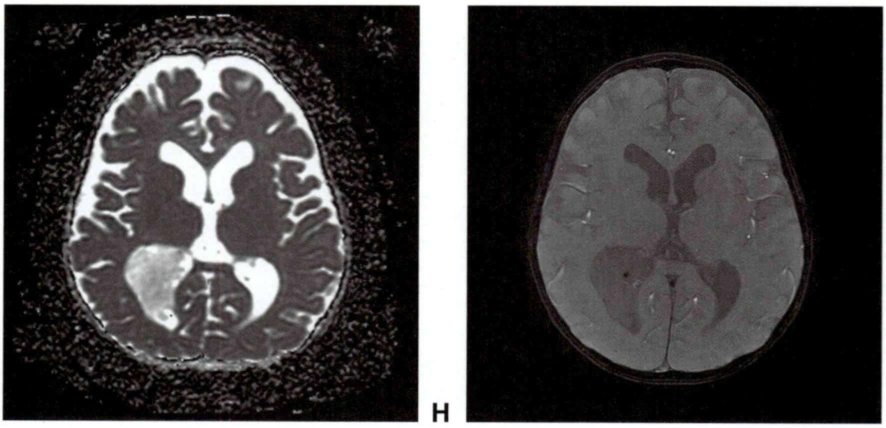

Figure 16.1. ***(continued)*** **G**. Apparent diffusion coefficient (ADC): Mildly increased diffusion. **H**. SWI: Punctate of calcium.

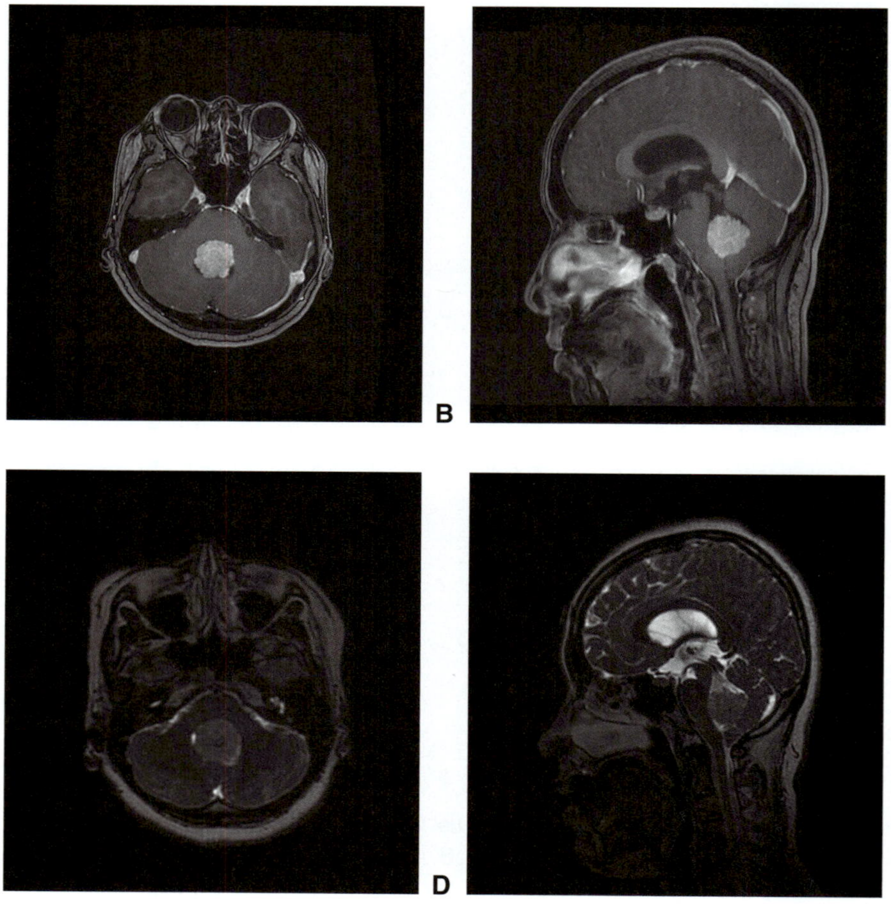

Figure 16.2. Imaging of Choroid Plexus Papilloma in an adult. A. Axial T1-post-contrast: Avidly enhancing fourth ventricular mass. **B**. Sagittal T1-postcontrast: Avidly enhancing fourth ventricular mass. **C**. Axial T2: Isointense to brain. **D**. Sagittal T2 FSE: Isointense to brain.

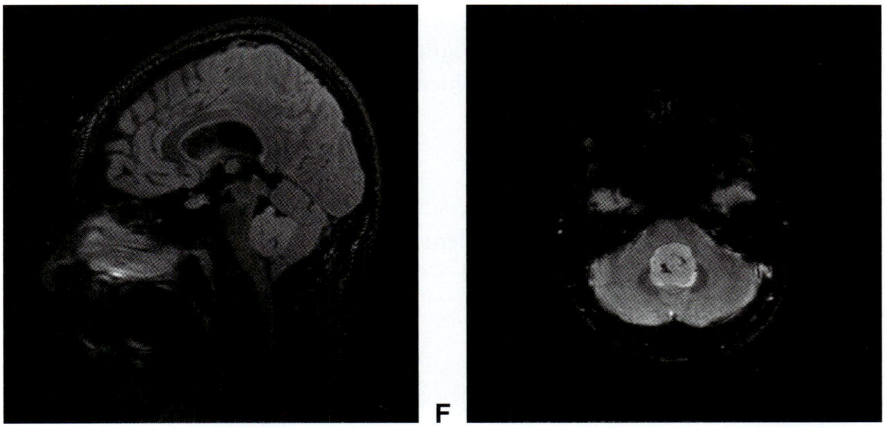

Figure 16.2. ***(continued)*** **E**. Sagittal FLAIR: Hyperintense to surrounding brain. **F**. Axial Susceptibility-weighted imaging (SWI): Central areas of susceptibility due to calcium.

Choroid Plexus Carcinoma

Definition: Choroid plexus carcinoma is a highly malignant, hypervascular, intraventricular tumor arising from choroid plexus, most commonly occurring in the lateral ventricle in infants and toddlers and often invading surrounding brain structures and metastasizing or seeding via the cerebrospinal fluid.

Epidemiology: Choroid plexus carcinoma (CPC) primarily affects infants and toddlers, is a very rare central nervous system (CNS) tumor comprising less than 1% of all brain tumors, and comprises about 14% of all tumors occurring in the first decade of life and 34% of all tumors involving the choroid plexus. Similar to choroid plexus papilloma, most CPCs occur sporadically, except in two hereditary syndromes—Aicardi syndrome (defect in X chromosome leading to malformations) and Li–Fraumeni syndrome (autosomal dominant syndrome linked to germline mutations of *p53* tumor suppressor gene).

Affected age group: The vast majority of CPCs occur within and around the lateral ventricle.

Molecular and genetic profile: About 40% of CPCs are associated with germline *TP53* mutations and Li–Fraumeni syndrome. CPCs have also been associated with a familial cancer syndrome, a rhabdoid tumor predisposition syndrome, caused by germline mutation in the *SMARCB1* gene.

CSF markers: None.

Clinical features and standard therapy: Extent of surgical resection is the key factor impacting long-term survival since currently there is no effective chemotherapy and radiation therapy is for short-term tumor control. Compared to CPPs, CPCs are highly malignant, both histologically and clinically, and tend to recur and spread widely throughout brain and spine via CSF.

Imaging

Overall, imaging features of CPCs are similar to those of CPPs, but CPCs tend to show more prominent vasogenic edema, frank invasion of neighboring brain, and higher propensity for CSF spread.

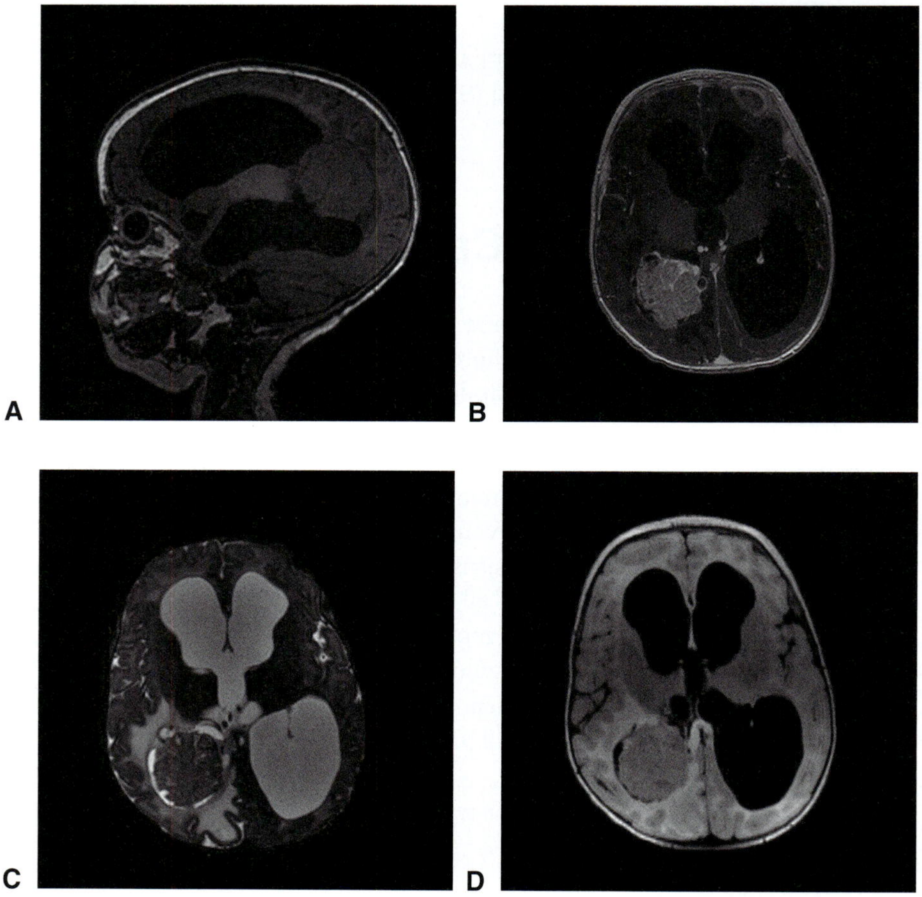

Figure 16.3. Imaging of Choroid Plexus Carcinoma in a child. A. Sagittal T1-precontrast: Hypo- or isointense to surrounding brain; hyperintense when the cystic component contains proteinaceous material. **B**. T1-postcontrast: Avid but heterogeneous enhancement except in areas of cyst or calcium. **C**. T2 FSE: Hypo- or isointense to brain with surrounding vasogenic edema. **D**. FLAIR: Isointense to brain.

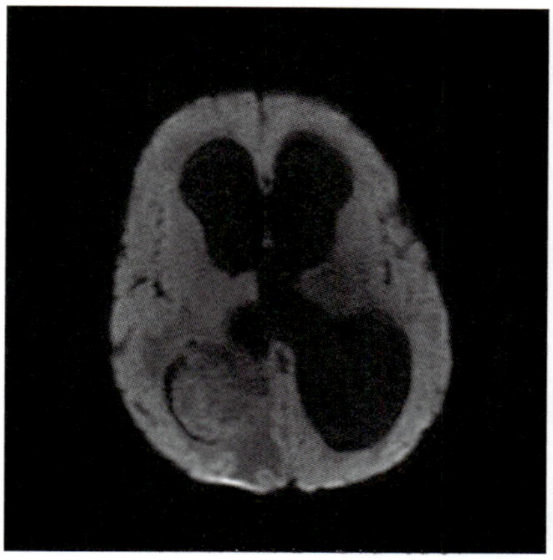

E

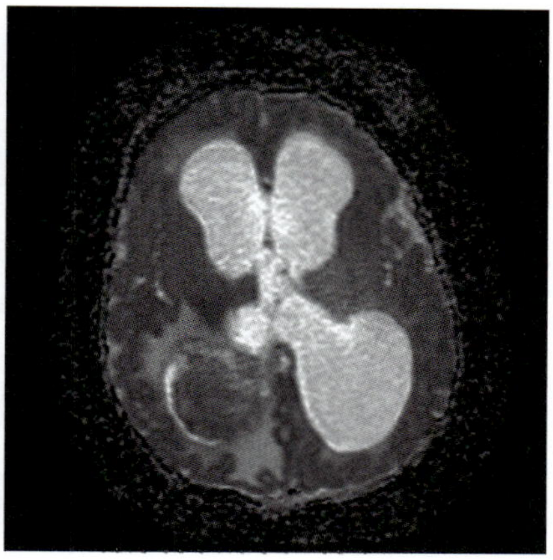

F

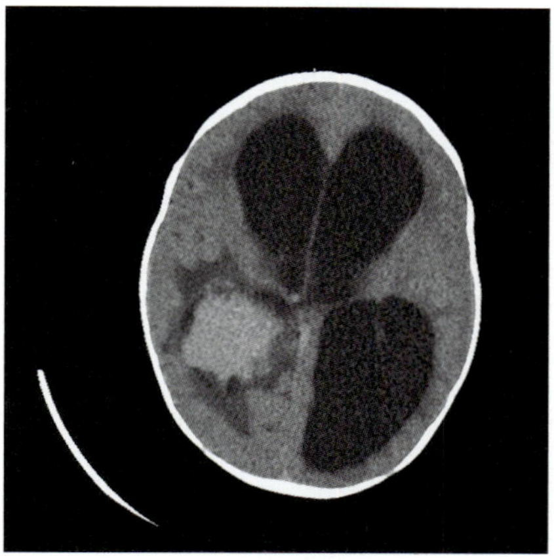

G

Figure 16.3. ***(continued)*** **E**. Diffusion-weighted imaging (DWI): Similar to normal brain. **F**. ADC: Similar to normal brain. **G**. CT: Hyperdense solid mass.

Bibliography

Gopal P, Parker JR, Debski R, Parker JC. Choroid plexus carcinoma. *Arch Pathol Lab Med.* 2008;132:1350–1354.

Gozali AE, Britt B, Shane L, et al. Choroid plexus tumors; management, outcome, and association with the Li-Fraumeni syndrome: the Children's Hospital Los Angeles (CHLA) experience, 1991–2010. *Pediatr Blood Cancer*. 2012;58:905–909.

Jaiswal AK, Jaiswal S, Sahu RN, et al. Choroid plexus papilloma in children: diagnostic and surgical considerations. *J Pediatr Neurosci*. 2009;4:10–16.

Taylor MB, Jackson RW, Hughes DG, Wright NB. Magnetic resonance imaging in the diagnosis and management of choroid plexus carcinoma in children. *Pediatr Radiol.* 2001;31:624–630.

17 Neuronal and Mixed Glioneuronal Tumors

Overview

	Age range (median age in years)	Female: male ratio	Cell of origin	WHO Grade	Molecular/ genetic markers	Prognosis
Dysembryoplastic neuroepithelial tumor	0–20	1:1.5	Glioneuronal cells	I	S100, NeuN, synaptophysin, GFAP	Good
Ganglioglioma	0–70	1:1.5	Ganglion cells	I	*BRAF V600E*	Favorable
Desmoplastic infantile astrocytoma (DIA) and ganglioglioma (DIG)	0–2	1:1	Astrocytes Mature neuronal cells	I	GFAP, vimentin, *MAP2* (DIG) BRAF	Favorable
Dysplastic cerebellar gangliocytoma (Lhermitte–Duclos disease)	30–50	1:1	Ganglion cells	I	PTEN germline loss; PTEN/AKT/mTOR pathway	Guarded
Rosette-forming glioneuronal tumor	6–79 (27)	1.3:1	Pluripotent cells of subependymal plate	I	Undefined	Favorable
Diffuse leptomeningeal glioneuronal tumor	0.5–46 (5)	1:1	Oligodendroglial-like cells	I	*KIAA1549-BRAF* fusion, 1p deletion	Guarded
Central neurocytoma	20–40 (29)	1:1	Mature neurocytes	II	Synaptophysin, NeuN, *MAP-2*, *MYCN*, loss of *BIN1*	Favorable
Extraventricular neurocytoma	5–76 (34)	1:1	Mislocated neural progenitor cells	II	Undefined	Good
Paraganglioma	9–75 (46)	1:1.5	Neural crest cells of paraganglia	I	*SDHD*, *SDHA*, *SDHAF2*, *SDHC*, *SDHB*	Good

AKT, Ak strain transforming; PTEN, Phosphatase and TENsin homolog; TOR, Target of rapamycin.

Dysembryoplastic Neuroepithelial Tumor

Definition: Dysembryoplastic neuroepithelial tumor (DNET) is a benign, mixed glioneuronal neoplasm affecting pediatric and young adult age groups and predominantly involving the cortical location with multinodular architecture composed of columns of axonal bundles oriented perpendicularly to the cortical surface. Seizure is the most common presenting symptom.

Epidemiology: This tumor accounts for 1.2% of all primary intracranial neuroepithelial tumors in patients aged <20 years and for 0.2% in patients aged >20 years.

Molecular and genetic profile: *BRAF* V600E mutations have been seen in up to 30% of all DNETs and associated with activation of mTOR signaling pathway. Rare association with neurofibromatosis type 1 or XYY syndrome has been noticed.

Clinical features and standard therapy: Gross total resection ensures favorable prognosis, but subtotal resection can lead to slow recurrence and malignant transformation in very rare instances, especially after radiation therapy or chemotherapy.

Imaging

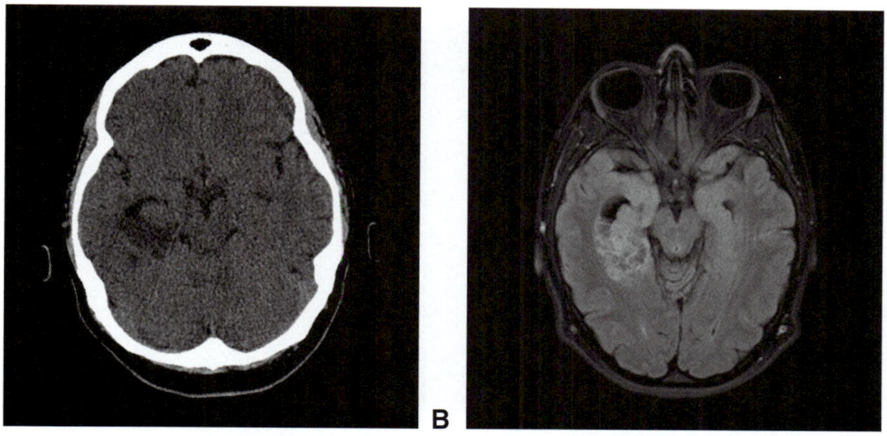

A B

Figure 17.1. Imaging of DNET, right temporal lobe. A. Axial CT unenhanced: Low-density lesion in the right posterior hippocampus. **B.** Axial fluid-attenuated inversion recovery (FLAIR): Heterogeneously hyperintense lesion.

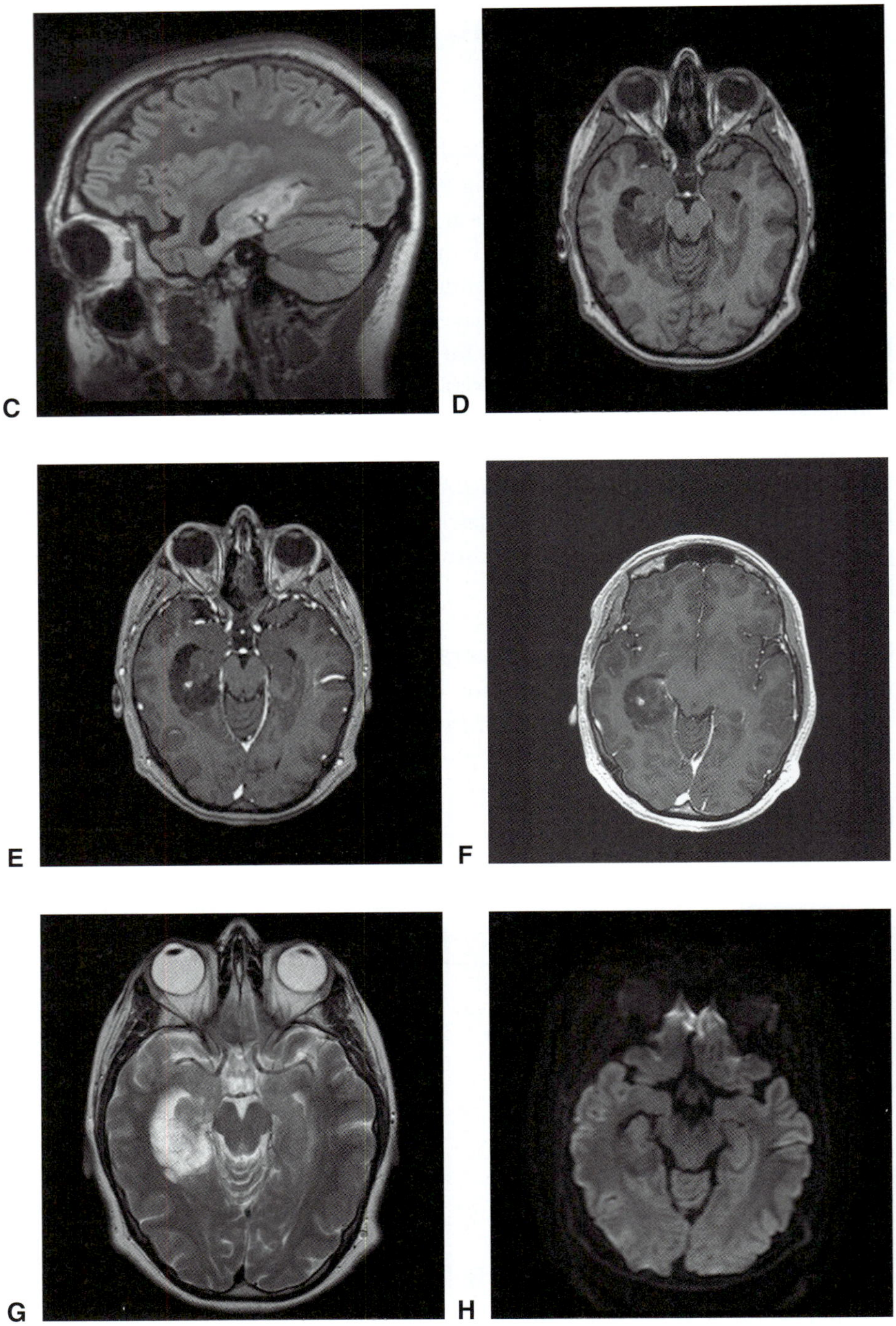

Figure 17.1. ***(continued)*** **C.** Sagittal FLAIR: Heterogeneously hyperintense lesion. **D.** Axial T1 precontrast: Hypointense lesion. **E.** Axial T1 postcontrast: Small focal area of enhancement within the lesion. **F.** Axial T1 postcontrast: Small focal area of enhancement within the lesion. **G.** Axial T2: Hyperintense lesion. **H.** Axial diffusion-weighted imaging (DWI): Hypointense lesion.

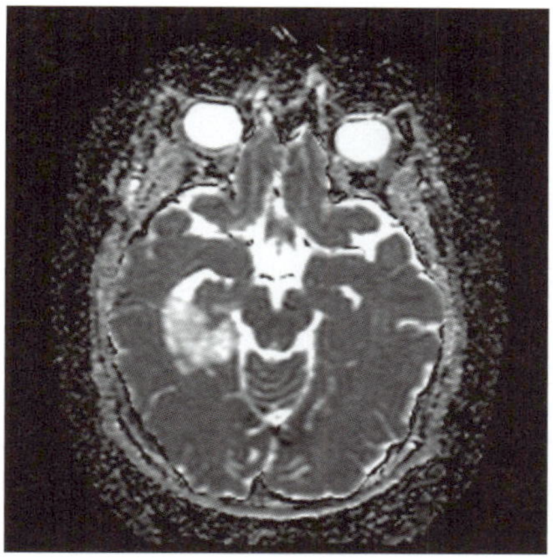

Figure 17.1. ***(continued)*** **I.** Axial apparent diffusion coefficient (ADC): No reduced diffusion within the lesion.

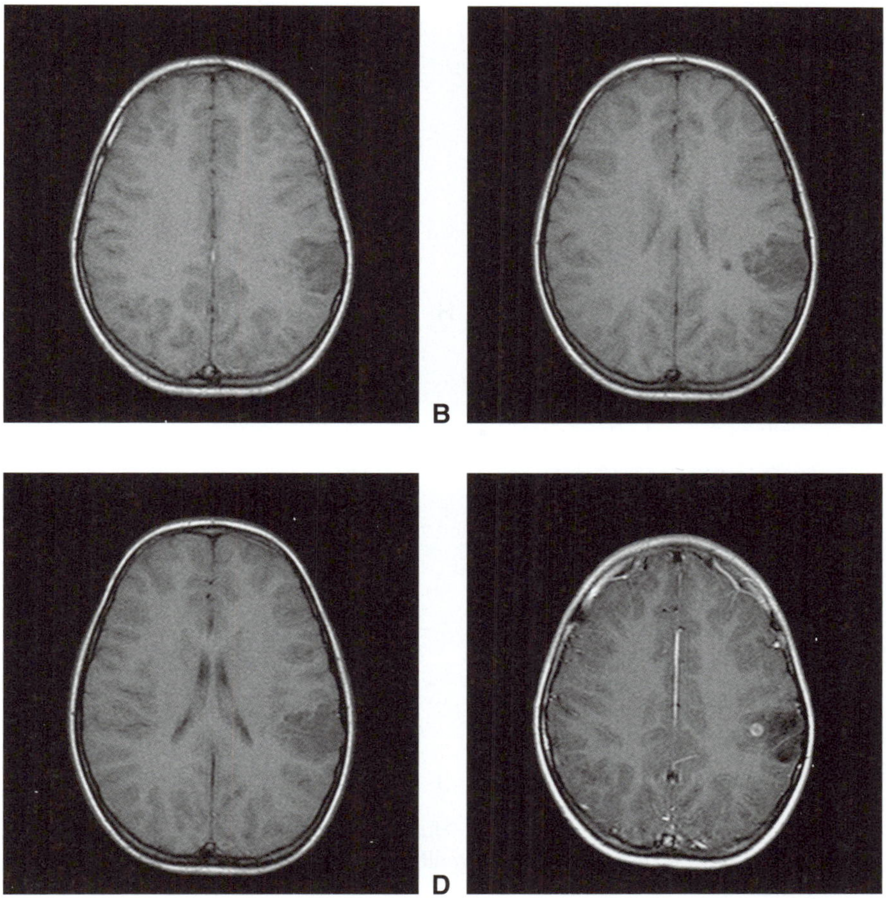

Figure 17.2. Imaging of DNET, left frontal lobe. A–C. Axial T1 precontrast: Heterogeneous hypointense multicystic lesion. **D–F.** Axial T1 postcontrast: Small focal enhancement in the deep aspect of the lesion.

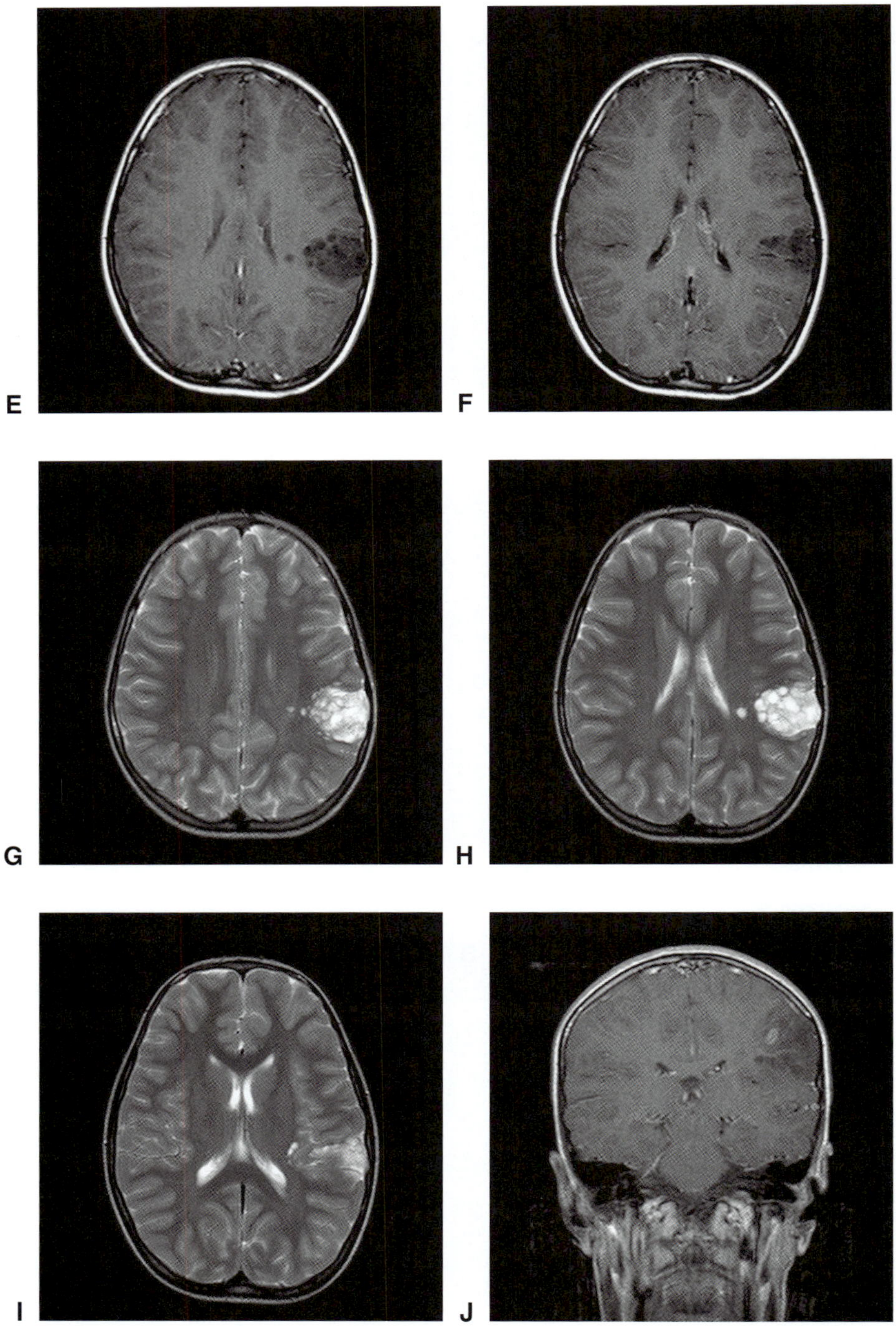

Figure 17.2. ***(continued)*** **G–I.** Axial T2: "Bubbly" pattern of multicystic hyperintense lesion. **J–L.** Coronal T1 postcontrast: Small focal enhancement in the deep aspect of the lesion.

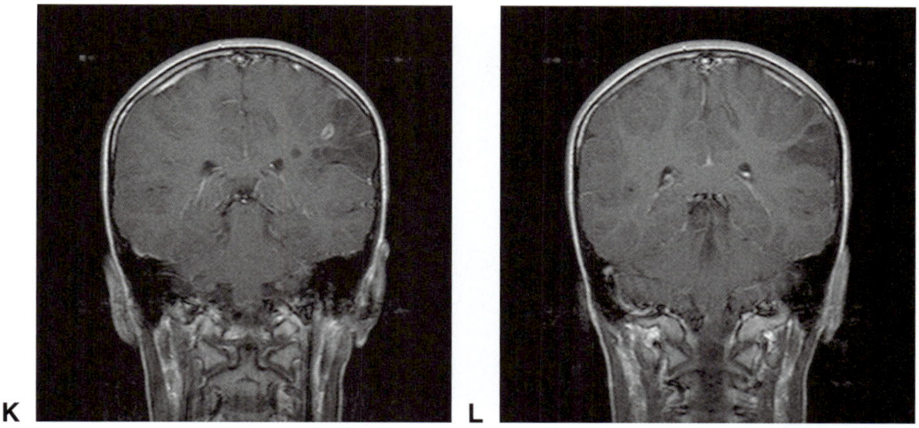

Figure 17.2. ***(continued)***

Ganglioglioma

Definition: Ganglioglioma is a slow-growing, low-grade glioneuronal neoplasm composed of dysplastic and cytologically atypical ganglion cells, with predilection for temporal lobes.

Epidemiology: Less than 2% of all primary central nervous system (CNS) tumors, ganglioglioma primarily affects children and young adults, mostly in the age range of 8.5 to 25 years, with a slight male predominance (~52%).

Molecular and genetic profile: Up to 60% of gangliogliomas have *BRAF* V600E mutations and one third show gain of chromosome 7.

Clinical features and standard therapy: Surgery is the first line of therapy and gross total resection ensures favorable prognosis, but recurrence is not uncommon in the setting of subtotal resection. Anaplastic ganglioglioma may require adjuvant radiation therapy and chemotherapy.

Imaging

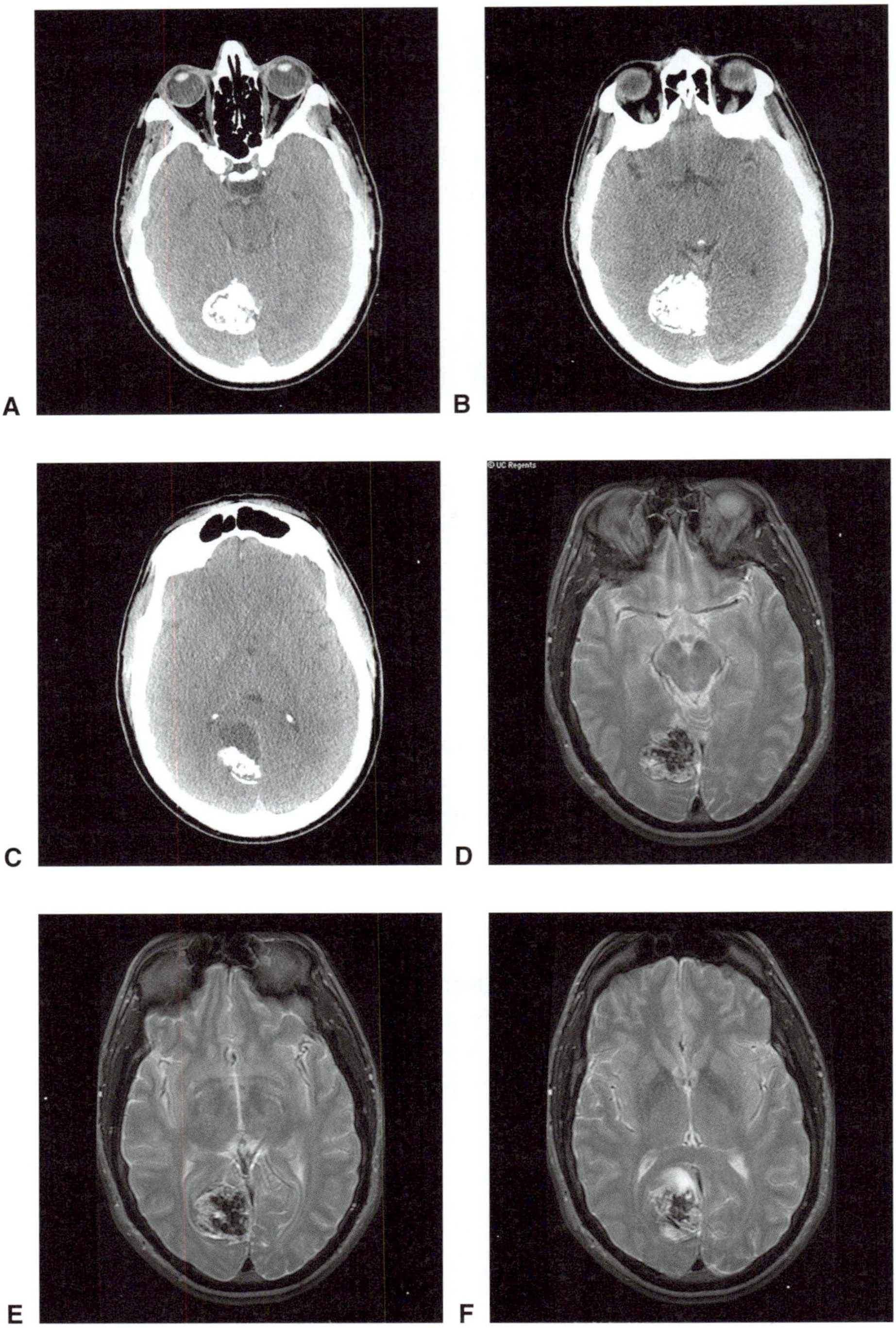

Figure 17.3. **Imaging of Ganglioglioma. A–C.** Axial CT unenhanced: Heavily calcified right parietal mass with anterior cystic component. **D–F.** Axial T2: Heterogeneously hypointense mass with anterior cystic component with high-signal intensity.

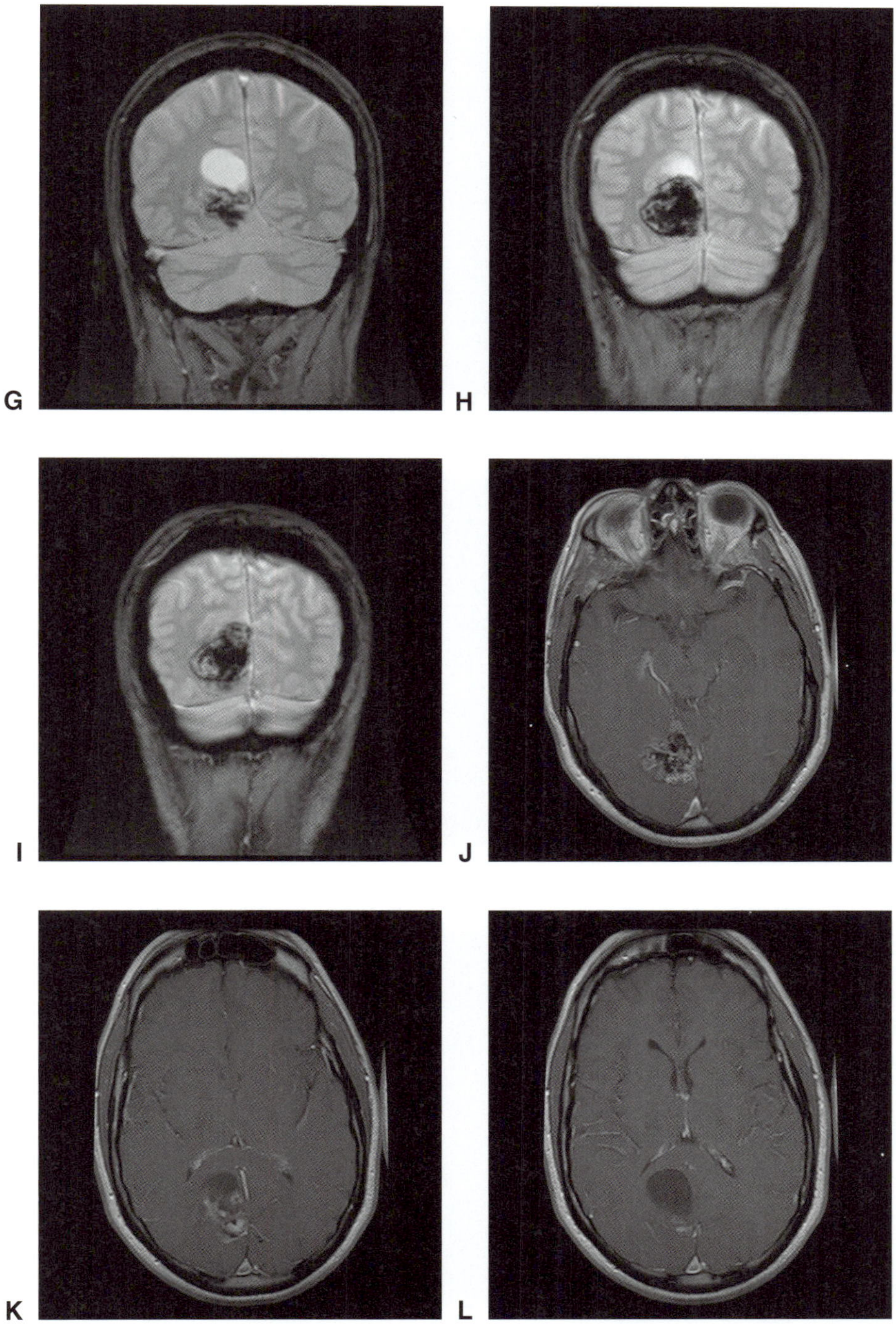

Figure 17.3. ***(continued)*** **G–I.** Coronal gradient echo: Susceptibility blooming due to calcium and circumscribed superior cystic component. **J–L.** Axial T1 postcontrast: Peripheral nodular enhancement.

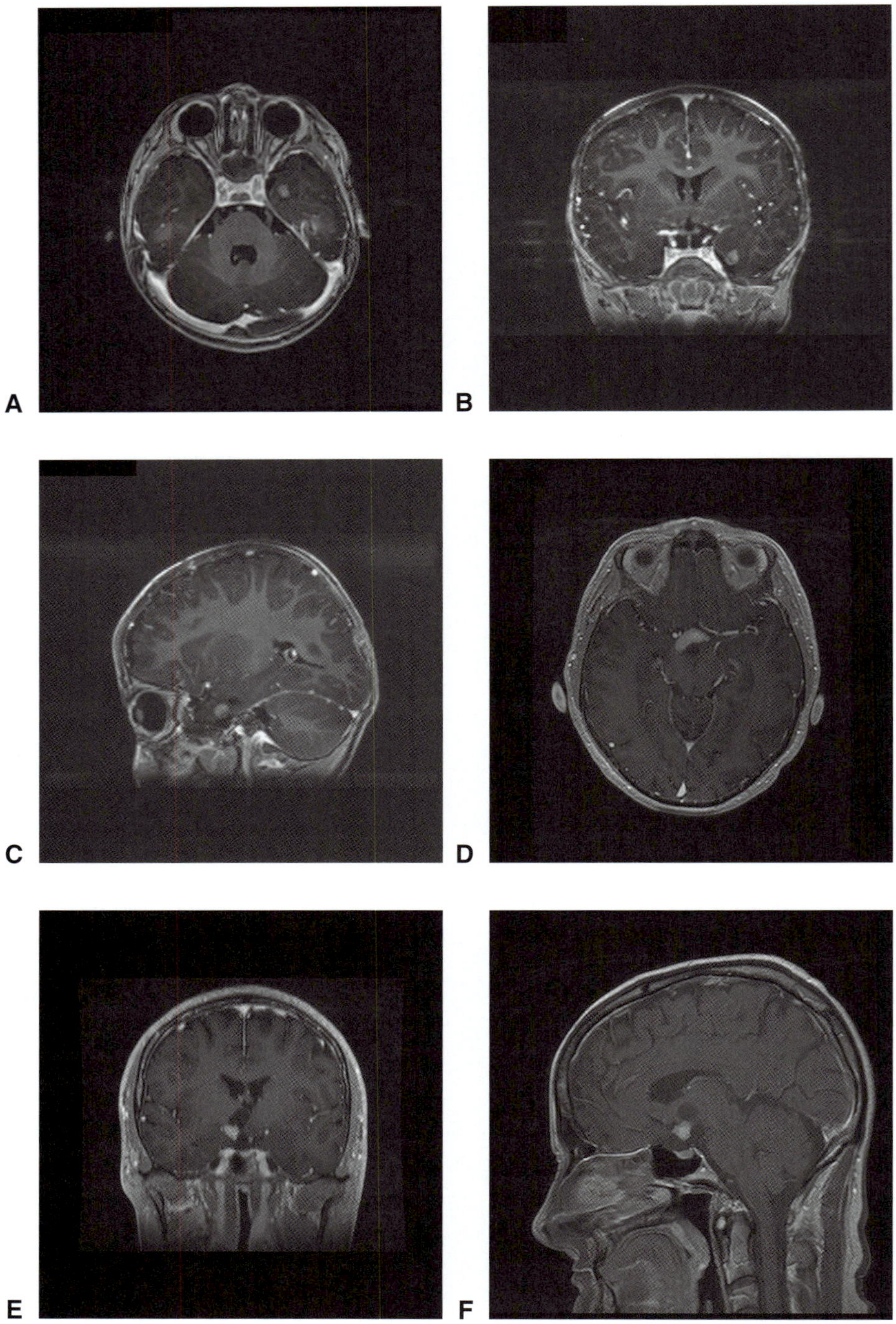

Figure 17.4. **Imaging of Gangliogliomas, four different patients, postcontrast T1-weighted Imaging. A–C.** Left medial temporal ganglioglioma: Small enhancing nodule in the left medial temporal lobe. **D–F.** Hypothalamic ganglioglioma: Enhancing nodule in the hypothalamus with inferior extension in the suprasellar cistern and a superior cystic component causing mass effect on the third ventricle.

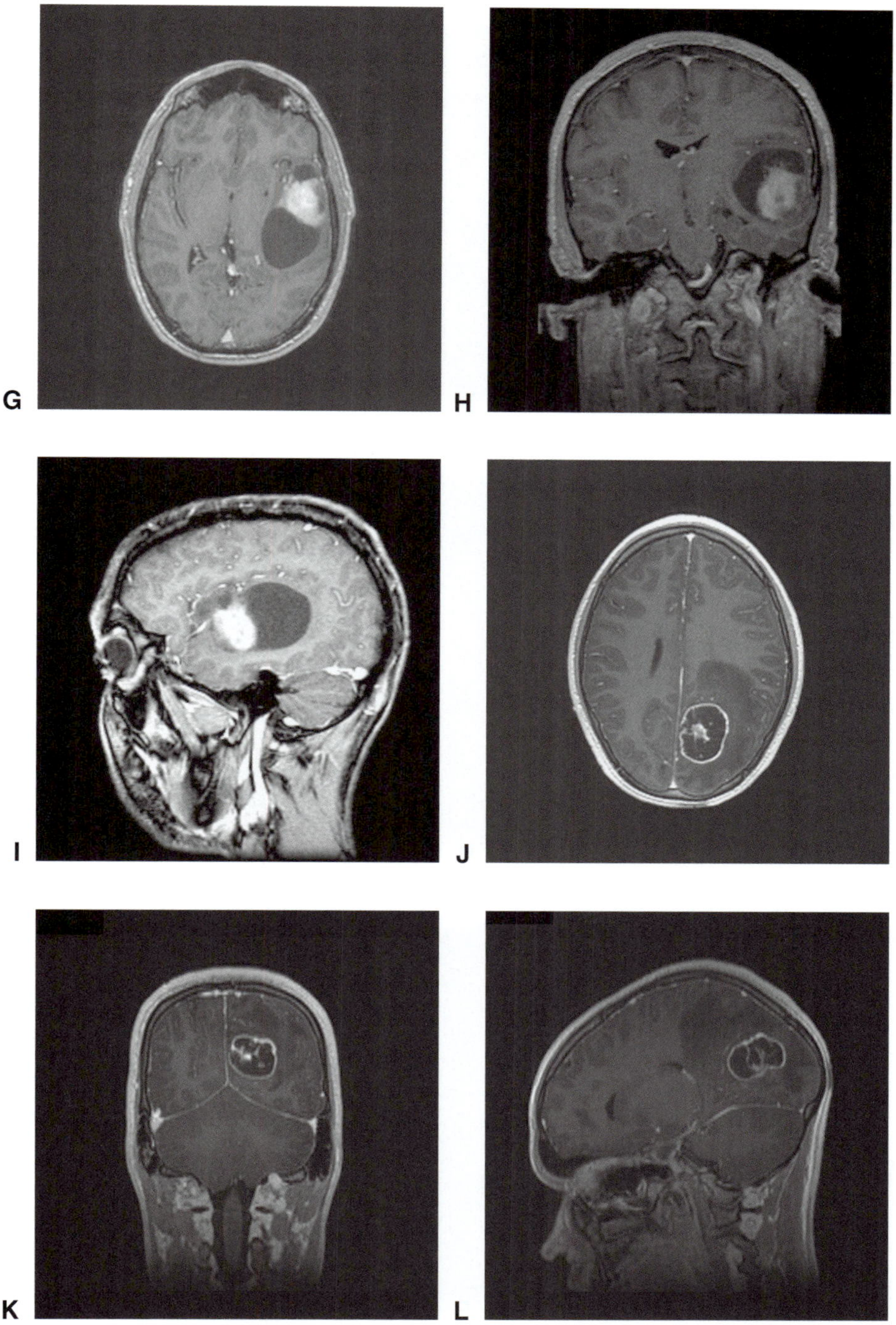

Figure 17.4. *(continued)* **G–I.** Left temporal ganglioglioma: Large cystic and solid nodular mass with mild mass effect but no surrounding edema. **J–L.** Left occipital anaplastic ganglioglioma: Circumscribed mass with rim enhancement and internal stellate nodule and marked surrounding edema.

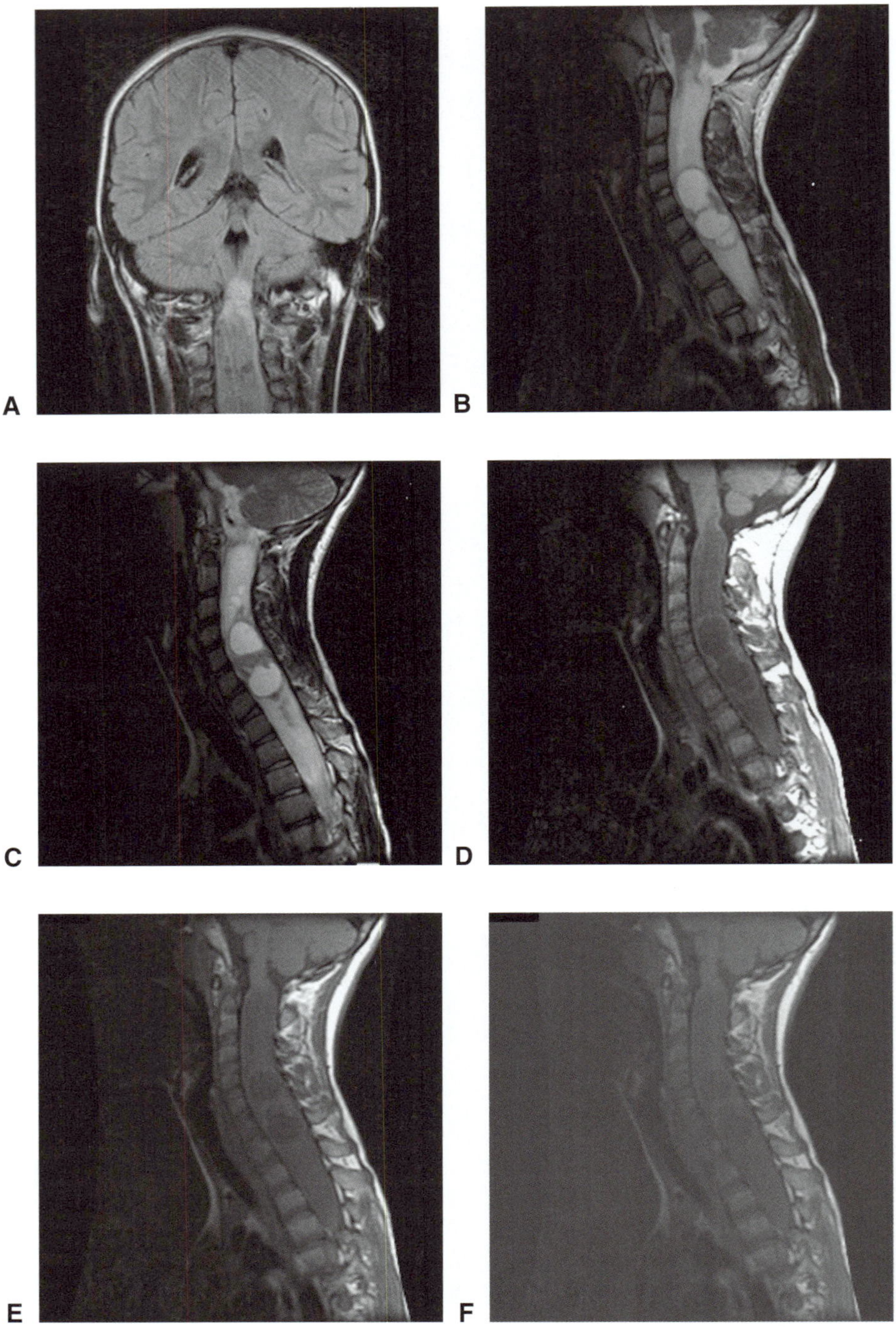

Figure 17.5. **Imaging of Spinal Ganglioglioma. A.** Coronal FLAIR: Expansile hypointense medullary and cervical spinal cord mass. **B–C.** Sagittal T2: Hyperintense mass with circumscribed cystic component from C4 to C7 levels and central solid tissue at C5–C6. **D–F.** Sagittal T1 precontrast: Expansile hypointense mass with circumscribed cystic component from C4 to C7 levels and central solid tissue at C5–C6.

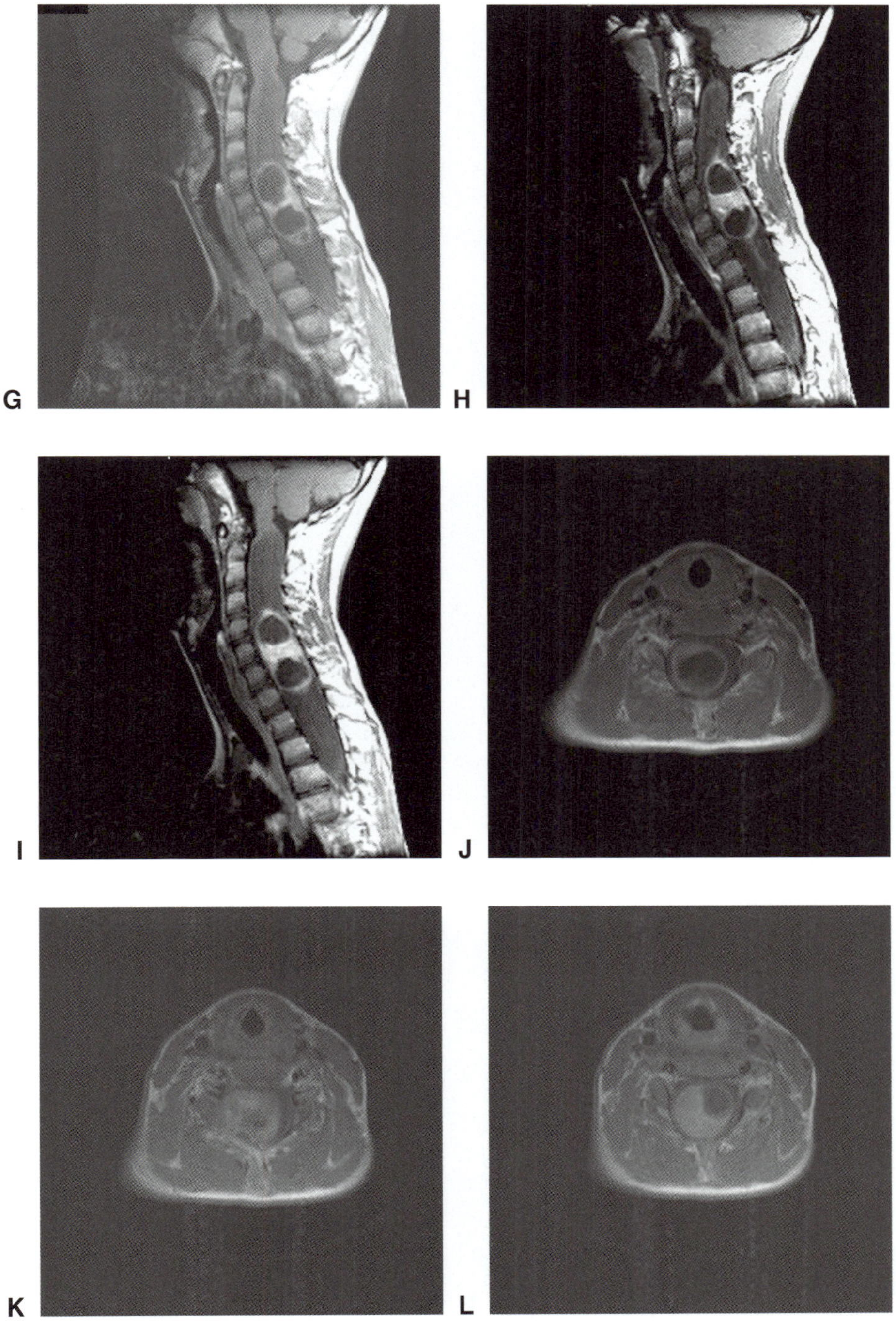

Figure 17.5. ***(continued)*** **G–I.** Sagittal T1 postcontrast: Avid peripheral and central enhancement within the circumscribed cystic component. **J–L.** Axial T1 postcontrast: Thin peripheral and bulky eccentric enhancement.

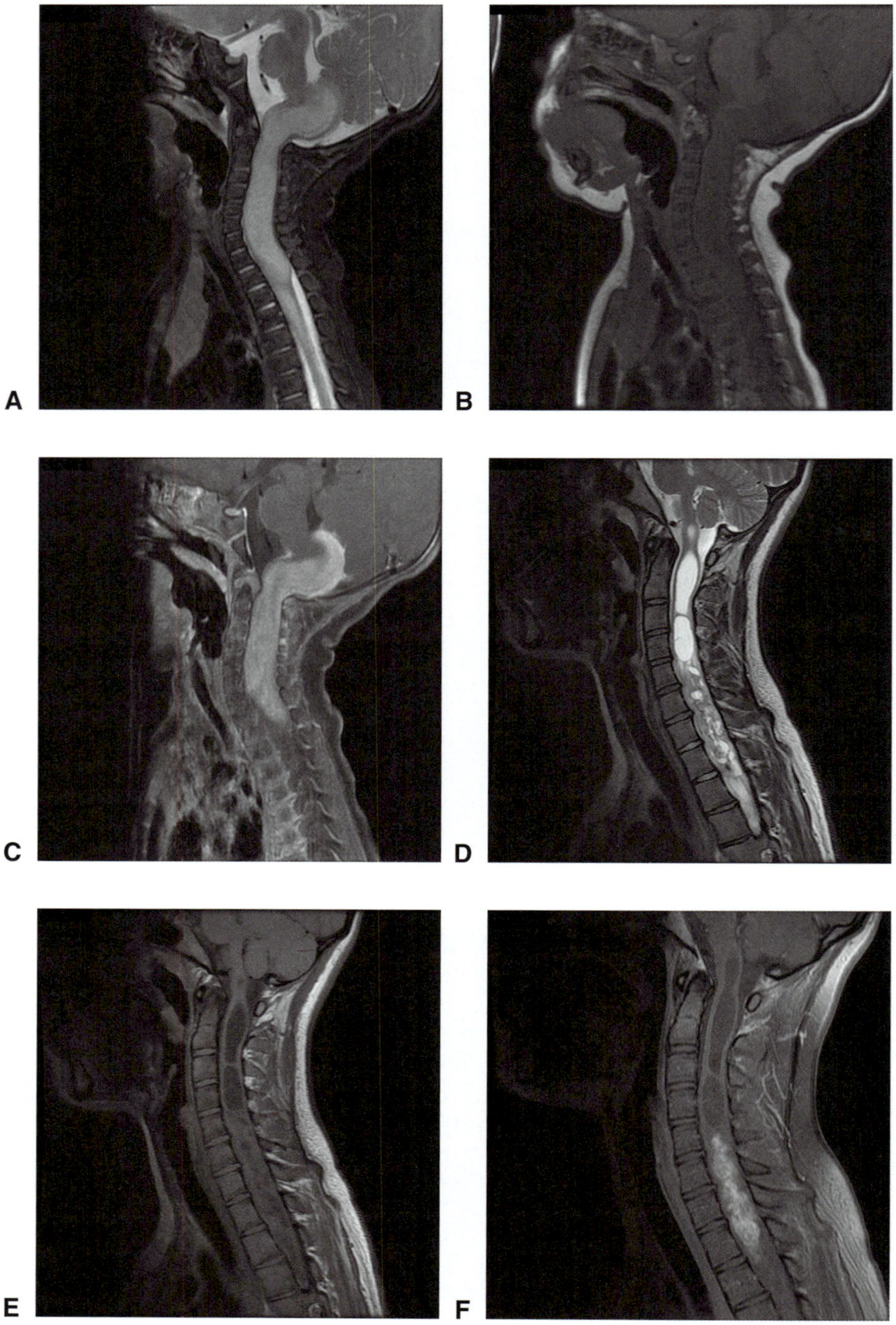

Figure 17.6. Imaging of Spinal Ganglioglioma, two different patients. **A–C.** Cervicomedullary ganglioglioma. **A.** Sagittal T2: Expansile homogeneously hyperintense intramedullary mass. **B.** Sagittal T1 precontrast: Expansile homogeneously hypointense intramedullary mass. **C.** Sagittal T1 postcontrast: Avid enhancement. **D–F.** Lower cervical ganglioglioma. **D.** Sagittal T2: Long segment multiloculated intramedullary cystic mass with syrinx from C1 to C4. **E.** Sagittal T1 precontrast: Heterogeneous hypointense mass. **F.** Sagittal T1 postcontrast: Heterogeneous enhancement of tumor from C5 to T1.

Desmoplastic Infantile Astrocytoma and Ganglioglioma

Definition: Desmoplastic infantile astrocytoma and ganglioglioma are low-grade and rare neuroepithelial tumors of infancy composed of neoplastic astrocytes without or with mature neuronal components, including ganglion cells in a background of prominent desmoplastic stroma. These tumors have previously been described by a variety of names, including "superficial cerebral astrocytomas attached to dura" and "desmoplastic supratentorial neuroepithelial tumors of infancy with divergent differentiation." Desmoplastic infantile astrocytoma (DIA) refers to tumor cells composed of neoplastic astrocytes without neuronal component, and desmoplastic infantile ganglioglioma (DIG) refers to tumor cells composed of both neoplastic astrocytes and mature neoplastic neuronal cells. DIA and DIG are considered a single molecular genetic entity with a spectrum of histological features and are placed in the same category in the current WHO classification of CNS tumors.

Epidemiology: Rare tumors of infancy or early childhood, DIA and DIG account for less than 20% of all CNS tumors of infants with the age range of 1–24 months, with a median age of 6 months and with male dominance (1.5:1)

Molecular and genetic profile: Due to the small number of cases with available cytogenetic analysis, characteristic molecular genetic features of DIA and DIG remain undefined.

Clinical features and standard therapy: Gross total resection results in long-term survival but recurrence is expected in subtotally resected tumors.

Imaging

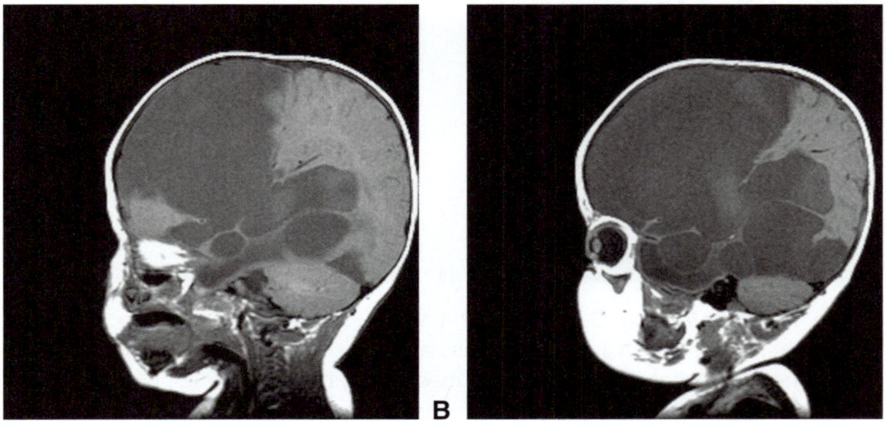

A B

Figure 17.7. Imaging of Desmoplastic Infantile Ganglioglioma. A–C. Sagittal T1 precontrast: Large cystic mass filling much of the left cerebral hemisphere.

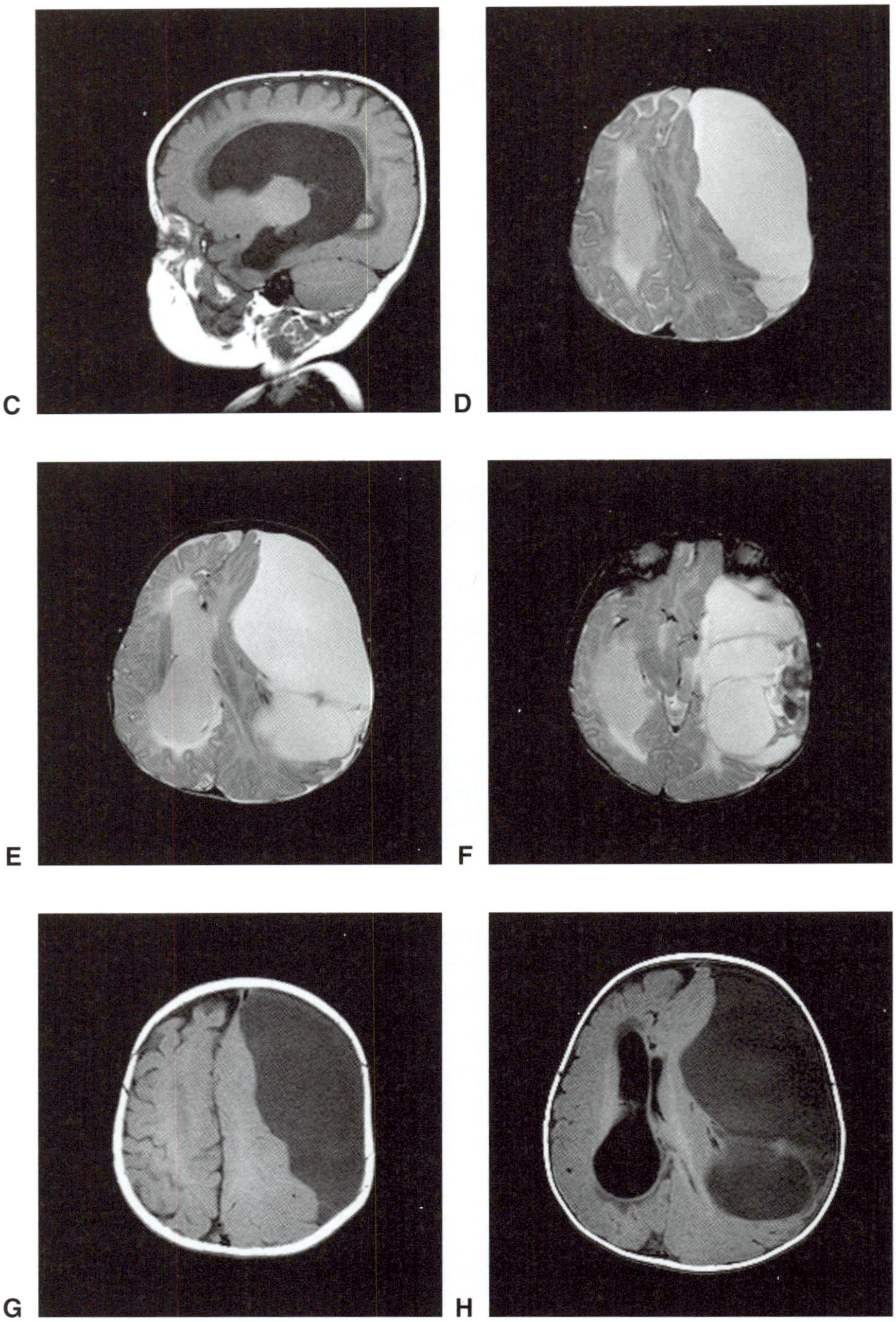

Figure 17.7. ***(continued)*** **D–F.** Axial T2: Large cystic mass filling much of the left cerebral hemisphere with linear septations and superficial solid nodular component. **G–L.** Axial T1 precontrast: Large cystic mass filling much of the left cerebral hemisphere with linear septations and hypointense superficial solid nodular component.

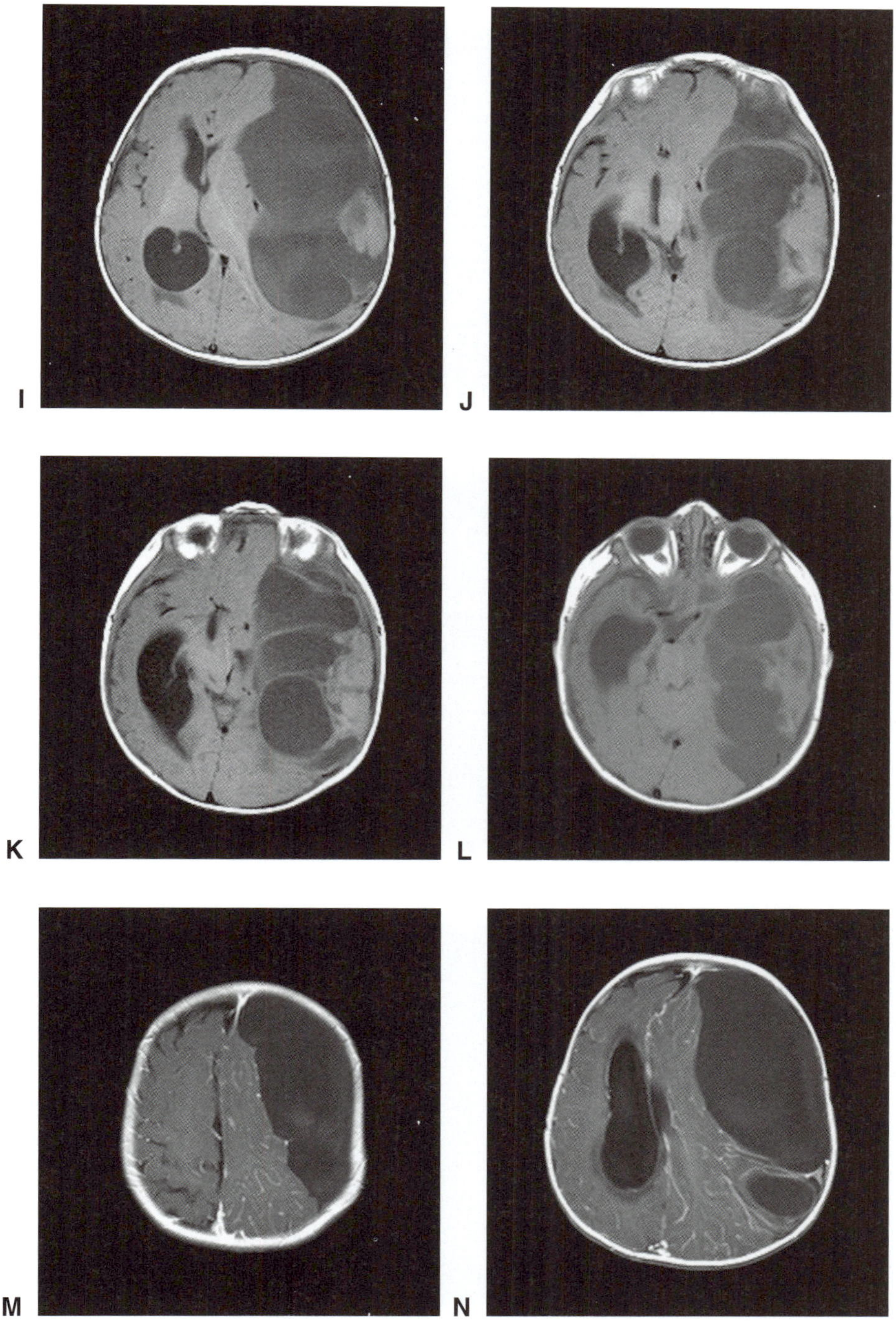

Figure 17.7. ***(continued)*** **M–R.** Axial T1 postcontrast: Large cystic mass filling much of the left cerebral hemisphere with enhancement of the linear septations and superficial solid nodular component.

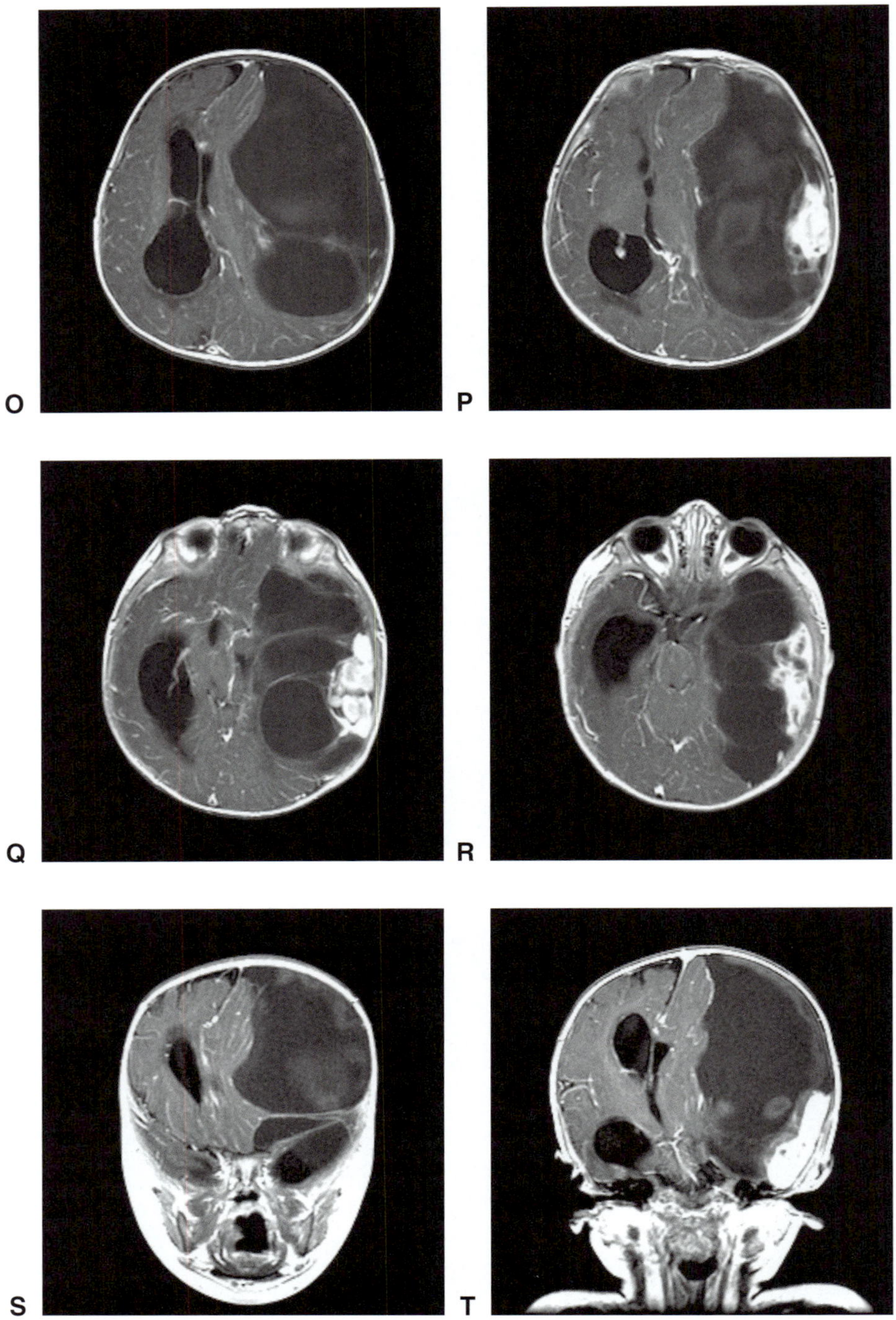

Figure 17.7. ***(continued)*** **S–U.** Coronal T1 postcontrast: Large cystic mass filling much of the left cerebral hemisphere with enhancement of the linear septations and superficial solid nodular component.

U

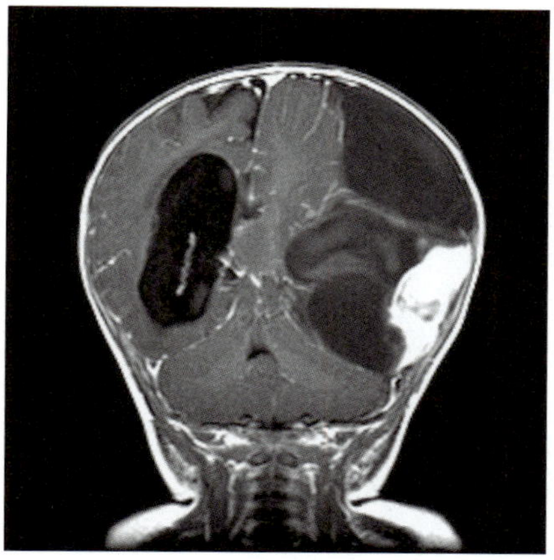

Figure 17.7. *(continued)*

Dysplastic Cerebellar Gangliocytoma (Lhermitte–Duclos Disease)

Definition: Dysplastic cerebellar gangliocytoma is a rare, benign hamartomatous growth in cerebellar hemisphere composed of dysplastic ganglion cells that conform to the existing cortical architecture; it is strongly associated with Cowden syndrome, an autosomal dominant condition characterized by multiple, noncancerous growths or hamartomas on various parts of the body.

Epidemiology: Pediatric and adult individuals can be affected, with the age range of 3 to 80 years old. PTEN mutations are identified in virtually all adults with lhermitte-Duclos disease (LDD) but not in children with LDD, suggesting that the cytogenetics and biology of the two are different. Up to one third of patients with Cowden syndrome can develop LDD.

Molecular and genetic profile: Germline mutation in PTEN is the most frequent cytogenic abnormality in adult-onset LDD, including intragenic mutations, promoter mutations, and large deletions/rearrangements.

Clinical features and standard therapy: Dysmetria and other cerebellar signs are the most common presenting symptoms. Surgical biopsy is the definitive approach to make the diagnosis, and there is no established standard of care therapy for LDD. Surveillance imaging and clinical assessment are the mainstay of clinical management because there is no effective therapy.

Imaging

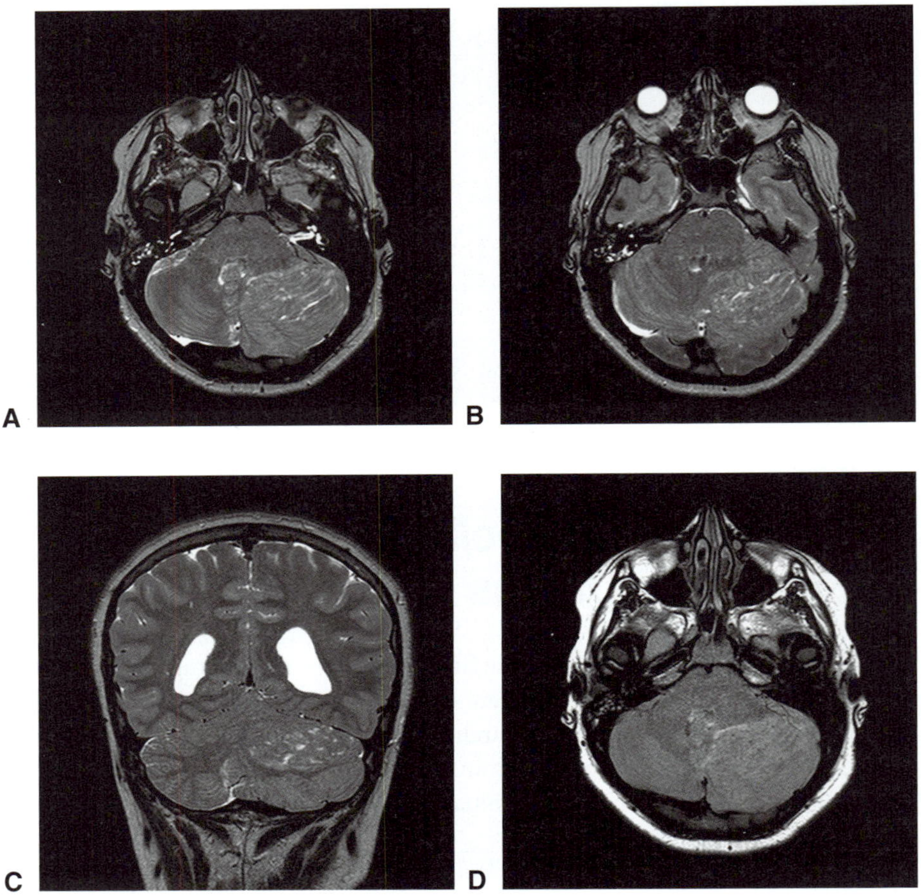

Figure 17.8. Imaging of Dysplastic Cerebellar Gangliocytoma (Lhermitte–Duclos Disease). A. Axial T2: Expansile isointense left cerebellar mass with distinct striated pattern and widened cerebellar folia. **B.** Axial T2: Expansile isointense left cerebellar mass with relative preservation of cortical striations. **C.** Coronal T2: Multifocal areas of widened cerebellar folia within the mass. **D.** Axial FLAIR: Expansile isointense left cerebellar mass with distinct striated pattern and widened cerebellar folia.

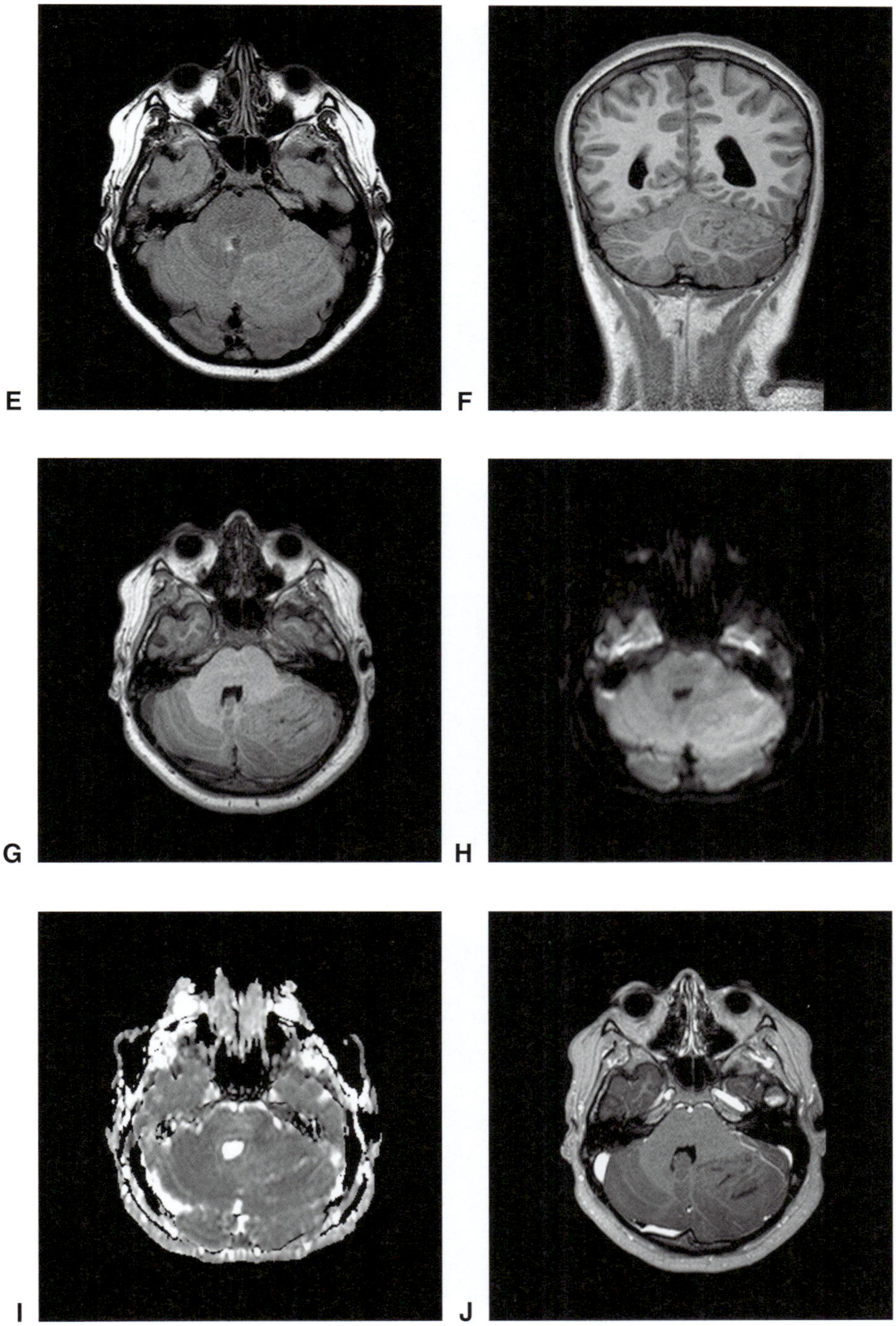

Figure 17.8. ***(continued)*** **E.** Axial FLAIR: Expansile isointense left cerebellar mass with relative preservation of cortical striations. **F.** Coronal T1 precontrast: Expansile hypointense left cerebellar mass with disorganized striated pattern. **G.** Axial T1 precontrast: Expansile hypointense left cerebellar mass with disorganized striated pattern. **H.** Axial DWI: No areas of reduced diffusion within the mass. **I.** Axial ADC: No areas of reduced diffusion within the mass. **J–L.** Axial T1 postcontrast: No abnormal enhancement within the mass.

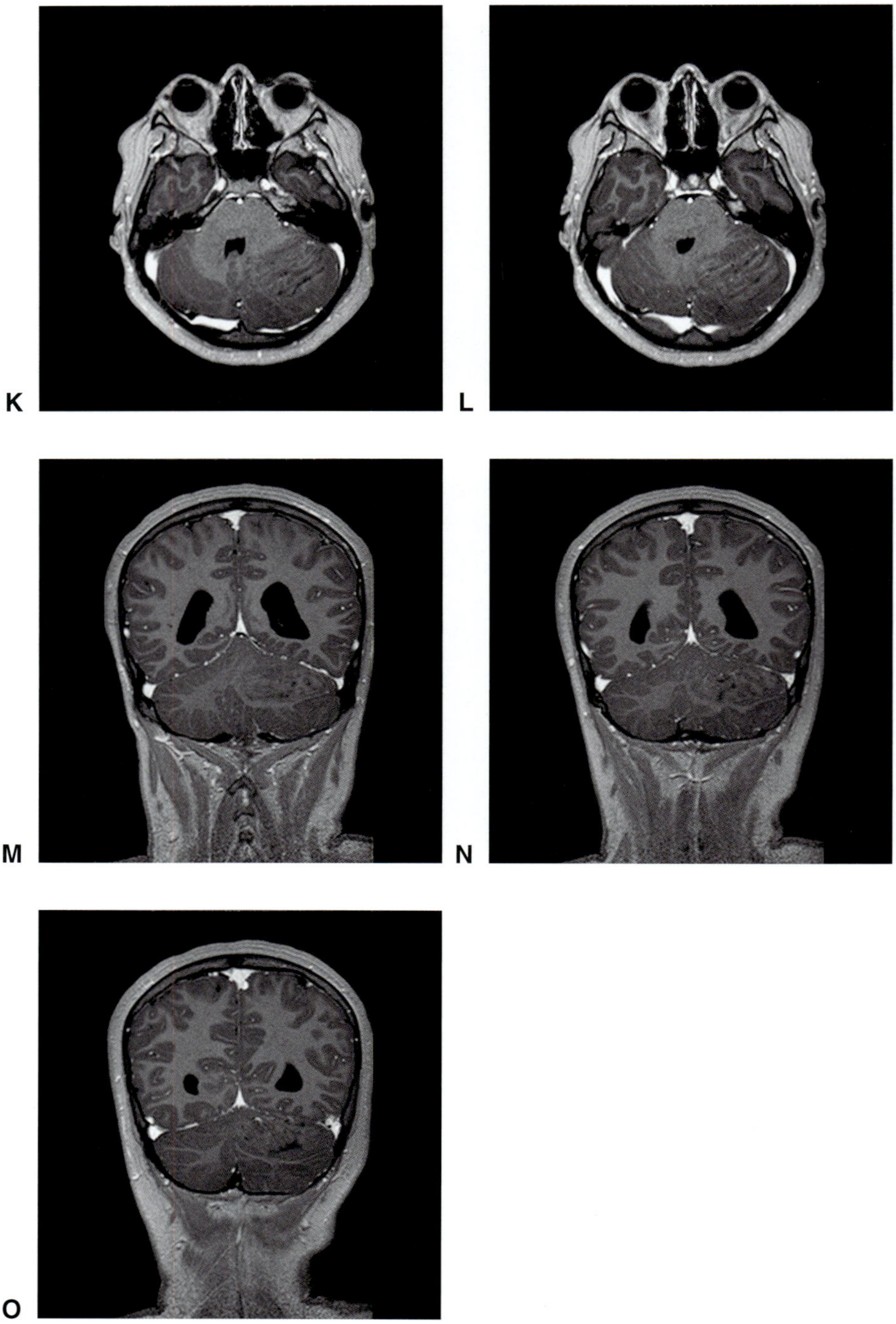

Figure 17.8. ***(continued)*** **M–O.** Coronal T1 postcontrast: No abnormal enhancement within the mass.

▸ Rosette-forming Glioneuronal Tumor

Definition: Dysplastic cerebellar gangliocytoma is a rare, benign, and slow-growing mixed glioneuronal tumor with predilection for fourth ventricular region and occurring predominantly in young adults.

Epidemiology: Due to its rarity, the specific population-based incidence rates are not available.

Molecular and genetic profile: Nuclear expression of thyroid transcription factor (*TTF1*) and strong immunoreactivity for S-100 protein can be seen.

Clinical features and standard therapy: Headache and ataxia are the two most common presenting symptoms related to obstructive hydrocephalus caused by tumor within the fourth ventricle. Surgical resection is the first line of therapy, but gross total resection may not always be possible due to intraventricular extension of tumor adherent to the wall or floor of the fourth ventricle. Radiation therapy and chemotherapy are ineffective and not recommended.

Imaging

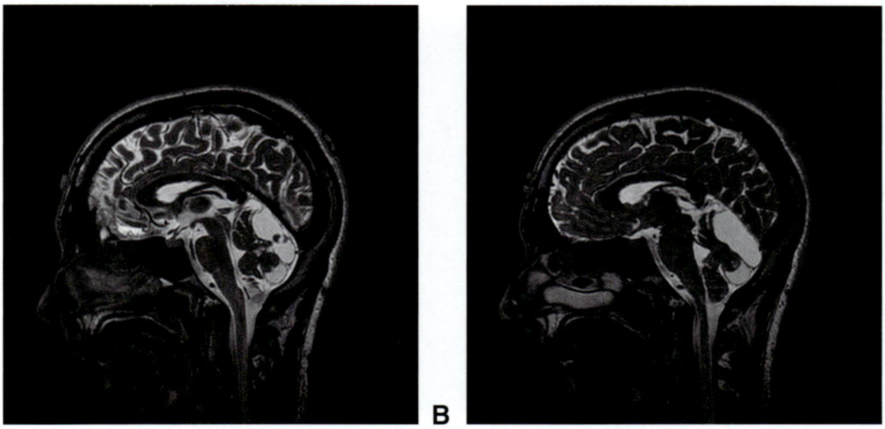
A B

Figure 17.9. Imaging of Rosette-forming Glioneuronal Tumor. A–C. Sagittal T2: Multicystic mass with isointense mural solid nodules.

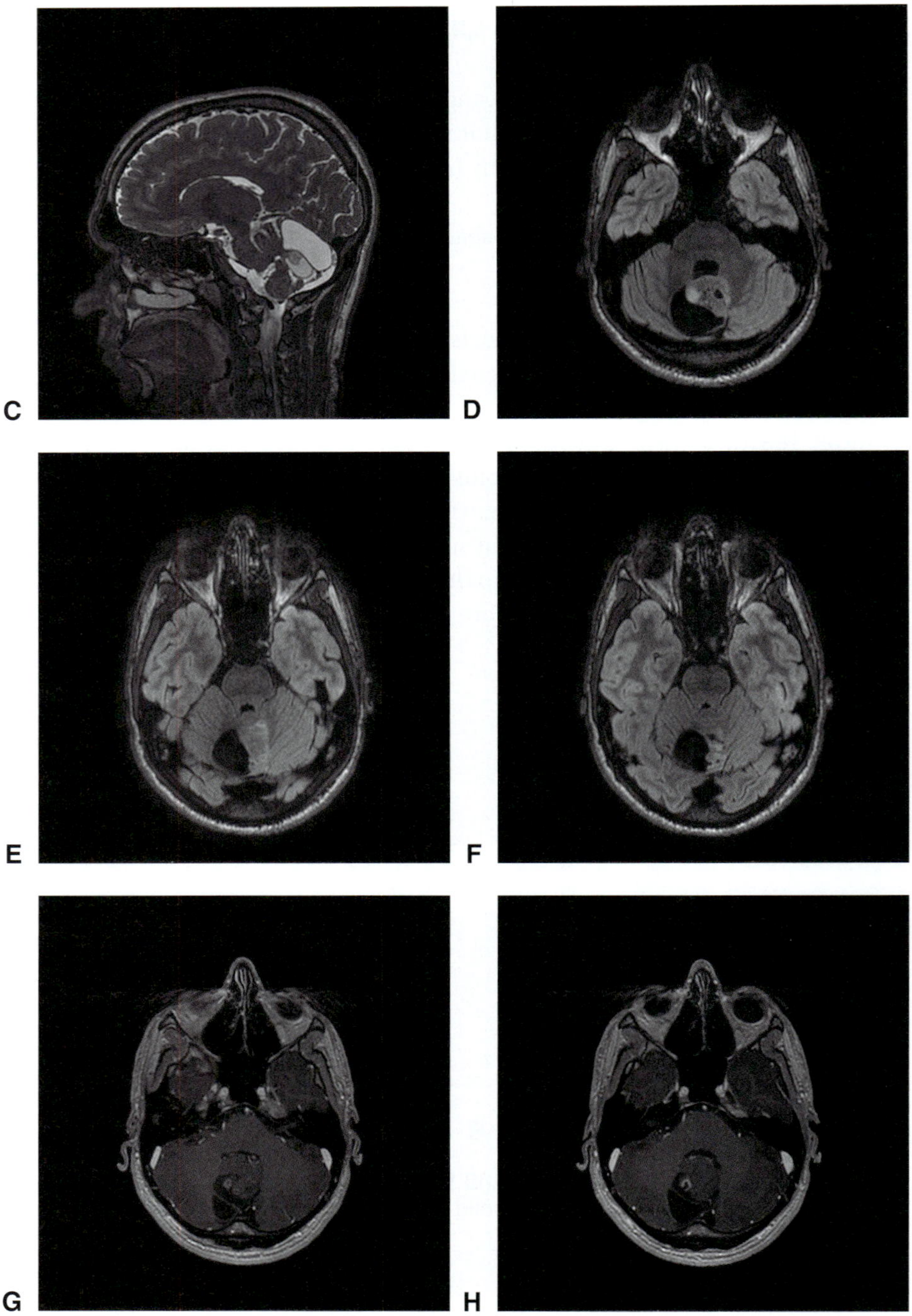

Figure 17.9. ***(continued)*** **D–F.** Axial FLAIR: Multicystic mass with hyperintense mural solid nodules. **G–L.** Axial T1 postcontrast: Multicystic components and isointense mural solid nodules with scattered rings and solid enhancement.

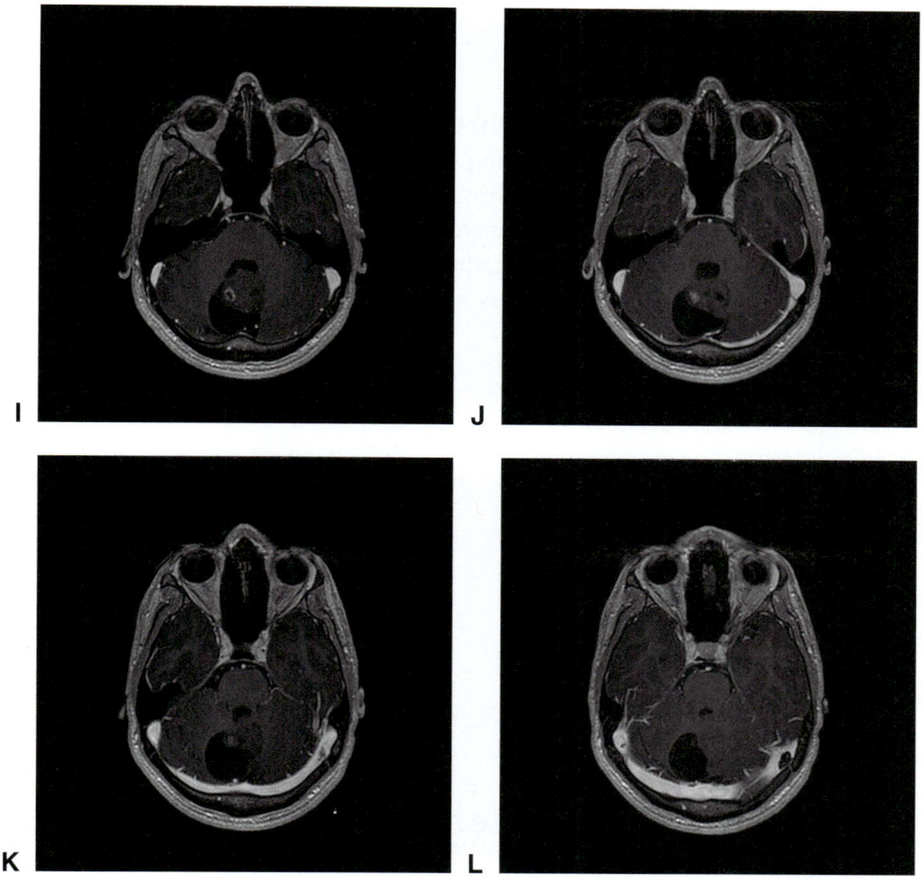

Figure 17.9. ***(continued)***

Diffuse Leptomeningeal Glioneuronal Tumor

Definition: Diffuse leptomeningeal glioneuronal tumor is a rare glioneuronal neoplasm with striking leptomeningeal growth and dissemination and extension into Virchow–Robin spaces and pial surface of the brain, an oligodendroglial-like cytology with neuronal differentiation, and primarily occurring in children and young adults. Although histologically low grade, widely disseminated disease of diffuse leptomeningeal glioneuronal tumor (DLGNTs) at presentation renders them clinically a high-grade neoplasm.

Epidemiology: Although the age range of affected patients is wide, from 5 months to 46 years, in the largest published series of 36 patients, the median age was 5 years and only 3 of the 36 were aged >18 years.

Molecular and genetic profile: *KIAA1549-BRAF* fusion and deletion of chromosomal arm 1p can be seen.

Clinical features and standard therapy: Acute presentation with symptoms of headache, nausea, and vomiting related to increased intracranial pressure or hydrocephalus is common. Gross total resection or substantial tumor debulking is not feasible due to leptomeningeal seeding and intramedullary or intraparenchymal tumor extension. Radiation therapy has been used to delay tumor progression with variable success, and there is no effective chemotherapy.

Imaging

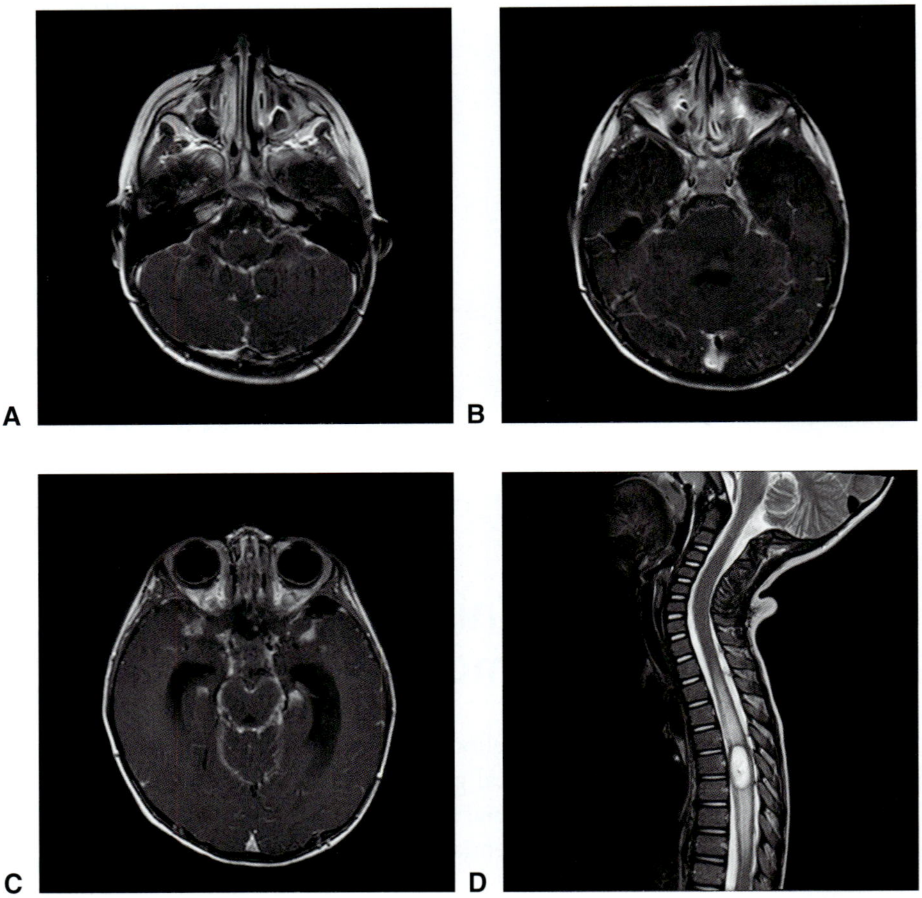

Figure 17.10. Imaging of Diffuse Leptomeningeal Glioneuronal Tumor. A–C. Axial T1 postcontrast: Diffuse leptomeningeal enhancement most prominently in the suprasellar, basilar, medullary cisterns. **D.** Sagittal T2: Circumscribed intramedullary mass centered at T6 level with surrounding cord edema.

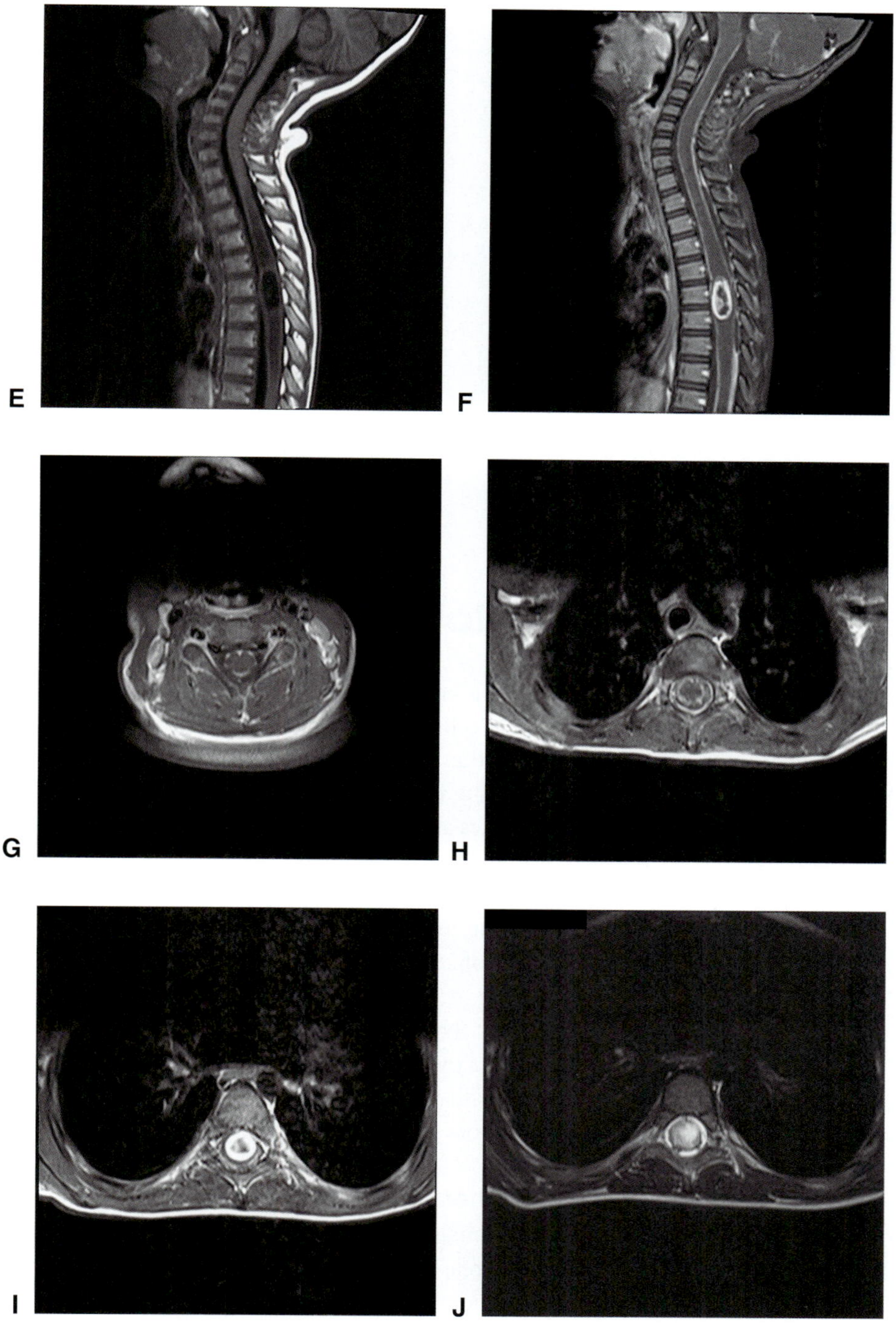

Figure 17.10. ***(continued)*** **E.** Sagittal T1 precontrast: Hypointense mass with isointense rim. **F.** Sagittal T1 postcontrast: Avid enhancement of the rim and diffuse circumferential pial surface enhancement coating the spinal cord, thickest along the dorsal cord from T8 to T10. **G–H.** Axial T1 postcontrast: Circumferential pial surface enhancement coating the spinal cord. **I.** Axial T1 postcontrast: Thick and avid rim enhancement of the intramedullary mass. **J–L.** Axial T2: Hyperintense intramedullar mass and inferior cord edema.

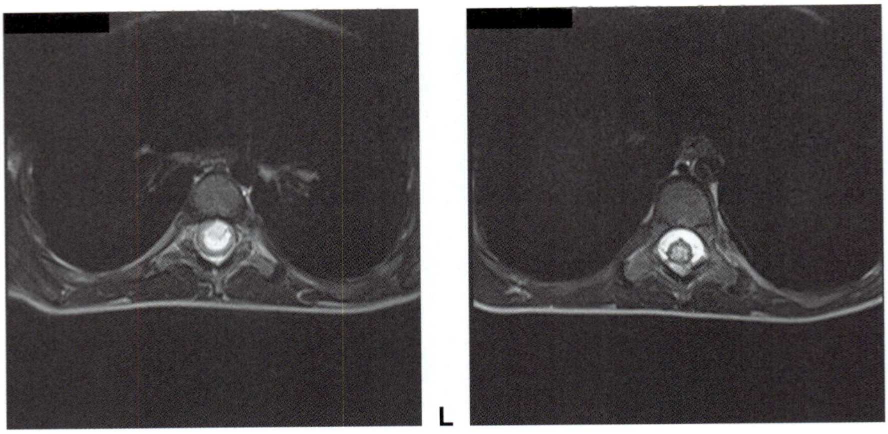

K L

Figure 17.10. ***(continued)***

Central Neurocytoma

Definition: Central neurocytoma is a benign, slow-growing, intraventricular tumor composed of mature neuronal cells and often inseparable from the septum pellucidum and located within the lateral ventricle near the foramen of Monro. Histologically similar-appearing tumors can occur in the cerebral cortex, spinal cord, or non-ventricular sites and are termed *extraventricular neurocytoma.*

Epidemiology: Young adults are the most commonly affected, with the age range of 20 to 40 years and mean age of 28.5 years with no gender predilection.

Molecular and genetic profile: Numerous DNA copy number alterations including MYCN gain as well as overexpression of genes involved in the wingless-related integration site (WNT) signaling pathway, calcium function, and homeostasis of neuronal progenitors have been reported.

Clinical features and standard therapy: Due to its proximity to the foramen of Monro, symptoms of hydrocephalus can be seen, but nonspecific symptoms such as headaches related to increased intracranial pressure are common. Extent of surgical resection has a major impact on prognosis and recurrence. Gross total resection may not always be achieved due to tight tumor adherence to the septum pellucidum or intraoperative hemorrhage. Radiation therapy is often considered following subtotal resection to prevent or delay tumor recurrence. There is no effective chemotherapy.

Imaging

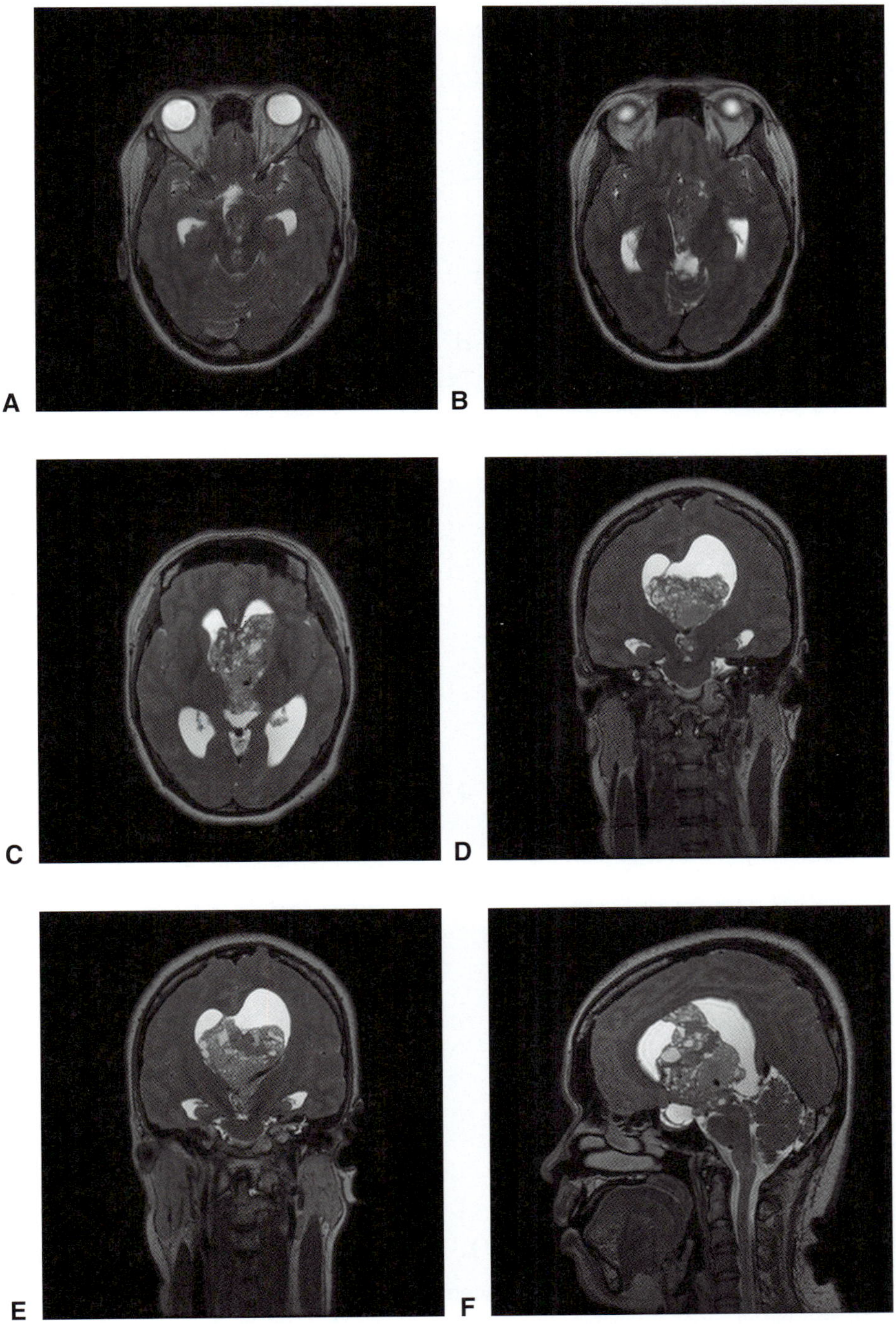

Figure 17.11. Imaging of Central Neurocytoma. A–C. Axial T2: Heterogeneous mixed intensity but mostly hypointense intraventricular mass with microcystic components. **D–E.** Coronal T2: Heterogeneous mixed intensity but mostly hypointense intraventricular mass attached to the septum pellucidum and obstructing foramen of Monroe with resultant hydrocephalus. **F.** Sagittal T2: Heterogeneous mixed intensity but mostly hypointense intraventricular mass attached to the septum pellucidum and obstructing foramen of Monroe with resultant hydrocephalus.

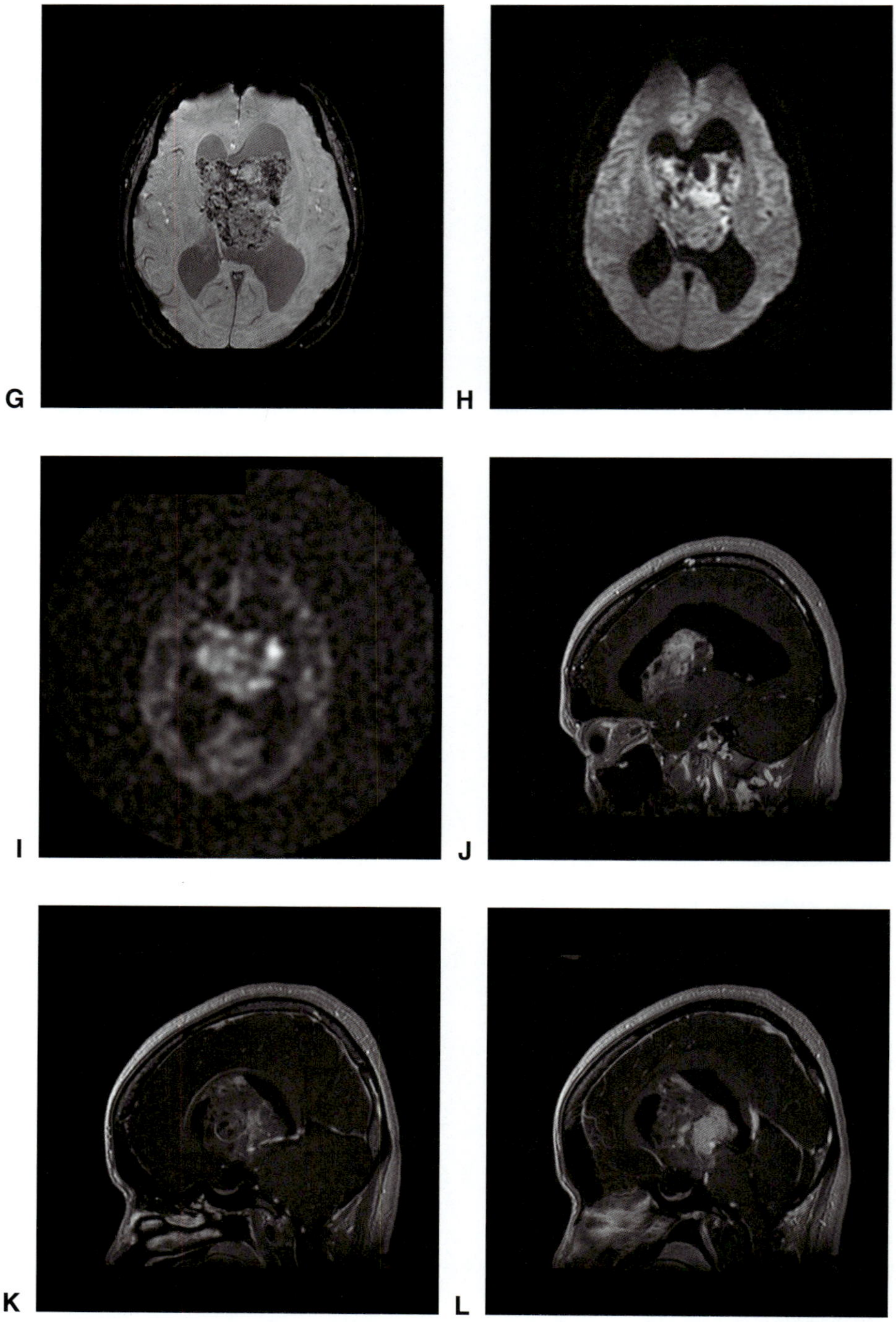

Figure 17.11. ***(continued)*** **G.** Axial susceptibility-weighted imaging (SWI): Diffuse scattered blood products within the mass. **H.** Axial DWI: Patchy areas of reduced diffusion within the mass. **I.** Axial arterial spin labeling (ASL): Hypervascular mass. **J–L.** Sagittal T1 postcontrast: Heterogeneous enhancement within the mass with areas of more solid enhancement.

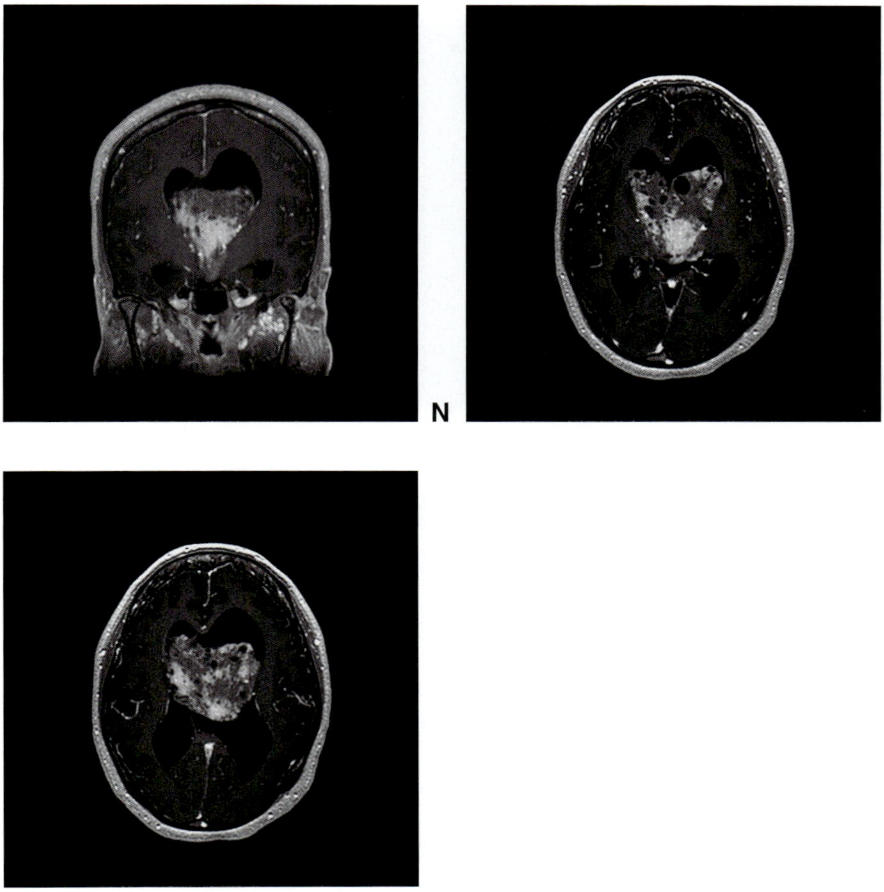

M N O

Figure 17.11. ***(continued)*** **M.** Coronal T1 postcontrast: Heterogeneous enhancement within the mass with areas of more solid enhancement inferiorly. **N–O.** Axial T1 postcontrast: Heterogeneous enhancement within the mass with areas of more solid enhancement.

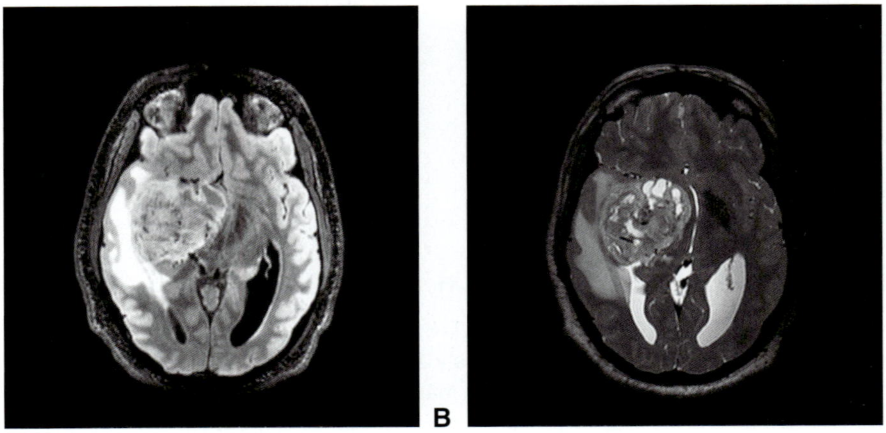

A B

Figure 17.12. Imaging of Extraventricular Neurocytoma. A. Axial FLAIR: Heterogeneously hypointense mass centered in the right insula and basal forebrain. **B.** Axial T2: Heterogeneously mixed intensity mass compressing the third and right lateral ventricle and trapping the left lateral ventricle.

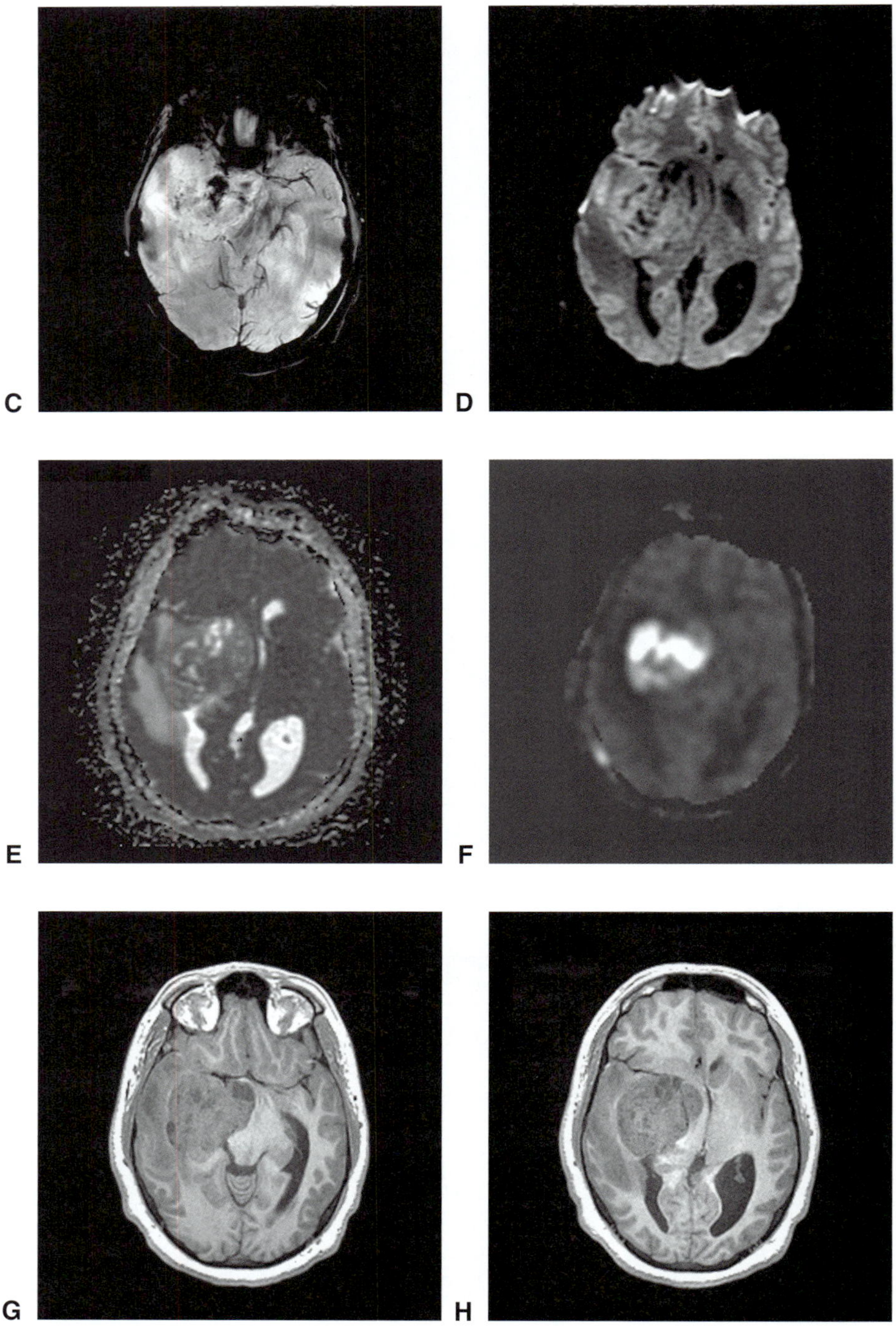

Figure 17.12. ***(continued)*** **C.** Axial SWI: Scattered areas of blood products within the mass. **D.** Axial DWI: Heterogeneously and mildly hyperintense mass. **E.** Axial ADC: Mildly reduced diffusion within the mass. **F.** Axial ASL: Marked hyperperfusion within the mass. **G–I.** Axial T1 precontrast: Heterogeneously hypointense mass.

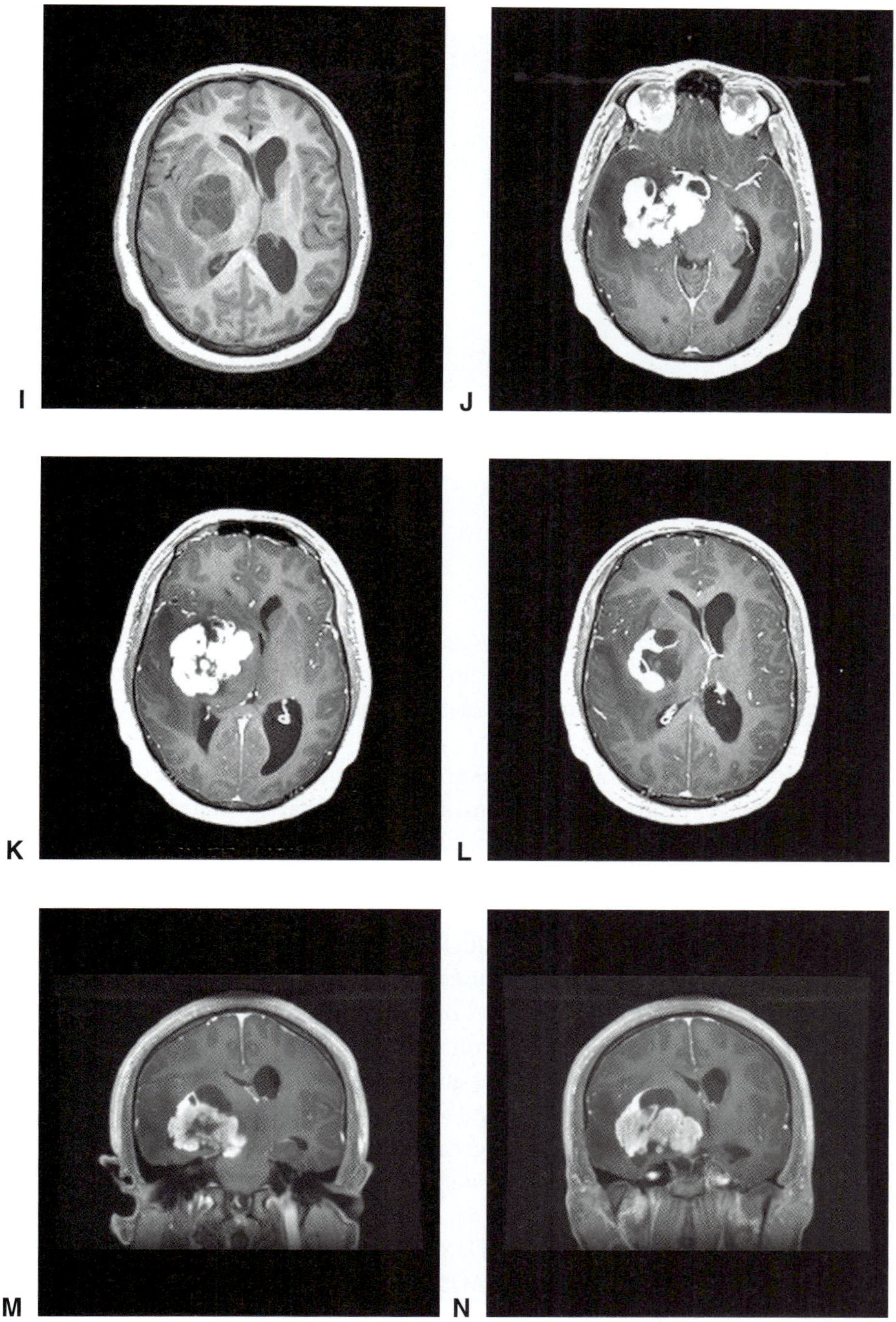

Figure 17.12. ***(continued)*** **J–L.** Axial T1 postcontrast: Avidly enhancing mass with medial peripheral cystic lesions. **M–O.** Coronal T1 postcontrast: Avidly enhancing mass with prominent cystic or necrotic areas.

O
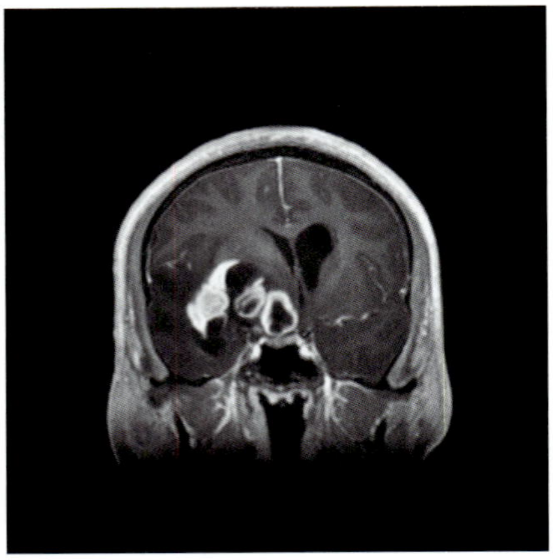

Figure 17.12. ***(continued)***

Paraganglioma

Definition: Paraganglioma is an encapsulated and benign neuroendocrine tumor arising in neural crest cells associated with paraganglia and in the CNS, primarily affecting the cauda equina, filum terminale, and jugulotympanic regions.

Epidemiology: CNS paragangliomas are uncommon and most present in the filum terminale or cauda equina regions, affecting primarily adults in the fourth to sixth decades of life, but they can occur in children and adults with the age range of 9 to 75 years and mean age of 46 years, with slight male predominance.

Molecular and genetic profile: Single benign CNS paraganglioma usually does not indicate underlying genetic susceptibility or syndrome. However, multiple paragangliomas or an association of paraganglioma with another tumor such as pituitary adenoma or pheochromocytoma raises the possibility of a genetic syndrome. When paragangliomas and pheochromocytomas occur together, more than half of the adult-onset and >80% of the childhood-onset cases are associated with autosomal dominant germline mutations of >10 genes, including *VHL* (von Hippel–Lindau syndrome), *RET* (multiple endocrine dysplasia type 2), *NF1* (neurofibromatosis type 1), genes coding for subunits of the succinate dehydrogenase enzyme—*SDHD*, *SDHA*, *SDHAF2*, *SDHC*, and *SDHB*—and the tumor suppressor genes *TMEM127* and *MAX*.

Clinical features and standard therapy: Similar to other more common spinal tumors, the clinical presentation of filum or cauda equina paragangliomas is nonspecific, low back pain and sciatica being the most common symptoms. Endocrinologically active spinal paragangliomas are exceedingly rare. Jugulotympanic paragangliomas can present with pulsatile tinnitus when they extend into the intracranial cavity. Surgical resection is the first line of therapy and subtotal resection can lead to slow recurrence. Endovascular tumor embolization can be used to decrease the tumor bulk and vascularity prior to surgery, which can increase the chance of gross total resection. Chemotherapy, radiotherapy, and use of octreotide and other somatostatin are occasionally used, but their effectiveness remains unknown.

Imaging

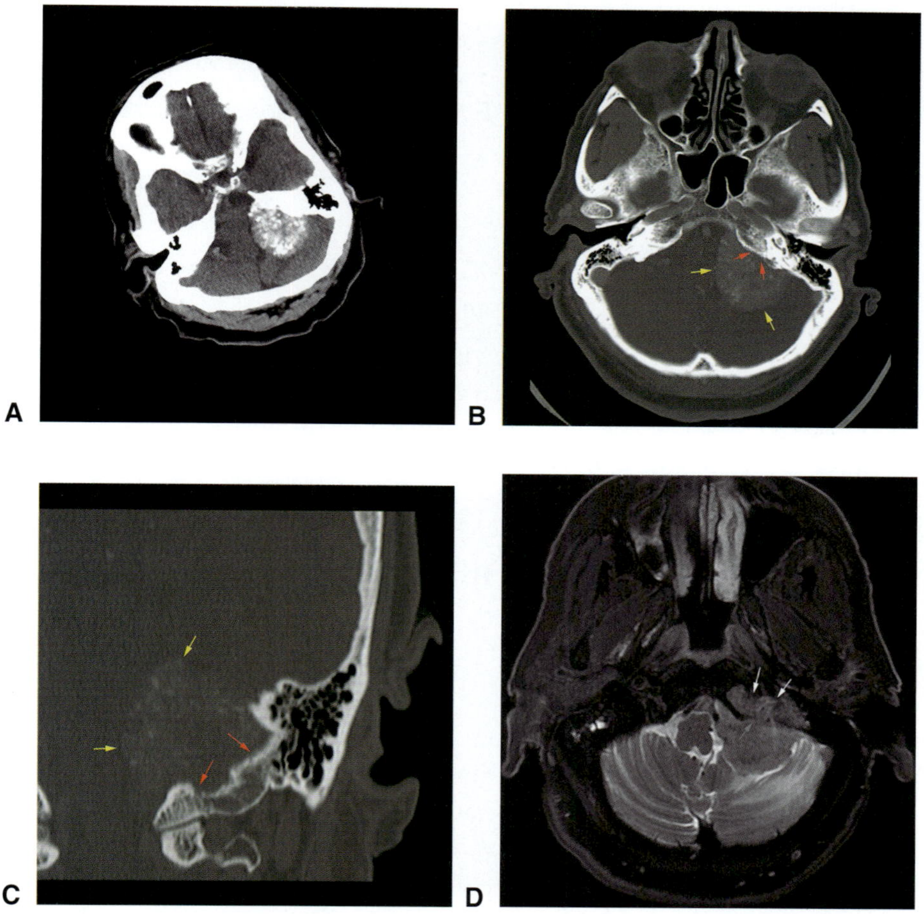

Figure 17.13. Imaging of Posterior Fossa Paraganglioma. A. Axial CT enhanced: Heterogeneously enhancing left cerebellopontine angle cistern mass with numerous stippled calcium. **B.** Axial CT bone window: Circumscribed tumor (yellow arrows) with subtle bony erosion of petrous bone (red arrows). **C.** Coronal CT bone window: Circumscribed tumor (yellow arrows) with subtle bony erosion of petrous bone (red arrows). **D–F.** Axial T2: Homogeneously hypointense extra-axial mass in the left cerebellopontine angle with bony destruction (red arrow) and intraosseous involvement of the left skull base and petrous bone (white arrows).

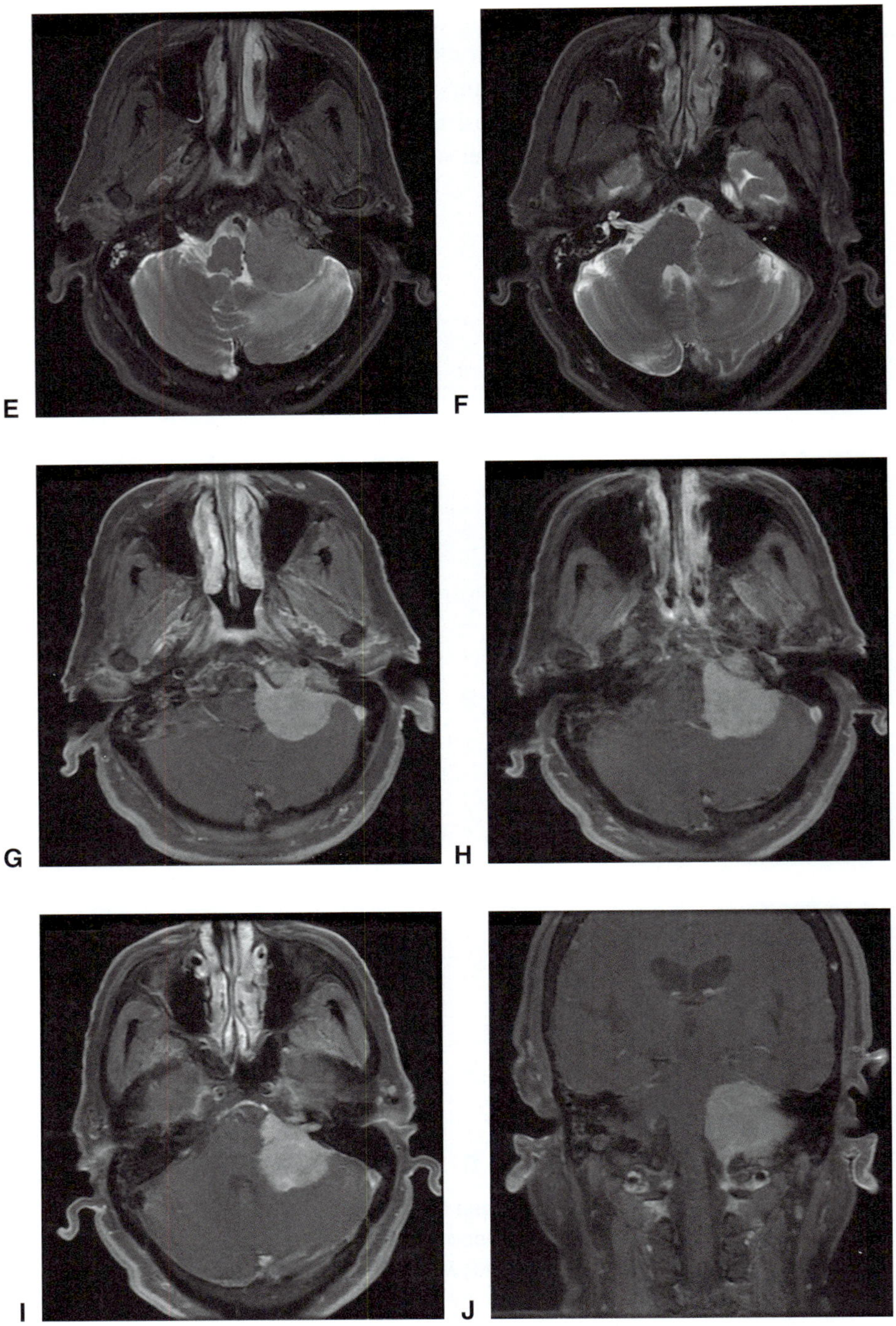

Figure 17.13. ***(continued)*** **G–I.** Axial T1 postcontrast fat saturated: Avid enhancement within the mass. **J–L.** Coronal T1 postcontrast fat saturated: Avid enhancement within the mass.

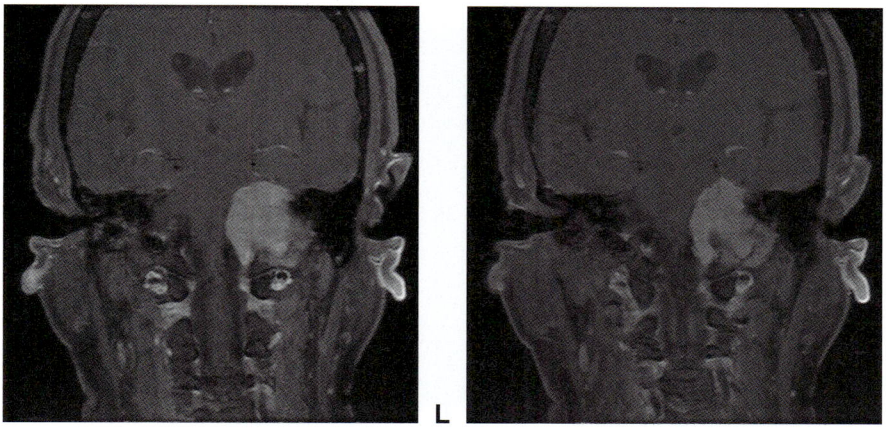

K L

Figure 17.13. ***(continued)***

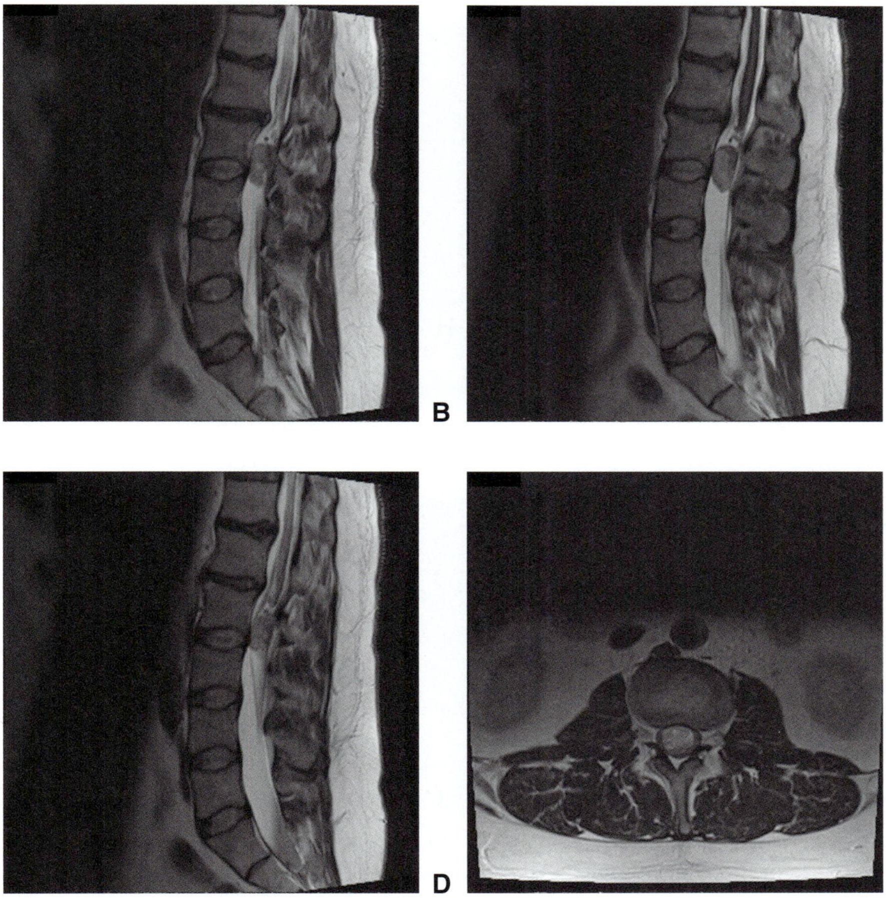

A B C D

Figure 17.14. Imaging of Spinal Paraganglioma. A–C. Sagittal T2: Hypointense cauda equina intradural extramedullary mass at L2. **D–F.** Axial T2: Hypointense cauda equina intradural extramedullary mass, centrally located and displacing intrathecal nerve roots.

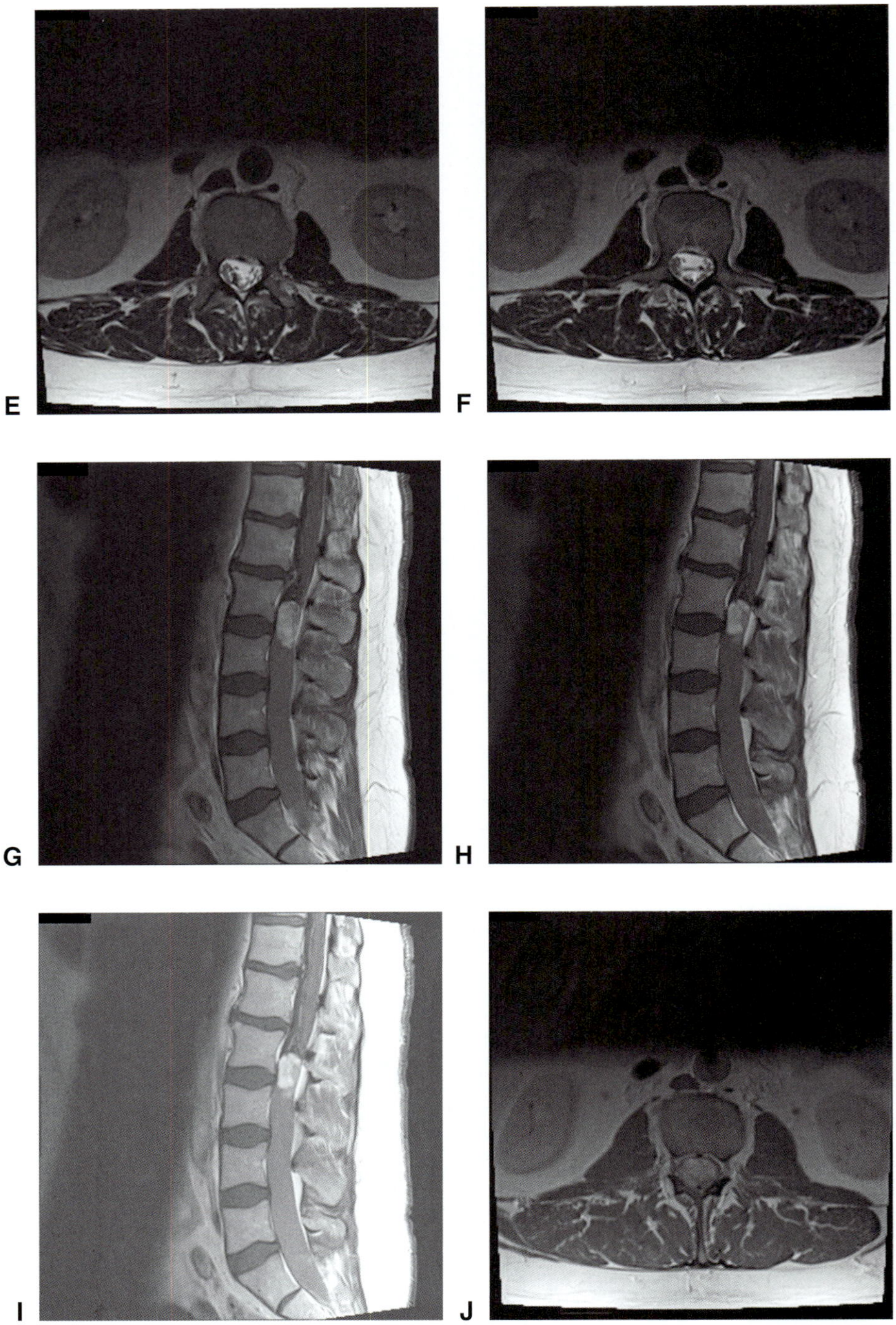

Figure 17.14. ***(continued)*** **G–I.** Sagittal T1 postcontrast: Avid enhancement within the mass. **J–L.** Axial T1 postcontrast: Avid enhancement within the mass.

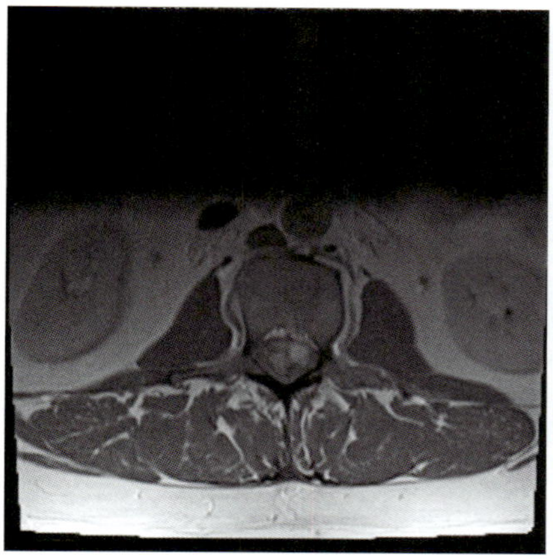

K

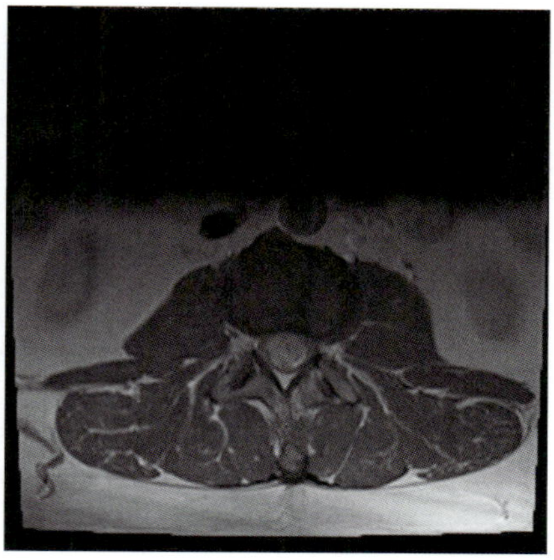

L

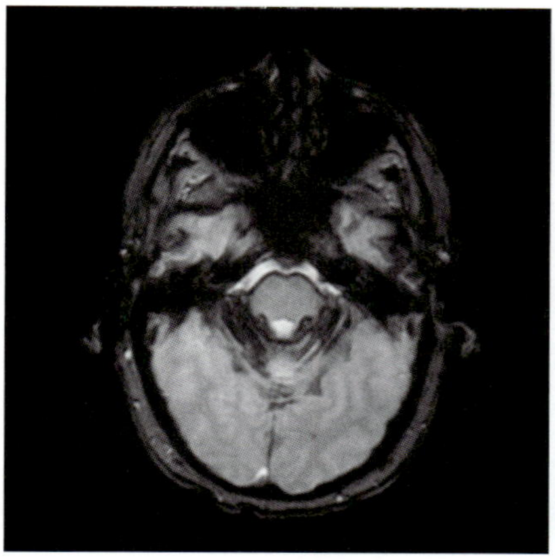

M

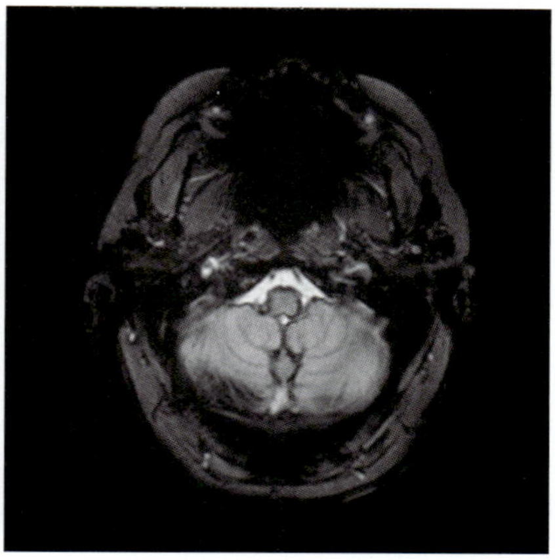

N

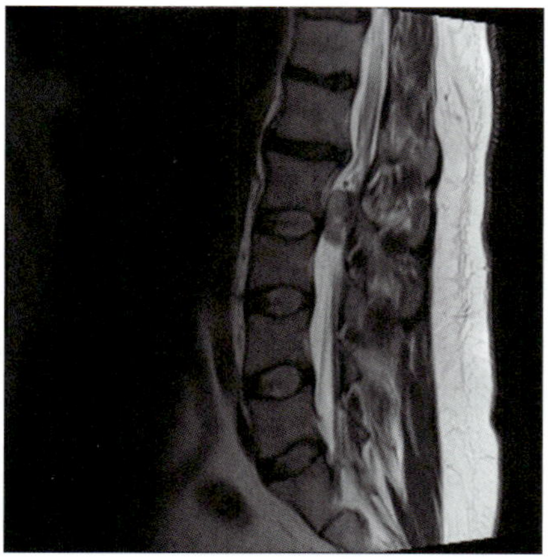

O

Figure 17.14. ***(continued)*** **M–O.** Axial SWI: Extensive superficial siderosis in the brain due to chronic hemorrhage due to the spinal paraganglioma.

Bibliography

Abel TW, Baker SJ, Fraser MM, et al. Lhermitte-Duclos disease: a report of 31 cases with immunohistochemical analysis of the PTEN/AKT/mTOR pathway. *J Neuropathol Exp Neurol*. 2005;64:341–349.

Anyanwu CT, Robinson TM, Huang JH. Rosette-forming glioneuronal tumor: an update. *Clin Transl Oncol*. 2020;22:623–630.

Bonney PA, Boettcher LB, Krysiak RS 3rd, Fung KM, Sughrue ME. Histology and molecular aspects of central neurocytoma. *Neurosurg Clin N Am*. 2015;26:21–29.

Cho HJ, Myung JK, Kim H, et al. Primary diffuse leptomeningeal glioneuronal tumors. *Brain Tumor Pathol*. 2015;32:49–55.

Donoho D, Zada G. Imaging of central neurocytomas. *Neurosurg Clin N Am*. 2015;26:11–19.

Furtado A, Arantes M, Silva R, et al. Comprehensive review of extraventricular neurocytoma with report of two cases, and comparison with central neurocytoma. *Clin Neuropathol*. 2010;29:134–40.

Hsu C, Kwan G, Lau Q, et al. Rosette-forming glioneuronal tumour: imaging features, histopathological correlation and a comprehensive review of literature. *Br J Neurosurg*. 2012;26:668–73.

Jain N, Chauhan U, Goel V, Puri SK. Lhermitte-Duclos disease: diagnosis on MRI, MR spectroscopy, CT and positron emission tomography. *J Clin Diagn Res*. 2015;9:TJ01–TJ02.

Luzzi S, Elia A, Del Maestro M, et al. Dysembryoplastic neuroepithelial tumors: what you need to know. *World Neurosurg*. 2019;127:255–265.

Pérez-Núñez A, Lagares A, Benítez J, et al. Lhermitte-Duclos disease and Cowden disease: clinical and genetic study in five patients with Lhermitte-Duclos disease and literature review. *Acta Neurochir (Wien)*. 2004;146:679–690.

Thomas B, Krishnamoorthy T, Radhakrishnan VV, Kesavadas C. Advanced MR imaging in Lhermitte-Duclos disease: moving closer to pathology and pathophysiology. *Neuroradiology*. 2007;49:733–738.

Wang AC, Jones DTW, Abecassis IJ, et al. Desmoplastic infantile ganglioglioma/astrocytoma (DIG/DIA) are distinct entities with frequent BRAFV600 mutations. *Mol Cancer Res*. 2018;16:1491–1498.

Yang C, Li G, Fang J, et al. Clinical characteristics and surgical outcomes of primary spinal paragangliomas. *J Neurooncol*. 2015;122:539–547.

Yang GF, Wu SY, Zhang LJ, et al. Imaging findings of extraventricular neurocytoma: report of 3 cases and review of the literature. *AJNR Am J Neuroradiol*. 2009;30:581–585.

Yang SY, Jin YJ, Park SH, et al. Paragangliomas in the cauda equina region: clinicopathoradiologic findings in four cases. *J Neurooncol*. 2005;72:49–55.

Zaky W, Patil SS, Park M, et al. Ganglioglioma in children and young adults: single institution experience and review of the literature. *J Neurooncol*. 2018;139:739–747.

18

Metastatic Tumors to the Central Nervous System

Overview

The incidence of metastatic tumors to the central nervous system (CNS) is rising in part due to advances in therapy that result in longer survival of patients with systemic cancer. Despite the development of effective immunotherapy and molecularly targeted therapies, metastatic tumors to the CNS can cause considerable morbidity and mortality in patients. Metastatic tumors to the CNS can be subdivided into five types based on the location—intraparenchymal, leptomeningeal, dural, intraventricular, and osseous compartment. Hematogenous spread is considered the most common route of entry into the CNS by metastatic tumors. Leptomeningeal carcinomatosis is poorly understood in terms of pathogenesis and mechanism of spread and remains one of the most difficult forms of metastatic tumors to treat.

Central Nervous System Metastatic Tumors

Definition: Central nervous system (CNS) metastatic tumor is a cancer that has spread from the primary (original systemic) site of the tumor to the CNS via hematogenous spread or direct extension.

Epidemiology: CNS metastases are the most common CNS neoplasms in adults but account for less than 2% of all tumors in the pediatric age group. Up to 30% of adults and 10% of children with cancer develop CNS metastases during the course of lifetime. The overall incidence of CNS metastatic tumors is increasing due to two main factors: (1) longer life expectancy of systemic cancer patients due to improvement in therapy and (2) wider availability and use of MR imaging for detection of symptomatic and asymptomatic CNS metastasis. Tumors with a high propensity to metastasize to the brain are lung cancer, breast cancer, renal cell carcinoma, and melanoma. About 14% of men and 8% of women with CNS metastatic tumor show no clear primary tumor and thus are diagnosed as carcinoma of unknown primary.

Molecular and genetic profile: CNS metastatic tumors mirror the molecular and genetic profiles of the original primary tumor of the body. Some molecularly defined tumor subtypes are more likely to metastasize to the CNS, such as erythroblastic leukemia viral oncogene homolog 2 (ERBB2)-positive and triple-negative breast cancer.

Clinical features and standard therapy: Surgical resection is reserved for large metastasis causing significant edema and mass effect. Gamma knife radiosurgery is used for multiple CNS metastases <2.5 cm in size. Whole brain radiation therapy is used for innumerable CNS metastases or leptomeningeal/dural metastases. Brachytherapy is used for recurrent CNS metastases. Targeted chemotherapy is used for CNS metastases from systemic cancer with specific molecular genetic alterations.

Imaging

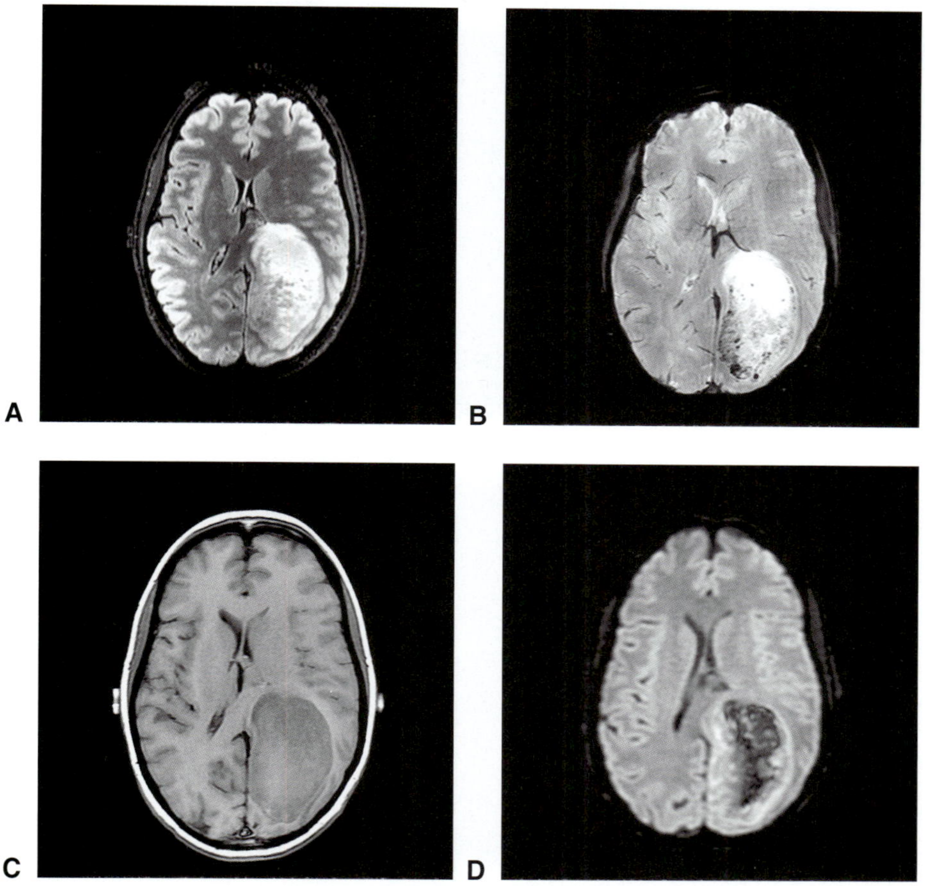

Figure 18.1. Imaging of intraparenchymal cervical cancer metastasis with minimal edema. A. Axial fluid-attenuated inversion recovery (FLAIR): Large heterogeneously hyperintense intraparenchymal mass in the left occipital lobe with minimal surrounding vasogenic edema. **B.** Axial susceptibility-weighted imaging (SWI): Scattered blood products within the mass. **C.** Axial T1-precontrast: Mixed hypointense and isointense mass. **D.** Axial diffusion-weighted imaging (DWI): Mostly increased diffusion within the mass with rim of reduced diffusion.

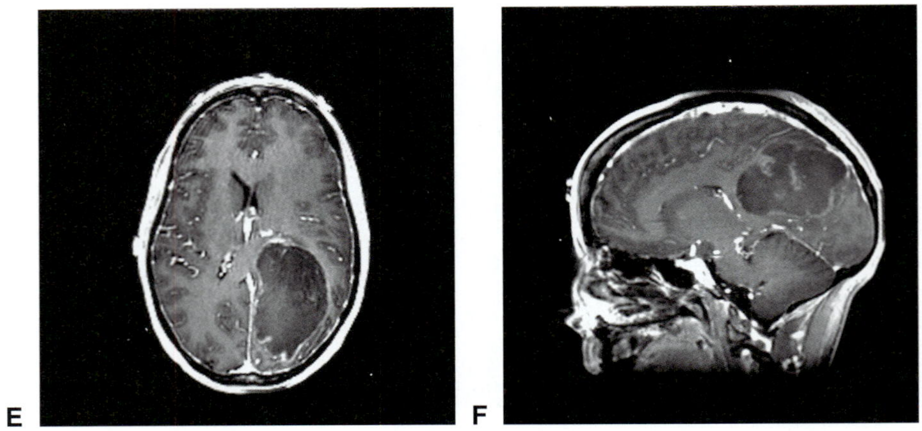

Figure 18.1. ***(continued)*** **E.** Axial T1-postcontrast: Minimal to mild rim enhancement. **F.** Sagittal T1-postcontrast: Minimal to mild rim enhancement.

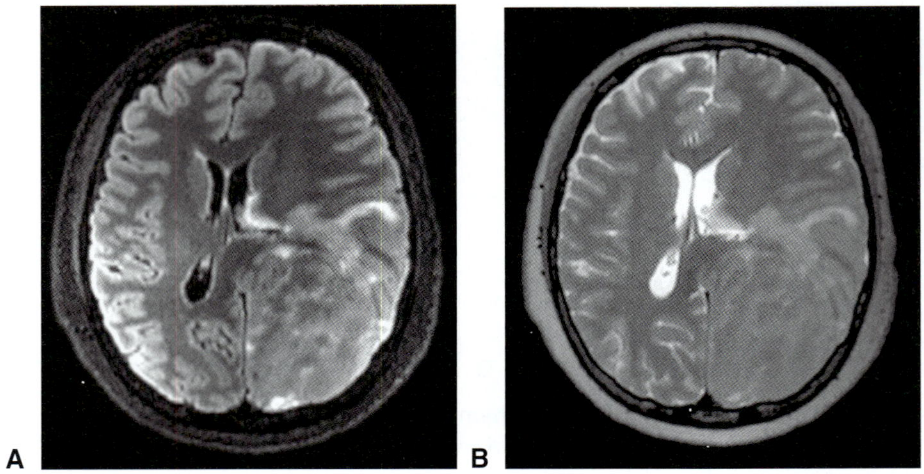

Figure 18.2. Imaging of intraparenchymal endometrial cancer metastasis with moderate edema. A. Axial FLAIR: Large heterogeneously hypointense intraparenchymal mass in the left occipital lobe with moderate surrounding vasogenic edema. **B.** Axial T2: Markedly hypointense mass.

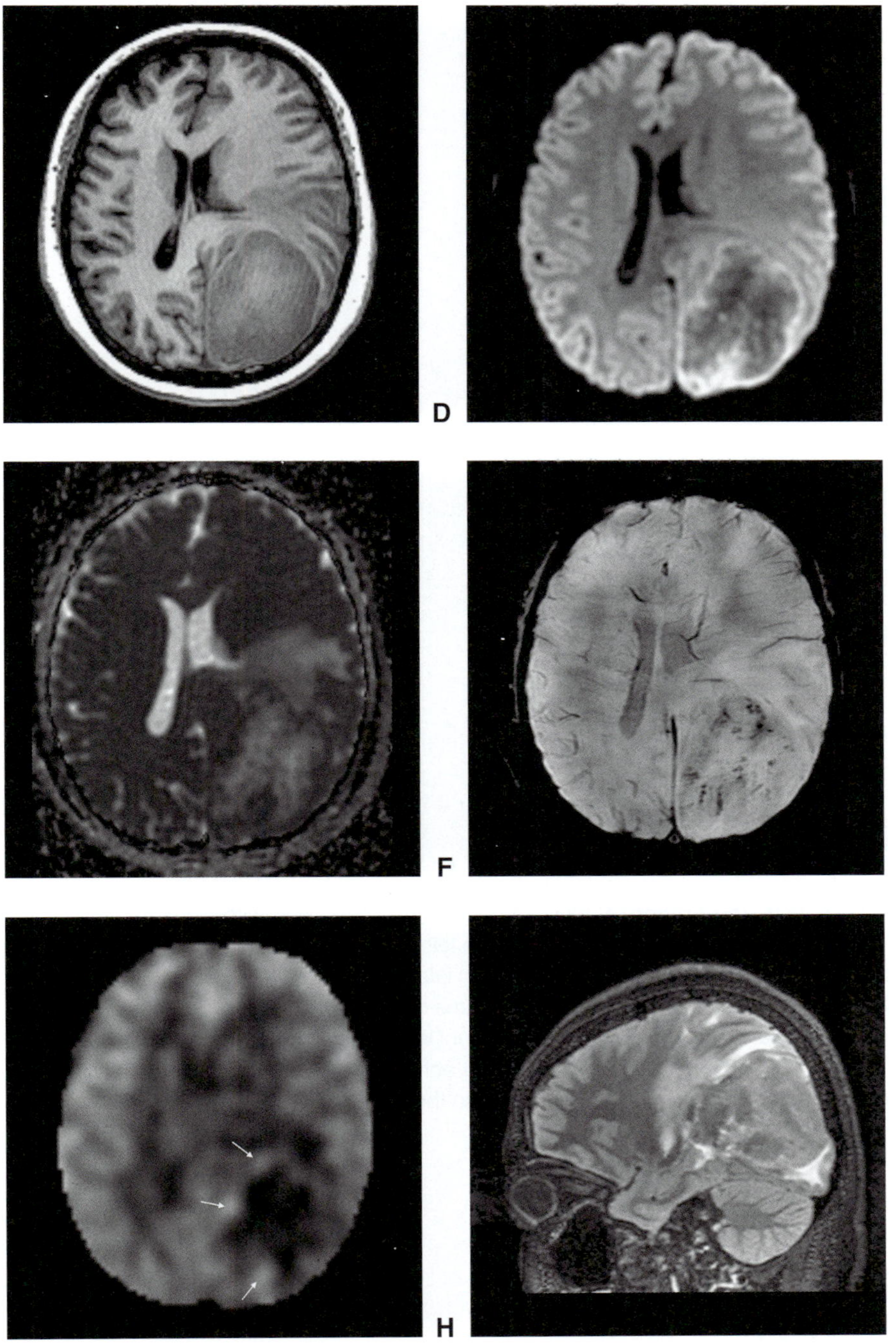

C D E F G H

Figure 18.2. ***(continued)*** **C.** Axial T1-precontrast: Mixed hypointense and isointense mass. **D.** Axial DWI: Mostly increased diffusion within the mass with rim of reduced diffusion. **E.** Axial apparent diffusion coefficient (ADC): Mostly increased diffusion within the mass with rim of reduced diffusion. **F.** Axial SWI: Scattered blood products within the mass. **G.** Axial arterial spin labeling (ASL): Scattered areas of hyperperfusion within the rim of the mass (white arrows). **H.** Sagittal FLAIR: Heterogeneously hypointense mass with moderate surrounding vasogenic edema.

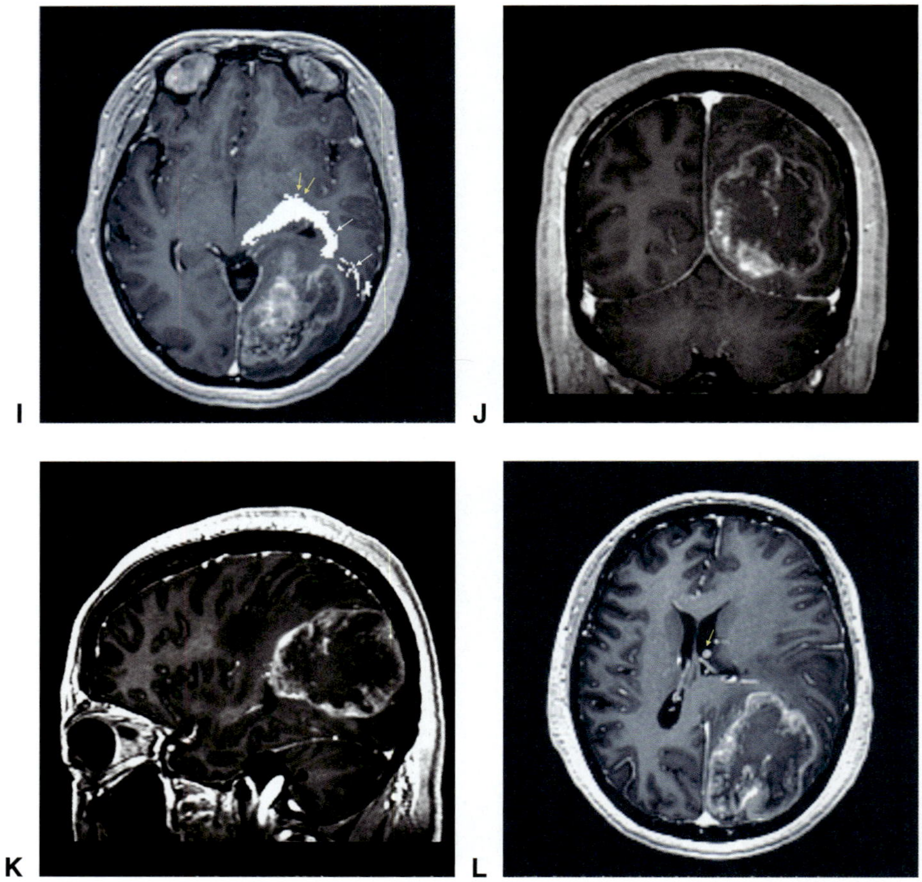

Figure 18.2. ***(continued)*** **I.** Axial T1-postcontrast overlayed with visual pathway tractography: Left occipital mass displaces the left lateral geniculate ganglion (yellow arrow) anteriorly and optic radiation (white arrows) laterally. **J.** Coronal T1-postcontrast: Irregular and nodular rim enhancement with large area of central necrosis. **K.** Sagittal T1-postcontrast: Irregular and nodular rim enhancement with large area of central necrosis. **L.** Axial T1-postcontrast: Irregular and nodular rim enhancement with large area of central necrosis and second enhancing nodule within the anterior lateral ventricle (yellow arrow).

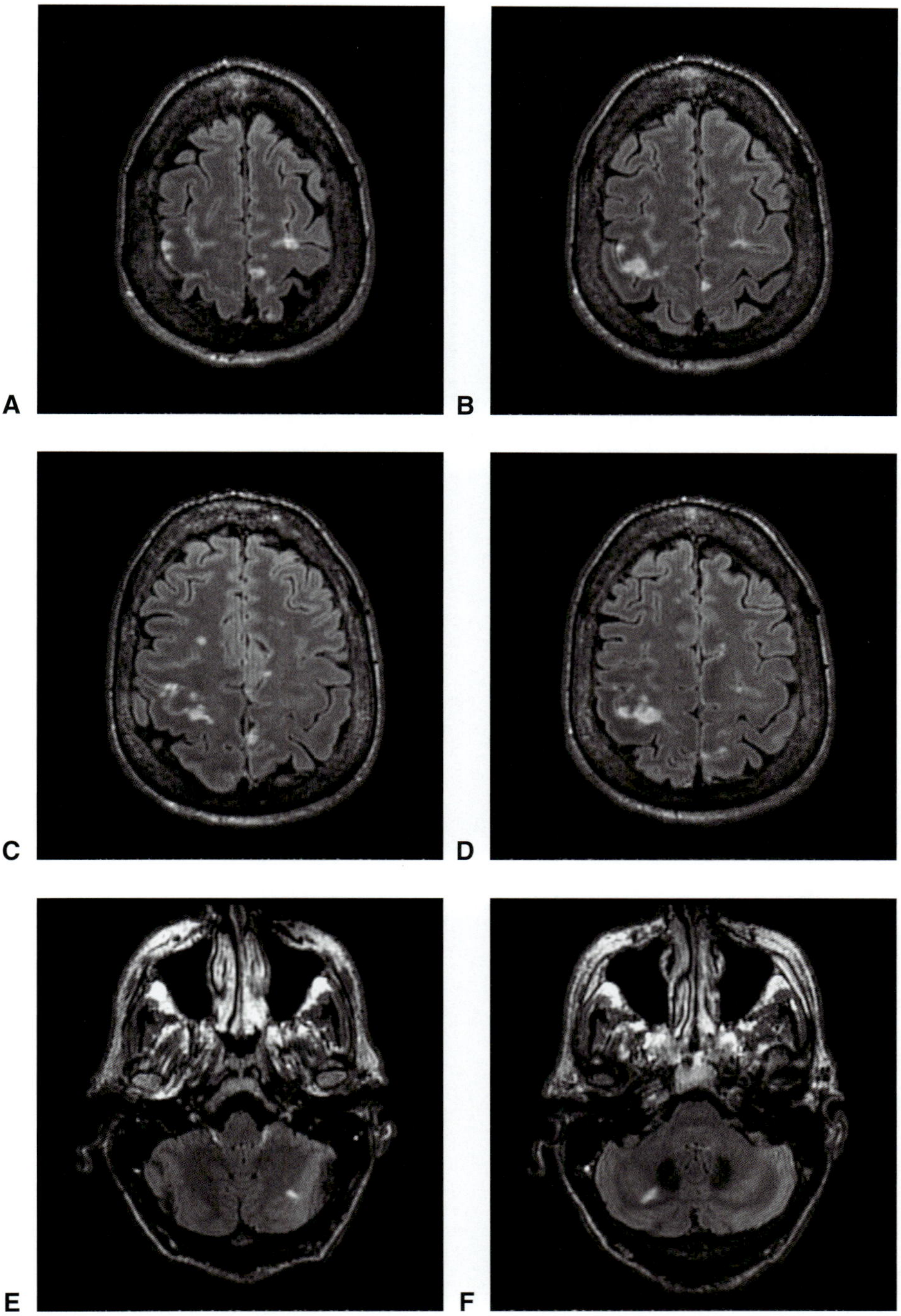

Figure 18.3. Imaging of pancreatic mucinous adenocarcinoma metastases. A–F. Axial FLAIR: Multiple foci of parenchymal and leptomeningeal hyperintense lesions diffusely involving supra- and infra-tentorial brain.

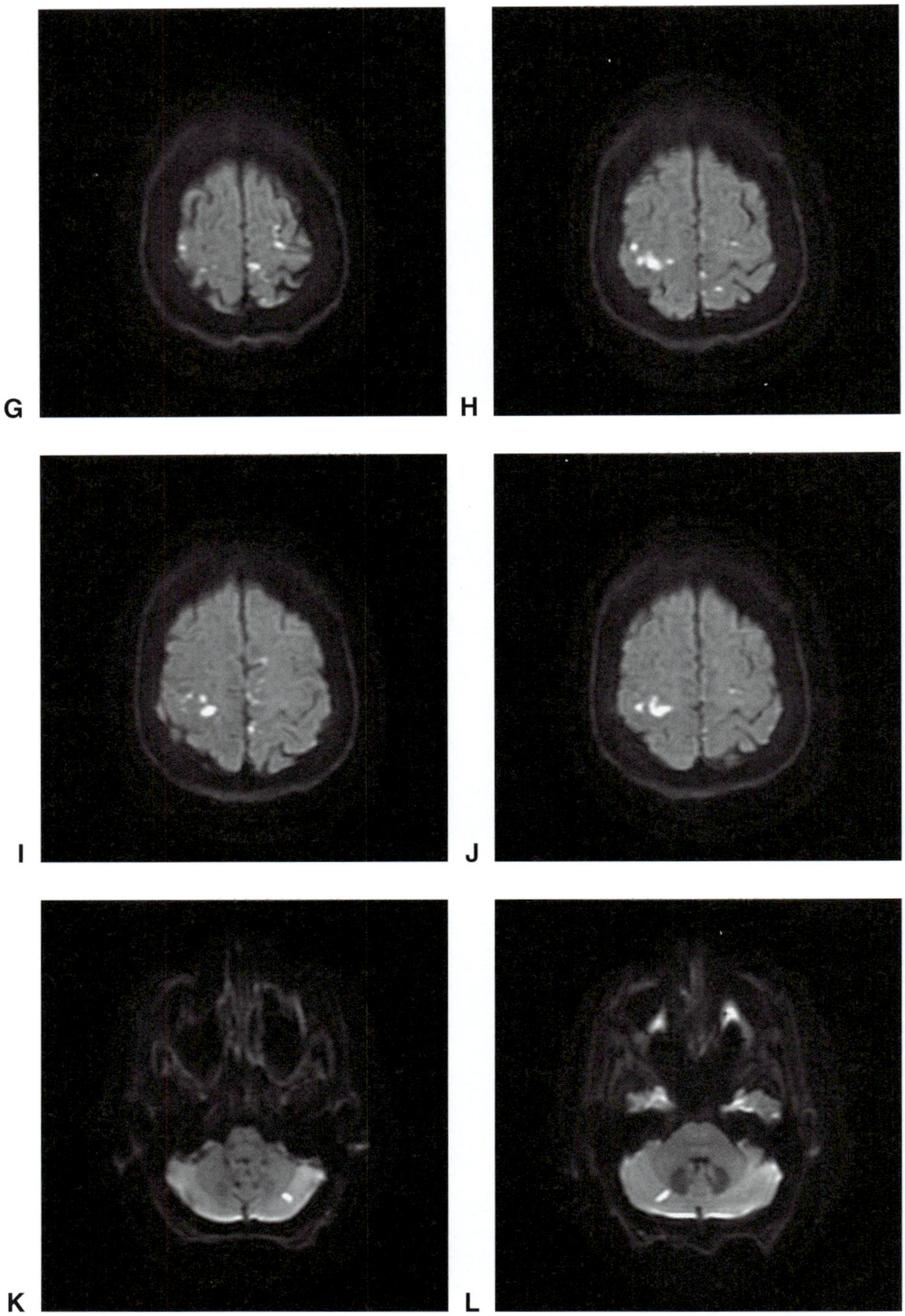

Figure 18.3. ***(continued)*** **G–L.** Axial DWI: Reduced diffusion corresponding to the multiple foci of parenchymal and leptomeningeal hyperintense FLAIR lesions diffusely involving supra- and infra-tentorial brain.

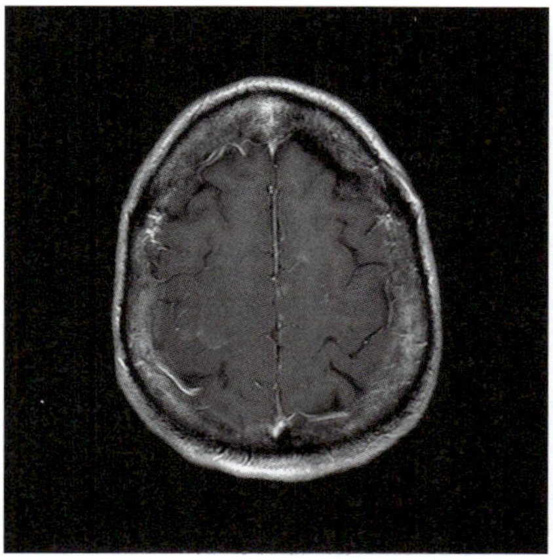
M

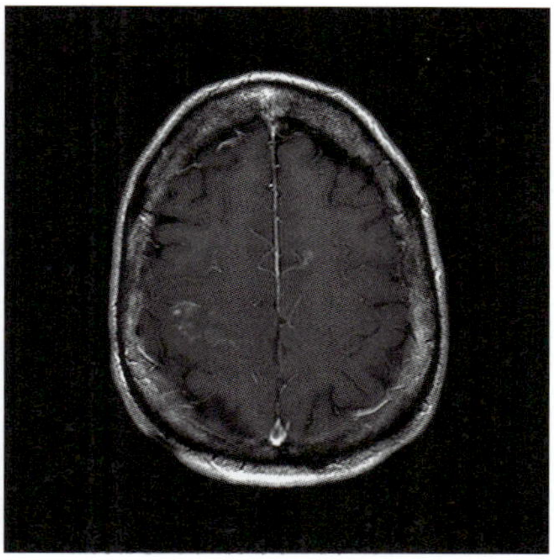
N

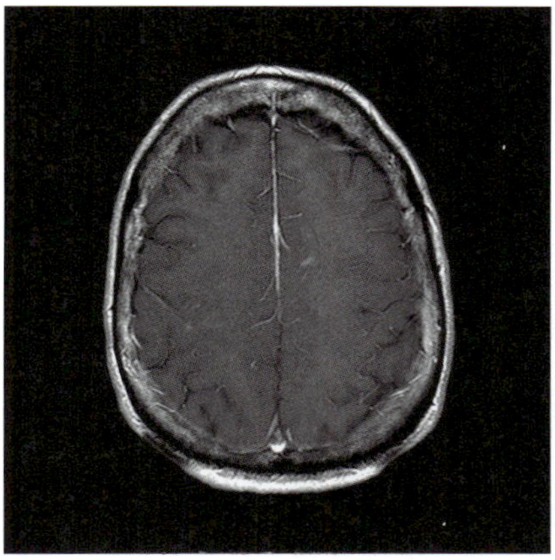
O

Figure 18.3. ***(continued)*** **M–O.** Axial T1-postcontrast: Minimal to mild enhancement associated with the multiple foci of parenchymal and leptomeningeal lesions.

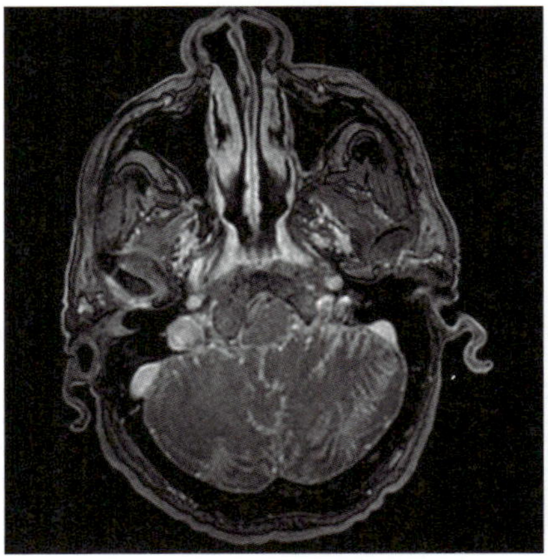
A

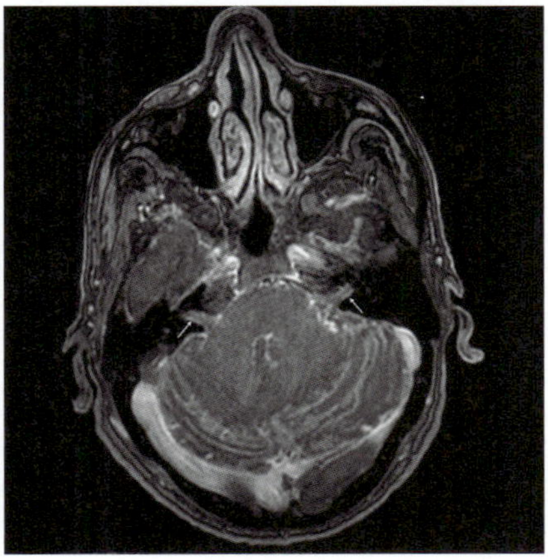
B

Figure 18.4. **Imaging of disseminated leptomeningeal esophageal cancer metastasis. A–C.** Axial T1-postcontrast: Diffuse leptomeningeal enhancement coating bilateral cerebellar hemispheres and superior vermis (arrows).

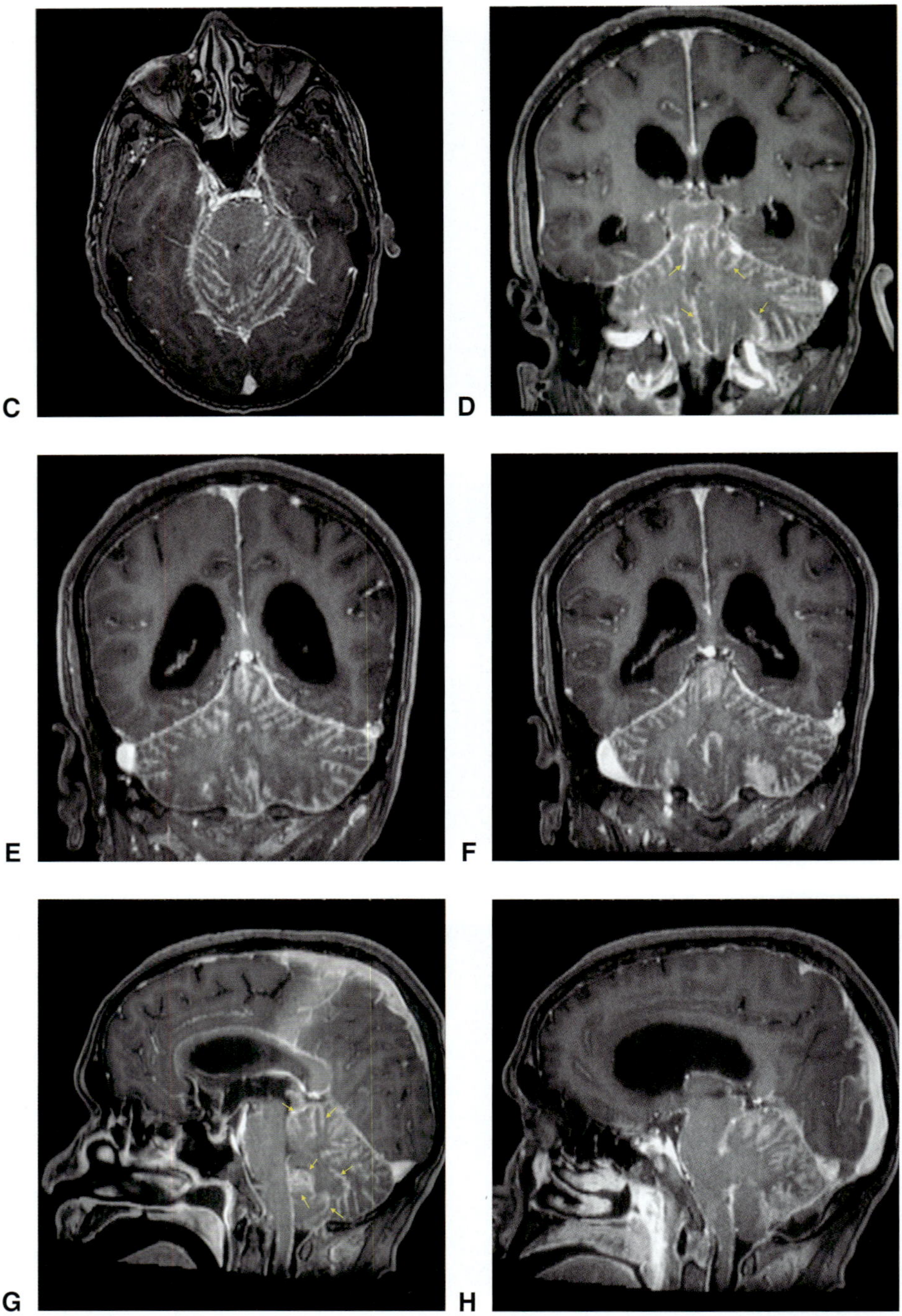

Figure 18.4. ***(continued)*** **D–F.** Coronal T1-postcontrast: Extensive enhancement along the cerebellar folia (arrows on **D**). **G–I.** Sagittal T1-postcontrast: Extensive leptome-ningeal disease (arrows on **G**) involving the entire posterior fossa.

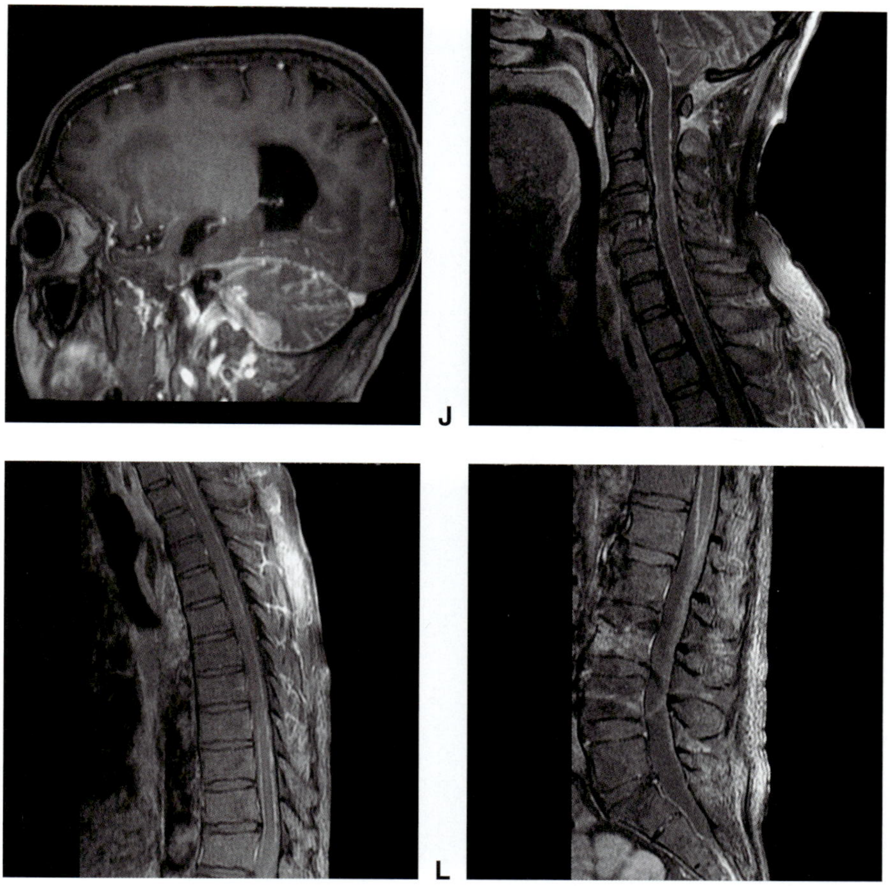

Figure 18.4. ***(continued)*** **J–L.** Sagittal T1-postcontrast-cervical (J), thoracic (K), and lumbar (L) spine: Diffuse leptomeningeal and pial enhancement coating the entire spinal cord.

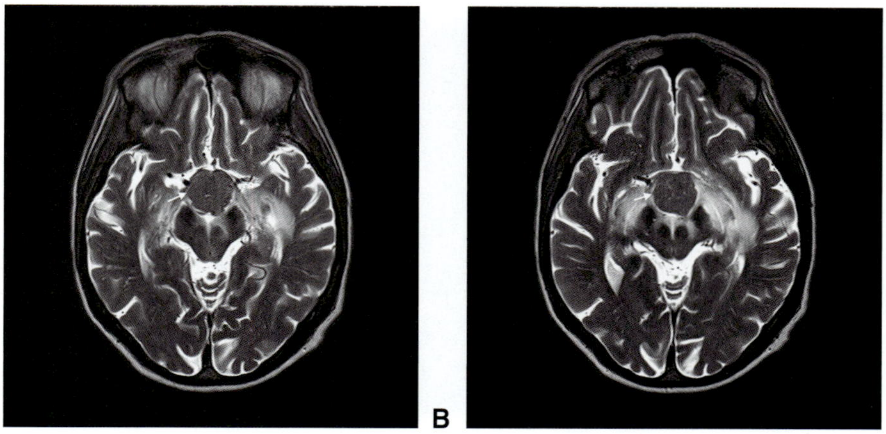

Figure 18.5. Imaging of pituitary metastasis from adenocarcinoma of unknown primary. A. Axial T2: Homogeneously hypointense suprasellar mass (white arrow) with surrounding edema. **B.** Axial T2: Homogeneously hypointense suprasellar mass (white arrow) with surrounding edema.

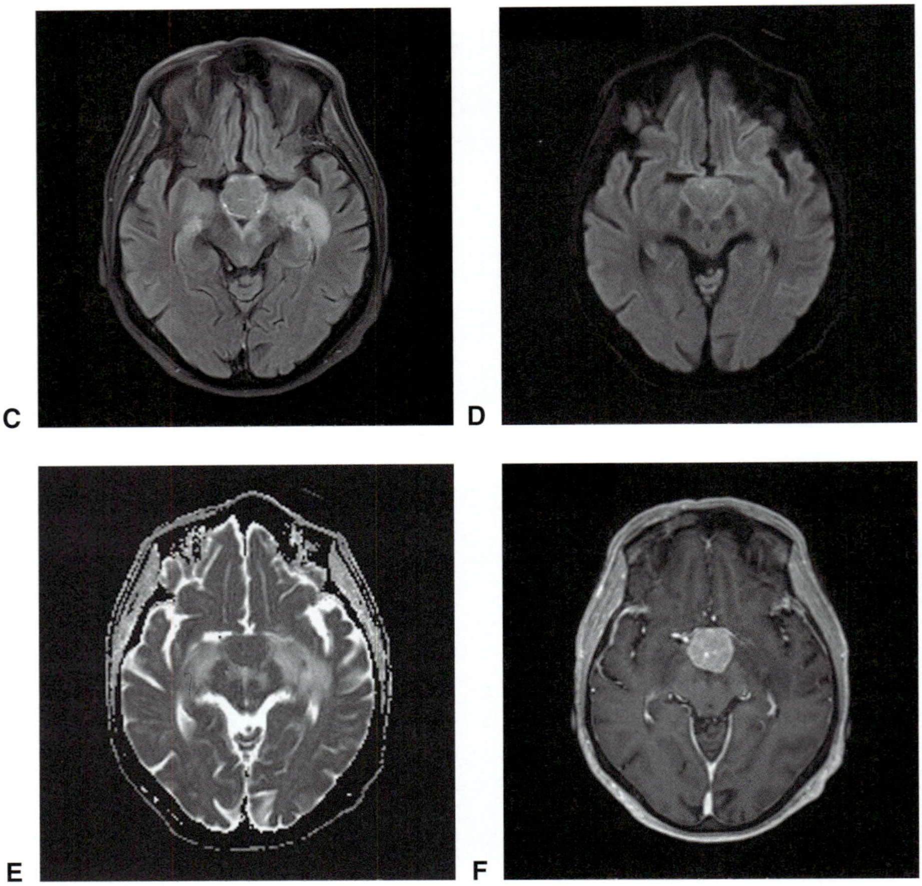

Figure 18.5. ***(continued)*** **C.** Axial FLAIR: Heterogeneously hypointense suprasellar mass. **D.** Axial DWI: Mild reduced diffusion within the mass. **E.** Axial ADC: Mild reduced diffusion within the mass. **F.** Axial T1-postcontrast: Avid enhancement within the mass.

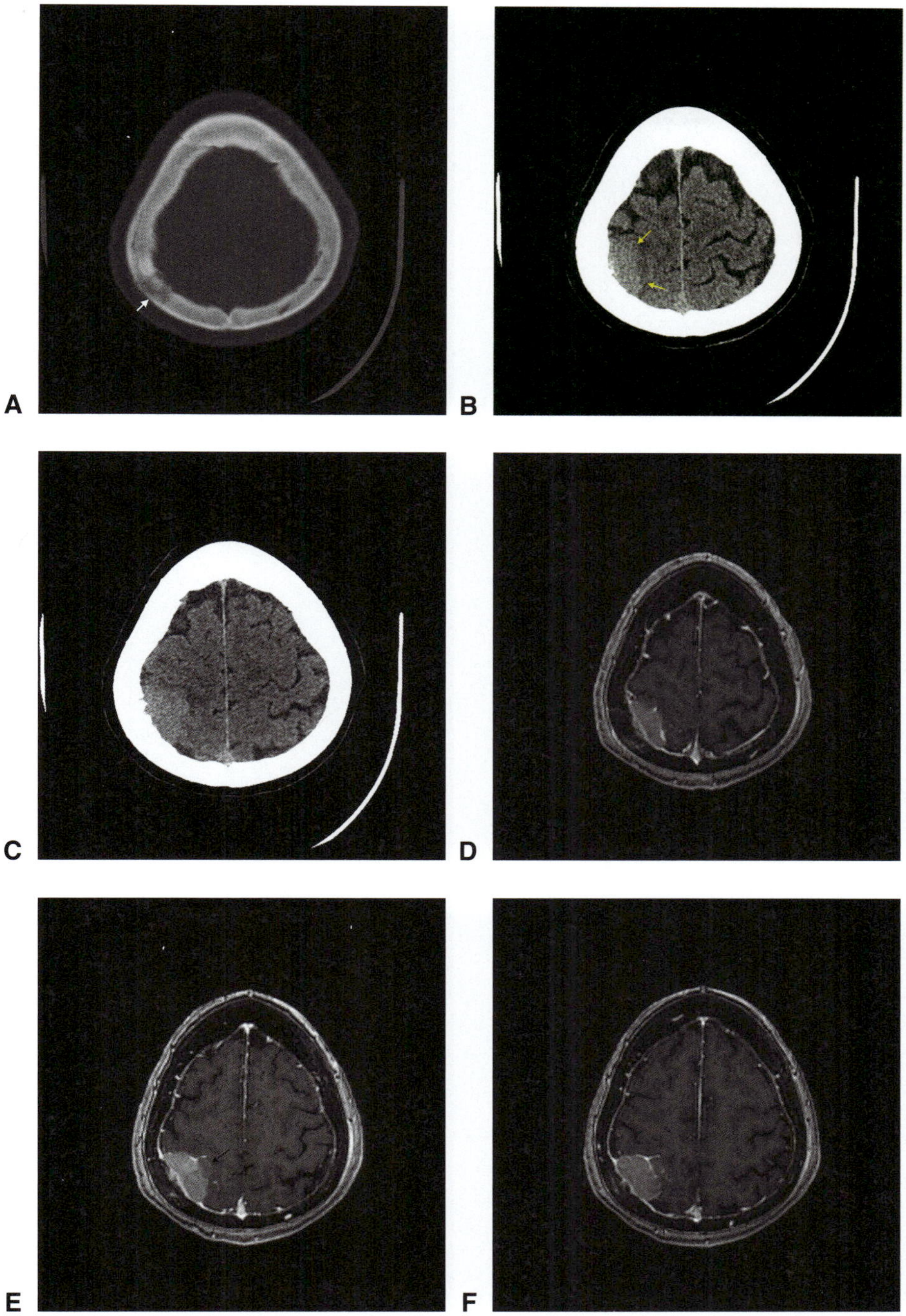

Figure 18.6. Imaging of skull and dural-based breast carcinoma metastasis. A–C. Axial CT unenhanced. Bone window (A) and brain window (B and C): Permeative pattern osseous destruction of right parietal skull (white arrow) and adjacent mildly hyperdense dural-based mass (yellow arrows). **D–F.** Axial T1-postcontrast: Heterogeneous but avid enhancement within the dural-based mass with minimal enhancement in the intraparenchymal component (black arrow).

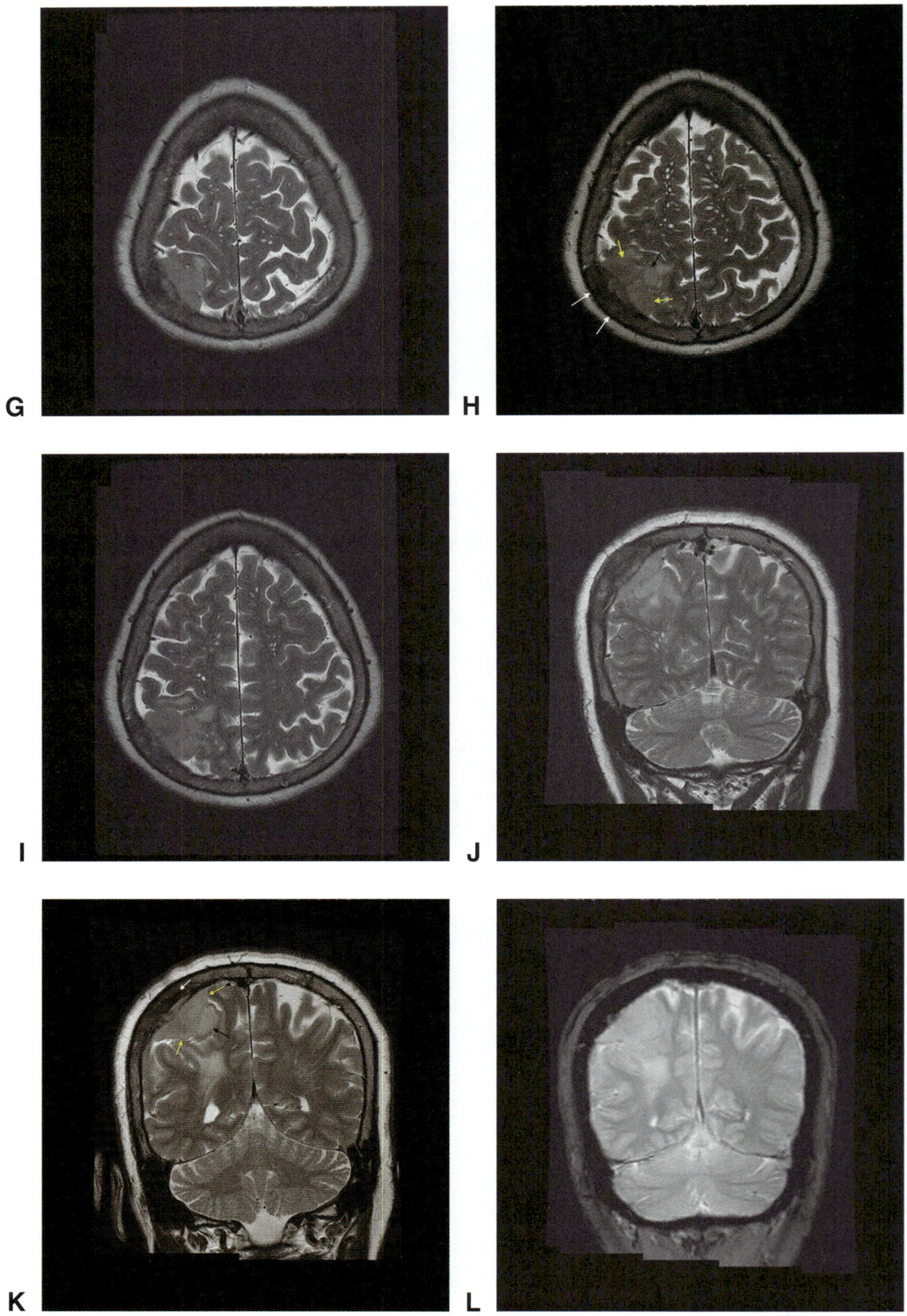

Figure 18.6. ***(continued)*** **G–I.** Axial T2: Heterogeneously hypointense skull lesion (white arrow) and mildly hypointense dural-based lesions (yellow arrows) and mildly hyperintense intraparenchymal component (black arrow). **J and K.** Coronal T2: Heterogeneously hypointense skull lesion (white arrow) and mildly hypointense dural-based lesions (yellow arrows) and mildly hyperintense intraparenchymal component (black arrow). **L.** Coronal gradient echo: no blood product is noted within the intracranial component of the mass.

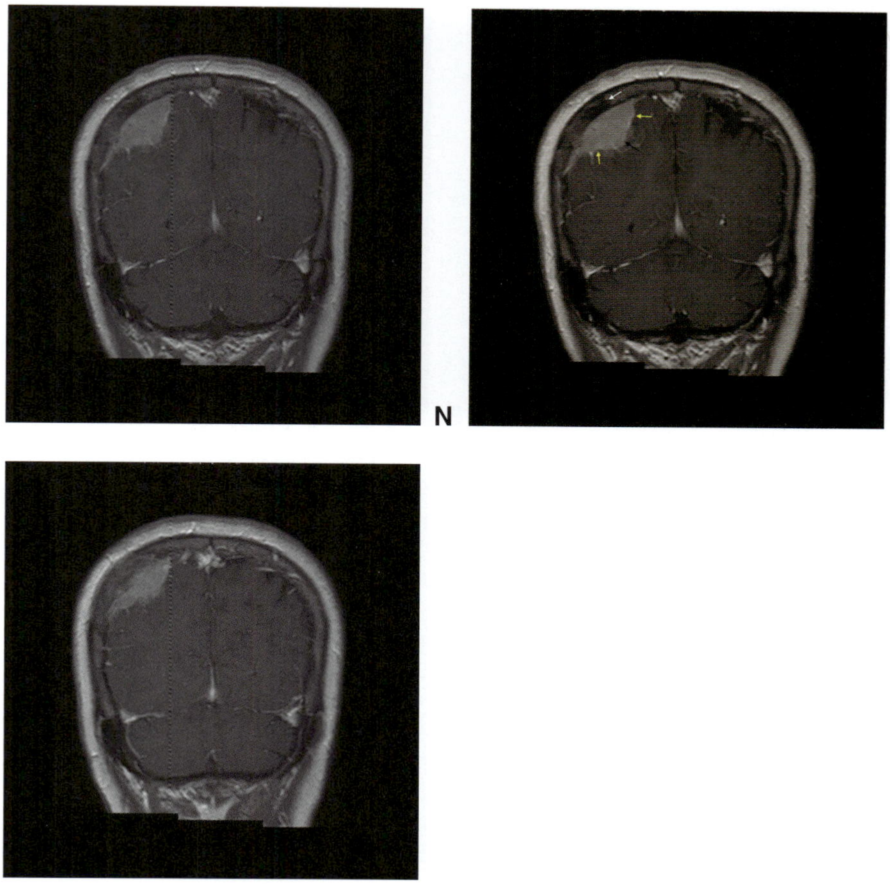

M N O

Figure 18.6. ***(continued)*** **M.** Coronal gradient echo: No blood products within the mass. **N and O.** Coronal T1-postcontrast: Heterogeneous but avidly enhancing dubbral-based lesion (yellow arrows), mildly enhancing intraparenchymal component (black arrow), and minimally enhancing skull lesion (white arrow).

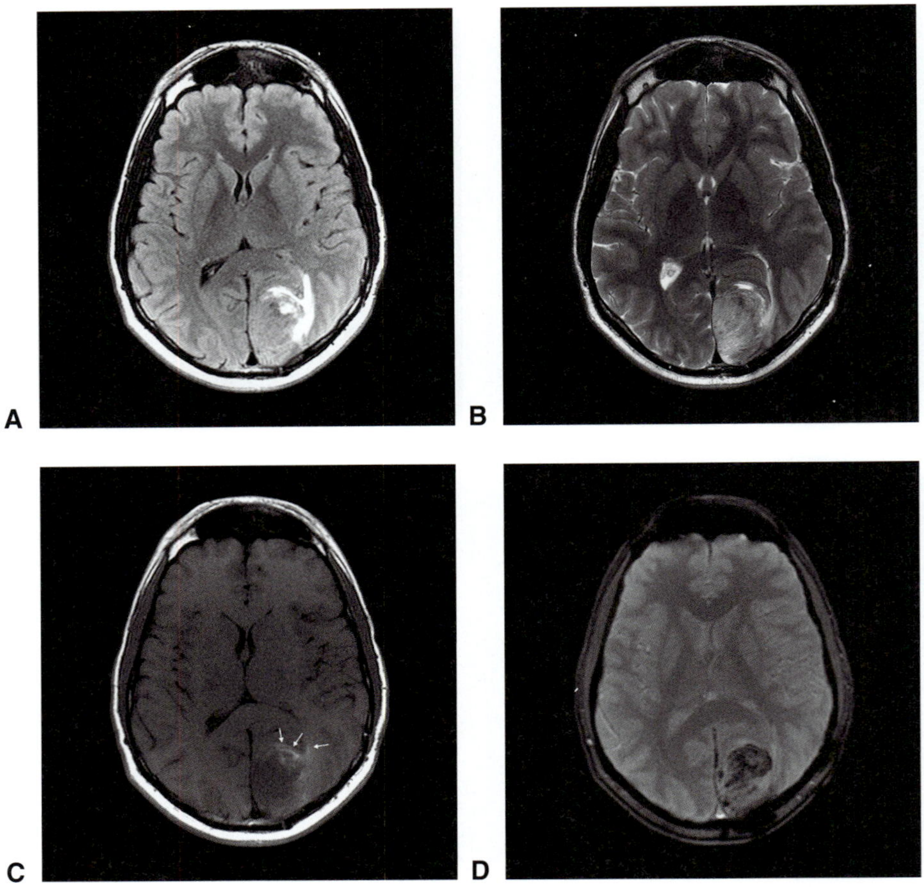

Figure 18.7. Imaging of dural and parenchymal testicular germ cell metastasis. **A.** Axial FLAIR: Heterogeneous hypointense left occipital dural and parenchymal mass with moderate surrounding vasogenic edema. **B.** Axial T2: Heterogeneous hyperintense left occipital dural and parenchymal mass with moderate surrounding vasogenic edema. **C.** Axial T1-precontrast: Heterogeneous hypointense left occipital dural component and wispy areas of T1 shortening in the deeper parenchymal component (white arrows). **D.** Axial SWI: Prominent blood products within the mass.

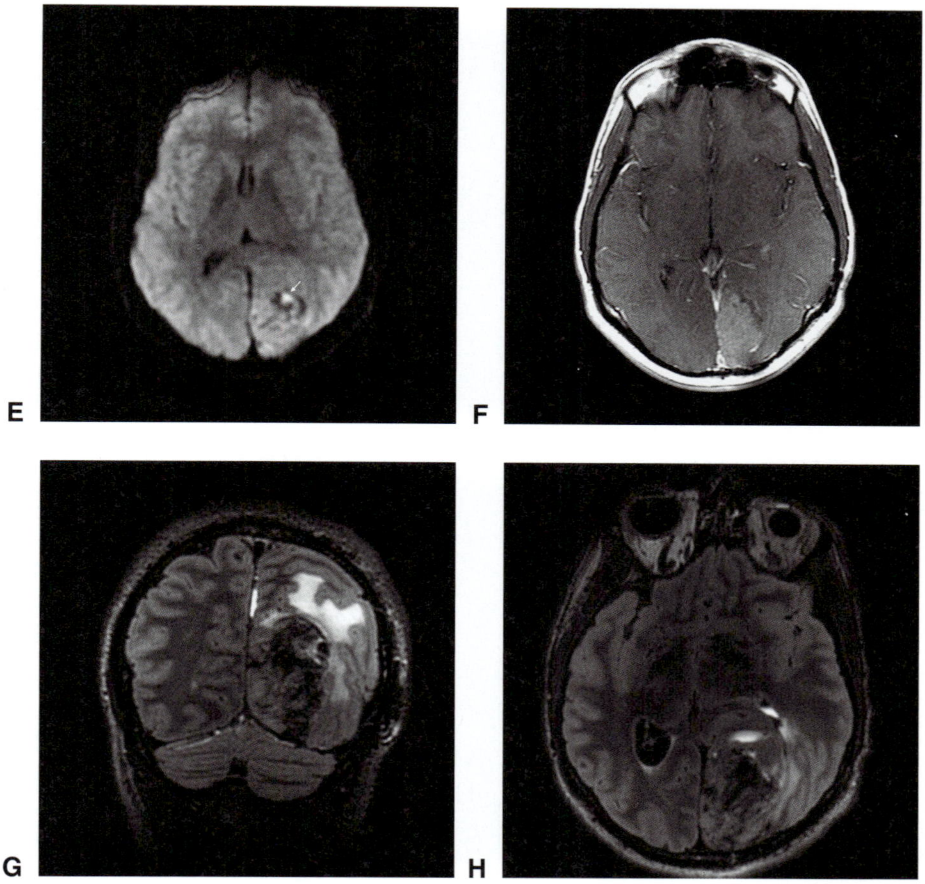

Figure 18.7. ***(continued)*** **E.** Axial DWI: Small nodular area of reduced diffusion in the deeper parenchymal component (white arrow). **F.** Axial T1-postcontrast: Mild homogeneous enhancement within the mass. **G–L.** Imaging obtained 10 days later. **G.** Coronal FLAIR: Marked interval increase in tumor size due to intratumoral hemorrhage. **H.** Axial FLAIR: Marked interval increase in tumor size due to intratumoral hemorrhage.

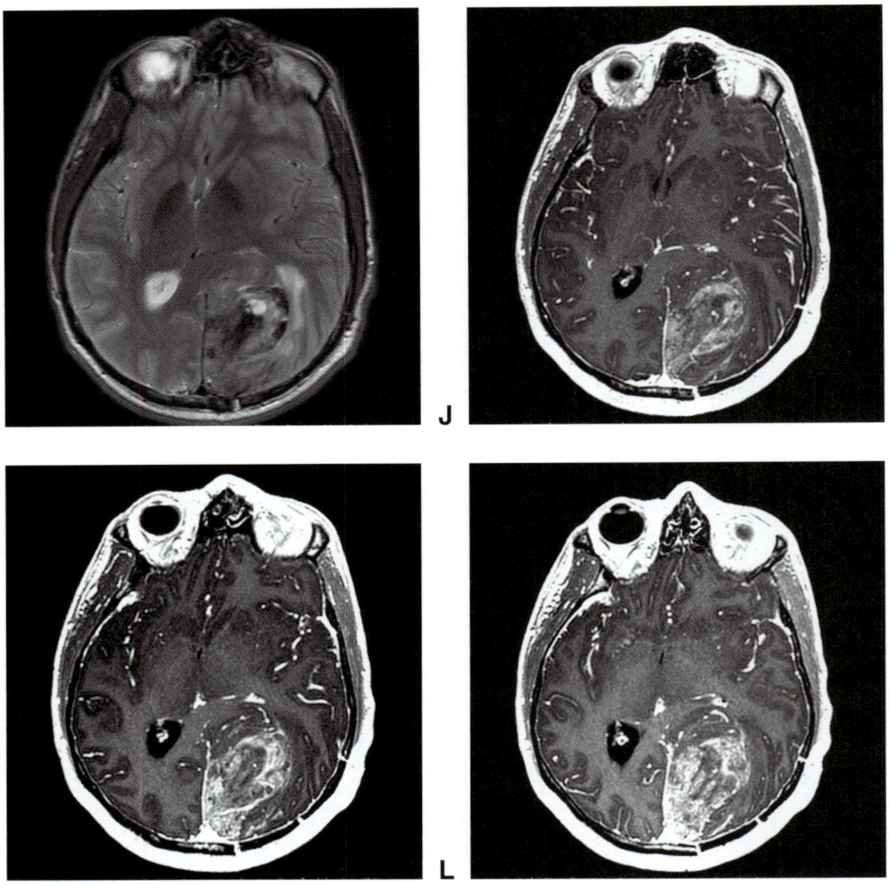

I J K L

Figure 18.7. ***(continued)*** **I.** Axial FLAIR: Marked interval increase in tumor size due to intratumoral hemorrhage. **J–L.** Axial T1-postcontrast: Heterogeneous enhancement within the hemorrhagic mass.

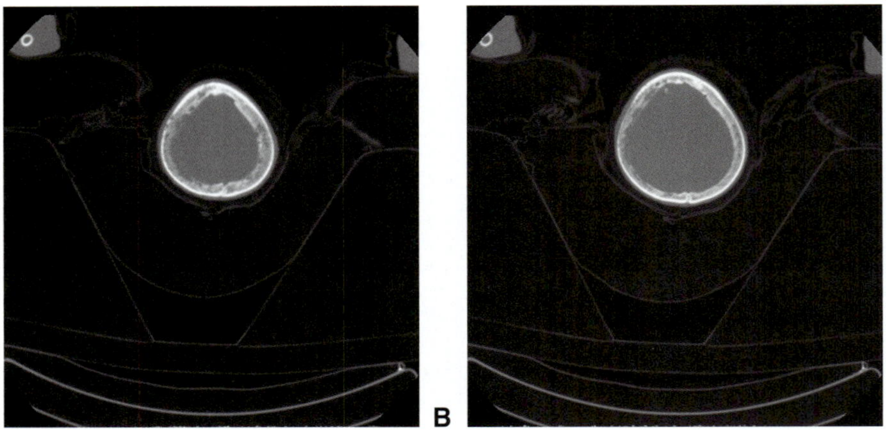

A B

Figure 18.8. Imaging of osseous skull metastases from gastric adenocarcinoma. A–C. Axial CT unenhanced, bone window: Diffuse permeative lytic destruction of the bilateral, right greater than left, frontal and parietal skull.

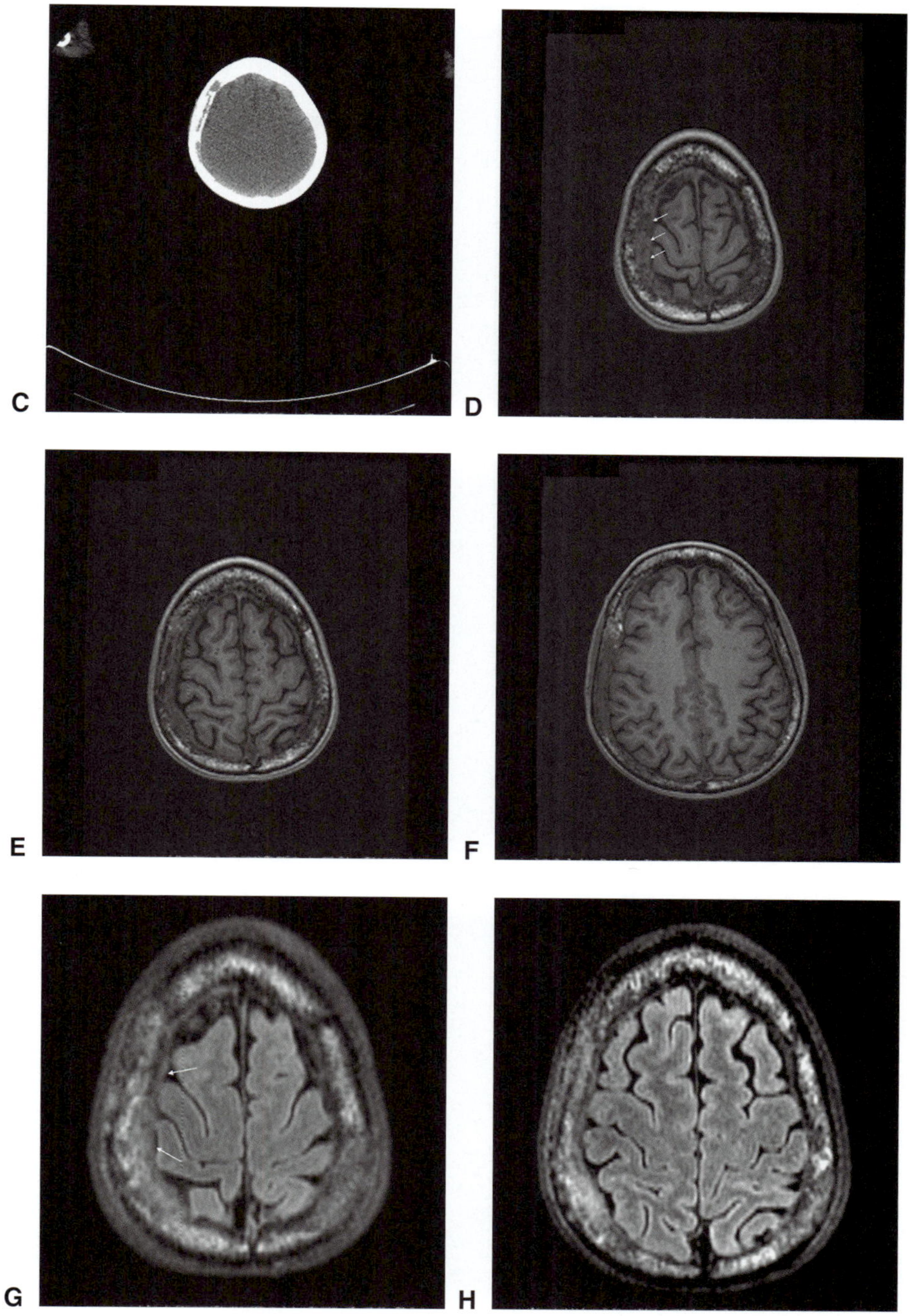

Figure 18.8. ***(continued)*** **D–F.** Axial T1-precontrast: Heterogeneous marrow replacement of involved skull with violation of inner table on the right with intracranial extension (white arrows). **G–I.** Axial FLAIR: Heterogeneous marrow replacement of involved skull with violation of inner table on the right with intracranial extension.

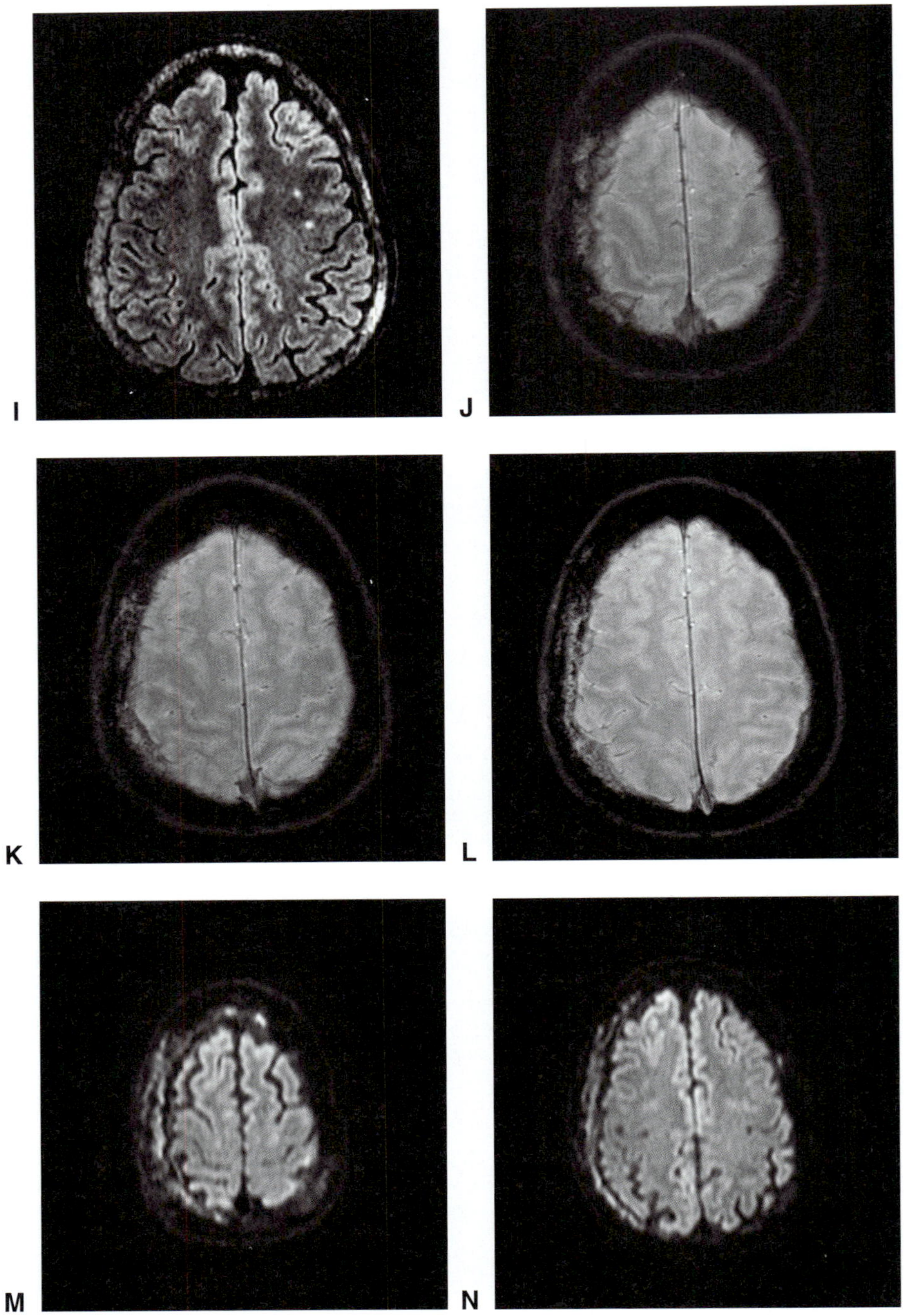

Figure 18.8. *(continued)* **J–L.** Axial SWI: Heterogeneous marrow replacement of involved skull with violation of inner table on the right with intracranial extension. **M–O.** Axial DWI: Heterogeneous marrow replacement of involved skull with violation of inner table on the right with intracranial extension.

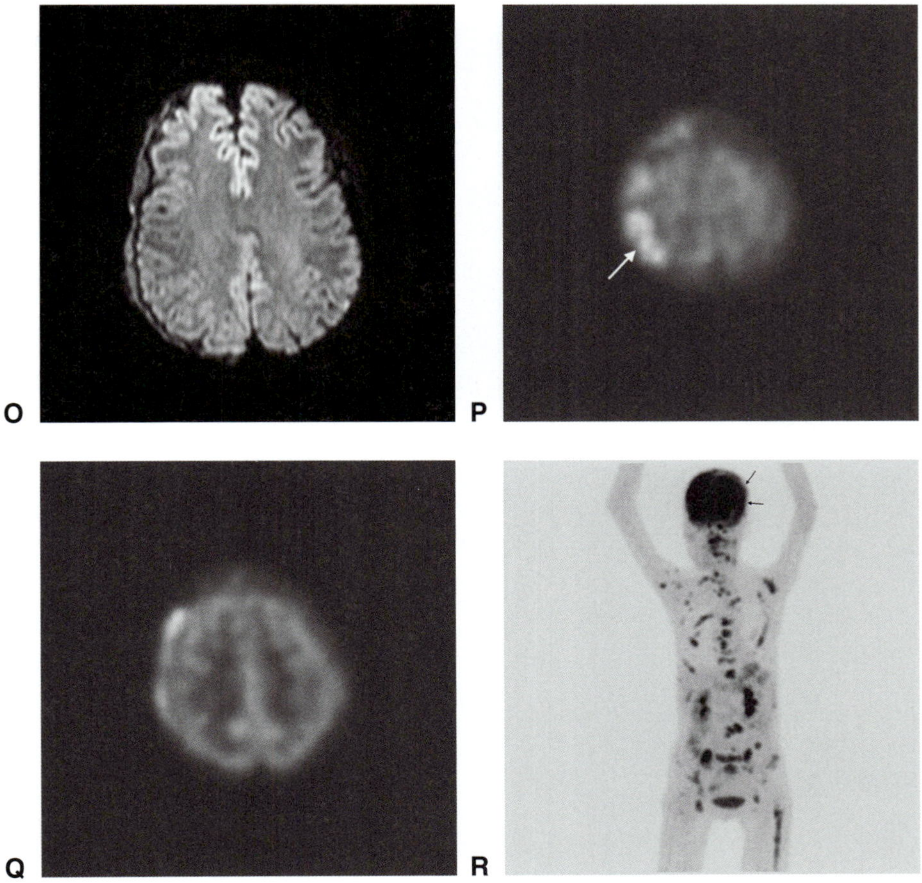

Figure 18.8. ***(continued)*** **P–R.** Fluorodeoxyglucose (FDG) PET: Hypermetabolic FDG uptake primarily within the right-sided skull lesion.

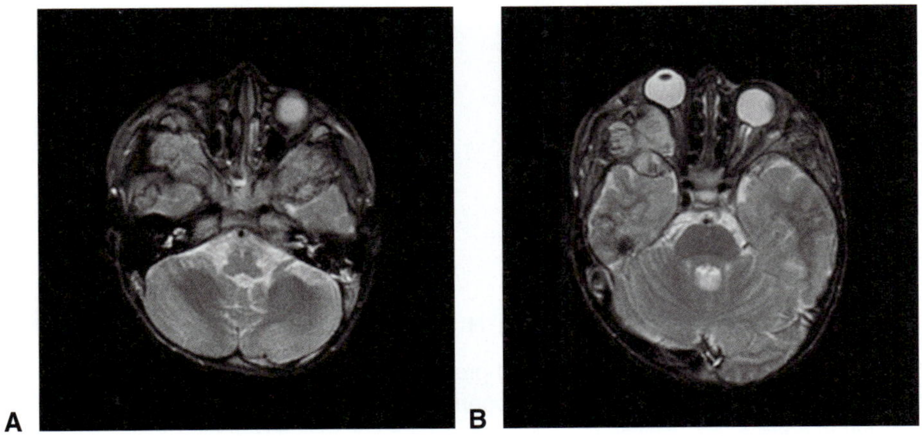

Figure 18.9. **Imaging of neuroblastoma metastases. A–C.** Axial T2: Multiple foci of bulky destructive osseous and extra-osseous heterogeneously hyperintense masses in bilateral sphenoid ridge and frontal skull, right greater than left, with intra-orbital extension on the right.

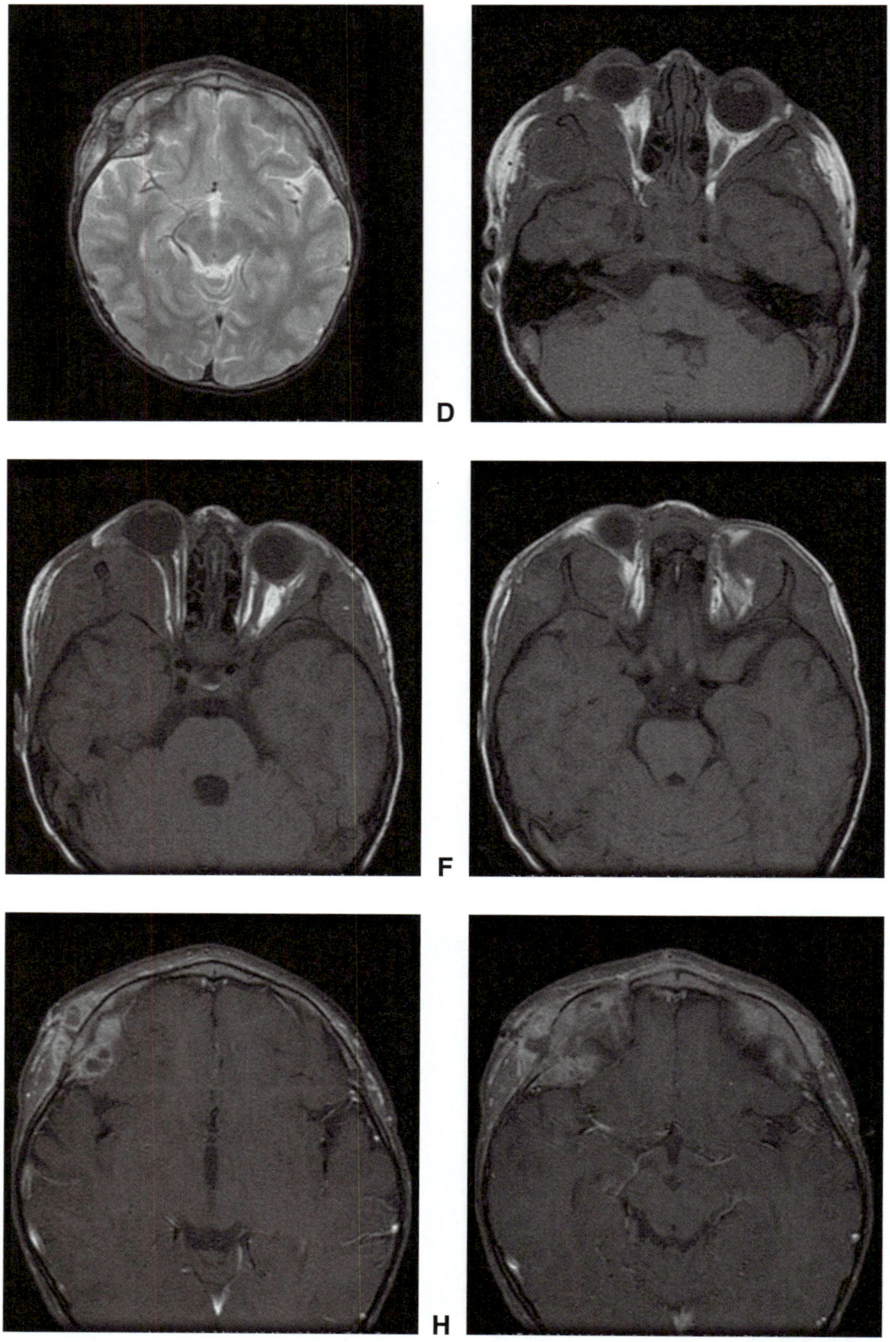

C D E F G H

Figure 18.9. ***(continued)*** **D–F.** Axial T1-precontrast: Multiple foci of bulky destructive osseous and extra-osseous heterogeneously hypointense masses in bilateral sphenoid ridge and frontal skull, right greater than left, with intraorbital extension on the right. **G–L.** Axial T1-postcontrast: Heterogeneous and avid enhancement of the multiple foci of bulky destructive osseous and extra-osseous masses.

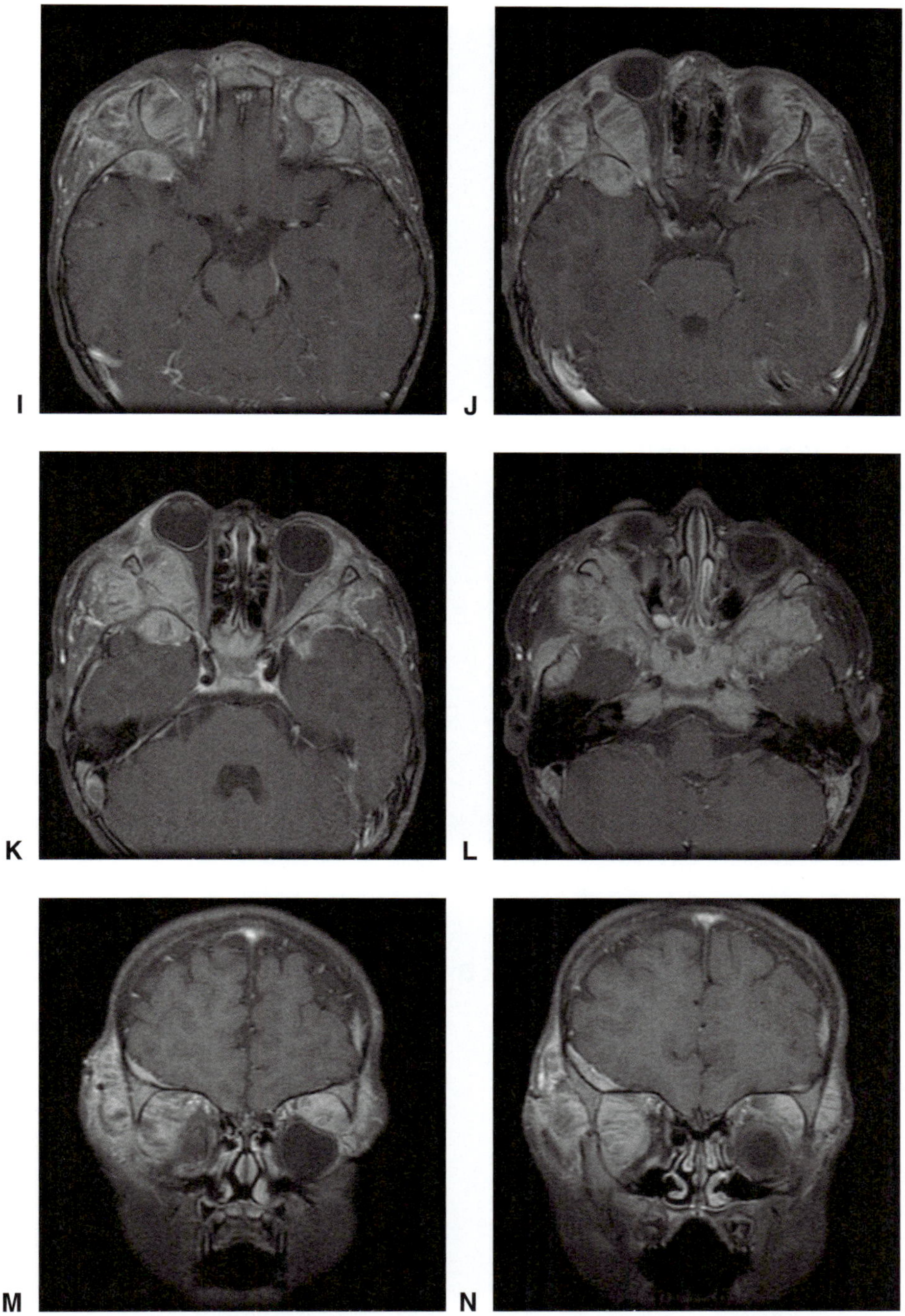

Figure 18.9. ***(continued)*** **M–O.** Coronal T1-postcontrast: Heterogeneous and avid enhancement of the multiple foci of bulky destructive osseous and extra-osseous masses.

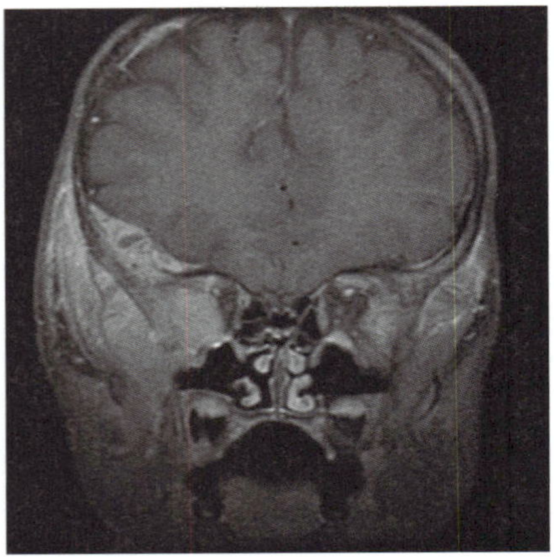

O

Figure 18.9. ***(continued)***

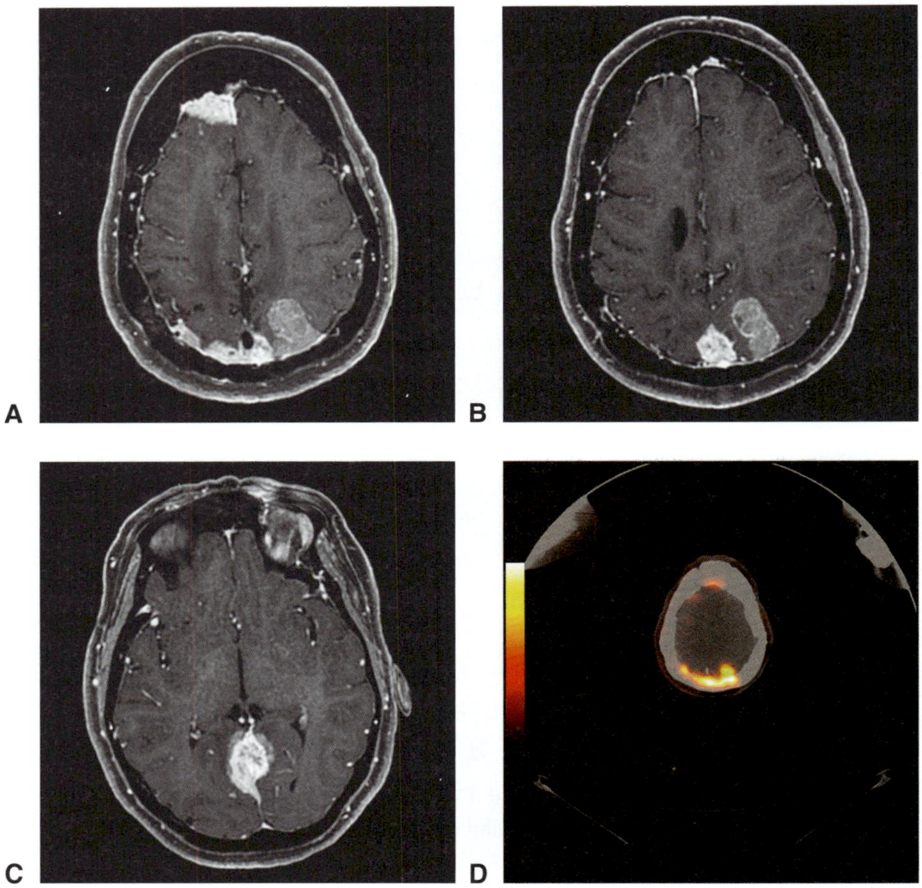

Figure 18.10. Imaging of meningioma metastasis to liver. A–C. Axial T1-post-contrast: Multiple meningiomas with avid enhancement. **D–F.** Axial positron emission tomography (PET)/computed tomography (CT), 68Ga-dotatate (DOTA)-Octreotate: Avid somatostatin receptor-positive uptake within the meningiomas.

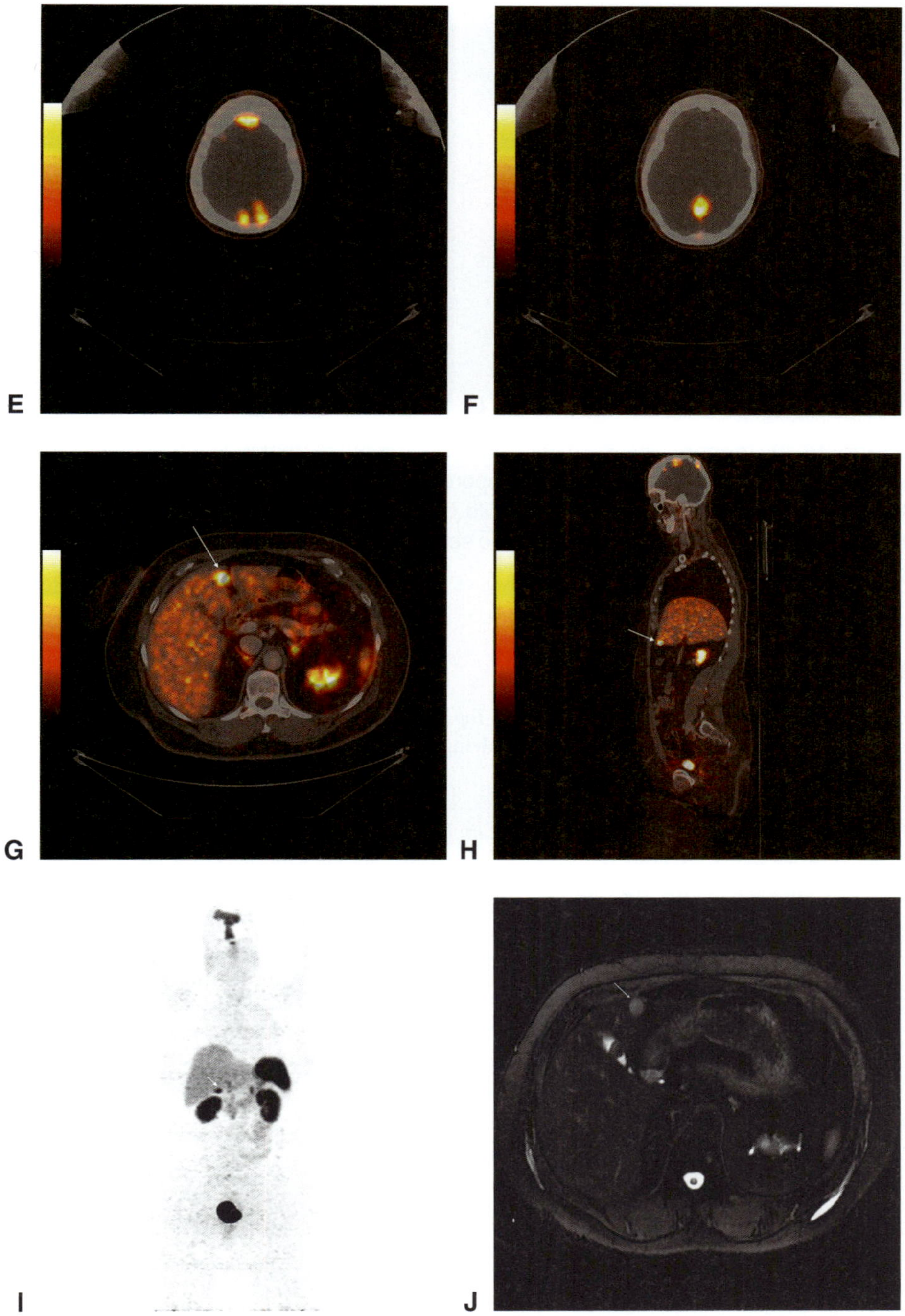

Figure 18.10. ***(continued)*** **G–I.** Axial PET–CT, 68Ga-DOTA-Octreotate: Abnormal somatostatin receptor-positive update in the hepatic segment IVb (arrows). **J.** Axial single-shot fast spin-echo (SSFSE) fat-saturated: Hyperintense meningioma metastasis in the hepatic segment IVb (white arrow) corresponding to the abnormality on the PET–CT.

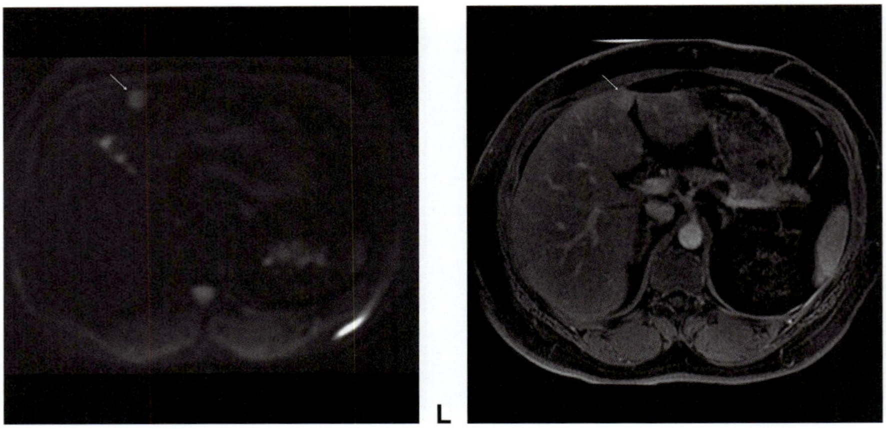

K L

Figure 18.10. ***(continued)*** **K.** Axial DWI: Hyperintense meningioma metastasis hepatic segment IVb (white arrow) corresponding to the abnormality on the PET–CT. **L.** Axial T1-postcontrast fat-saturated: Mild but homogeneous enhancement within the meningioma metastasis in the hepatic segment IVb (white arrow) corresponding to the abnormality on the PET-CT.

Bibliography

Cha S. Perfusion MR imaging of brain tumors. *Top Magn Reson Imaging*. 2004;15:279–289.

Fecci PE, Champion CD, Hoj J, et al. The evolving modern management of brain metastasis. *Clin Cancer Res*. 2019;25:6570–6580.

Fink KR, Fink JR. Imaging of brain metastases. *Surg Neurol Int*. 2013;4:209–219.

Pope WB. Brain metastases: neuroimaging. *Clin Neurol*. 2018;149:89–112.

Villanueva-Meyer JE, Magill ST, Lee JC, Umetsu SE, Flavell RR. Detection of metastatic meningioma to the liver using 68Ga-DOTA-Octreotate PET/CT. *Clin Nucl Med*. 2018;43:338–340.

19

Genetic Tumor Syndromes

Overview

	Inheritance	Mutation	Common tumors	Other features
Neurofibromatosis type 1	Autosomal dominant	*NF1* gene on chromosome 17	Neurofibromas Optic gliomas Pheochromocytomas	Lisch nodules
Neurofibromatosis type 2	Autosomal dominant	*NF2* gene on chromosome 22	Vestibular schwannomas Meningioma Ependymoma	Cataracts
Tuberous sclerosis complex	Autosomal dominant	*TSC1* gene on chromosome 9 *TSC2* gene on chromosome 16	Subependymal giant cell astrocytoma Cardiac rhabdomyoma Retinal angiomyolipoma	Infantile spasms Intellectual disability
von Hippel–Lindau Disease	Autosomal dominant	*VHL* gene on chromosome 3	Retinal and CNS hemangioblastoma Renal cell carcinomas Pheochromocytoma	Renal cyst Pancreatic cysts
Li–Fraumeni syndrome	Autosomal dominant	*TP53* gene on chromosome 17	Diffuse astrocytoma Medulloblastoma Choroid plexus carcinoma Breast cancer Osteosarcoma Soft tissue sarcoma Adrenocortical carcinoma Leukemia	-

CNS: central nervous system.

Neurofibromatosis Type 1

Definition: Neurofibromatosis (NF) type 1 is one of the most common inherited disorders and the most common neurocutaneous syndrome. NF1, also known as von Recklinghausen disease, is an autosomal dominant disorder due to genetic mutations of the *NF1* gene on chromosome 17q11.2 and characterized by neurofibromas, multiple café-au-lait spots, axillary and inguinal freckling, optic gliomas, osseous lesions, and iris hamartomas. Slightly increased risk for malignant nerve sheath tumor, gastrointestinal stromal tumor, rhabdomyosarcoma, juvenile chronic myeloid leukemia, duodenal carcinoids, medullary thyroid carcinomas, and pheochromocytoma has been noticed.

Epidemiology: Prevalence of NF1 is approximately 1 in 3,000–3,500 births, regardless of ethnic and racial background, and about 50% of the cases are familial; the remaining cases are de novo mutations occurring primarily in paternally derived chromosomes.

Molecular and genetic profile: Mutational inactivation of the *NF1* gene locus on chromosome 19q11.2 can be seen.

Clinical features and standard therapy: Multiple sites and organ systems may be involved in NF1, with the central and peripheral nervous system, the skin, the eyes, and the bones being the most common sites. Café-au-lait spots are generally the heralding feature of NF1 and bring the patient for medical examination. The first step in management of patients with NF1 is genetic counseling. It is essential to examine parents to determine whether they are affected. Regular medical appointments to a multidisciplinary clinic with annual examinations are necessary. Imaging studies are indicated only when patients are symptomatic. Surgery is currently the only treatment option for most NF1 lesions, and chemotherapy is helpful with optic pathway gliomas and higher grade astrocytomas. No effective chemotherapy is available to treat plexiform neurofibromas.

Imaging

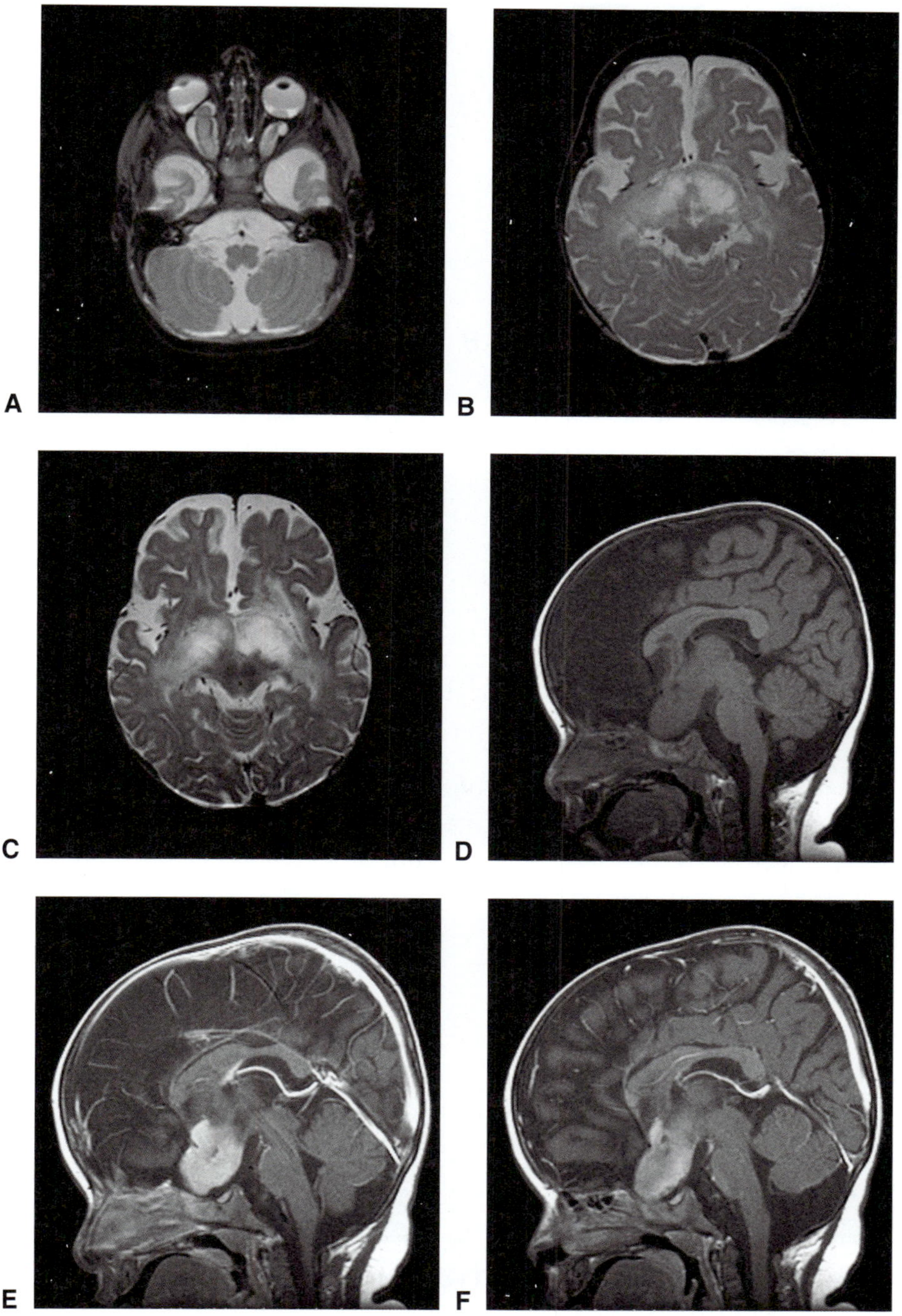

Figure 19.1. Imaging of optic glioma, NF type 1. A–C. Axial T2: Expansile mass involving bilateral optic nerves from intraorbital to optic tracks. **D.** Sagittal T1-precontrast: Isointense mass centered in the optic chiasm. **E and F.** Sagittal T1-postcontrast: Heterogeneous but avid enhancement within the mass.

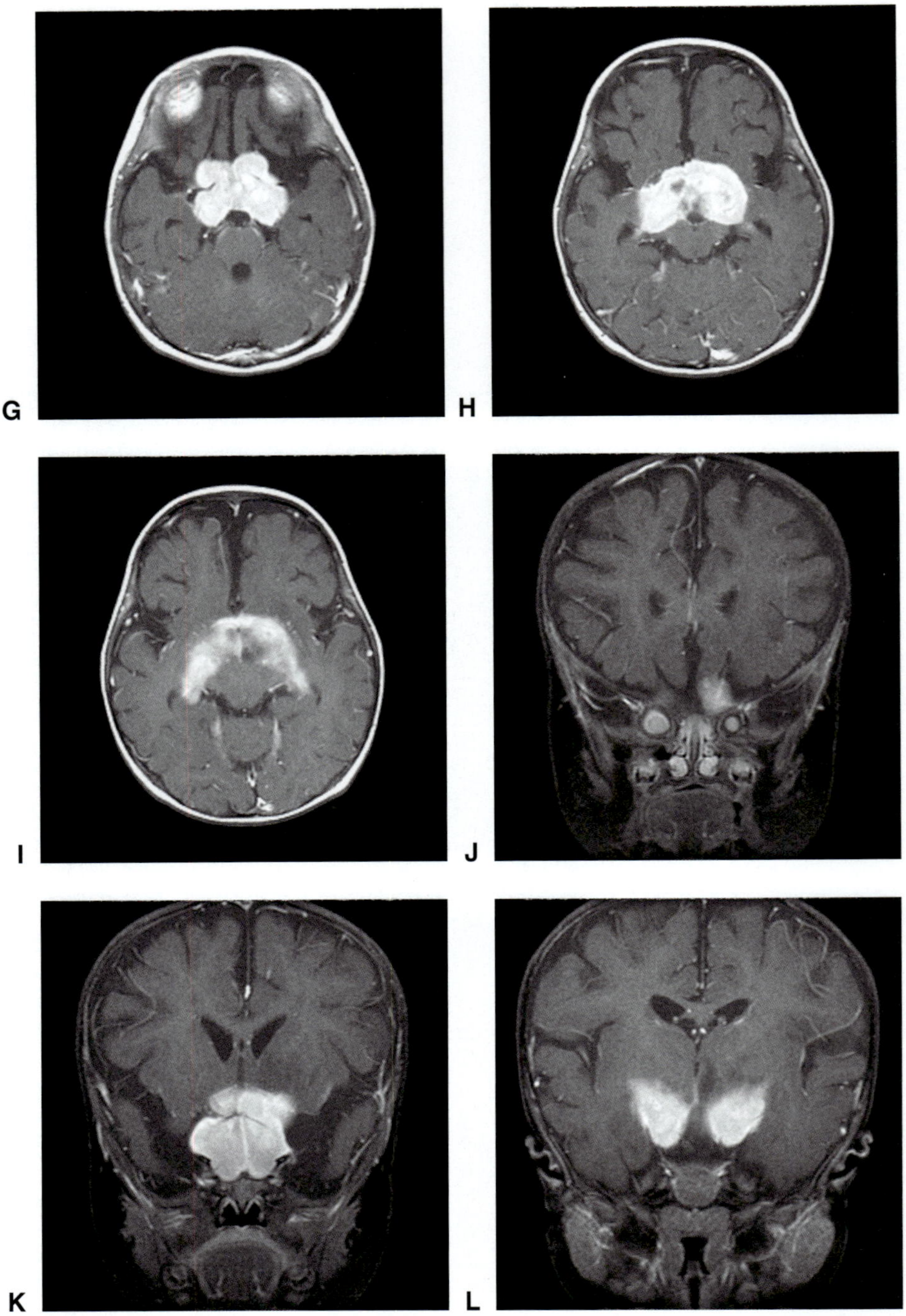

Figure 19.1. ***(continued)*** **G–I.** Axial T1-postcontrast: Heterogeneous but avid enhancement within the mass. **J–L.** Coronal T1-postcontrast: Heterogeneous but avid enhancement within the mass.

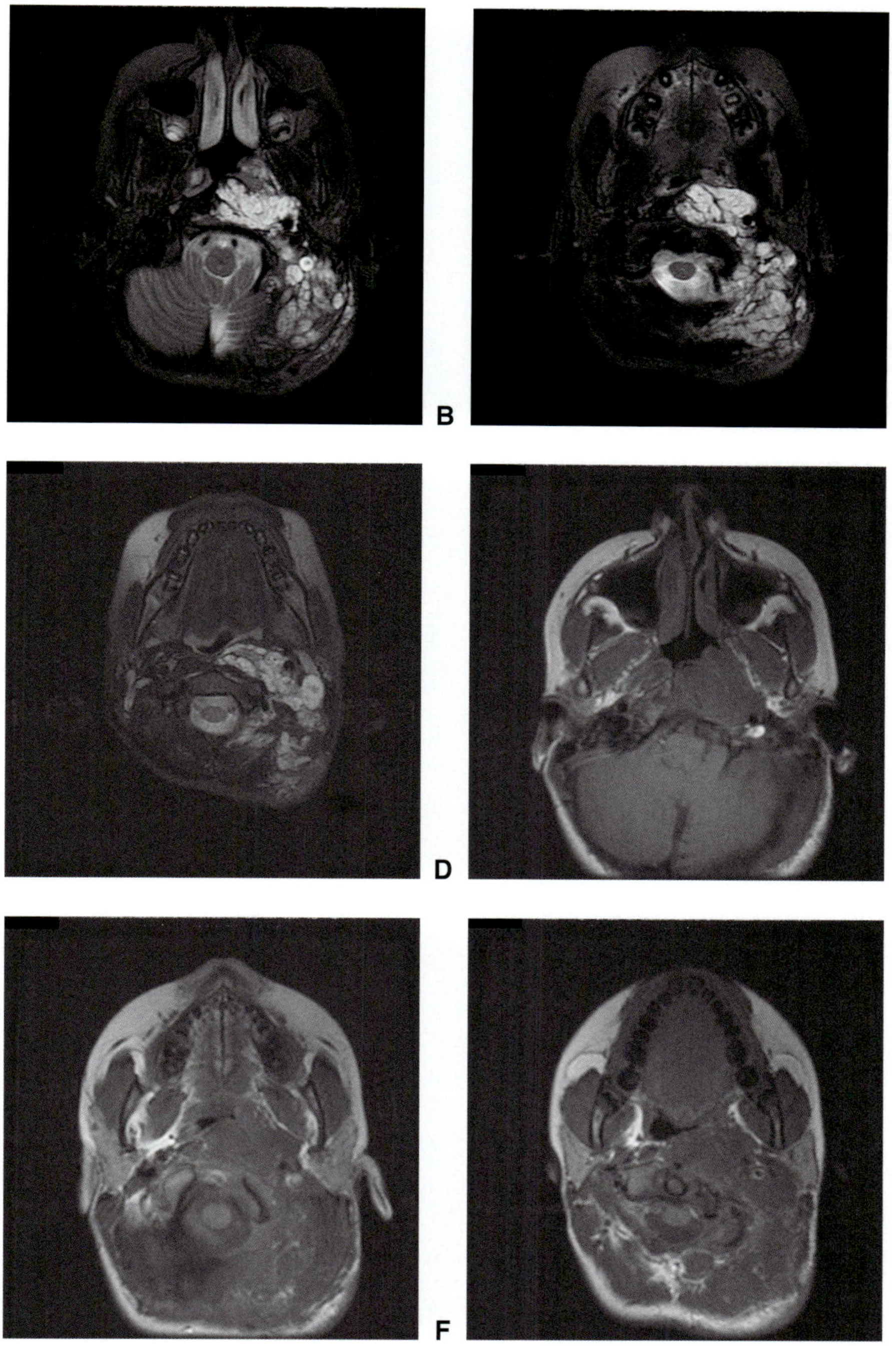

A B C D E F

Figure 19.2. Imaging of plexiform neurofibroma, NF type 1. A–C. Axial T2-fat-saturated: Heterogeneously hyperintense right parapharyngeal mass. **D–F.** Axial T1-pre-contrast: Hypointense mass.

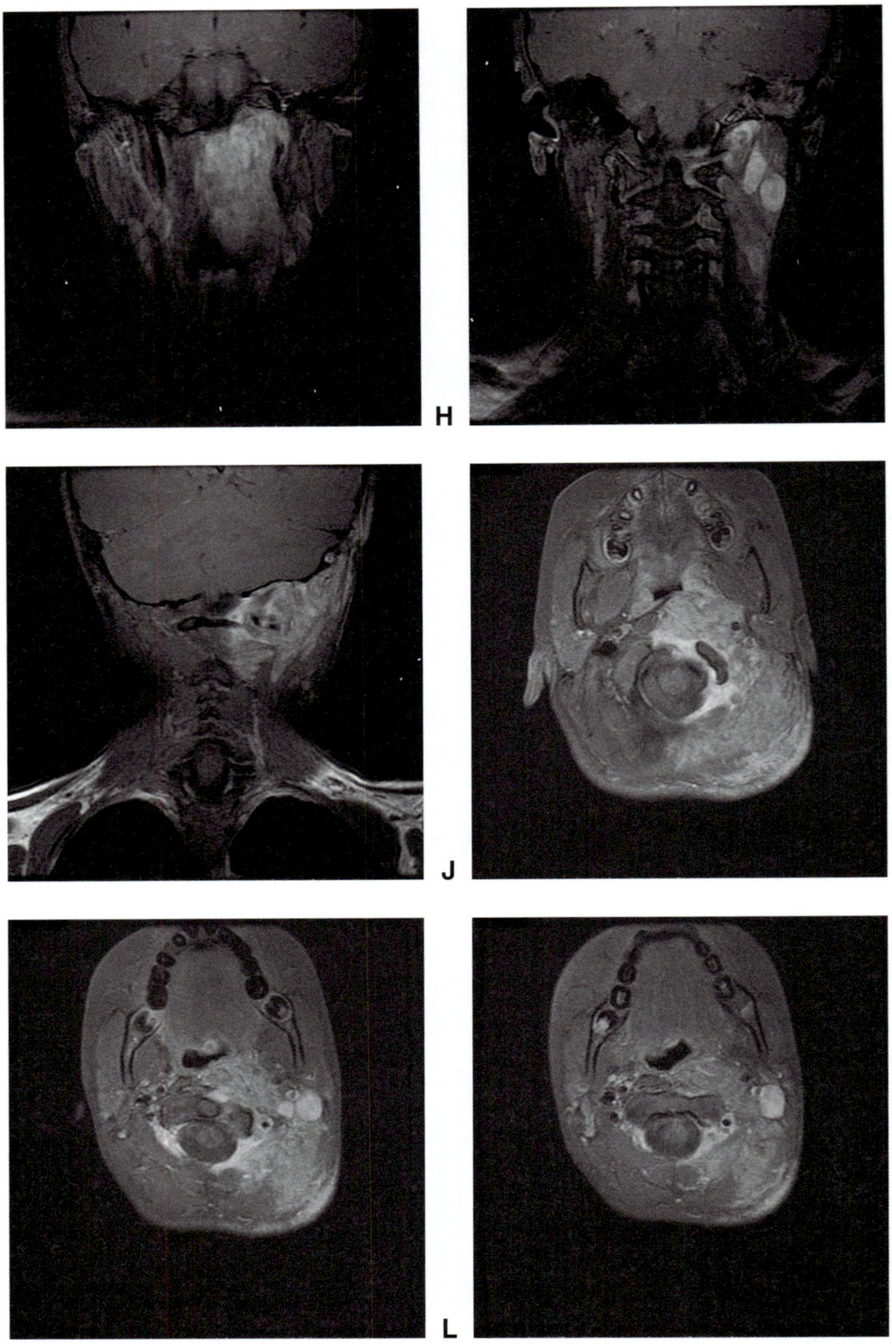

Figure 19.2. ***(continued)*** **G–I.** Coronal T1-postcontrast: Heterogeneous enhancement with distinct areas of nodularity. **J–L.** Axial T1-postcontrast: Heterogeneous enhancement with distinct areas of nodularity.

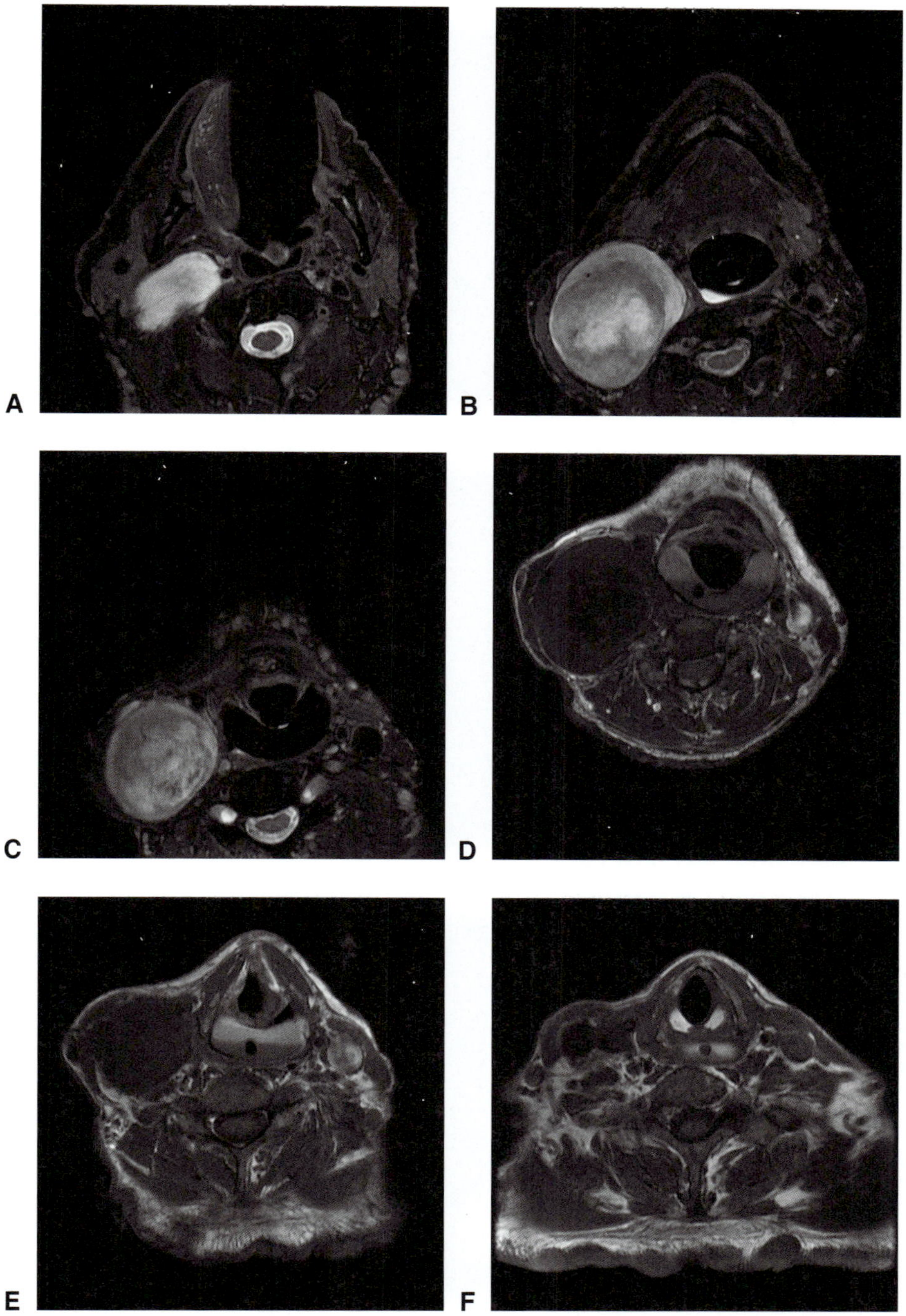

Figure 19.3. Imaging of malignant peripheral nerve sheath tumor, NF type 1. A–C. Axial T2-fat-saturated: Bulky hyperintense solid mass in the left prevertebral and lateral neck with multinodular architecture. **D–F.** Axial T1-precontrast: Hypointense mass. **G–I.** Coronal T1-postcontrast: Heterogeneous enhancement with intratumoral necrosis (yellow arrow).

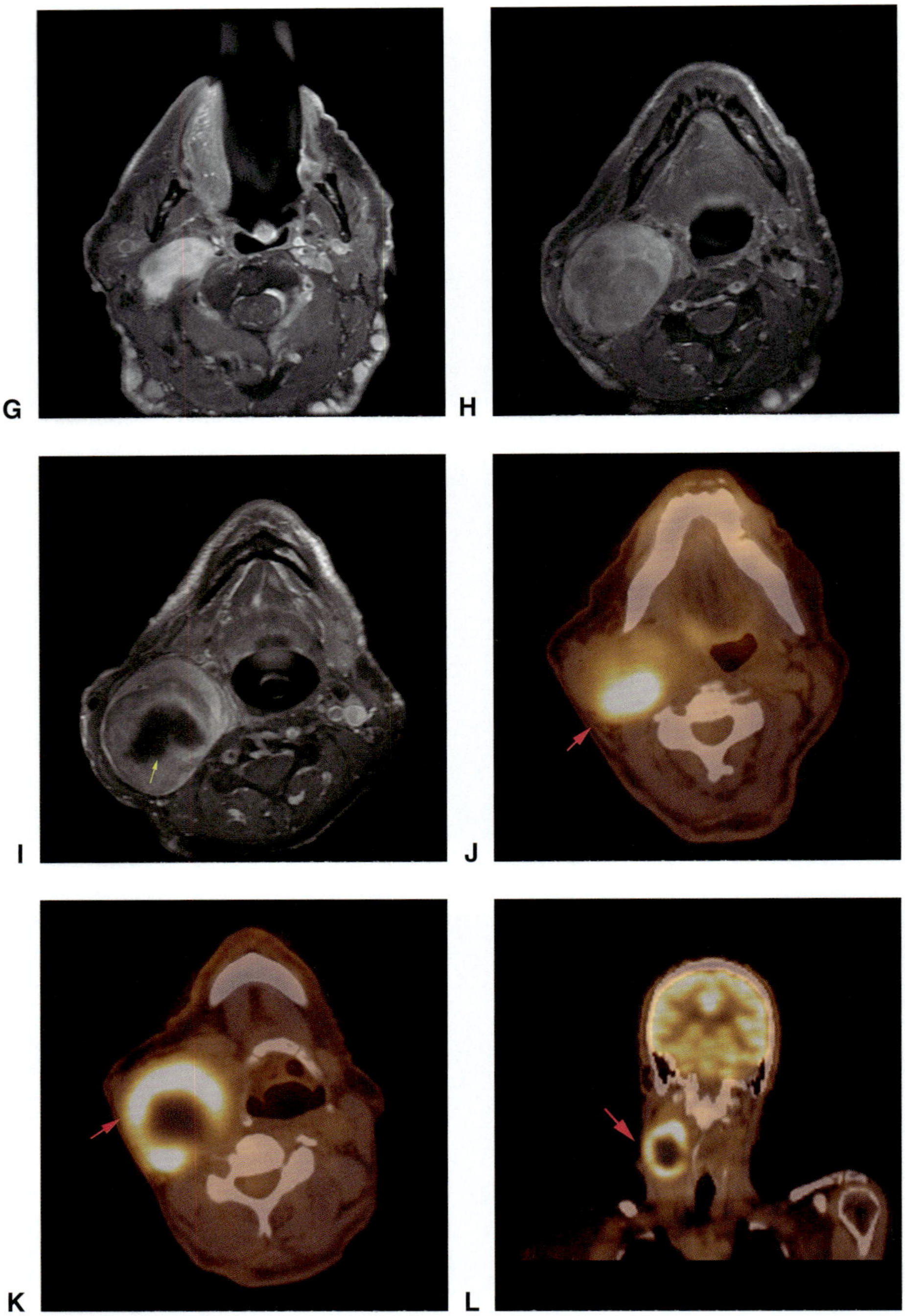

Figure 19.3. ***(continued)*** **J–L.** Fluorodeoxyglucose (FDG)-positron emission tomography (PET)-computed tomography (CT) (FDG-PET-CT): Marked hypermetabolism within the peripheral aspect (red arrows) of the mass except in the area of necrosis.

▶ Neurofibromatosis Type 2

Definition: Neurofibromatosis type 2 is a rare, autosomal dominant disorder caused by mutations of *NF2* gene on chromosome 22q12 and characterized by noncancerous neoplastic and dysplastic lesions that primarily affect the nervous system, with bilateral vestibular schwannomas as a diagnostic hallmark. Schwannomas can occur involving other cranial nerves, spinal and peripheral nerves, intracranial and spinal meningiomas and ependymomas, and a variety of nonneoplastic and dysplastic/hamartomatous lesions such as meningioangiomatosis, glial hamartomas, ocular abnormalities, and neuropathy.

Epidemiology: Prevalence is around 1 in 60,000.

Molecular and genetic profile: NF2 is inherited as an autosomal dominant trait in some patients or de novo mutation in the *NF2* gene, which is located in the long arm of chromosome number 22 (22q12.2). The *NF2* gene encodes for the protein known as merlin, which is found in the Schwann cells in the nervous system and acts as a tumor suppressor gene.

Clinical features and standard therapy: Signs and symptoms usually appear during adolescence or early in the second decade, with hearing loss, tinnitus, and balance problems being the most common. For those patients with bilateral vestibular schwannomas, a major goal of treatment is to preserve the hearing for as long as possible. Surgery is usually done in patients who have lost hearing, and radiation therapy can be done for any residual tumor. Recently, bevacizumab (Avastin), a humanized antivascular endothelial growth factor monoclonal antibody that interferes with blood vessel formation, has been shown to slow the growth of vestibular schwannomas and to partially restore hearing in some patients and holds promise that other drugs may be proven effective as well.

Imaging

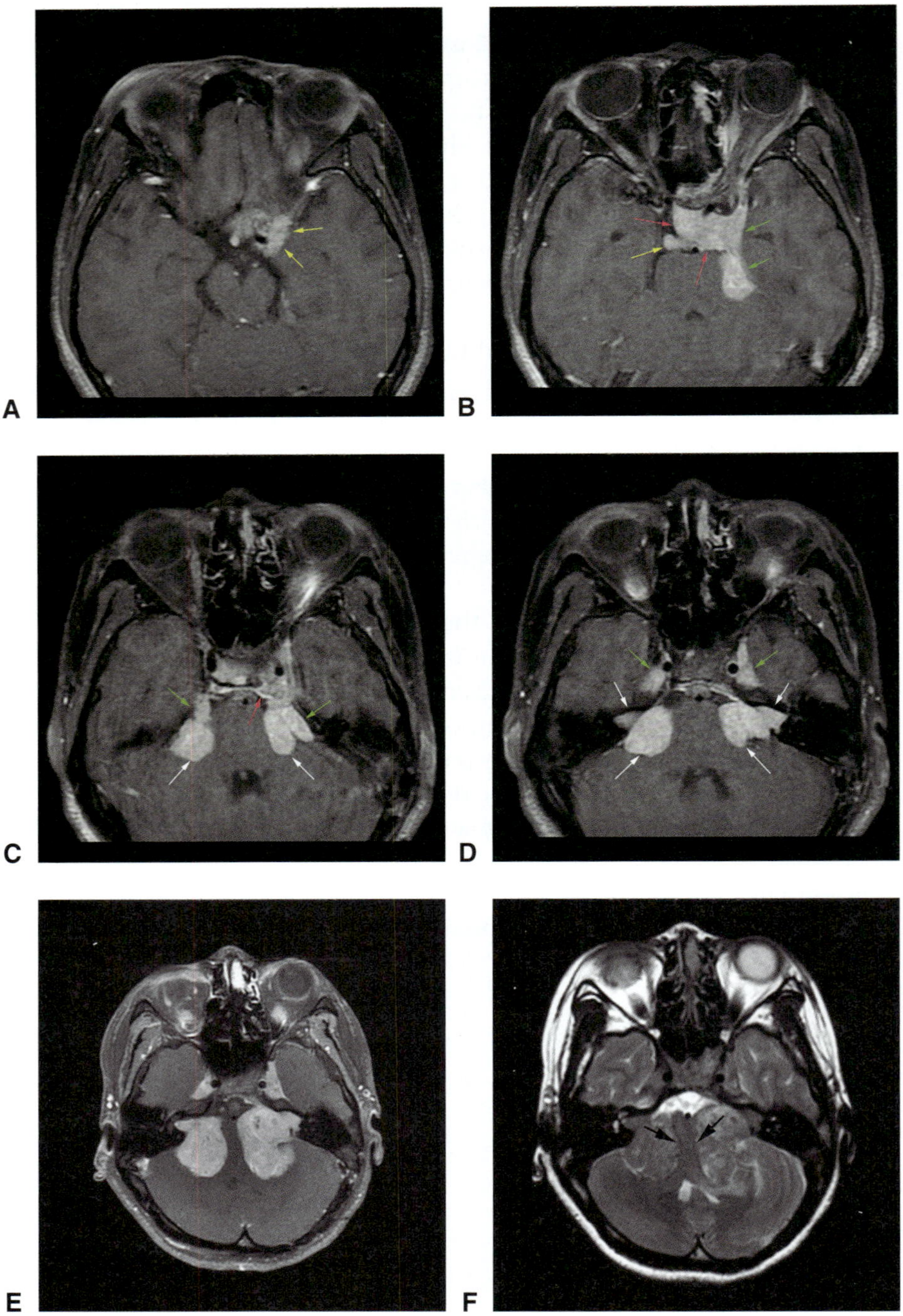
A B C D E F

Figure 19.4. Imaging of NF type 2, multiple schwannomas and meningiomas. **A–E.** Axial T1-postcontrast: Bilateral oculomotor schwannomas (yellow arrows), trigeminal schwannomas (green arrows), and bilateral vestibular schwannomas (white arrows), and cavernous sinus meningioma (red arrows). **F.** Axial T2: Mixed intensity bilateral vestibular schwannomas causing marked mass effect on pons (black arrows).

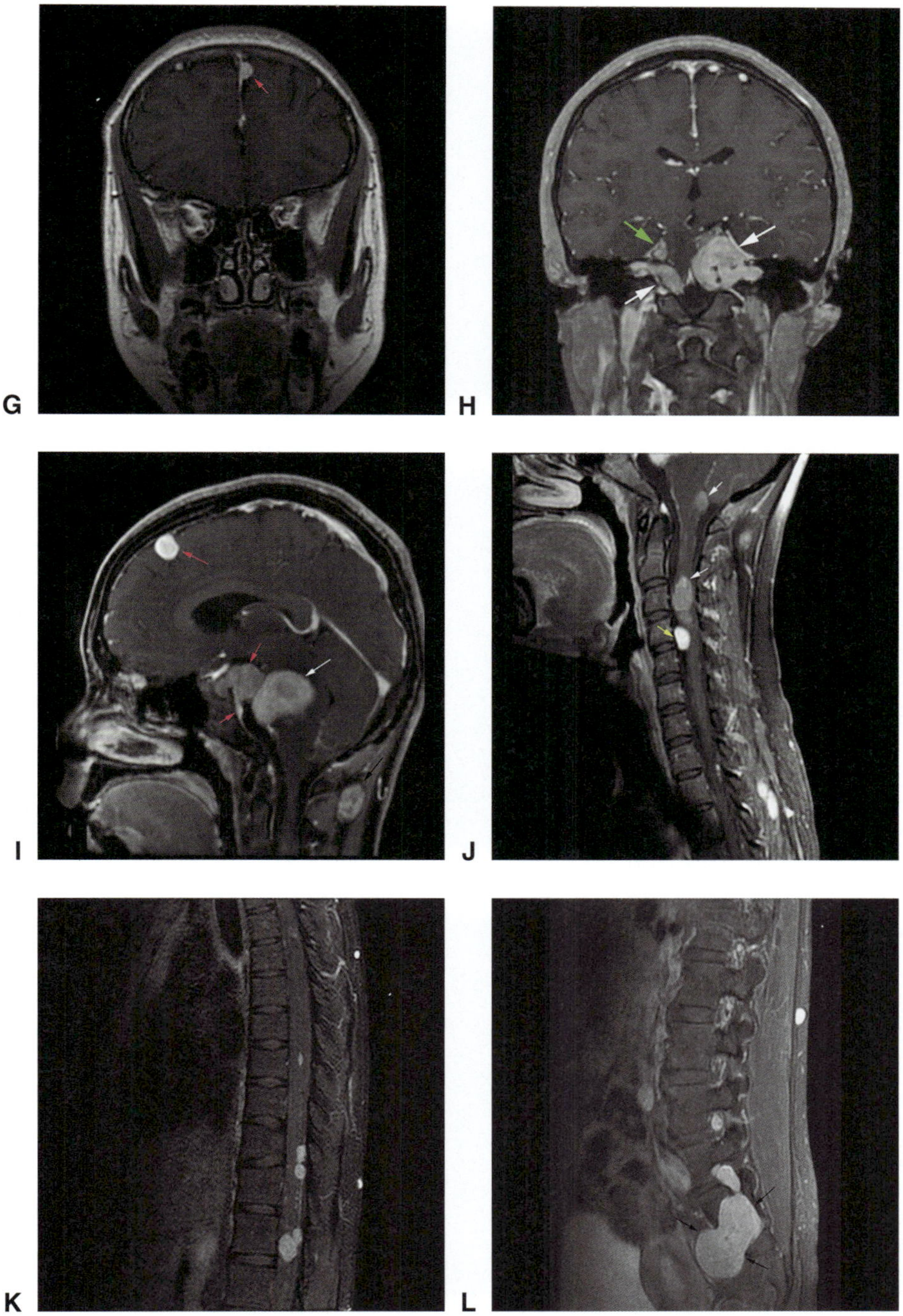

Figure 19.4. ***(continued)*** **G and H.** Coronal T1-postcontrast: Left falcine meningioma (red arrow), trigeminal schwannomas (green arrow), and bilateral vestibular schwannomas (white arrows). **I.** Sagittal T1-postcontrast: Left falcine meningioma and cavernous meningioma with retroclival dural tail (red arrows) and vestibular schwannoma filling the cerebellopontine angle cistern (white arrows). **J–L.** Sagittal T1-postcontrast: Multiple schwannomas in the spine with intramedullary lesions (white marrows) distinct from extramedullary lesion (yellow arrow) and a large extraforaminal sacral schwannoma (black arrows).

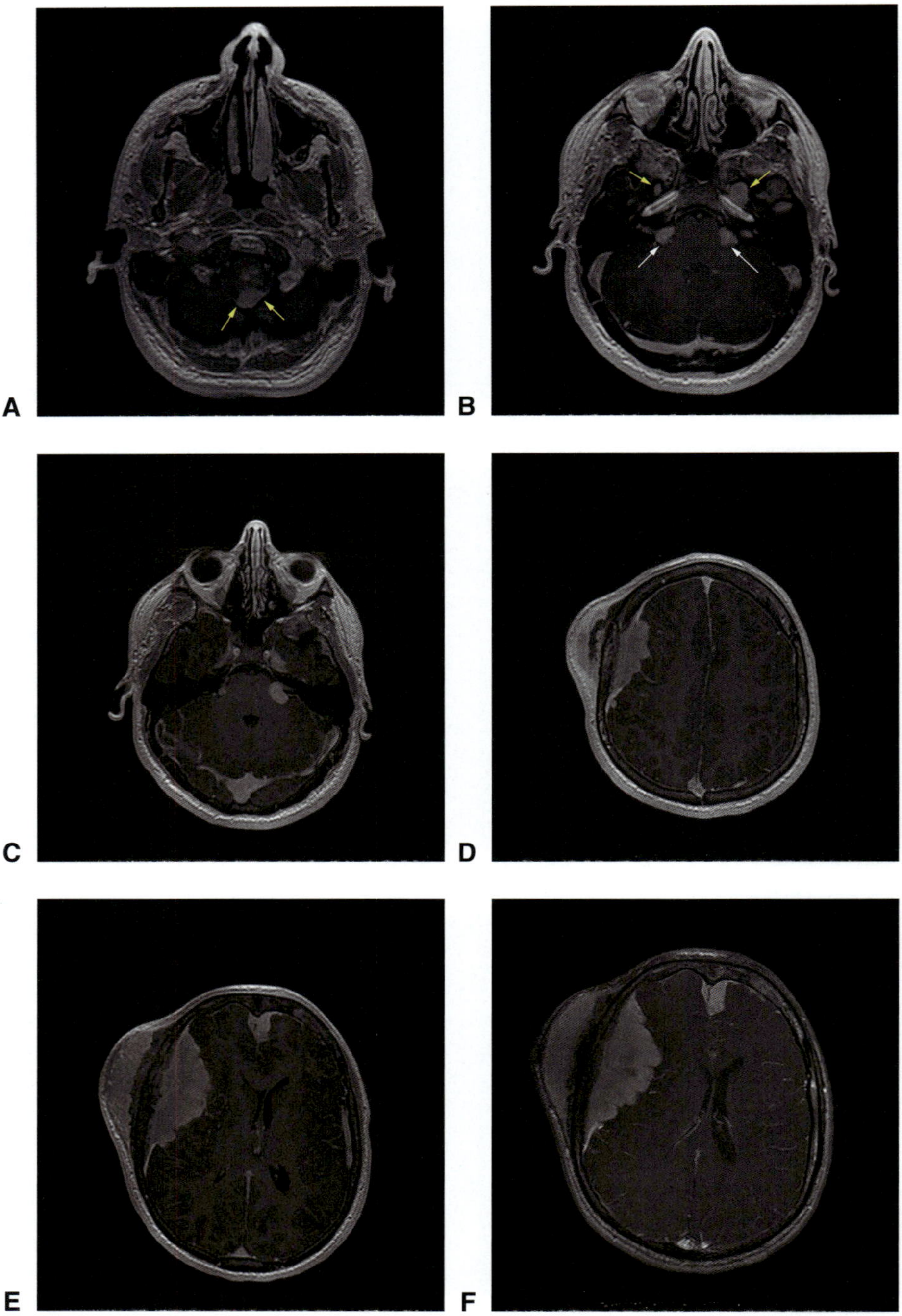

Figure 19.5. Imaging of NF type 2, multiple meningiomas and schwannomas. A. Axial T1-postcontrast: Dorsal foramen magnum meningioma (yellow arrows). **B and C.** Axial T1-postcontrast: Bilateral vestibular schwannomas (white arrows) and bilateral trigeminal schwannomas (yellow arrows). **D–F.** Axial T1-postcontrast: Large right frontal convexity meningioma involving dura, skull, and scalp as well as additional meningiomas along the left anterior falx and superior frontal convexity.

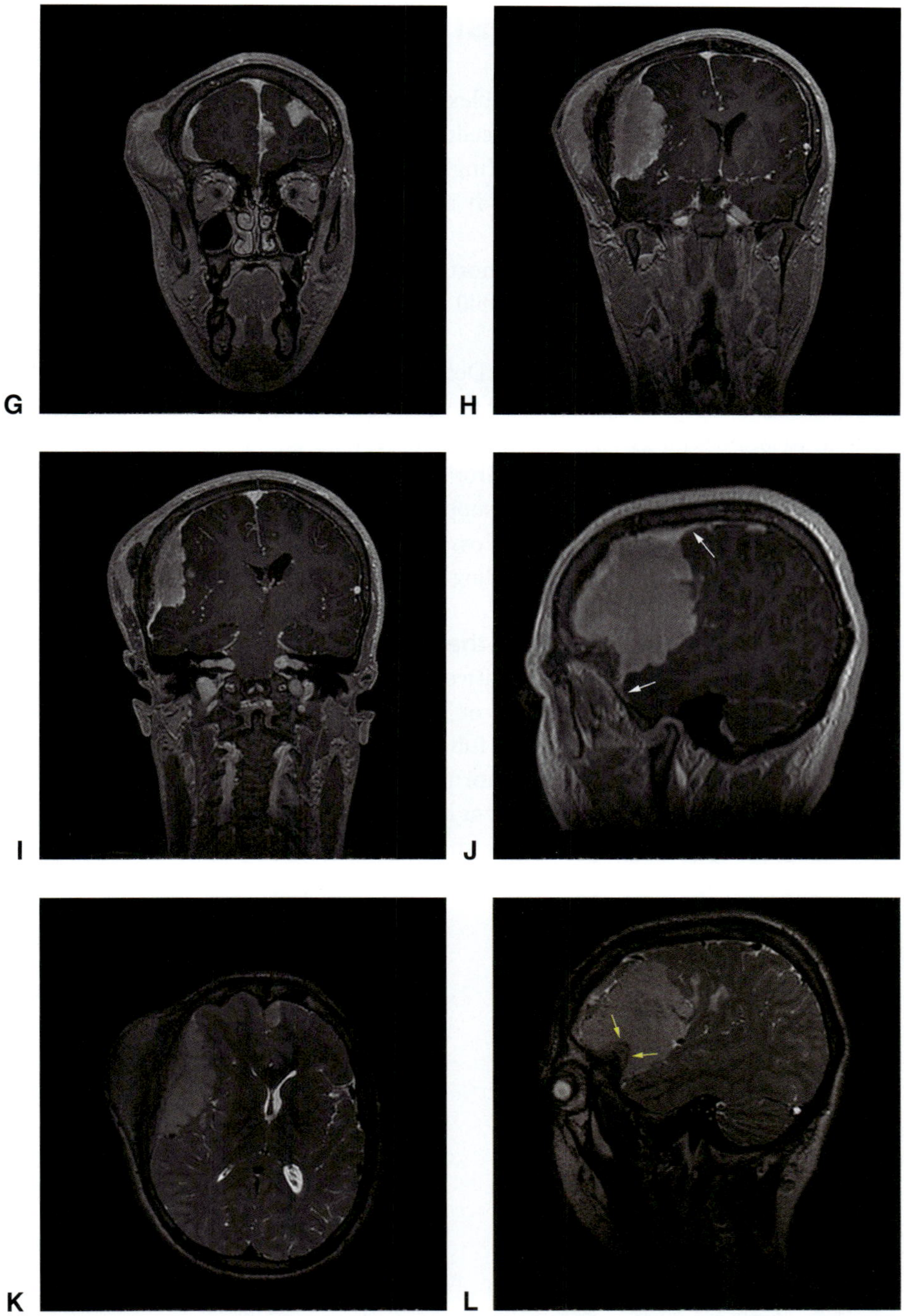

Figure 19.5. ***(continued)*** **G–I.** Coronal T1-postcontrast: Large right frontal convexity meningioma involving dura, skull, and scalp. **J.** Sagittal T1-postcontrast: Large right frontal convexity meningioma with dural tail of enhancement (white arrows). **K.** Axial T2: Heterogeneous and varying signal intensity among different compartments of the large right frontal meningioma. **L.** Sagittal T2: Homogeneously isointense mass with prominent intraosseous involvement (yellow arrows).

Tuberous Sclerosis Complex

Definition: Tuberous sclerosis complex (TSC) is a multisystem, autosomal dominant, genetic disorder affecting cellular differentiation, proliferation, and migration early in development, resulting in a variety of benign tumors or hamartomatous lesions throughout the body including the brain.

Epidemiology: TSC is the second most common neurocutaneous disease after NF1, with incidence rate of 1 in 6,000 newborns in the United States.

Molecular and genetic profile: Defects or mutations on two genes are detected—*TSC1* and *TSC2*. Only one of the genes needs to be affected for tuberous sclerosis to be present. The *TSC1* gene is on chromosome 9 and produces a protein hamartin and the *TSC2* gene on chromosome 16 produces a protein tuberlin. Hamartin and tuberlin act as growth suppressors by inhibiting the activation of target of rapamycin (mTOR) protein. Loss of regulation of mTOR occurs in cells lacking either hamartin or tuberlin, leading to benign tumors throughout the body.

Clinical features and standard therapy: Most patients with TSC have epilepsy; one half or more have cognitive deficits, learning disabilities, behavioral issues, psychosocial difficulties, or autistic spectrum disorder related to glioneuronal hamartomas (also called tubers), subependymal giant cell astrocytomas, and complex white matter abnormalities. Although there is no cure for TSC, there are many effective treatment options for most symptoms related to underlying CNS lesions. Antiepileptic medications can help treat and control infantile spasms and other types of seizures associated with TSC.

Imaging

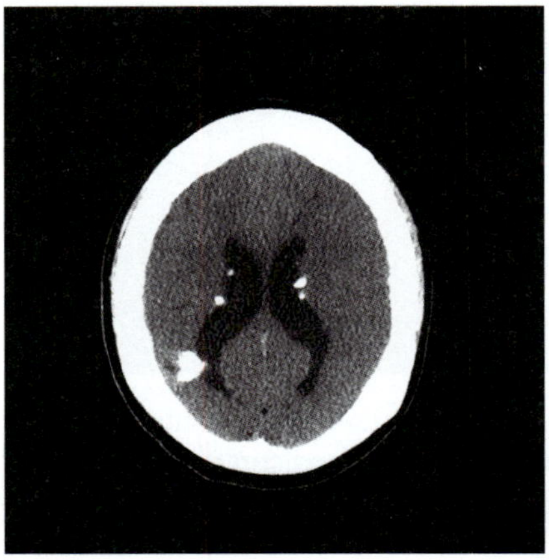
A

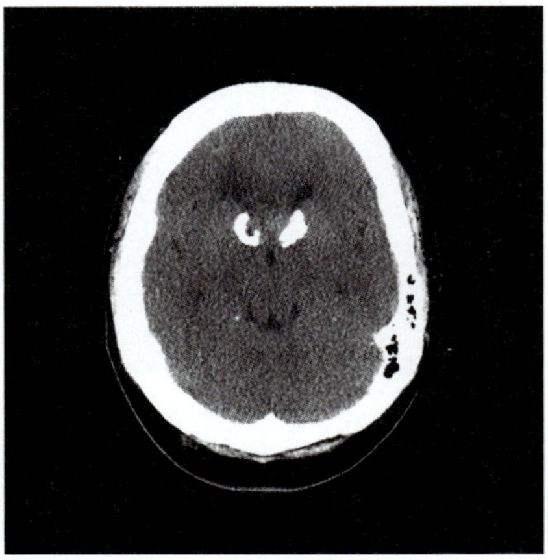
B

Figure 19.6. Imaging of tuberous sclerosis complex, bilateral subependymal giant cell astrocytomas. A–C. Axial CT, unenhanced: Numerous subependymal calcified nodules including bilateral lesions near the foramen of Monro.

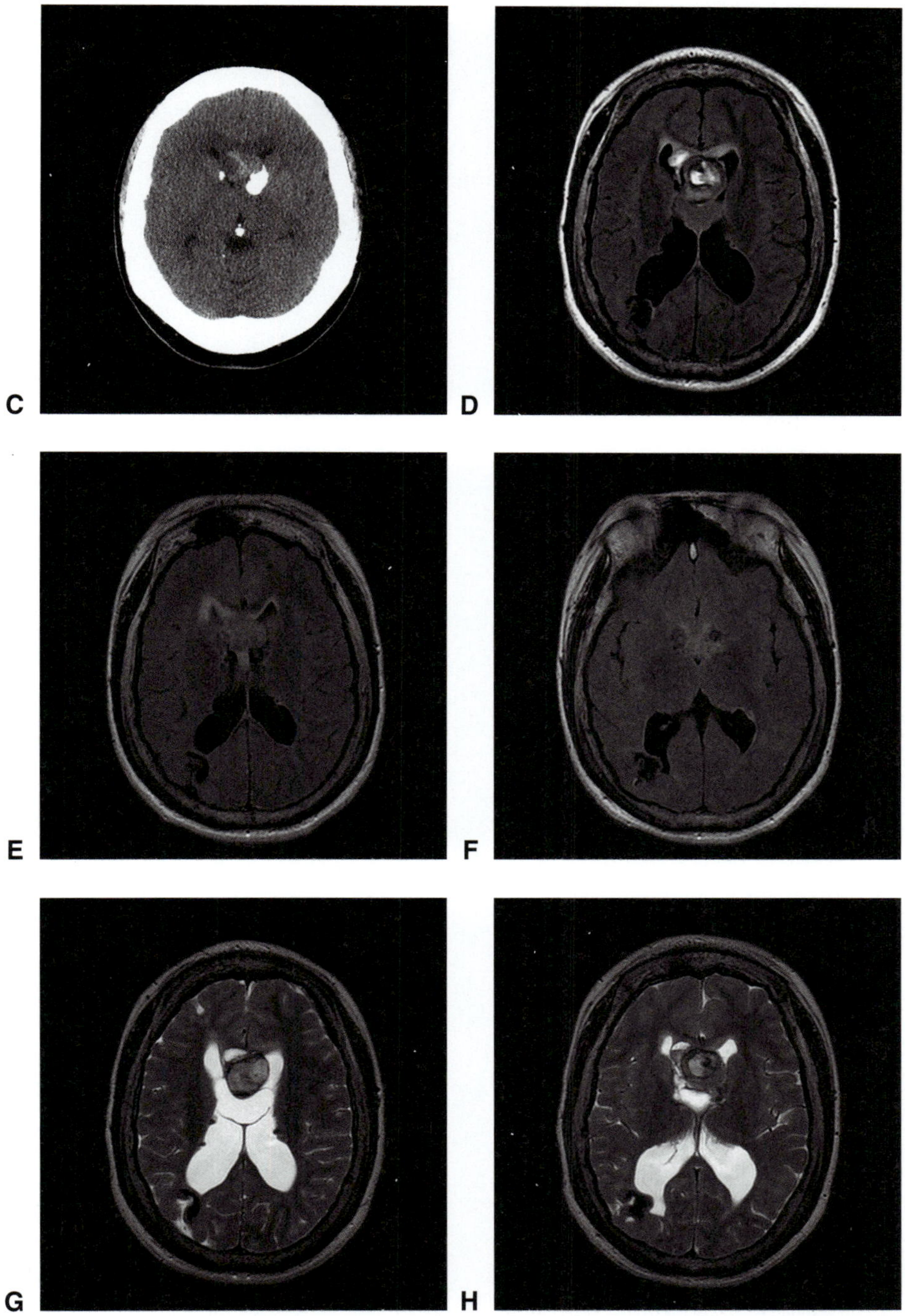

Figure 19.6. ***(continued)*** **D–F.** Axial fluid-attenuated inversion recovery (FLAIR): Heterogeneously hypointense nodules. **G–I.** Axial T2: Heterogeneously hypointense nodules.

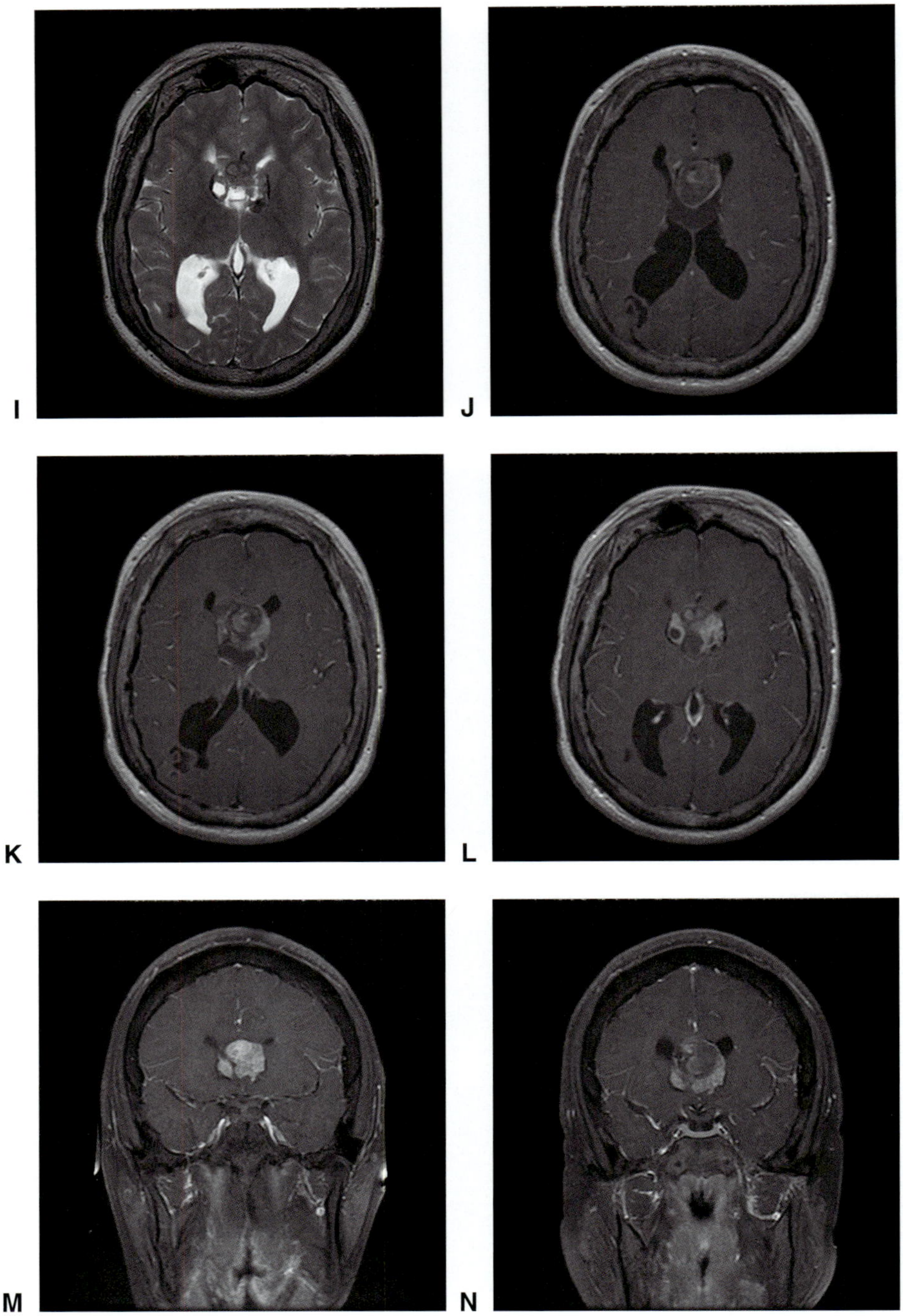

Figure 19.6. ***(continued)*** **J–L.** Axial T1-postcontrast: Heterogeneous enhancement within bilateral subependymal nodules near the foramen of Monro, subependymal giant cell astrocytomas. **M–O.** Coronal T1-postcontrast: Heterogeneous enhancement within bilateral subependymal nodules near the foramen of Monro, subependymal giant cell astrocytomas.

O 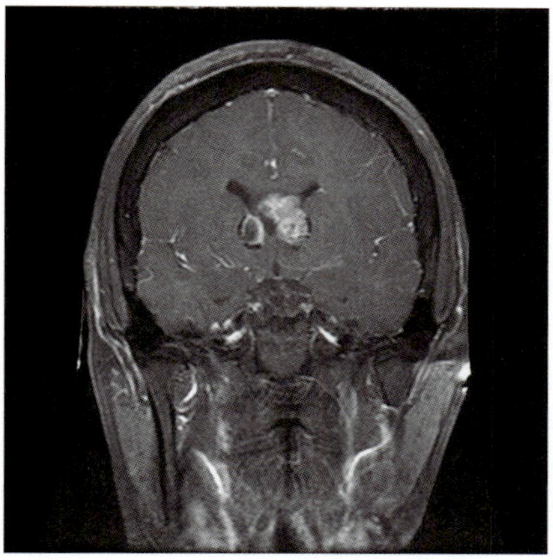

Figure 19.6. ***(continued)***

von Hippel–Lindau Disease

Definition: This autosomal dominant genetic condition results from a deletion or mutation in the *VHL* gene and is characterized by benign or cancerous tumors and visceral cysts in many parts of the body. Hemangioblastomas are the CNS hallmark of von Hippel–Lindau (VHL) disease, and they develop in the brain and spinal cord, or rarely, in the retina. Endolymphatic sac tumors of the inner ear can develop in up to 16% of patients, which can lead to severe and irreversible hearing loss.

Epidemiology: Incidence is 1 in 10,000 cases in the United States and 1 in 200,000 cases worldwide; 20% of patients are first-in-family or de novo cases. The mean age of onset is around 25 years without gender predilection.

Molecular and genetic profile: Heterozygous germline VHL pathogenic variant has been noticed.

Clinical features and standard therapy: Early detection and treatment are important and usually involve surgical removal of CNS hemangioblastomas. However, when there are numerous lesions, only the dominant or symptomatic lesions are removed and the remaining lesions are carefully followed or treated with radiation therapy.

Imaging

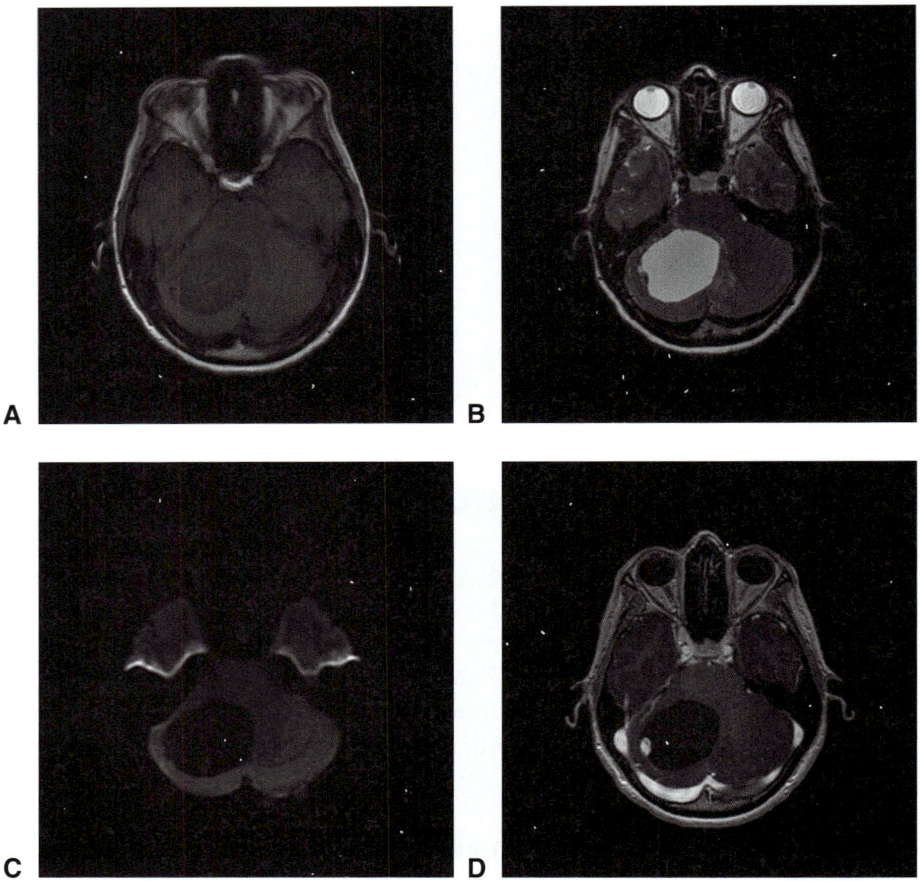

Figure 19.7. **Imaging of right cerebellar hemangioblastoma in von Hippel–Lindau Disease. A–F.** Right cerebellar hemangioblastoma, mostly cystic component with small pial nodule. **A.** Axial T1-precontrast: Primarily cystic mass with a small superficial pial nodule. **B.** Axial T2: Primarily cystic mass with a small superficial nodule and minimal surrounding edema. **C.** Axial DWI: Primarily cystic mass with a small superficial pial nodule. **D.** Axial T1-postcontrast: Avid enhancement within the small pial nodule.

E F

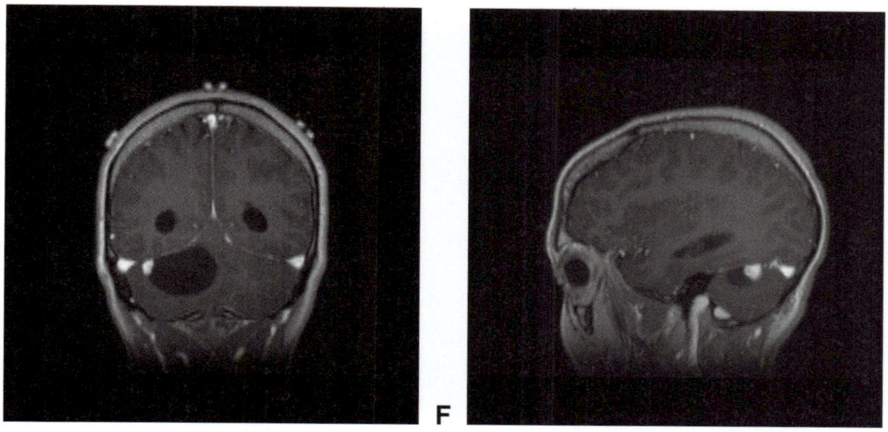

Figure 19.7. ***(continued)*** **E.** Coronal T1-postcontrast: Avid enhancement within the small pial nodule. **F.** Sagittal T1-postcontrast: Avid enhancement within the small pial nodule.

A B

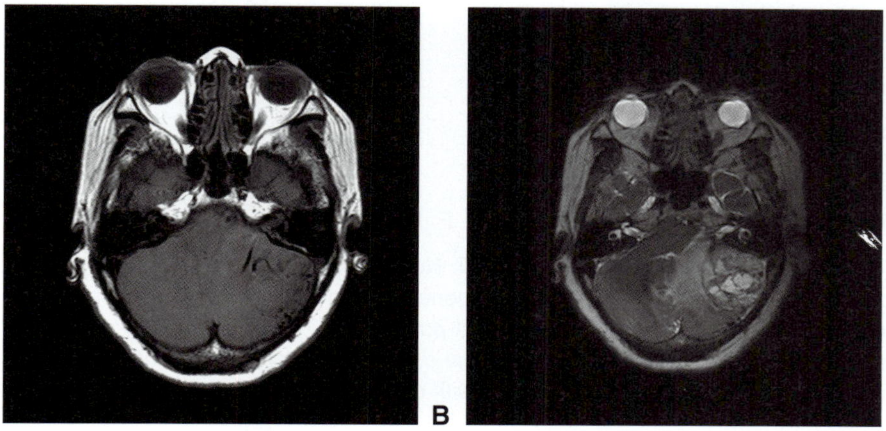

Figure 19.8. Imaging of left cerebellar hemangioblastoma in von Hippel–Lindau Disease. A. Axial T1-precontrast: Hypointense mass with prominent peripheral vessels. **B.** Axial T2: Heterogeneous solid and cystic mass with moderate surrounding edema.

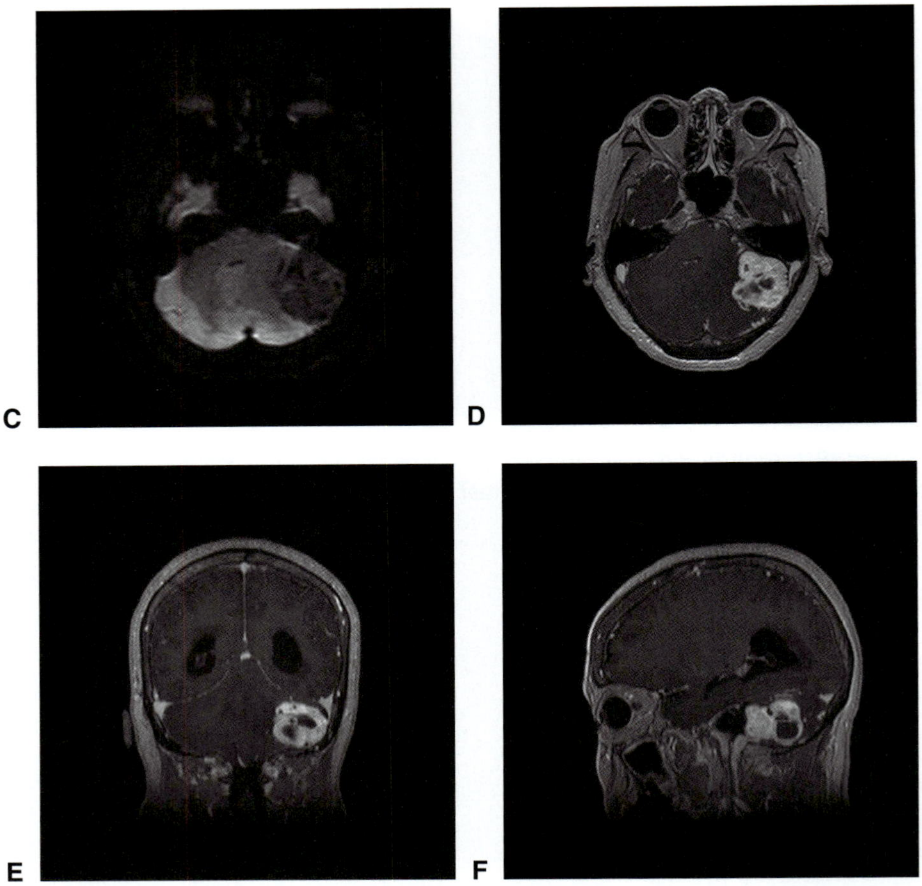

Figure 19.8. ***(continued)*** **C.** Axial DWI: No areas of reduced diffusion within the tumor. **D.** Axial T1-postcontrast: Heterogeneously and avidly enhancing mass with distinct intratumoral cysts. **E.** Coronal T1-postcontrast: Heterogeneously and avidly enhancing mass with distinct intratumoral cysts. **F.** Sagittal T1-postcontrast: Heterogeneously and avidly enhancing mass with distinct intratumoral cysts.

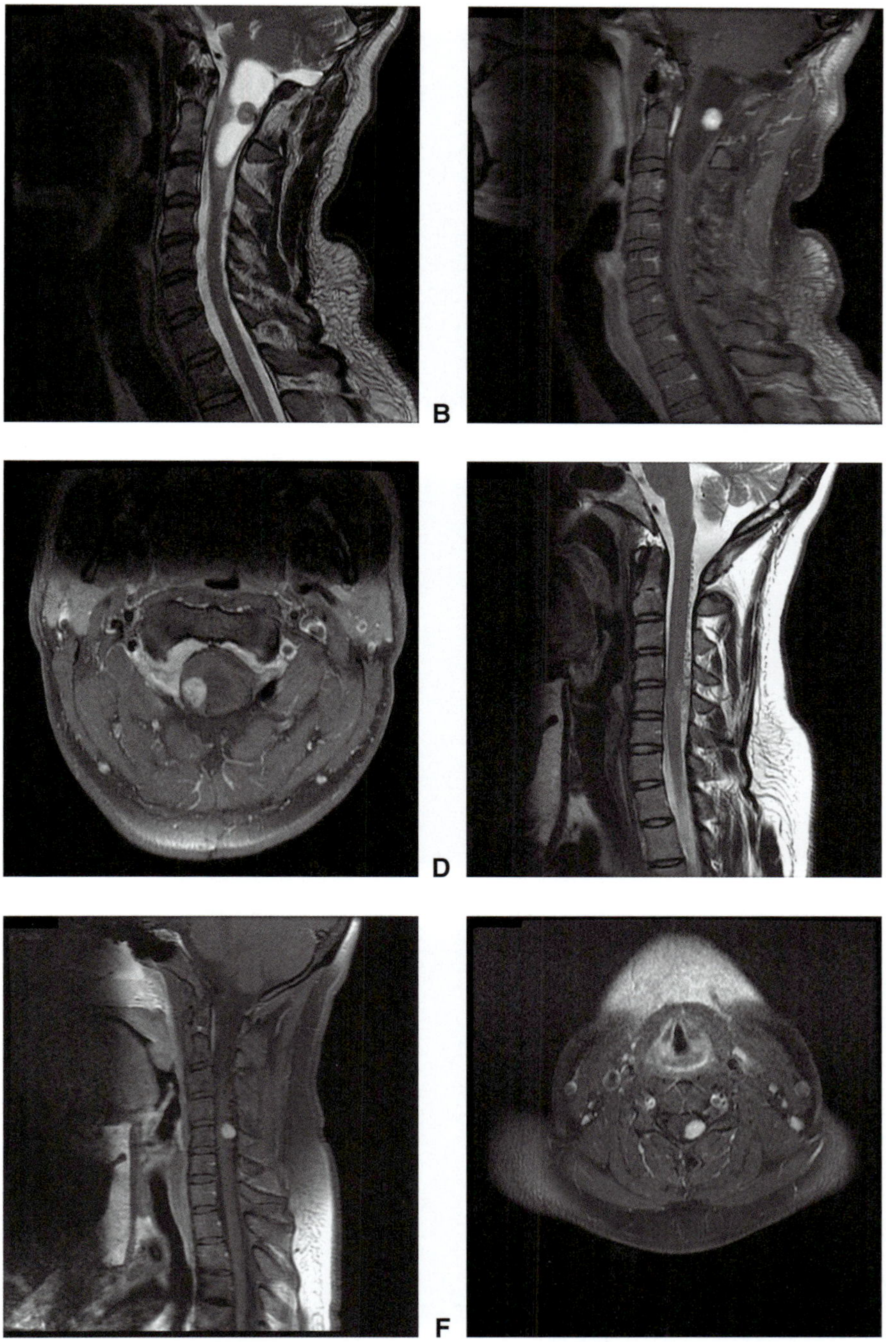

A B C D E F

Figure 19.9. **Imaging of spinal hemangioblastoma in von Hippel–Lindau disease, four different patients. A–C.** Cervicomedullary junction hemangioblastoma. **A.** Sagittal T2: Dorsal pial nodule within a large cystic mass. **B.** Sagittal T1-postcontrast: Avid enhancement within the pial nodule. **C.** Axial T1-postcontrast: Exophytic right dorsal pial nodule. **D–F.** Cervical hemangioblastoma. **D.** Sagittal T2: Dorsal pial nodule without associated cyst. **E.** Sagittal T1-postcontrast: Avid enhancement within the pial nodule. **F.** Axial T1-postcontrast: Exophytic left dorsal pial nodule.

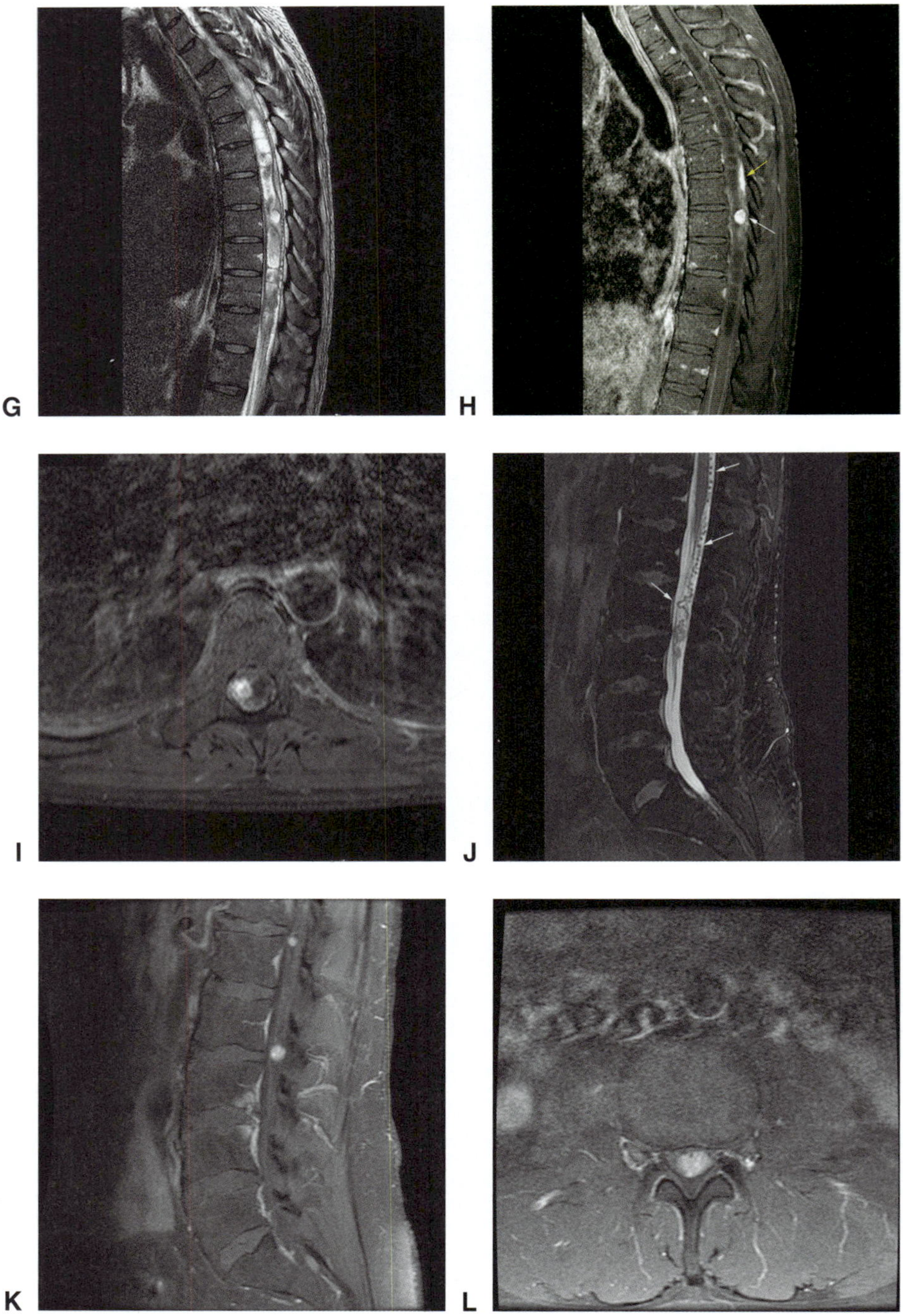

Figure 19.9. ***(continued)*** **G–I.** Thoracic hemangioblastoma. **G.** Sagittal T2: Dorsal pial nodule associated with extensive cysts and syrinx. **H.** Sagittal T1-postcontrast: Avid enhancement of the pial nodule (white arrow) and separate plaque-like enhancing lesion along the dorsal surface (yellow arrow). **I.** Axial T1-postcontrast: Exophytic right dorsal pial nodule. **J–L.** Lumbar hemangioblastoma. **J.** Sagittal T2: Prominent vessels along the nerve roots of cauda equina and dorsal pial surface (white arrows). **K.** Sagittal T1-postcontrast: Avid enhancement of nodule at L2–L3 thecal sac. **L.** Axial T1-postcontrast: Centrally located enhancing nodule.

Li–Fraumeni Syndrome

Definition: Li–Fraumeni syndrome (LFS) is an inherited autosomal dominant hereditary cancer predisposition syndrome in children and young adults due to germline mutations in the *TP53* gene. LFS is also known as the sarcoma, breast, leukemia, and adrenal gland (SBLA) cancer syndrome. In the CNS, diffuse astrocytoma, medulloblastoma, and choroid plexus carcinoma are the three most common tumors associated with LFS.

Epidemiology: Actual incidence is unknown, and approximately 400 reported families are found in the cumulative literature.

Molecular and genetic profile: Germline mutations in the *TP53* gene on chromosome 17p13, the genetic blueprint for p53 protein, are the hallmark of LFS. Less commonly, germline mutation in *CHEK2* has been implicated.

Clinical features and standard therapy: In most cases, cancers associated with LFS develop in children and young adults, usually before the age of 30 years. Diffuse astrocytomas are the most common CNS tumor associated with LFS, and up to 65% of patients with choroid plexus carcinoma have LFS. Surgical resection is the primary treatment for CNS tumors, and radiation therapy should be used with caution owing to concerns about increased risk for radiation-induced second primary tumors.

Imaging

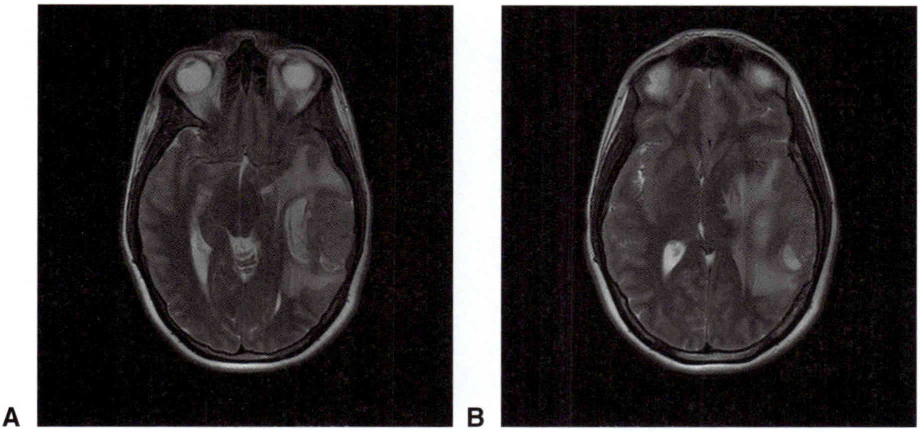

Figure 19.10. Imaging of glioblastoma in Li–Fraumeni syndrome. A–C. Axial T2: Hypointense solid mass with medial necrotic component and marked surrounding edema.

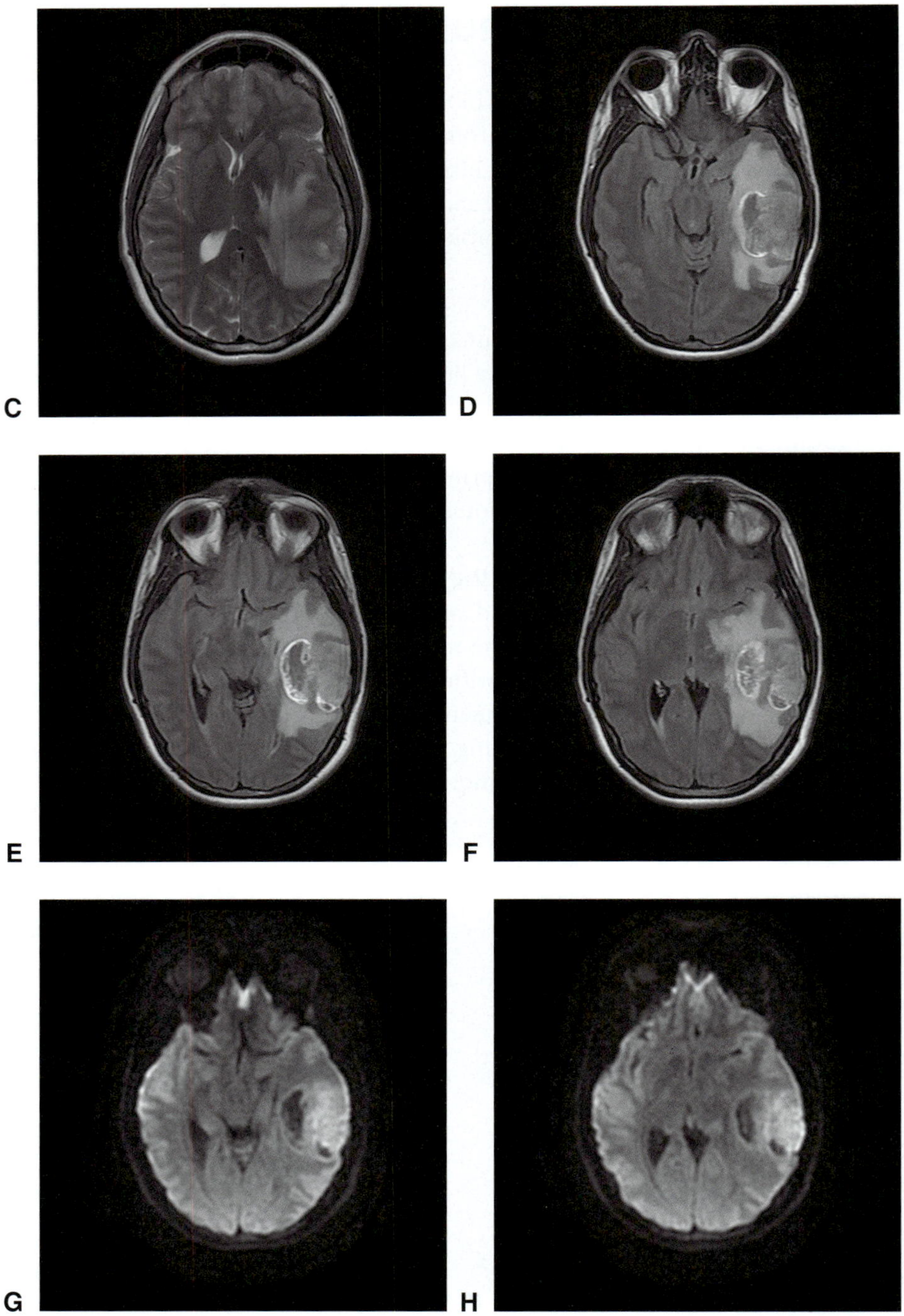

Figure 19.10. ***(continued)*** **D–F.** Axial FLAIR: Hypointense solid mass with medial necrotic component and marked surrounding edema. **G–I.** Axial DWI: Reduced diffusion within the solid mass.

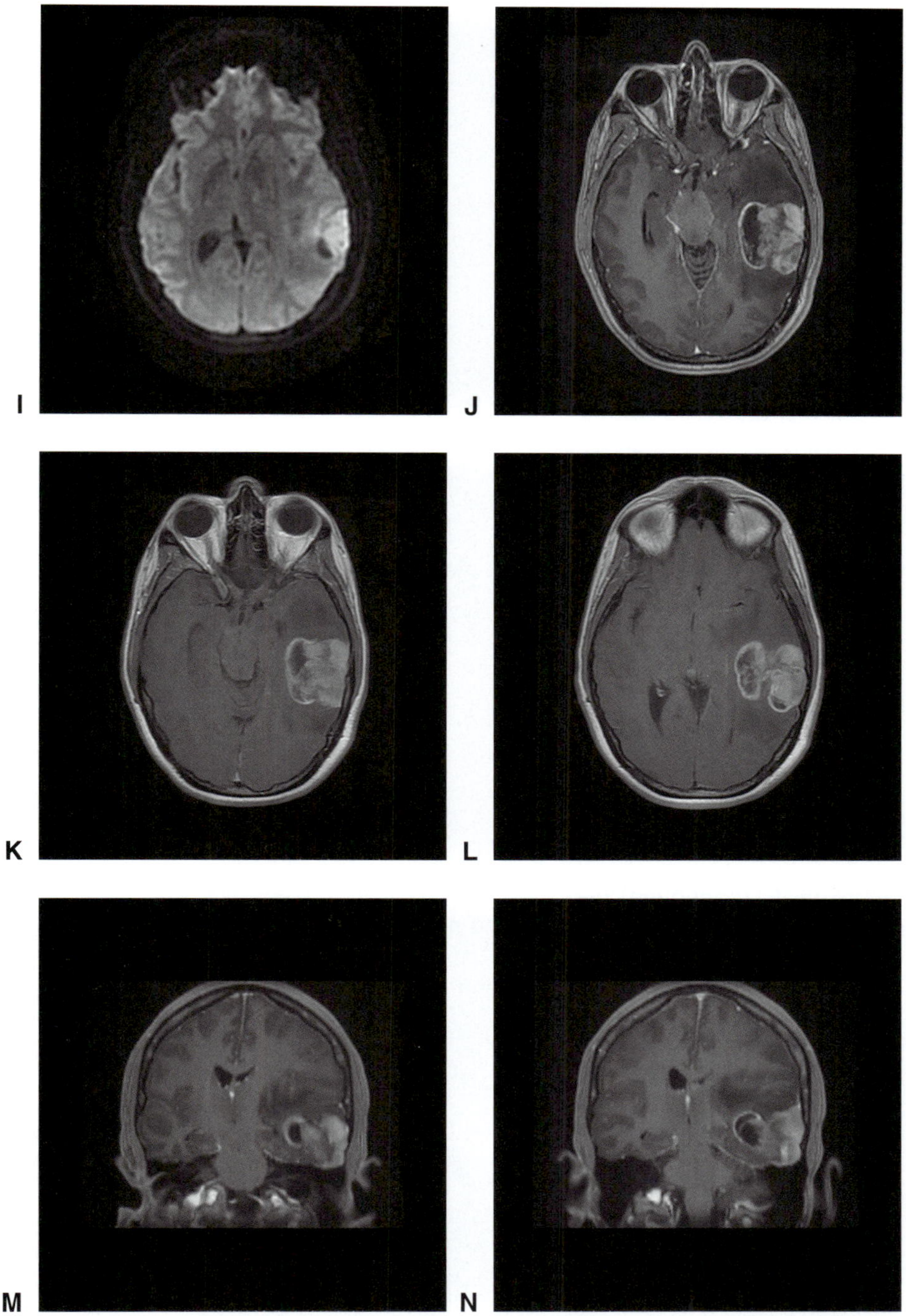

Figure 19.10. ***(continued)*** **J–L.** Axial T1-postcontrast: Avid but heterogeneous enhancement within the solid tumor and rim of enhancing encasing the necrotic component. **M–O.** Coronal T1-postcontrast: Avid but heterogeneous enhancement within the solid tumor and rim of enhancing encasing the necrotic component.

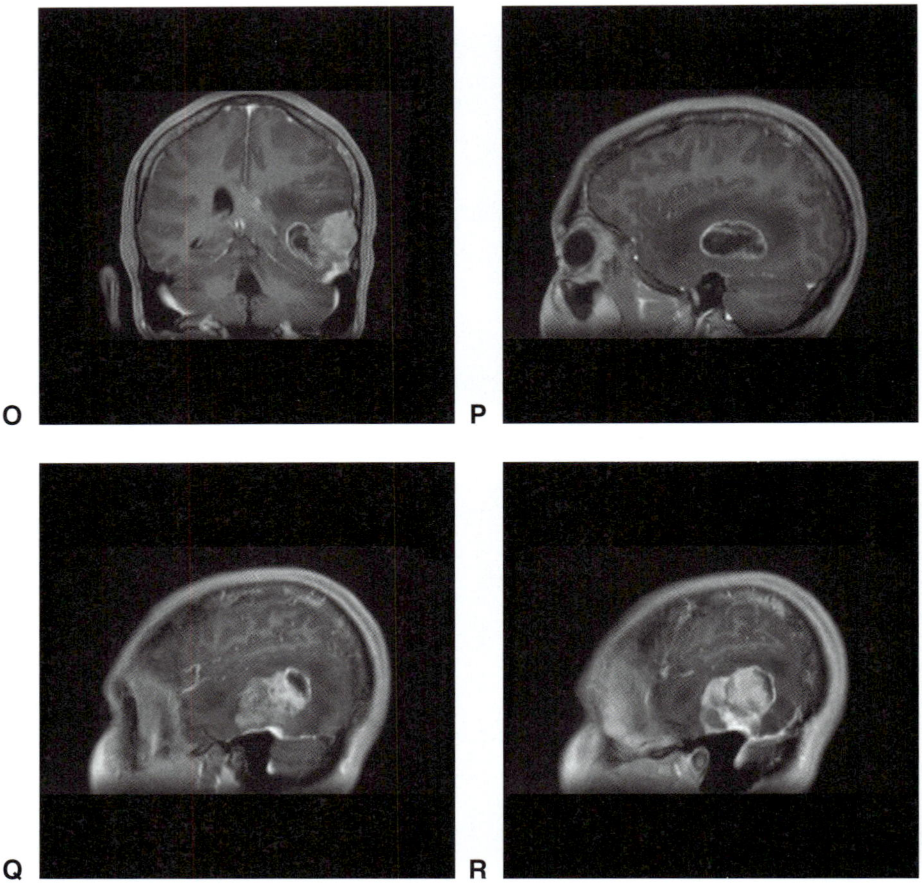

Figure 19.10. ***(continued)*** **P–R.** Sagittal T1-postcontrast: Avid but heterogeneous enhancement within the solid tumor and rim of enhancing encasing the necrotic component.

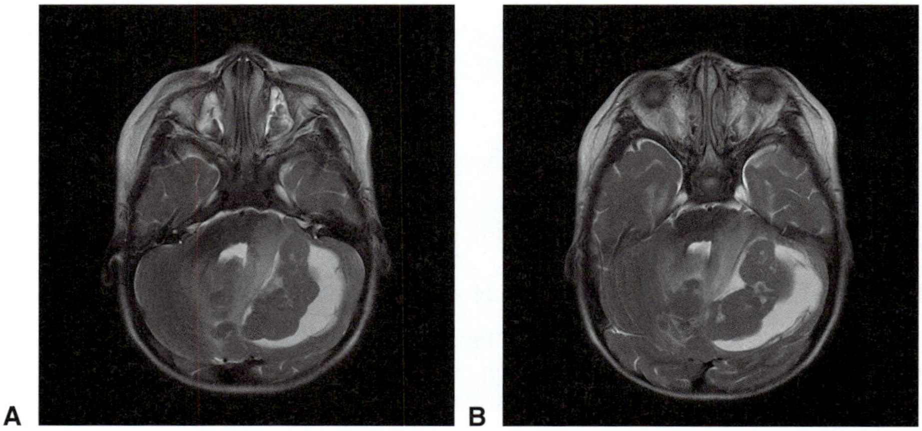

Figure 19.11. Imaging of medulloblastoma, sonic hedgehog (SHH)-activated, in Li–Fraumeni syndrome. A–C. Axial T2: Hypointense nodular mass in the left cerebellar hemisphere with prominent peripheral cystic component and surrounding edema.

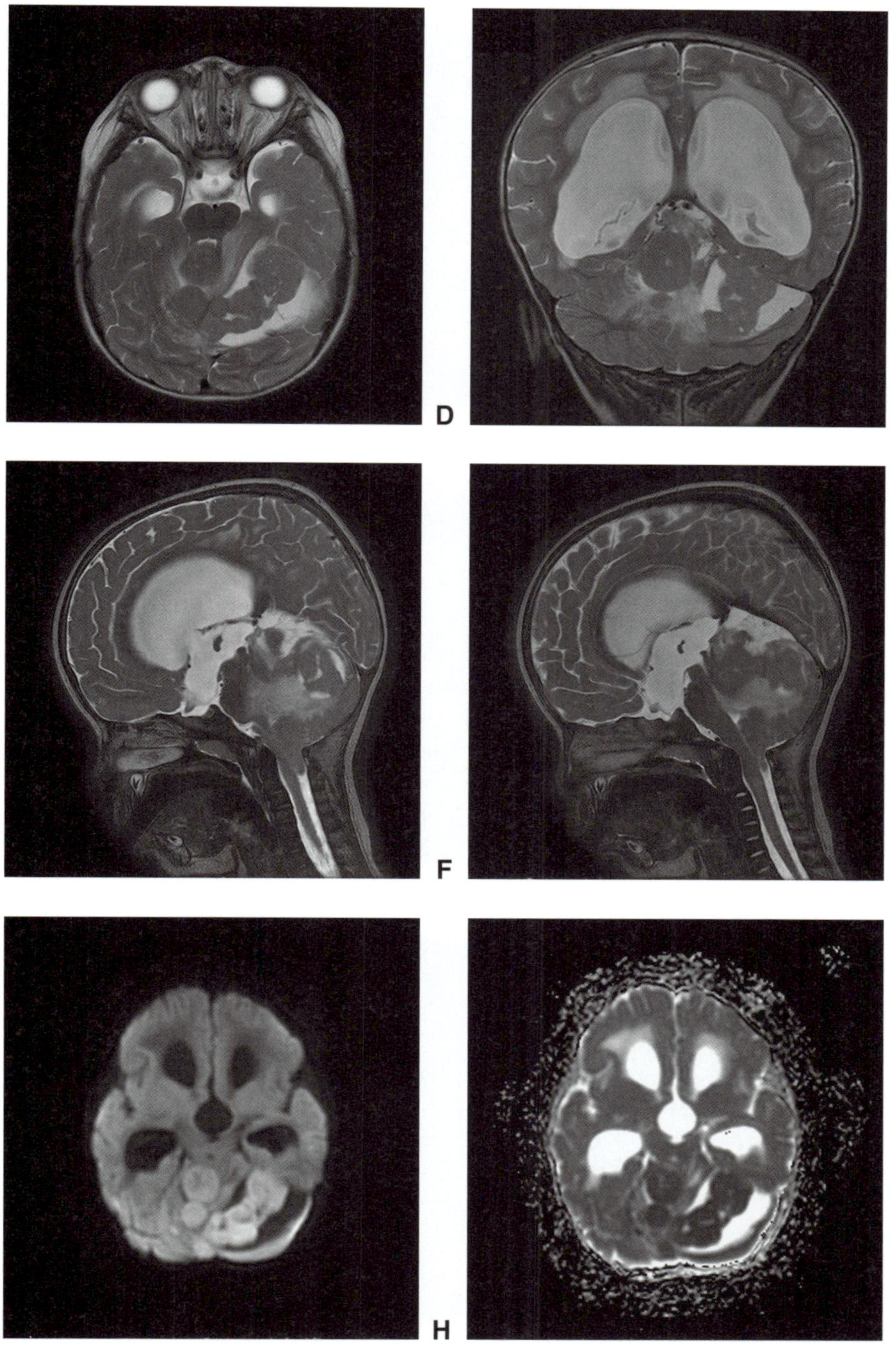

C D E F G H

Figure 19.11. ***(continued)*** **D.** Coronal T2: Hypointense nodular mass in the left cerebellar hemisphere with prominent peripheral cystic component and surrounding edema. **E and F.** Sagittal T2: Hypointense nodular mass in the left cerebellar hemisphere with prominent peripheral cystic component and surrounding edema. **G.** Axial diffusion-weighted imaging (DWI): Marked reduced diffusion within the nodular solid mass. **H and I.** Axial apparent diffusion coefficient (ADC): Marked reduced diffusion within the nodular solid mass.

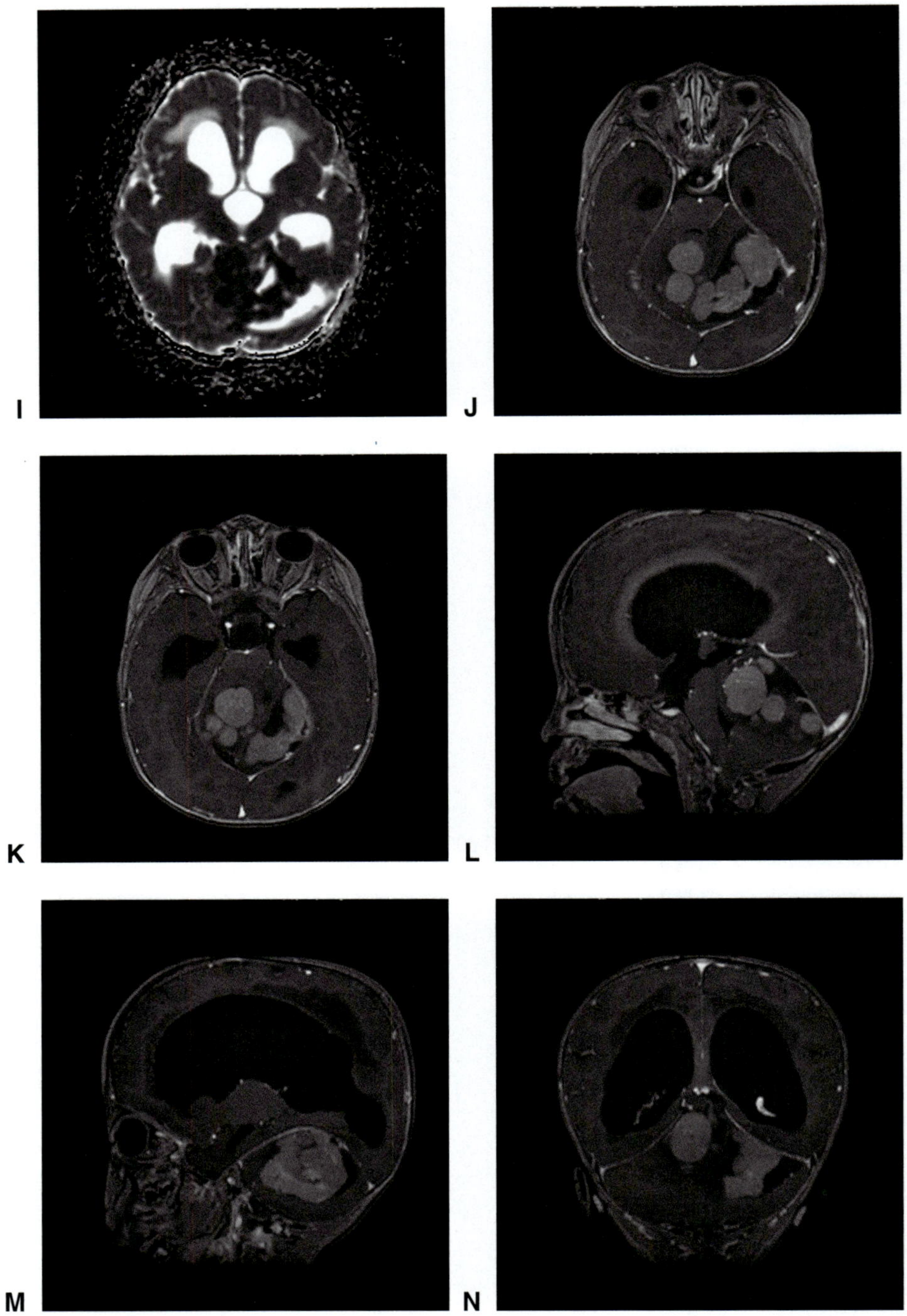

Figure 19.11. ***(continued)*** **J and K.** Axial T1-postcontrast: Avid enhancement within the nodular solid mass. **L and M.** Sagittal T1-postcontrast: Avid enhancement within the nodular solid mass. **N and O.** Coronal T1-postcontrast: Avid enhancement within the nodular solid mass.

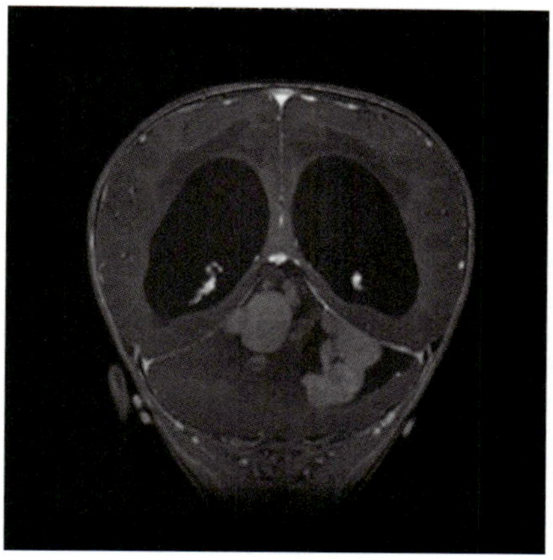

O

Figure 19.11. ***(continued)***

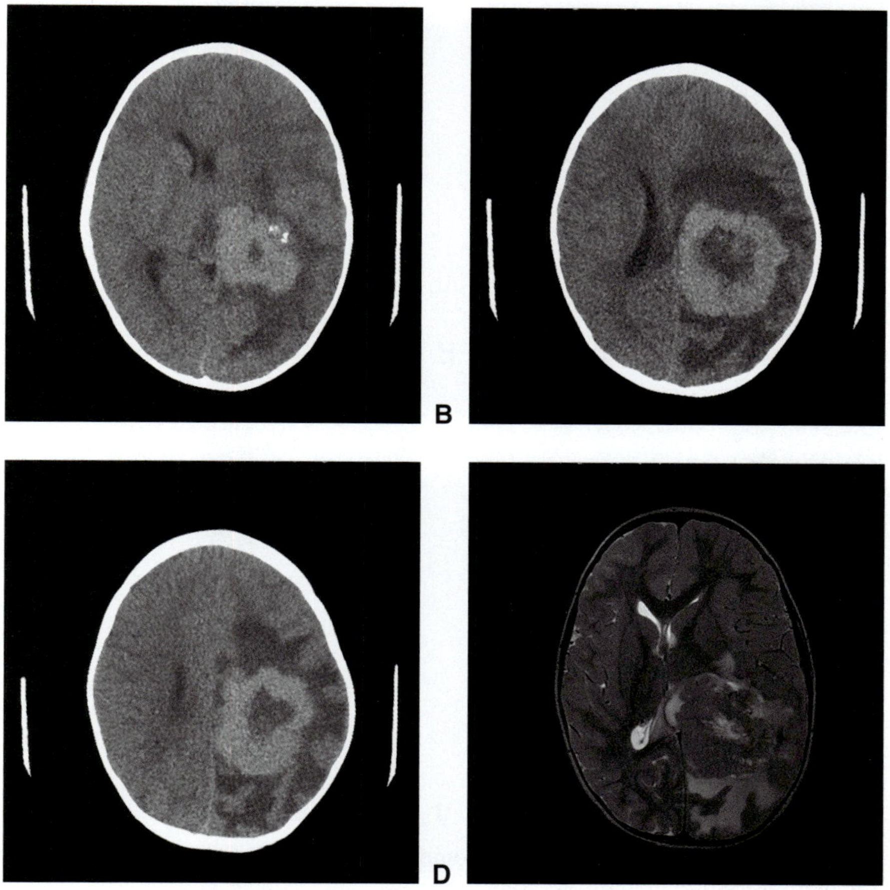

A B C D

Figure 19.12. **Imaging of choroid plexus carcinoma in Li–Fraumeni syndrome. A–C.** Axial CT, unenhanced: Lobulated hyperdense mass centered in the left atrium with peripheral calcium, central necrosis, and marked surrounding edema. **D–F.** Axial T2: Lobulated hypointense mass centered in the left atrium with central necrosis and marked surrounding edema.

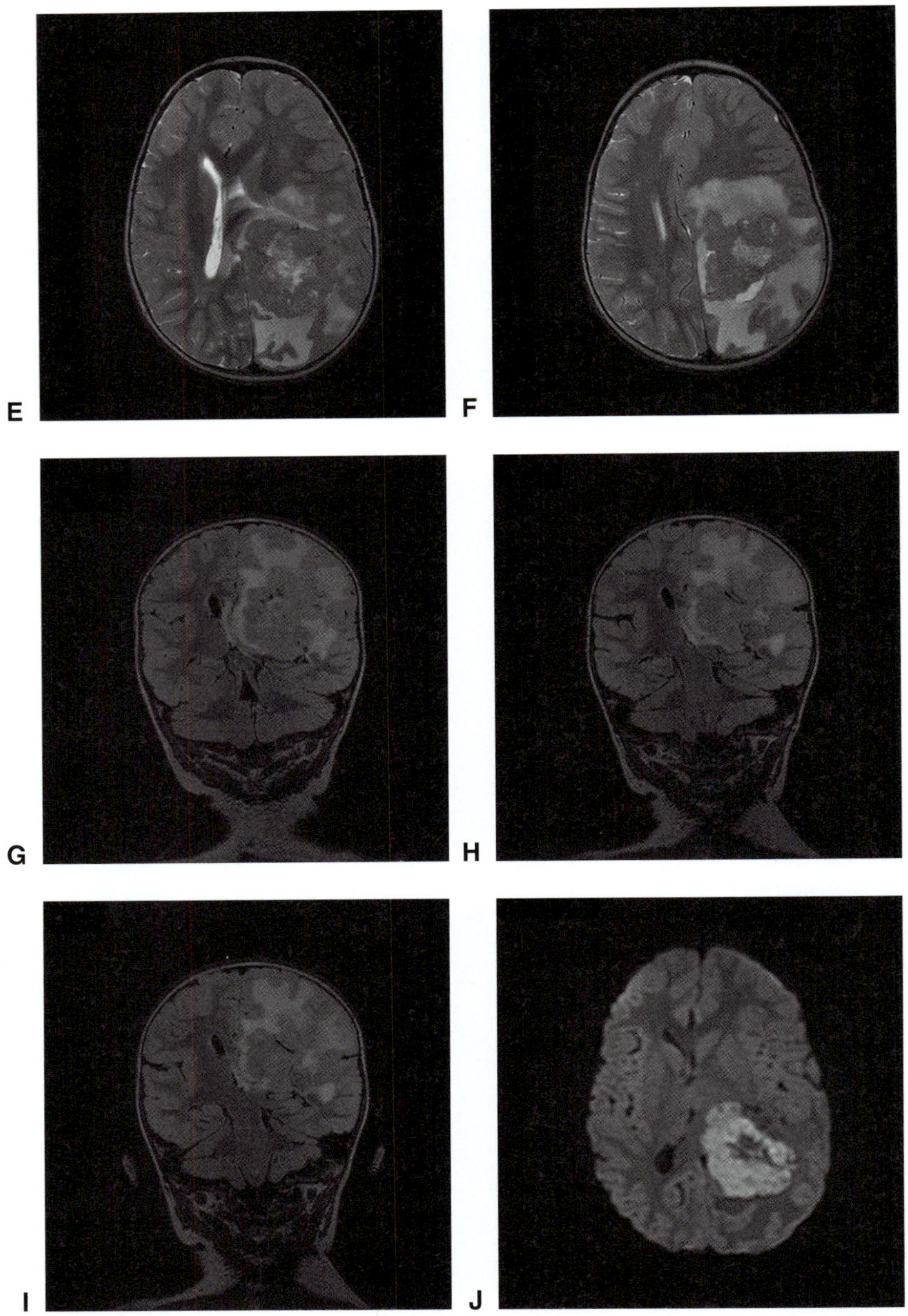

Figure 19.12. ***(continued)*** **G and I.** Coronal FLAIR: Lobulated hypointense mass centered in the left atrium with central necrosis and marked surrounding edema. **J–L.** Axial DWI: Marked reduced diffusion within the solid component.

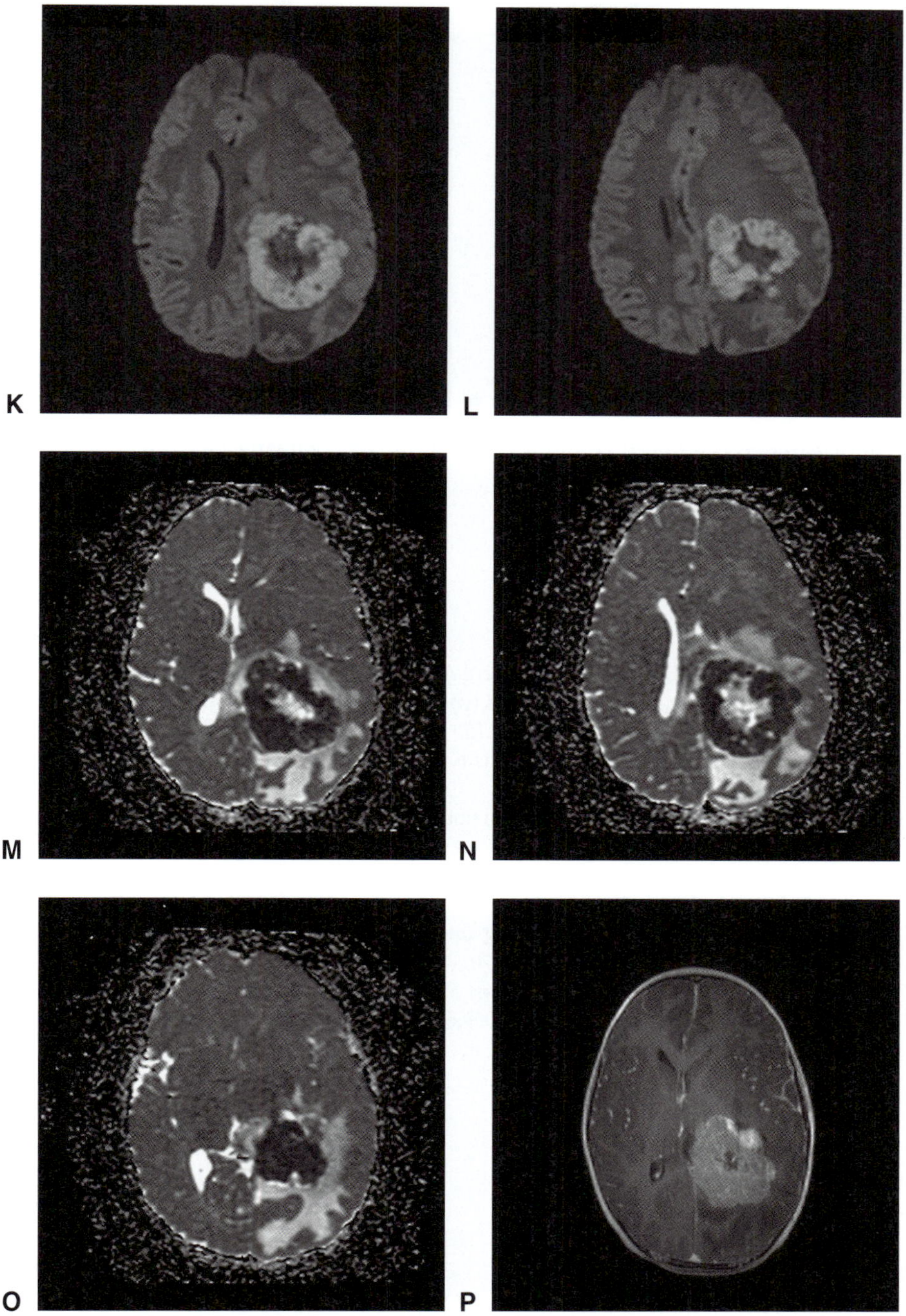

Figure 19.12. ***(continued)*** **M–O.** Axial ADC: Marked reduced diffusion within the solid component. **P.** Axial T1-postcontrast: Heterogeneous enhancement within the solid component.

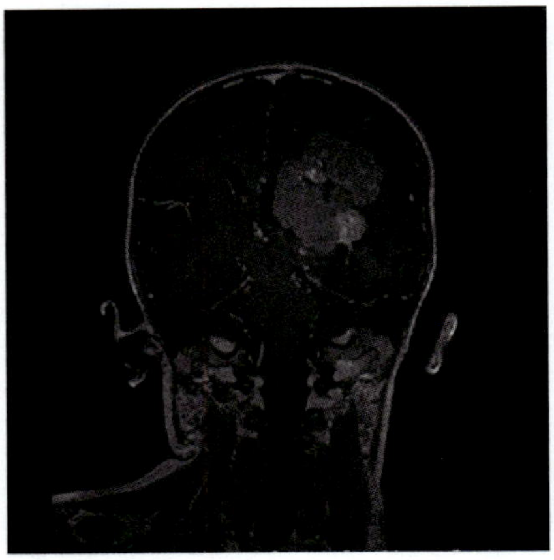

Q

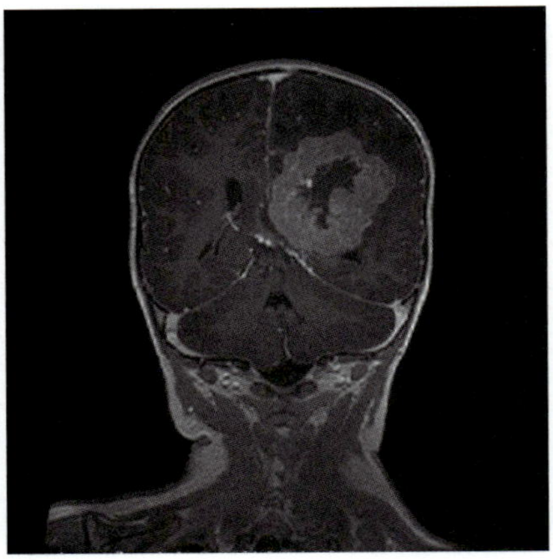

R

Figure 19.12. ***(continued)*** **Q and R.** Coronal T1-postcontrast: Heterogeneous enhancement within the solid component.

Bibliography

Ahlawat S, Blakeley JO, Langmead S, Berlzberg AJ, Faya LM. Current status and recommendations for imaging in neurofibromatosis type 1, neurofibromatosis type 2, and schwannomatosis. *Skeletal Radiol.* 2020;49:199–219.

Hirbe AC, Gutmann DH. Neurofibromatosis type 1: a multidisciplinary approach to care. *Lance Neurol.* 2014;13:834–843.

Orr BA, Clay MR, Pinto EM, Kesseran C. An update on the central nervous system manifestations of Li-Fraumeni syndrome. *Acta Neuropathol.* 2020;139:669–687.

Rad E, Tee AR. Neurofibromatosis type 1: fundamental insights into cell signaling and cancer. *Semin Cell Dev Biol.* 2016;52:39–46.

Rodriguez D, Poussaint TY. Neuroimaging findings in neurofibromatosis type 1 and 2. *Neuroimaging Clin N Am.* 2004;14:149–170.

Van Meerbeeck SFL, Verstraete KL, Janssens S, Mortier G. Whole body MR imaging in neurofibromatosis type 1. *Eur J Radiol.* 2009;69:236–242.

20

Central Nervous System Tumor Mimics

Overview

Nonneoplastic intracranial mass lesions that mimic brain tumors can be difficult to differentiate from true brain tumors based on clinical, laboratory, or imaging findings. Accurate preoperative differentiation between the two entities is essential for proper surgical and medical management of patients presenting with intracranial mass.

Central nervous system (CNS) tumor mimics fall into three general categories of disease process: infectious, inflammatory, and ischemic/vascular diseases. It is important to consider one of these entities as a possible diagnosis when an apparent brain tumor is suspected on imaging because both entities can look alike and radical surgical resection of a brain tumor mimic can potentially lead to a devastating outcome for the patient.

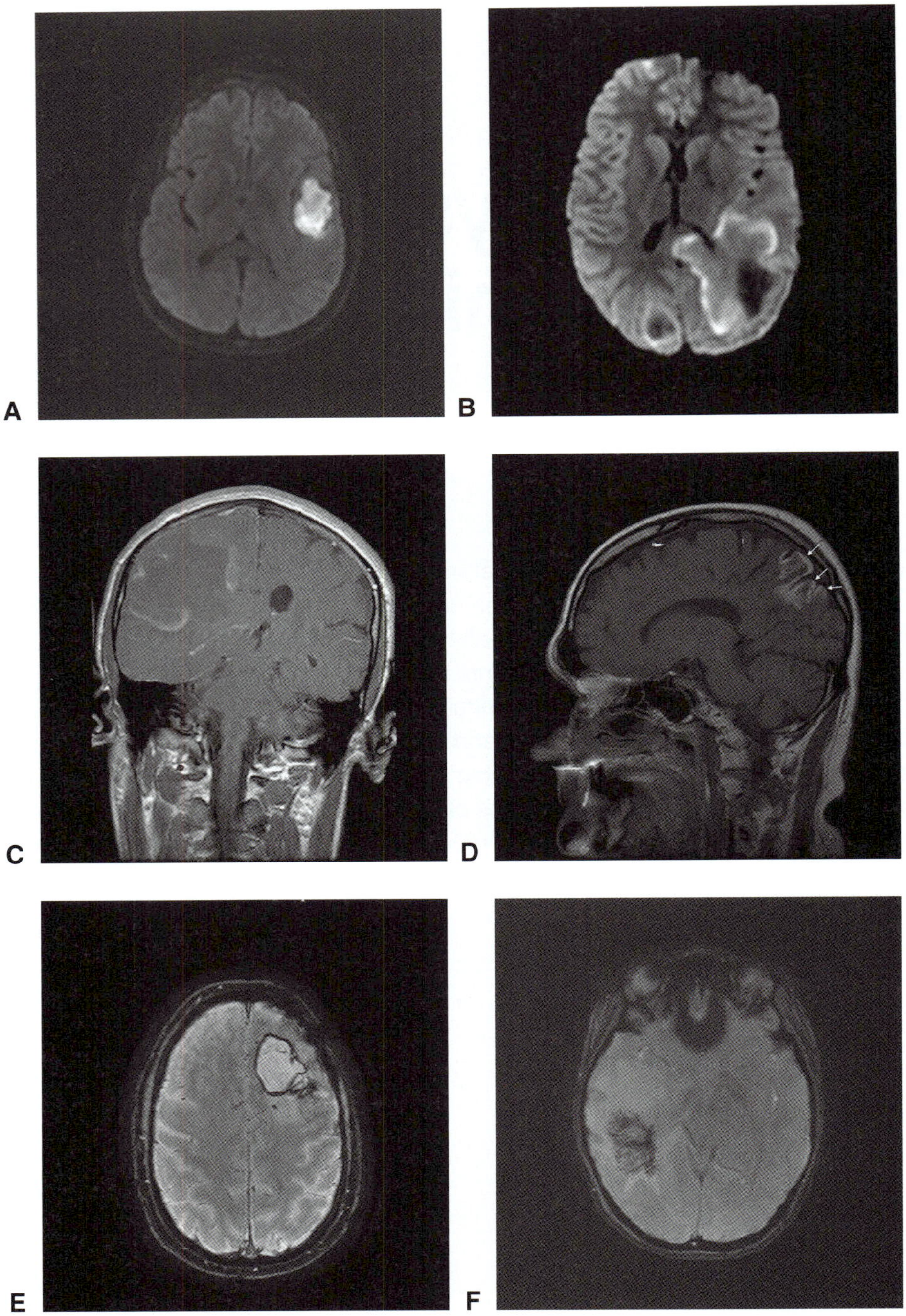

Figure 20.1. Six MR imaging features to identify brain tumor mimics. A. Axial DWI: Homogeneously reduced diffusion within a pyogenic abscess. **B.** Axial diffusion-weighted imaging (DWI): Peripheral incomplete rim of reduced diffusion of demyelinating lesions. **C.** Axial T1-postcontrast: Incomplete rim of enhancement of demyelinating lesion. **D.** Sagittal T1-precontrast imaging: Gyral form of T1 shortening in a subacute infarct. **E.** Axial T2: Thin complete rim of T2 shortening in a cavernous malformation. **F.** Axial SWI: Parallel stacked pattern of thrombosed vein in a region of venulitis.

Central Nervous System Infections

Central nervous system (CNS) infections are caused by various microbes, including but not limited to bacteria, viruses, fungi, parasites, protozoans, or prions, and manifested as meningitis, encephalitis/cerebritis, empyema, or brain abscess. The clinical signs and symptoms of CNS infection are often nonspecific and include headache, fever, altered mental status, and behavioral changes. A high index of suspicion, prompt diagnosis, and therapy of CNS infection are of utmost importance, which can positively impact clinical course and outcome. Delay in diagnosis and treatment of CNS infection, especially in cases of bacterial meningitis or herpes encephalitis, can lead to serious complications and negative outcomes.

Pyogenic abscesses of the brain are thought to result from a bacterial seeding of already devitalized tissue. Brain abscess can mimic malignant brain tumor but each requires vastly different urgent and long-term treatment. Neuroimaging of the two entities can appear very similar as well, but there are a few imaging findings that can help to distinguish brain abscess from the brain tumor. Homogeneously reduced diffusion or incomplete rim of reduced diffusion within a rim-enhancing mass suggests brain abscess although it is not definitive enough to exclude brain tumor. Neuroimaging findings need to be correlated with laboratory findings, especially cerebrospinal fluid (CSF) and white blood cell counts, as well as high index of suspicion for prompt and accurate diagnosis of CNS infection.

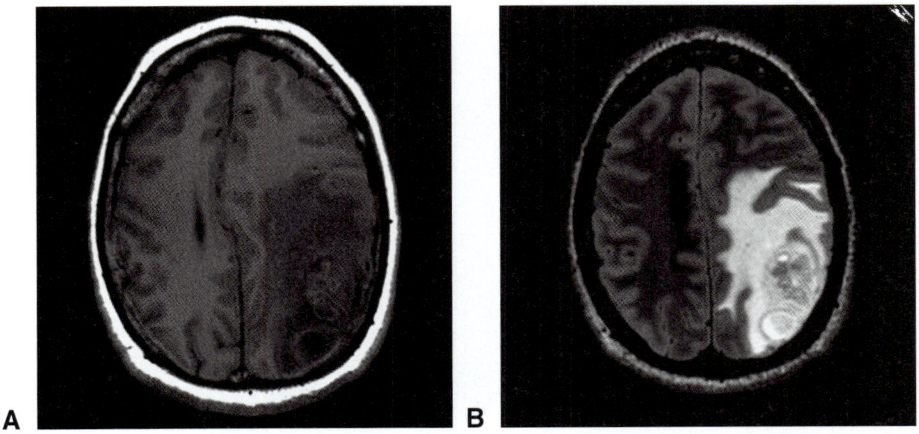

Figure 20.2. Imaging of CNS Infection, nocardia pyogenic abscess. A. Axial T1-precontrast: Large heterogeneously mixed intensity bi-lobed mass in the left parietal lobe. **B.** Axial fluid-attenuated inversion recovery (FLAIR): Heterogeneously mixed intensity mass with marked surrounding vasogenic edema.

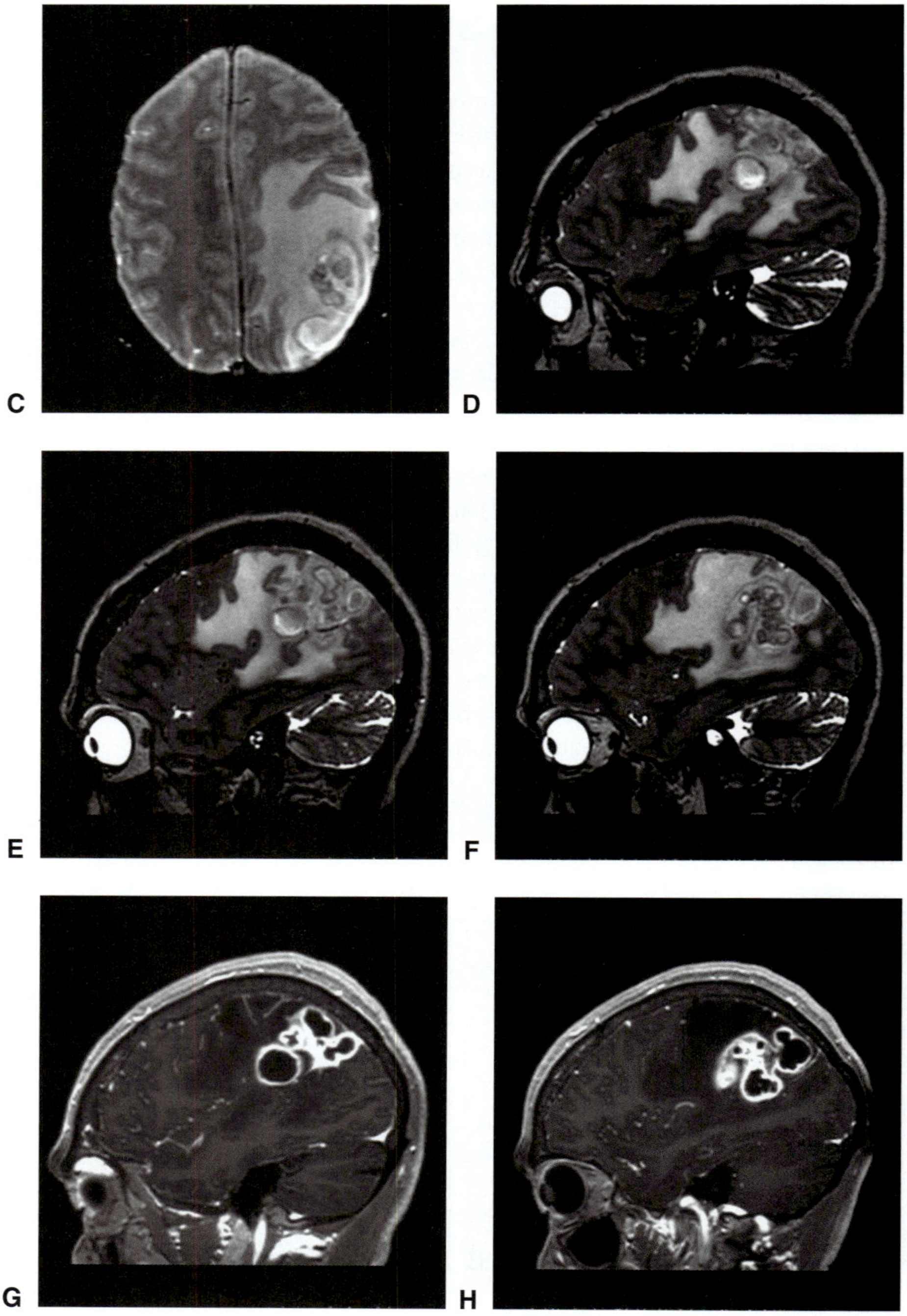

Figure 20.2. ***(continued)*** **C.** Axial susceptibility-weighted imaging (SWI): Nodular blood products within the anterior component. **D–F.** Sagittal T2: Multiple loculated collections in the left parietal lobe with severe surrounding vasogenic edema. **G–I.** Sagittal T1-postcontrast: Thick rim and nodular rim enhancement of the loculated collections.

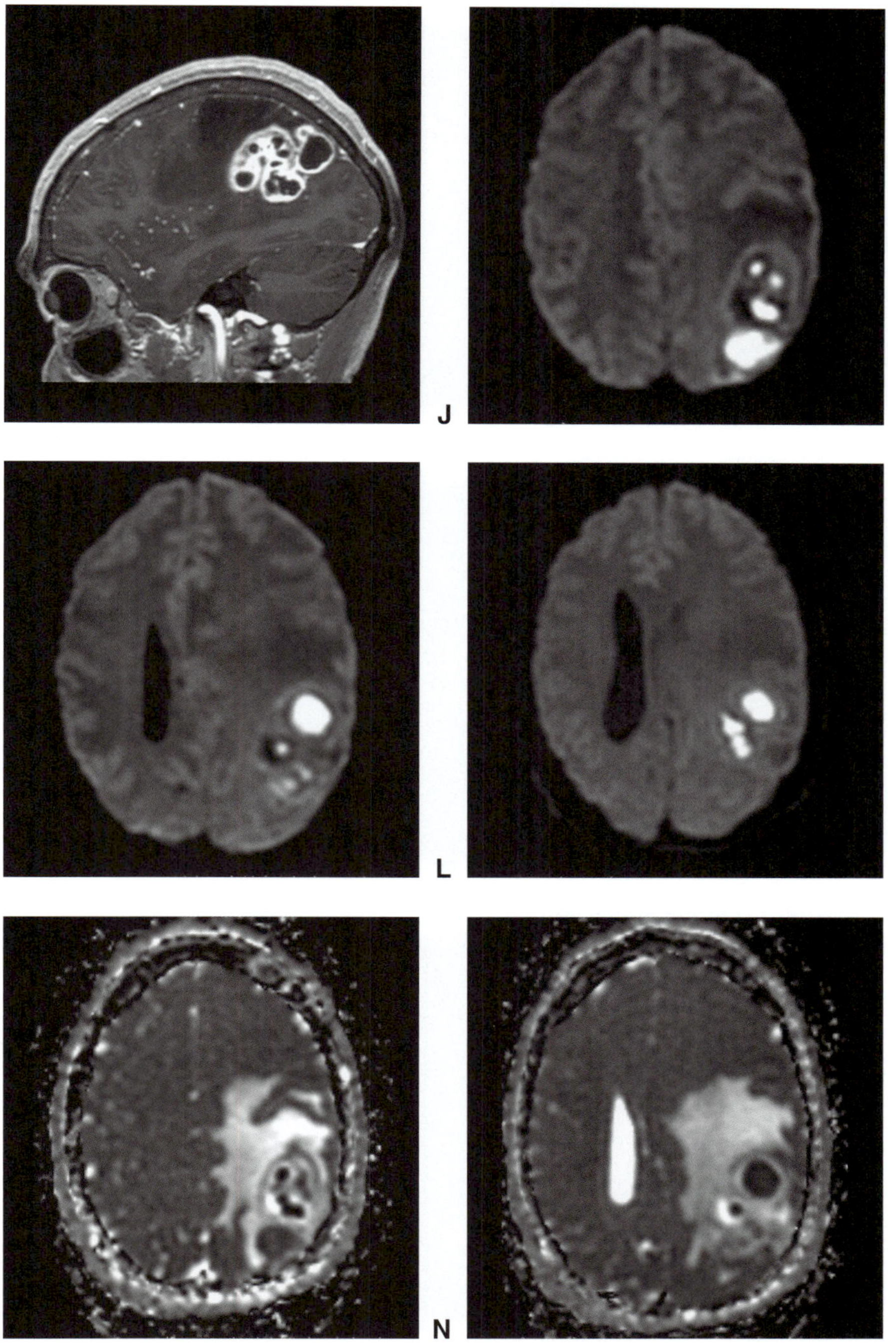

I J K L M N

Figure 20.2. ***(continued)*** **J–L.** Axial DWI: Marked reduced diffusion within several dominant loculated pyogenic collections. **M–O.** Axial apparent diffusion coefficient (ADC): Marked reduced diffusion within several dominant loculated pyogenic collections.

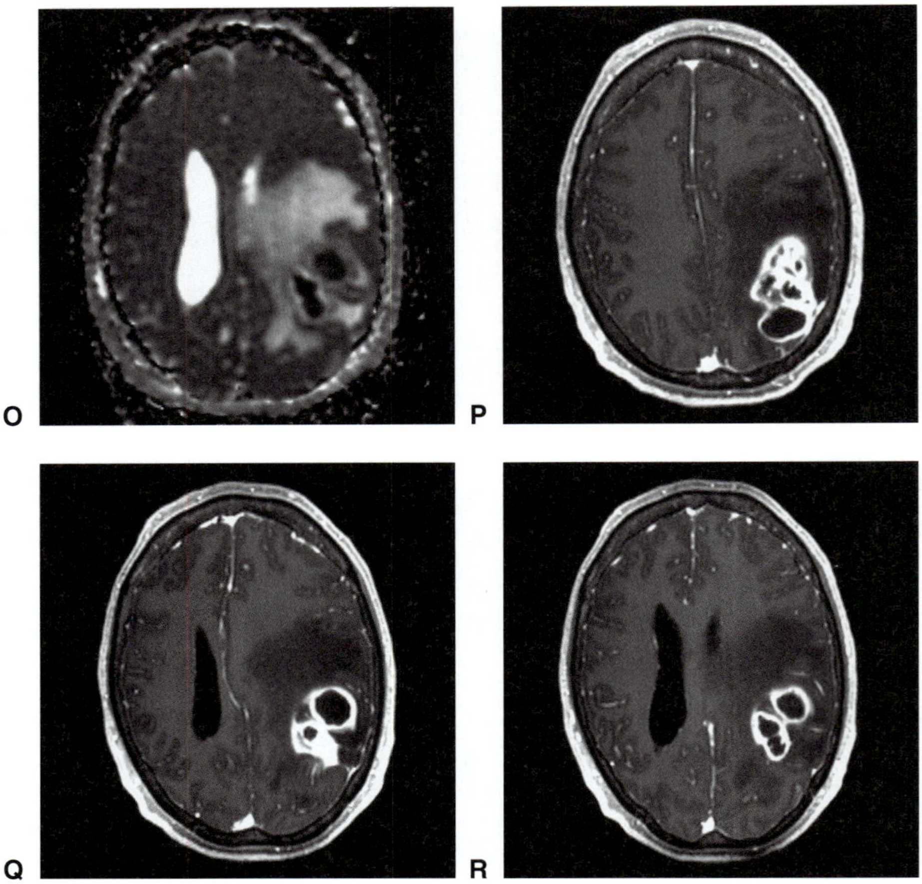

Figure 20.2. ***(continued)*** **P–R.** Axial T1-postcontrast: Thick rim and nodular rim enhancement of the loculated collections.

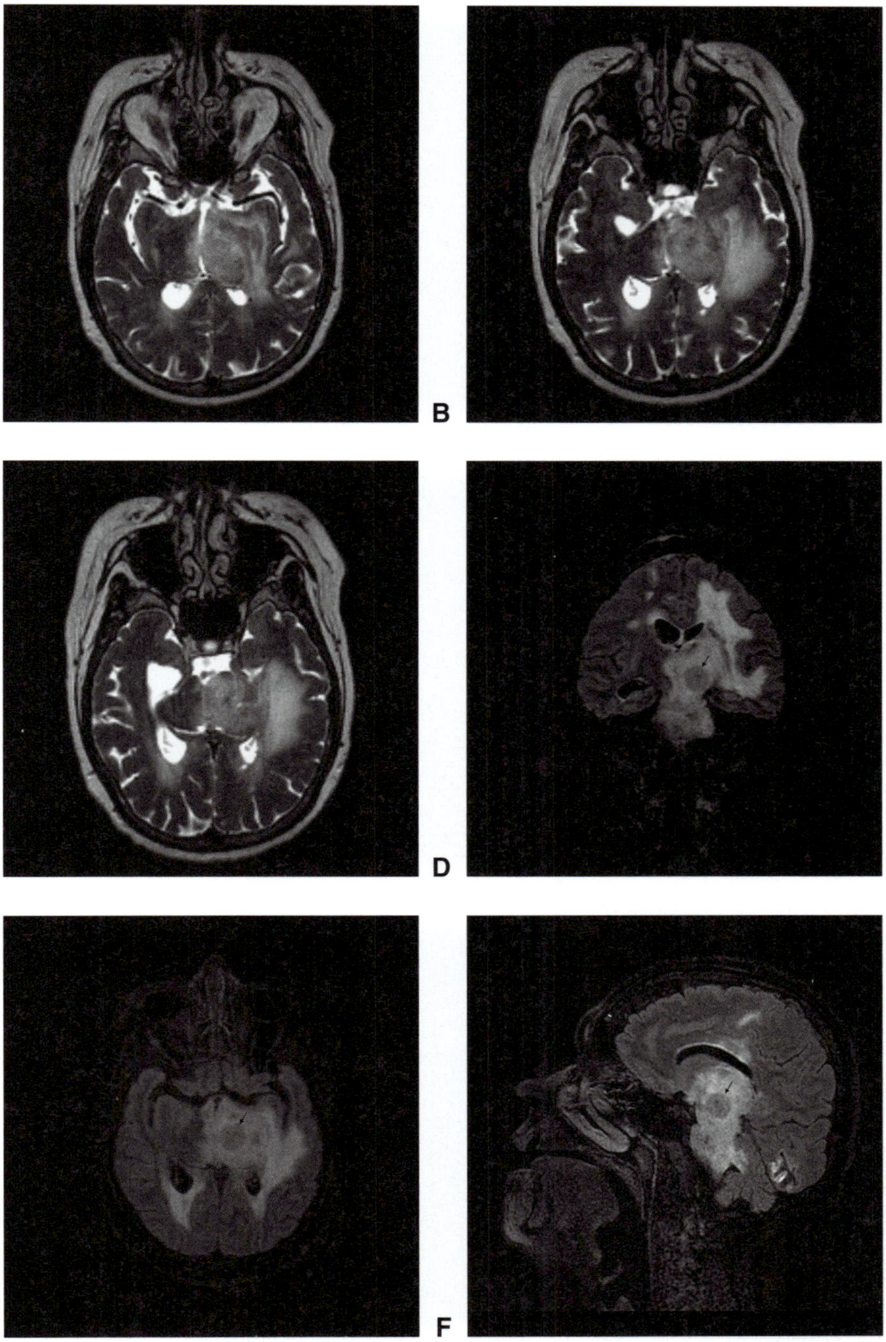

A B C D E F

Figure 20.3. Imaging of CNS infection, tuberculoma. A–C. Axial T2: Subtly outlined hypointense mass in the left thalamus and midbrain with marked surrounding edema. **D–F.** Axial (D), coronal (E), sagittal (F) FLAIR: Hypointense mass in the left thalamus and midbrain is bettered delineated (black arrows).

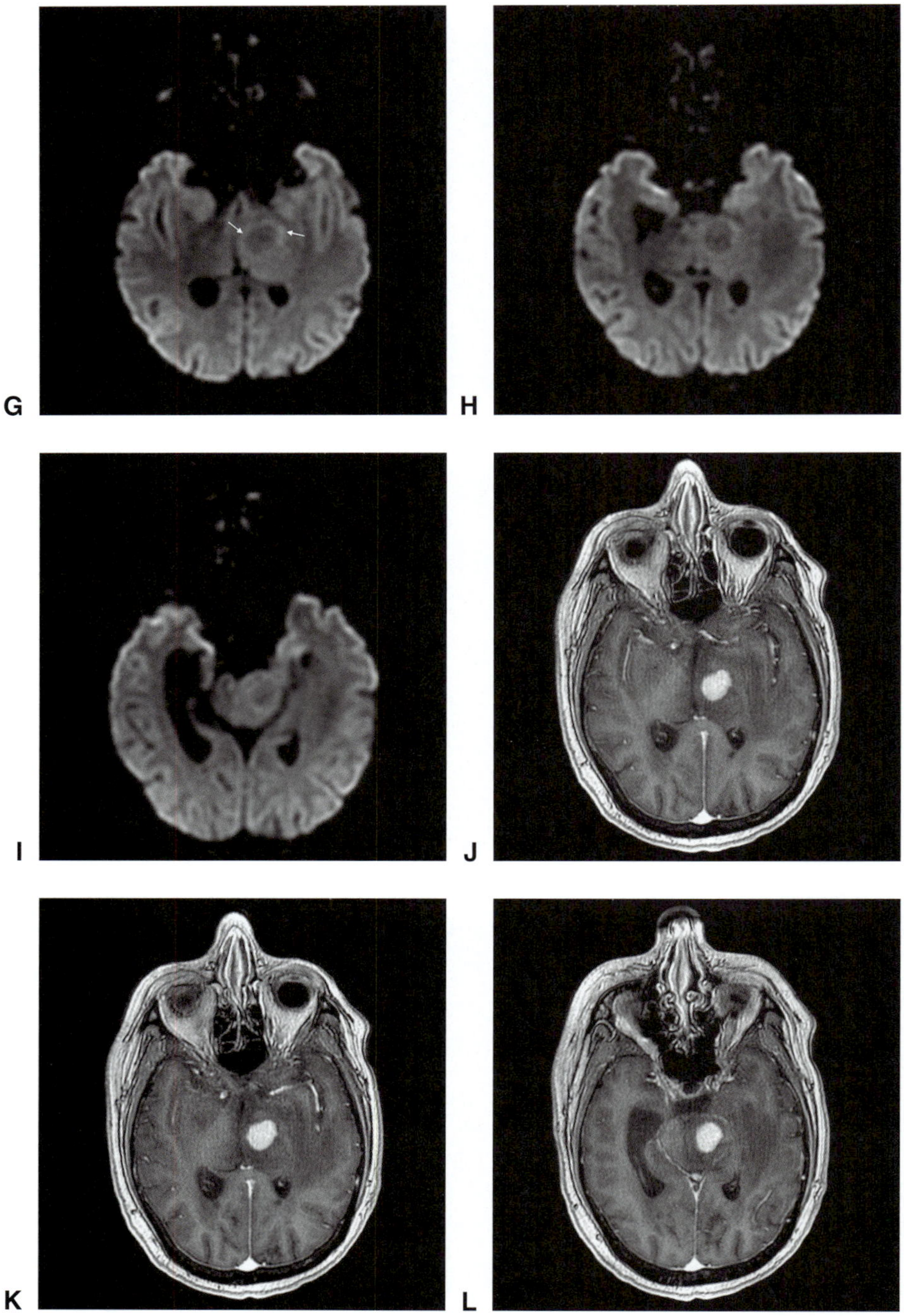

Figure 20.3. ***(continued)*** **G–I.** Axial DWI: Subtle incomplete rim (white arrows) of reduced diffusion. **J–L.** Axial T1-postcontrast: Avid and homogeneous enhancement within the mass.

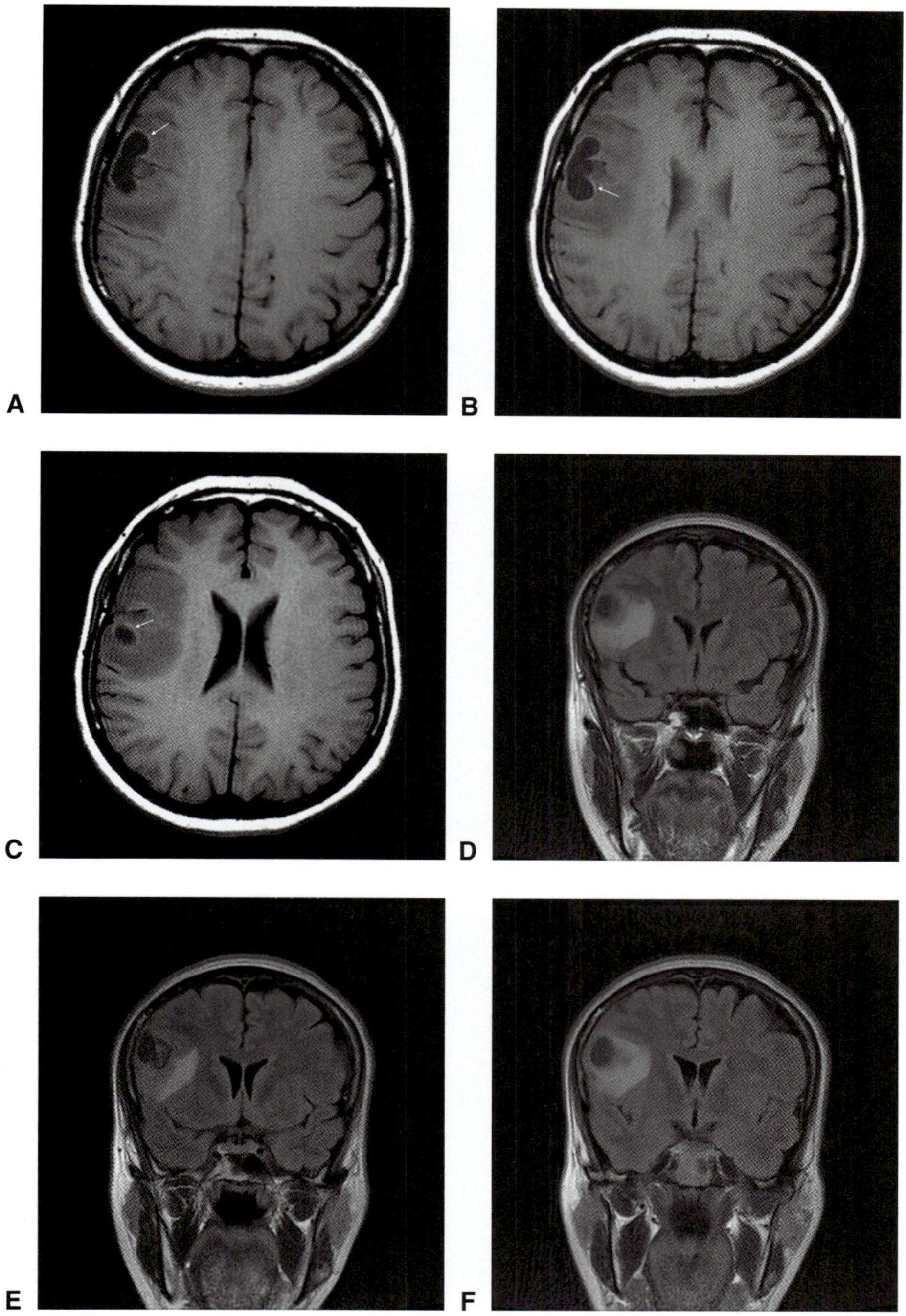

Figure 20.4. Imaging of CNS infection, neurocysticercosis. A–C. Axial T1-precontrast: Tri-lobed hypointense mass with subtle rim of T1 shortening (arrows). **D–F.** Coronal FLAIR: Homogeneously hypointense mass with marked surrounding edema.

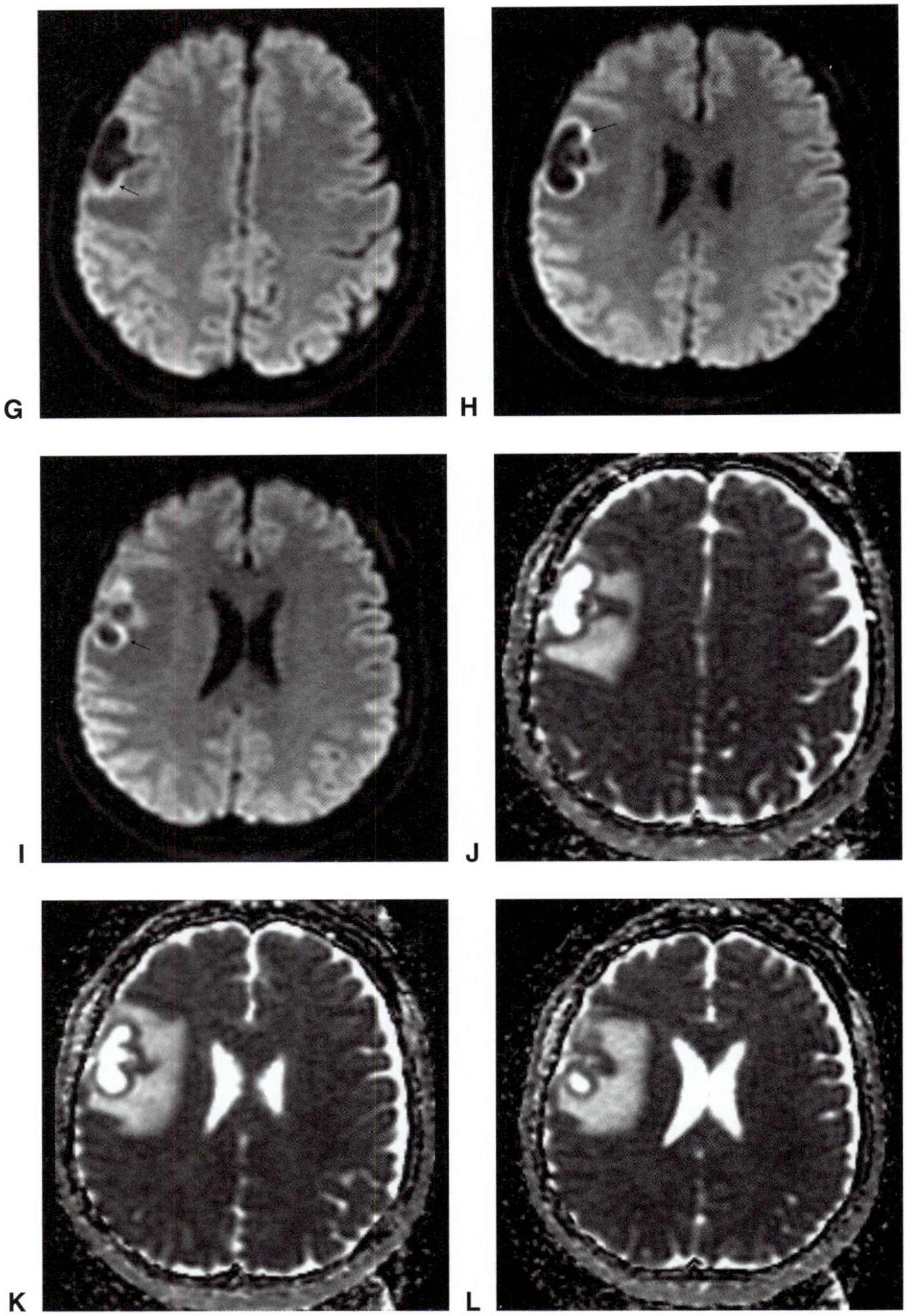

Figure 20.4. ***(continued)*** **G–I.** Axial DWI: Homogeneously hypointense mass with rim of reduced diffusion (black arrows). **J–L.** Axial ADC: Homogeneously hyperintense mass with rim of reduced diffusion.

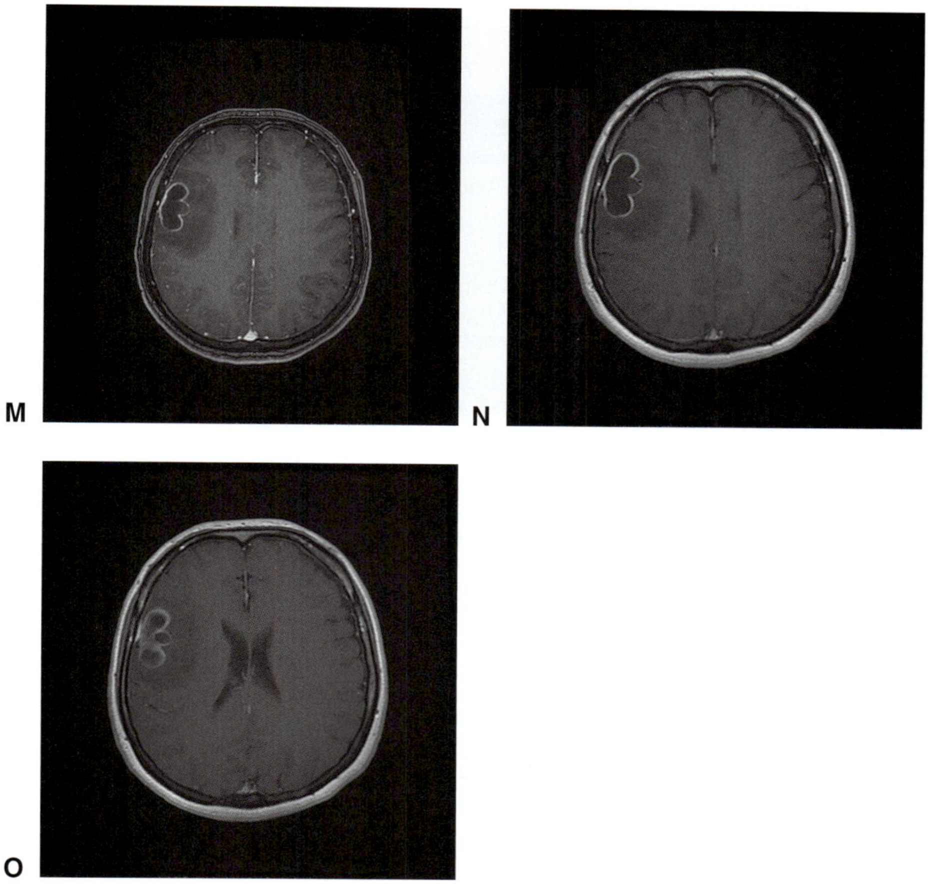

Figure 20.4. ***(continued)*** **M–O.** Axial T1-postcontrast: Thin rim of enhancement of the tri-lobed mass.

Central Nervous System Inflammatory (Noninfectious) Disease

Primary, noninfectious, neuroinflammatory disorders of the CNS are a heterogeneous group of diseases with varying causes and manifestations that include but are not limited to multiple sclerosis, tumefactive demyelinating disease, neuromyelitis optica, acute disseminated encephalomyelitis, primary angiitis, autoimmune limbic encephalitis, Susac's syndrome, neurosarcoidosis, systemic lupus erythematosus, giant cell arteritis, Behçet's disease, Sjögren's syndrome, and other vasculitides. During the acute inflammatory phase, CNS inflammatory disorders can present as mass lesions mimicking aggressive brain tumor with enhancement, hemorrhage, mass effect, and/or surrounding edema. It is

TABLE 20.1 Six MR Imaging Features to Identify Brain Tumor Mimics

MRI patterns of tumor mimics	Imaging sequence	Tumor mimics	Pitfall
Homogeneously reduced diffusion	Diffusion-weighted imaging	Pyogenic abscess	Hemorrhage
Peripheral incomplete rim of reduced diffusion	Diffusion-weighted imaging	Demyelinating lesion Angioinvasive aspergillosis	T2 shine through
Incomplete rim enhancement	T1-weighted postcontrast imaging	Demyelinating lesion Angioinvasive aspergillosis	Steroid therapy prior to imaging
Gyral form T1 shortening	T1-weighted precontrast imaging	Subacute or chronic infarct Subacute or chronic angiitis/vasculitis Subacute cortical hemorrhage	Prior steroid or radiation therapy
Thin rim of T2 shortening	Spin echo T2-weighted imaging	Subacute hematoma Cavernoma Foreign body granuloma	Melanoma metastasis
Branching or stacked pattern	Susceptibility-weighted imaging	Demyelinating lesion Vasculitis Angiitis Venulitis	-

essential to consider CNS inflammatory diseases in the differential diagnosis of any brain masses, especially those with one or more of the six imaging characteristics listed in Table 20.1.

Imaging

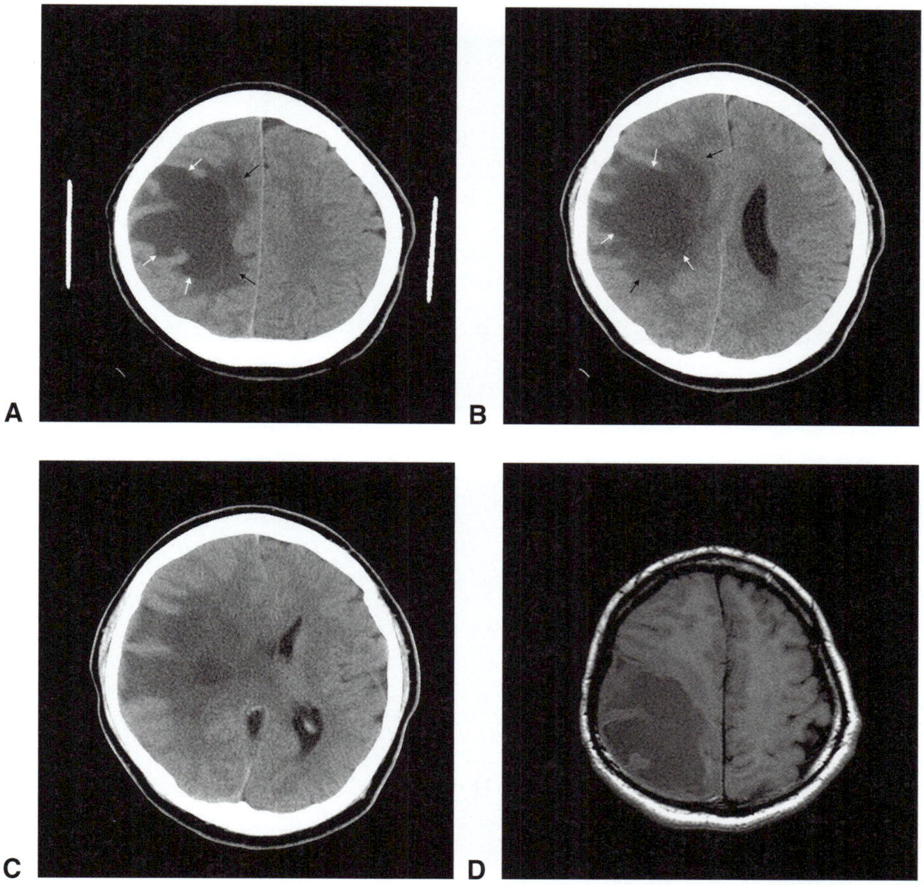

Figure 20.5. Imaging of tumefactive demyelinating disease, single lesion. A–C. Axial CT, unenhanced: Hypointense mass within the white matter (white arrows) with surrounding vasogenic edema (black arrows). **D.** Axial T1-precontrast: Hypointense mass within the white matter.

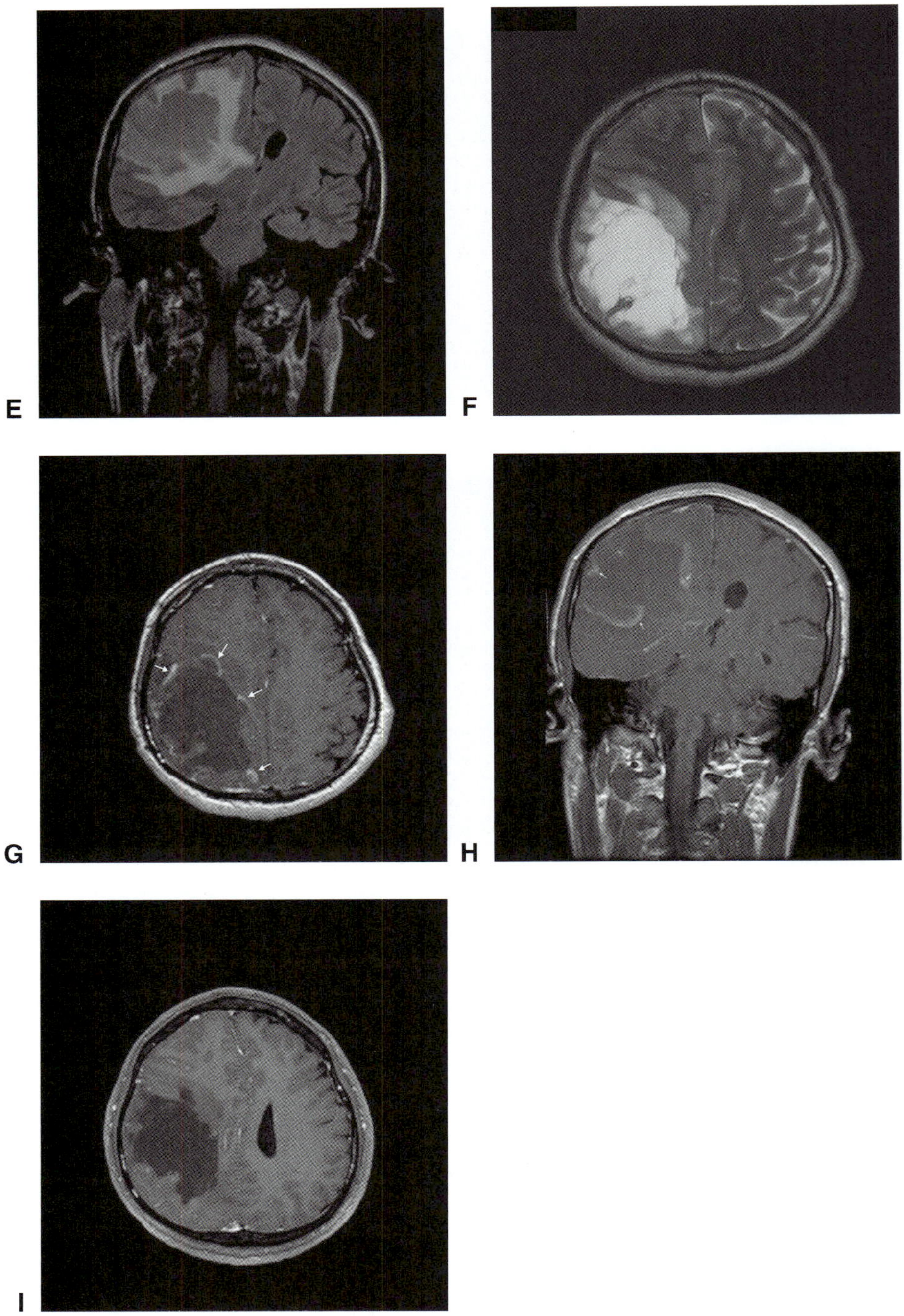

Figure 20.5. ***(continued)*** **E.** Coronal FLAIR: Hypointense mass with surrounding vasogenic edema. **F.** Axial T2: Homogeneously hyperintense mass. **G.** Axial T1-postcontrast: Discontinuous rim enhancement (white arrows). **H.** Coronal T1-postcontrast: Discontinuous rim enhancement (white arrows). **I.** Axial T1-postcontrast: Resolution of rim enhancement following 2 days of steroid therapy.

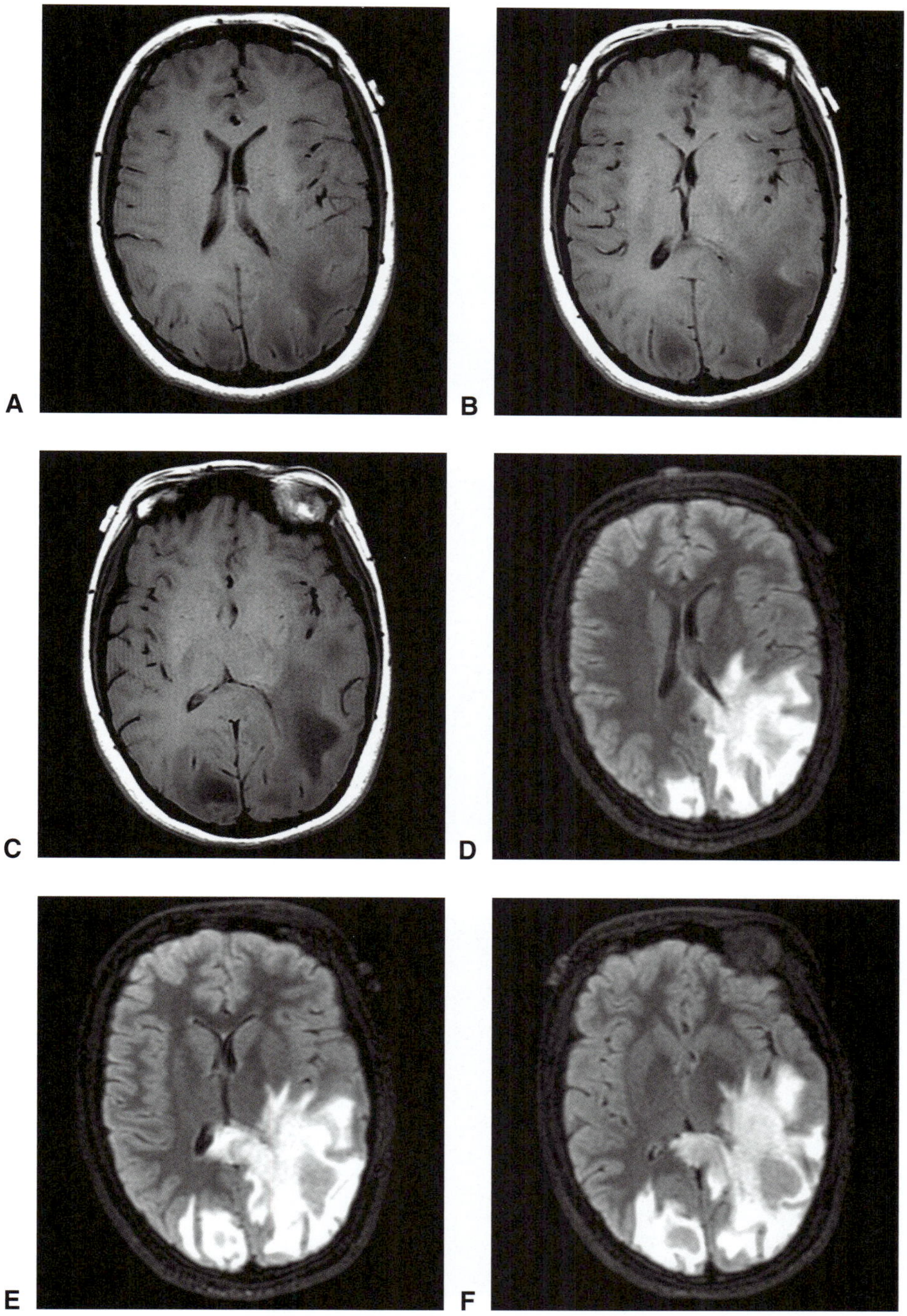

Figure 20.6. Imaging of tumefactive demyelinating disease, multiple lesions. **A–C.** Axial T1-precontrast: Ill-defined hypointense masses in right occipital and left parietal lobes. **D–F.** Axial FLAIR: Extensive vasogenic edema surrounding both masses.

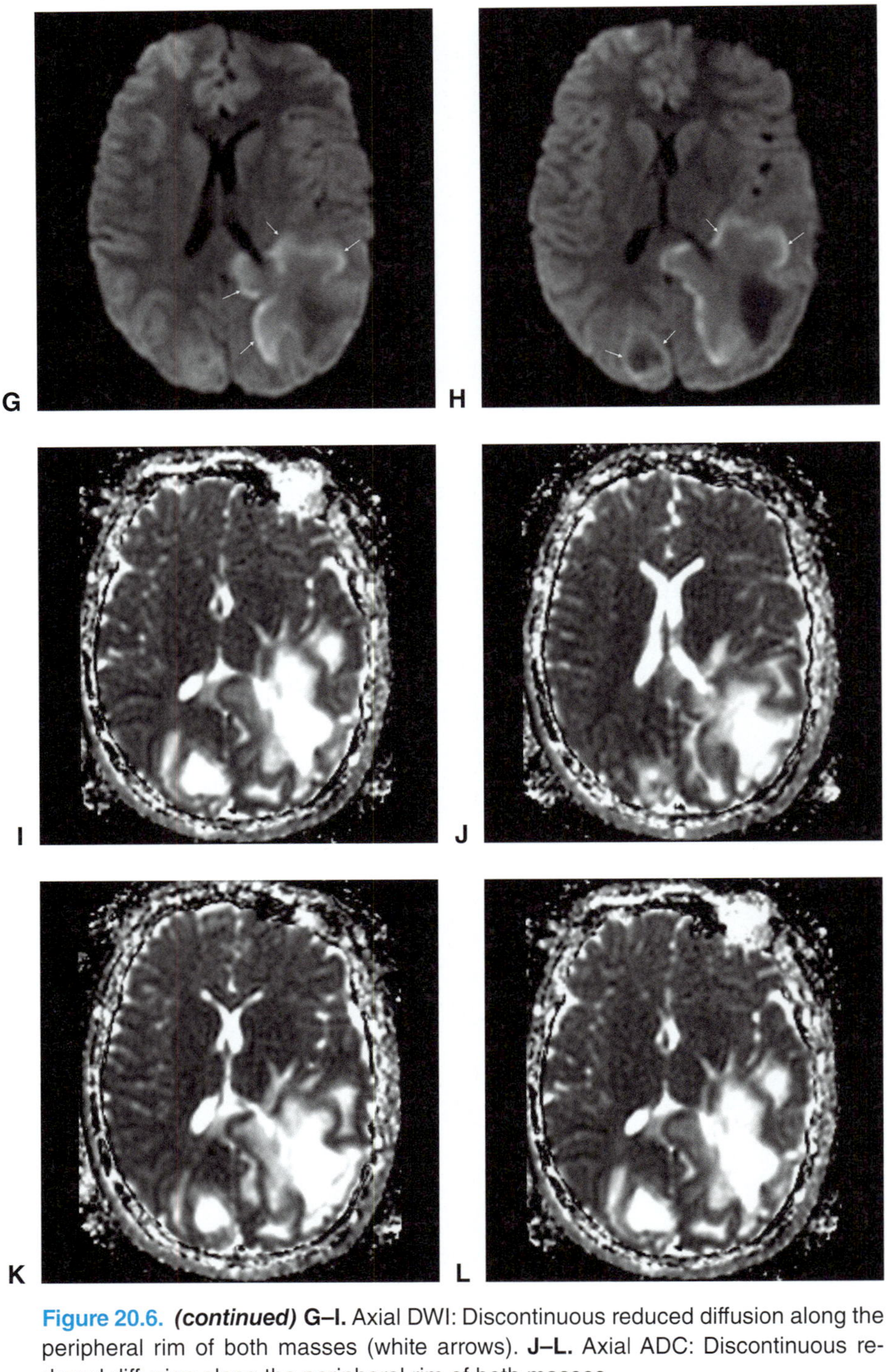

Figure 20.6. ***(continued)*** **G–I.** Axial DWI: Discontinuous reduced diffusion along the peripheral rim of both masses (white arrows). **J–L.** Axial ADC: Discontinuous reduced diffusion along the peripheral rim of both masses.

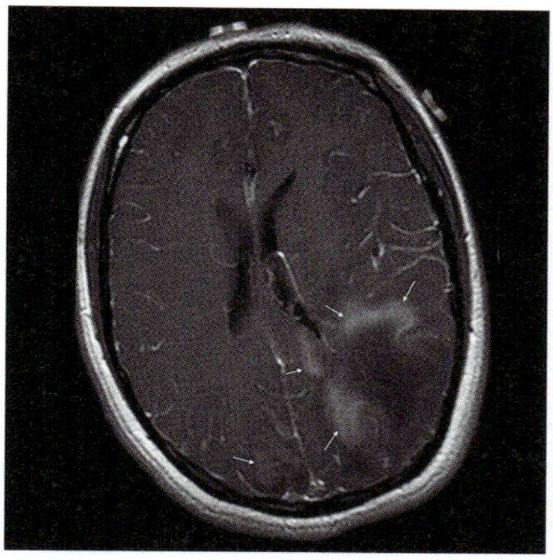

M

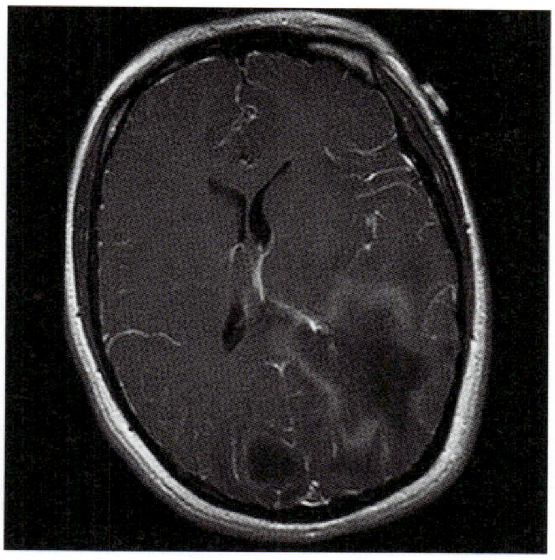

N

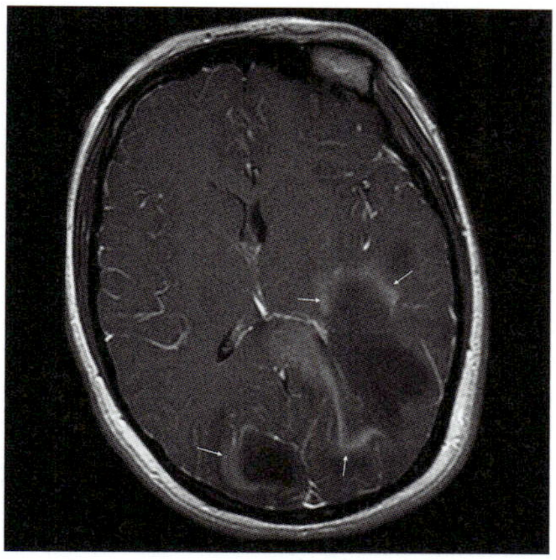

O

Figure 20.6. ***(continued)*** **M–O.** Axial T1-postcontrast: Discontinuous enhancement along the peripheral rim of both masses (white arrows).

Central Nervous System Ischemic Lesions

Focal ischemic lesions in the brain can simulate a brain tumor during the subacute stage of the disease process when there is alteration of the blood–brain barrier and reactive changes in the neighboring non-ischemic brain parenchyma. On MR imaging, subacute ischemic lesions often show irregular rim enhancement with a variable degree of surrounding edema and mass effect. Cortical laminar necrosis is the result of cortical neuronal death due to inadequate supply of oxygen and glucose due to ischemia and appears as a characteristic gyral pattern of T1 shortening.

Imaging

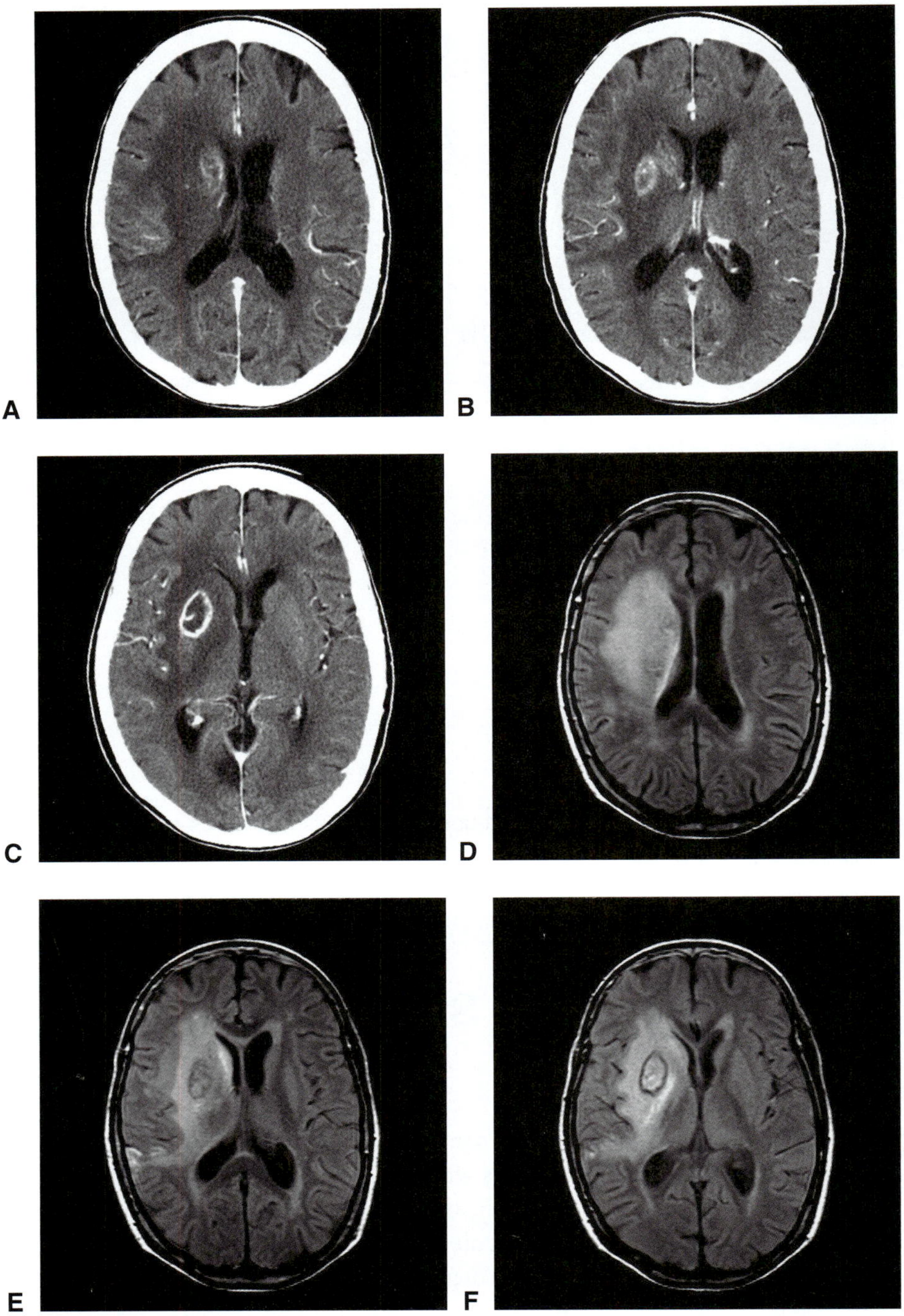

Figure 20.7. Imaging of subacute infarct. A–C. Axial CT, enhanced: Rim-enhancing, centrally necrotic mass in the right basal ganglia with surrounding edema. **D–F.** Axial FLAIR: Hyperintense mass with hypointense rim.

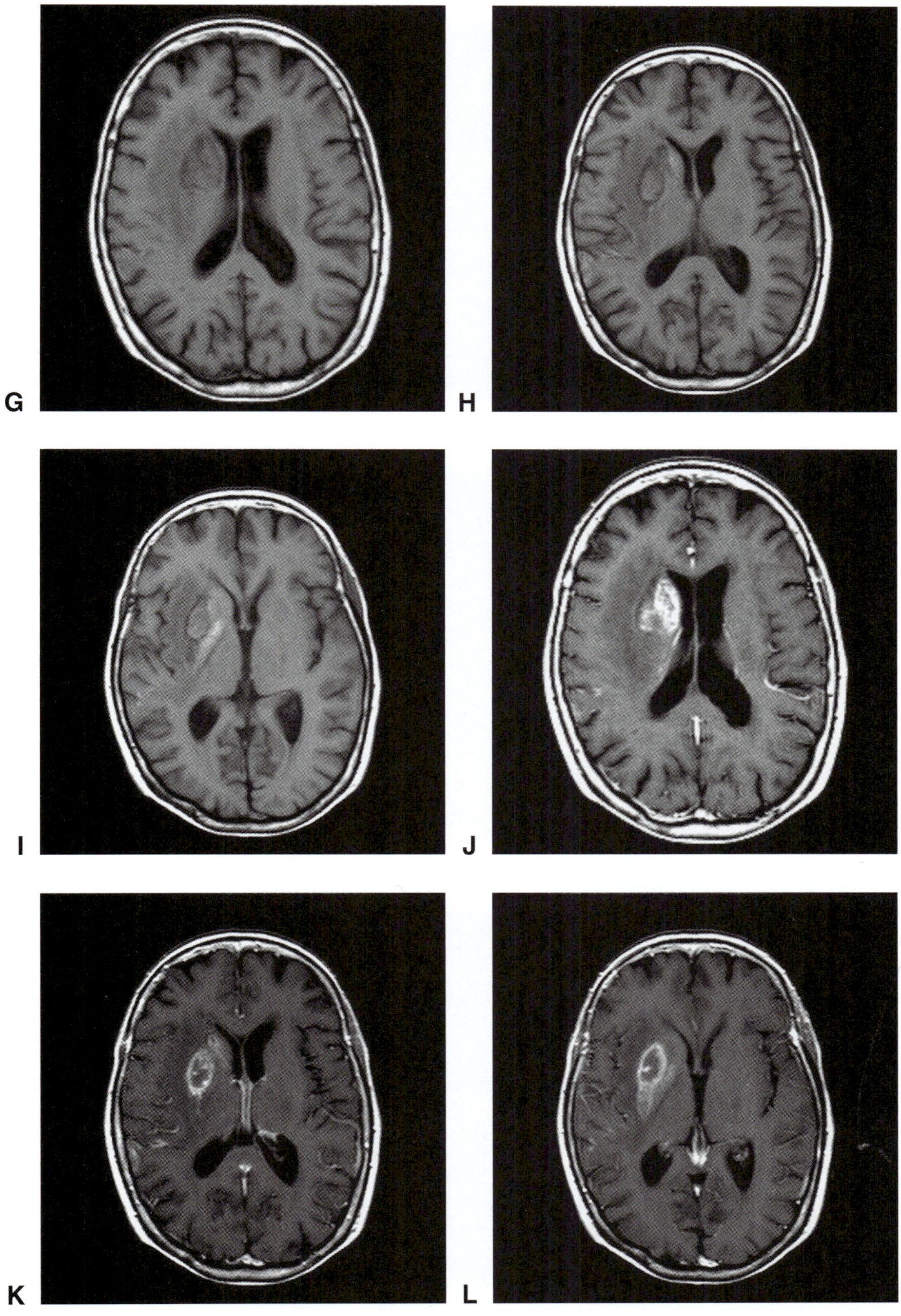

Figure 20.7. ***(continued)*** **G–I.** Axial T1-precontrast: Isointense mass with hypointense rim. **J–L.** Axial T1-postcontrast: Thick rim-enhancing, centrally necrotic mass.

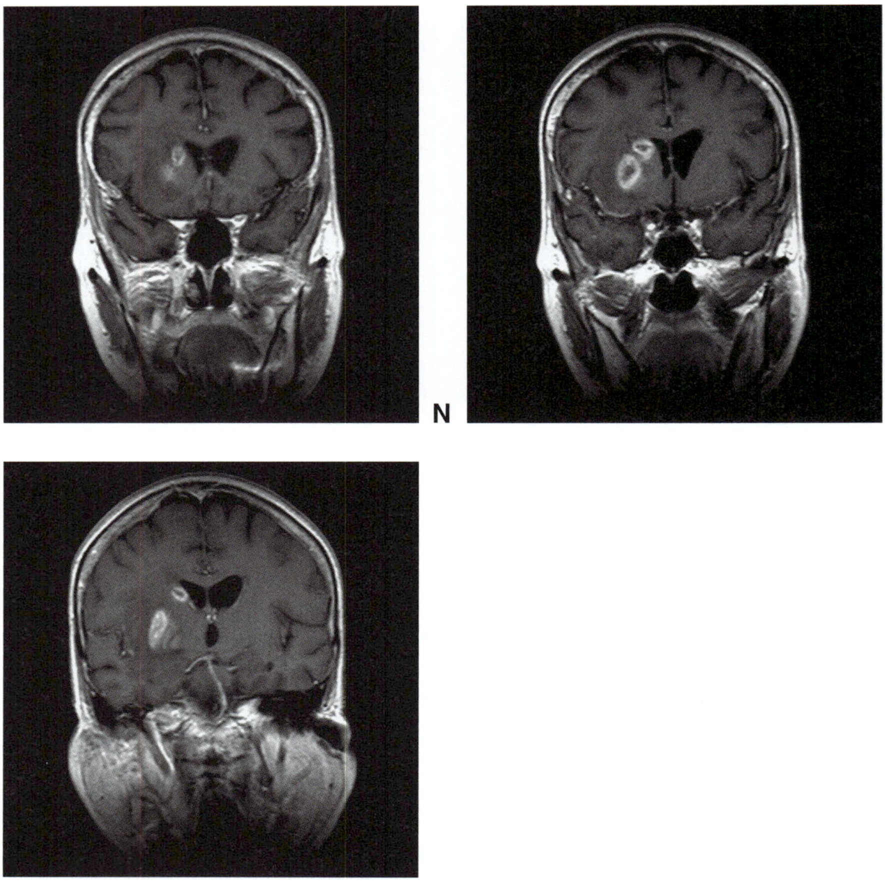

Figure 20.7. ***(continued)*** **M–O.** Coronal T1-postcontrast: Thick rim-enhancing, centrally necrotic mass.

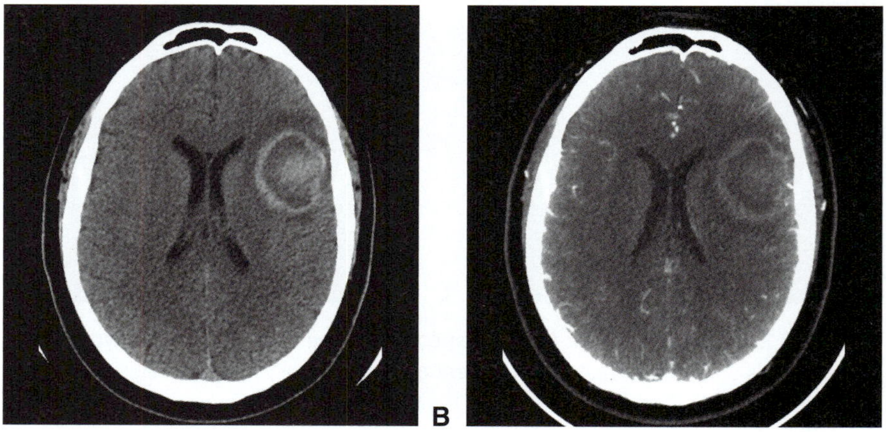

Figure 20.8. Imaging of cavernous malformation. A. Axial CT, unenhanced: Circumscribed mass with hyperdense rim and core in the left frontal lobe. **B.** Axial CT, enhanced: No enhancement within or around the mass.

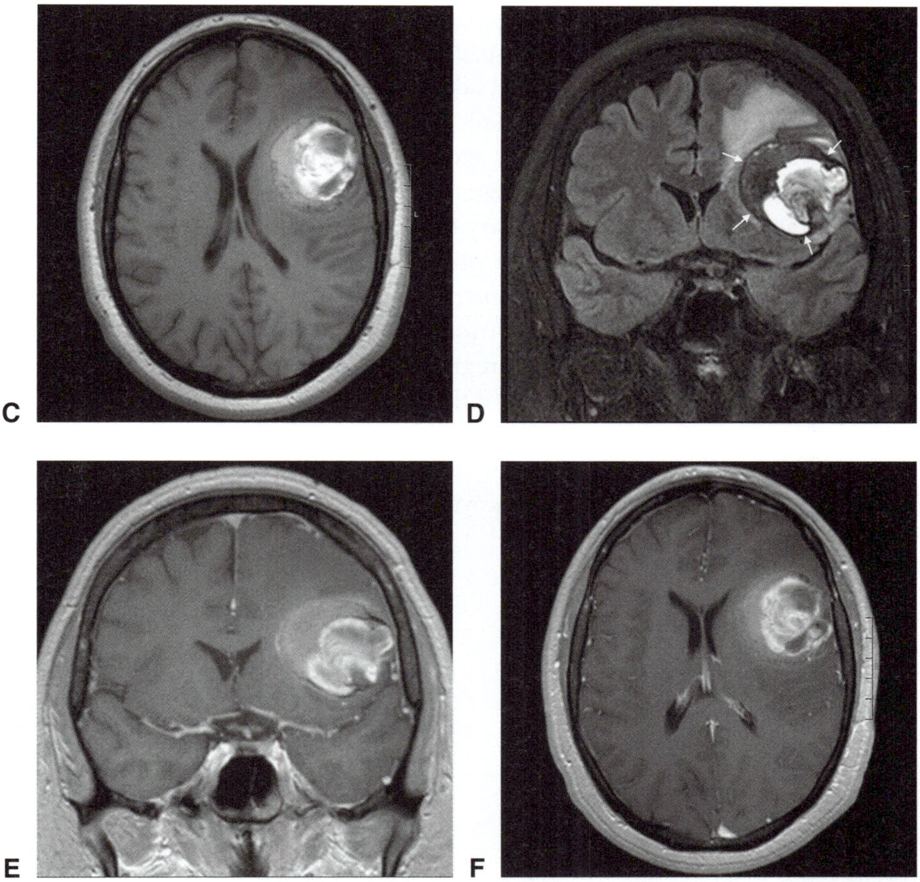

Figure 20.8. ***(continued)*** **C.** Axial T1-precontrast: Heterogeneously hyperintense mass. **D.** Coronal FLAIR: Heterogeneous mixed hyperintense and hypointense mass with thin hypointense rim (white arrows). **E.** Coronal T1-postcontrast: No robust enhancement within the mass. **F.** Axial T1-postcontrast: No robust enhancement within the mass.

Central Nervous System Vasculitis

Cerebral vasculitis is characterized by inflammation of the walls of blood vessels and may affect vessels of any size. The pathogenesis of vasculitis remains poorly understood. Vasculitis may affect large vessels (Takayasu arteritis and giant cell arteritis), medium-sized vessels (Kawasaki disease and polyarteritis nodosa), small vessels (immunoglobulin A vasculitis, microscopic polyangiitis, granulomatosis with polyangiitis, and eosinophilic granulomatosis with polyangiitis), or variable-sized vessels (Behçet disease and Cogan syndrome).

Primary angiitis of the CNS is an idiopathic disorder affecting the medium and small vessels of the CNS without evidence of generalized systemic inflammation. The clinical presentation of primary angiitis of central nervous system (PACNS) is broad and unspecific and the majority of the diagnostic approaches are hallmarked by a low specificity. Thus, PACNS is can be misdiagnosed as malignant brain tumor. In addition, due to its potential aggressive course, which may be altered by an adequate immunosuppressive treatment, delineation from other vasculopathies and PACNS mimics is crucial. CNS vasculitis may be secondary to systemic disease, infection, malignancy, drug use, or radiation therapy. Imaging findings vary from small ischemic changes to frank infarct, hemorrhage, and white matter edema and may show contrast enhancement. The cerebral arteries may demonstrate a beaded appearance with variable degrees of stenosis, occlusion, and contrast enhancement of the vessel wall. CNS venulitis is a rare entity where rapid progressive thrombosis and injury of small veins and venules lead to breakdown of the blood–brain barrier and present as a rim-enhancing, aggressive-appearing brain mass. During acute phase, CNS angiitis, vasculitis, or venulitis may present as a mass with enhancement, hemorrhage, and edema simulating an aggressive brain tumor.

Imaging

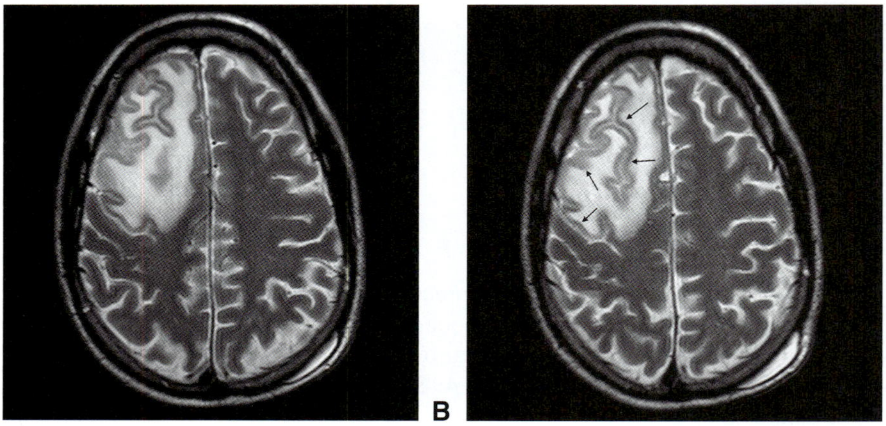
A B

Figure 20.9. Imaging of vasculitis. A–C. Axial T2: Large area of white matter hyperintensity with sparing of the overlying cortex (black arrows).

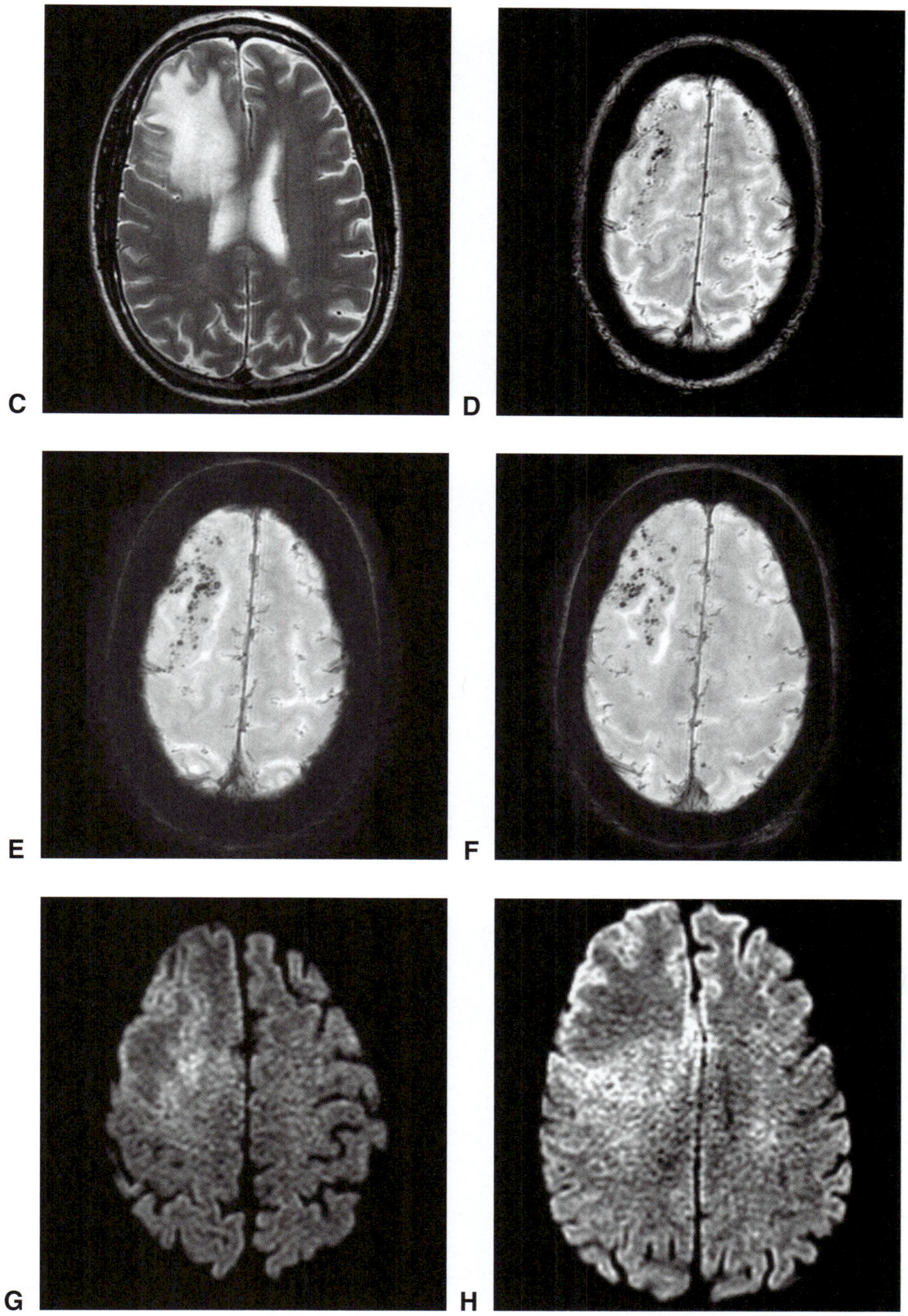

Figure 20.9. ***(continued)*** **D–F.** Axial SWI: Innumerable punctate blood products conforming to the subarachnoid vascular architecture. **G–I.** Axial DWI: No reduced diffusion within the white matter abnormality.

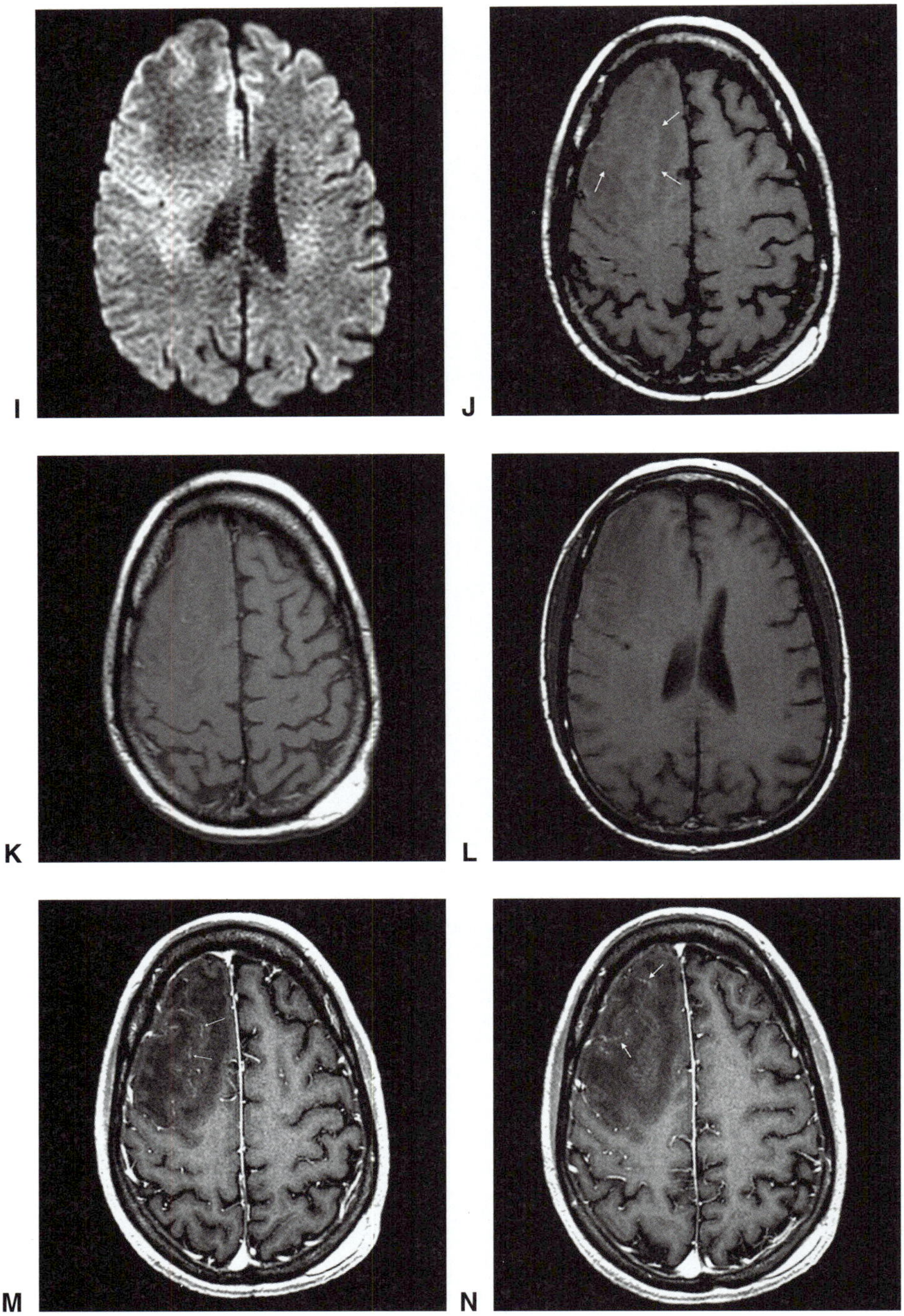

Figure 20.9. ***(continued)*** **J–L.** Axial T1-precontrast: Isointense white matter abnormality with faint cortical T1 shortening (white arrows). **M–O.** Axial T1-postcontrast: Prominent enhancement of sulcal vessels and absent enhancement within the white matter abnormality.

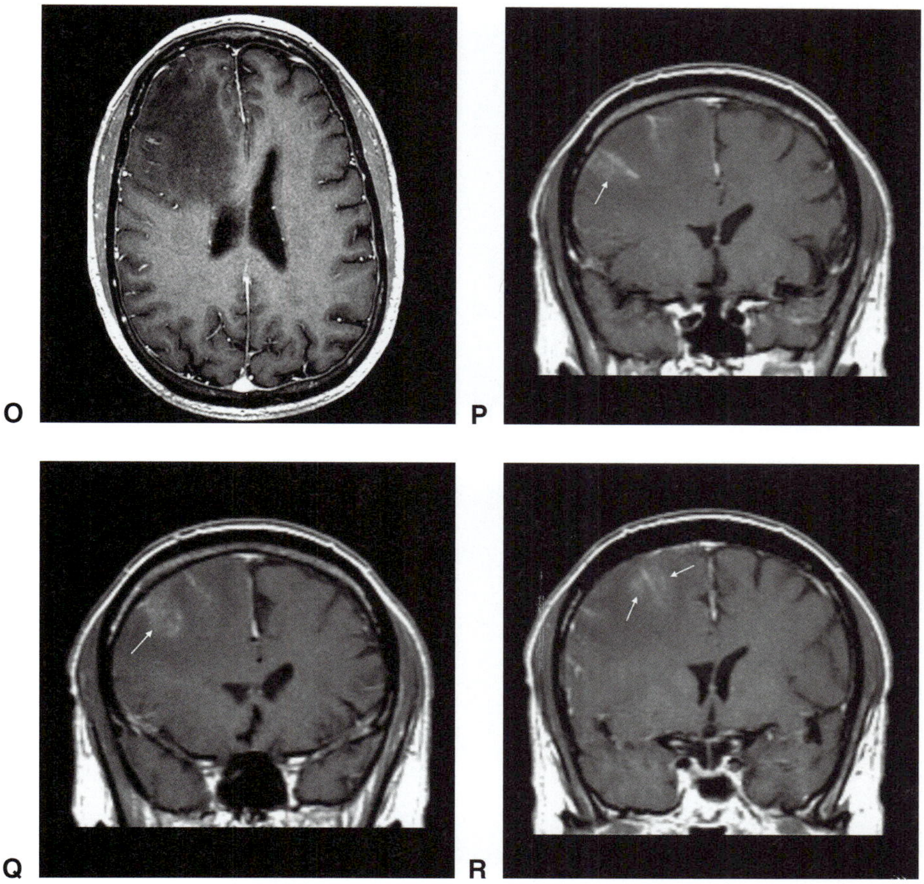

Figure 20.9. ***(continued)*** **P–R.** Coronal T1-postcontrast: Prominent enhancement of sulcal vessels and adjacent cortical smudgy enhancement (white arrows).

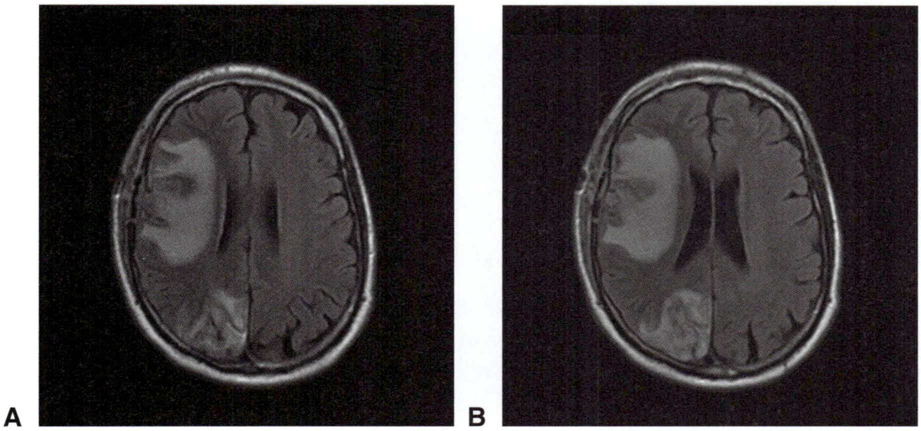

Figure 20.10. **Imaging of angiitis. A–C.** Axial FLAIR: Two separate discontiguous lesions in the right cerebral hemisphere with extensive surrounding edema.

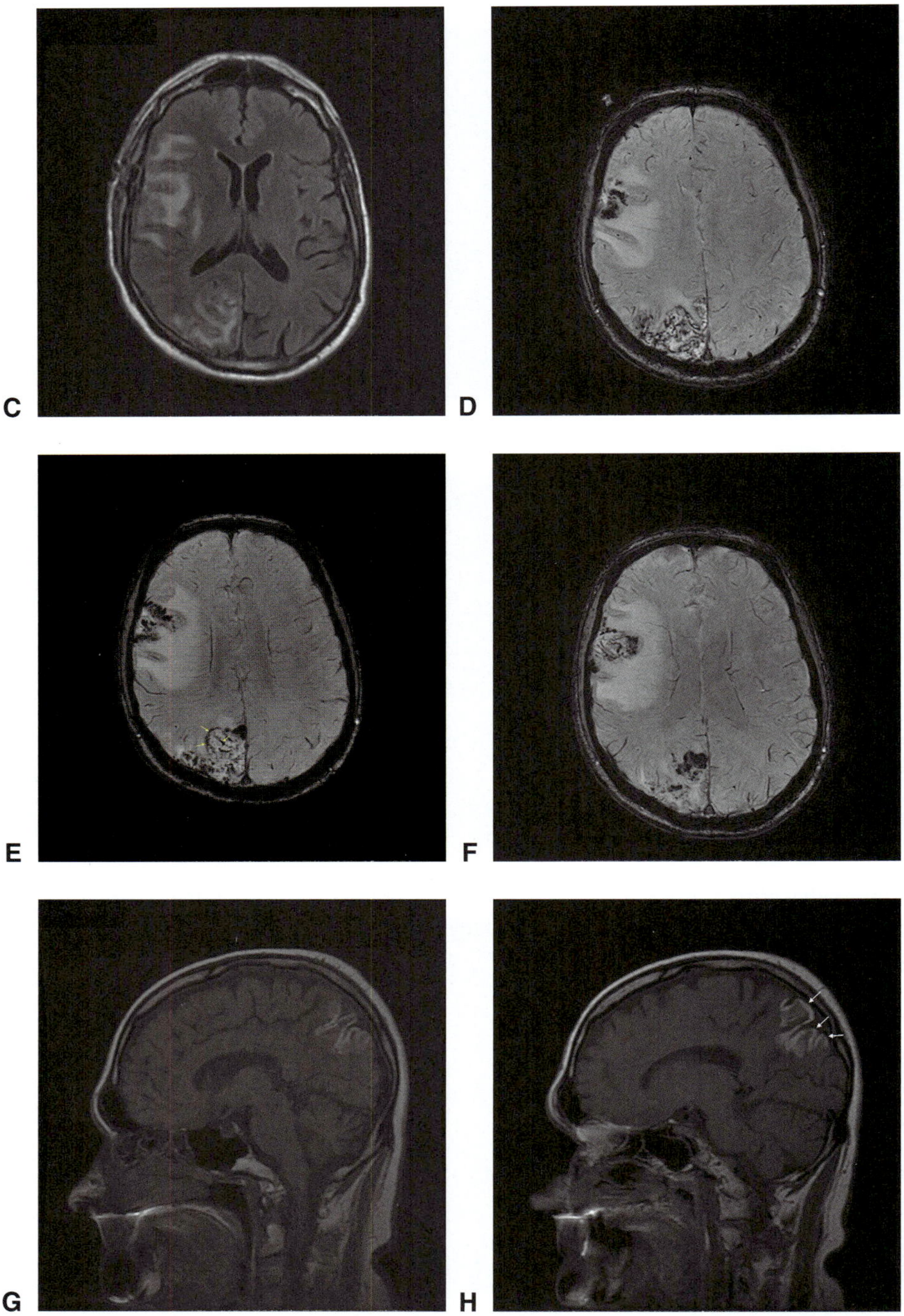

Figure 20.10. ***(continued)*** **D–F.** Axial SWI: Prominent blood products and thrombosed sulcal vessels (yellow arrows in **E**). **G–I**. Sagittal T1-precontrast: Striking cortical T1 shortening in a gyral pattern (white arrows in **H**).

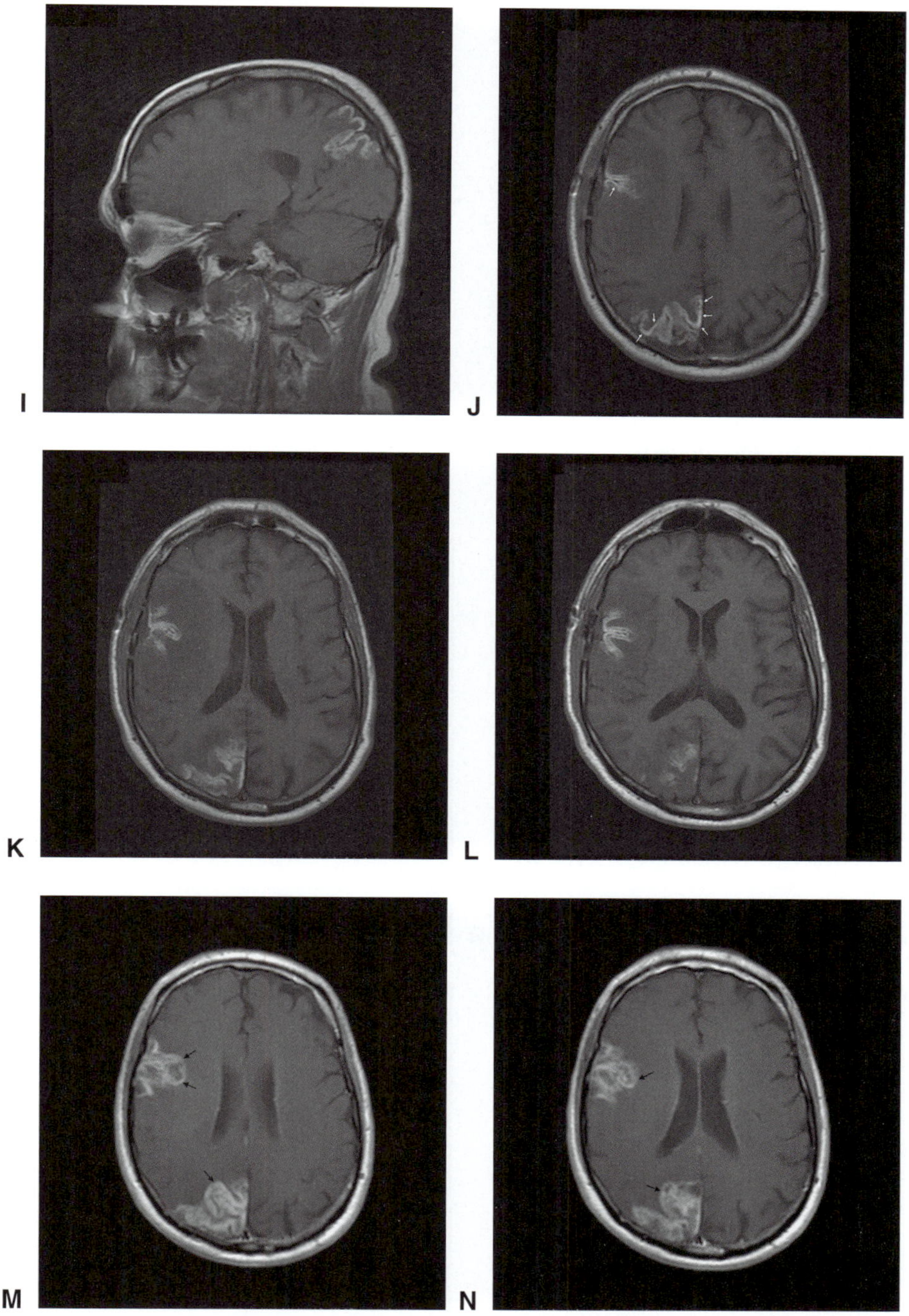

Figure 20.10. ***(continued)*** **J–L.** Axial T1-precontrast: Striking cortical T1 shortening in a gyral pattern (white arrows). **M–O.** Axial T1-postcontrast: Enhancement along the deep medial margin of each lesion (black arrows).

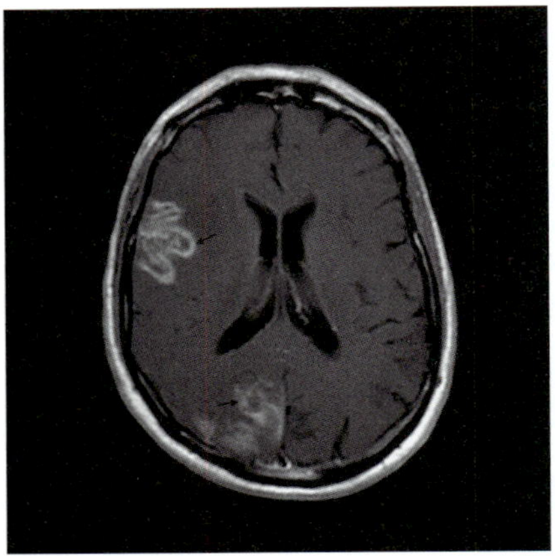

Figure 20.10. ***(continued)***

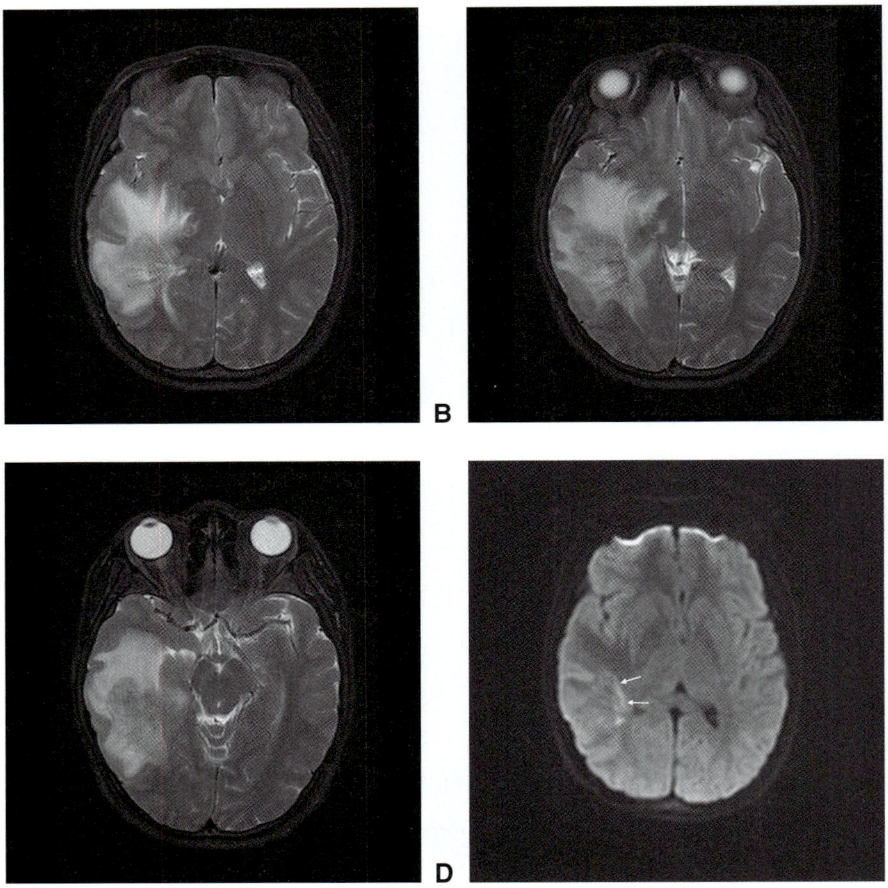

Figure 20.11. Imaging of venulitis. A–C. Axial T2: Ill-defined lesion in the right posterior temporal lobe with surrounding edema. **D–F.** Axial DWI: Leading edge reduced diffusion (white arrows) along the medial margin of the lesion.

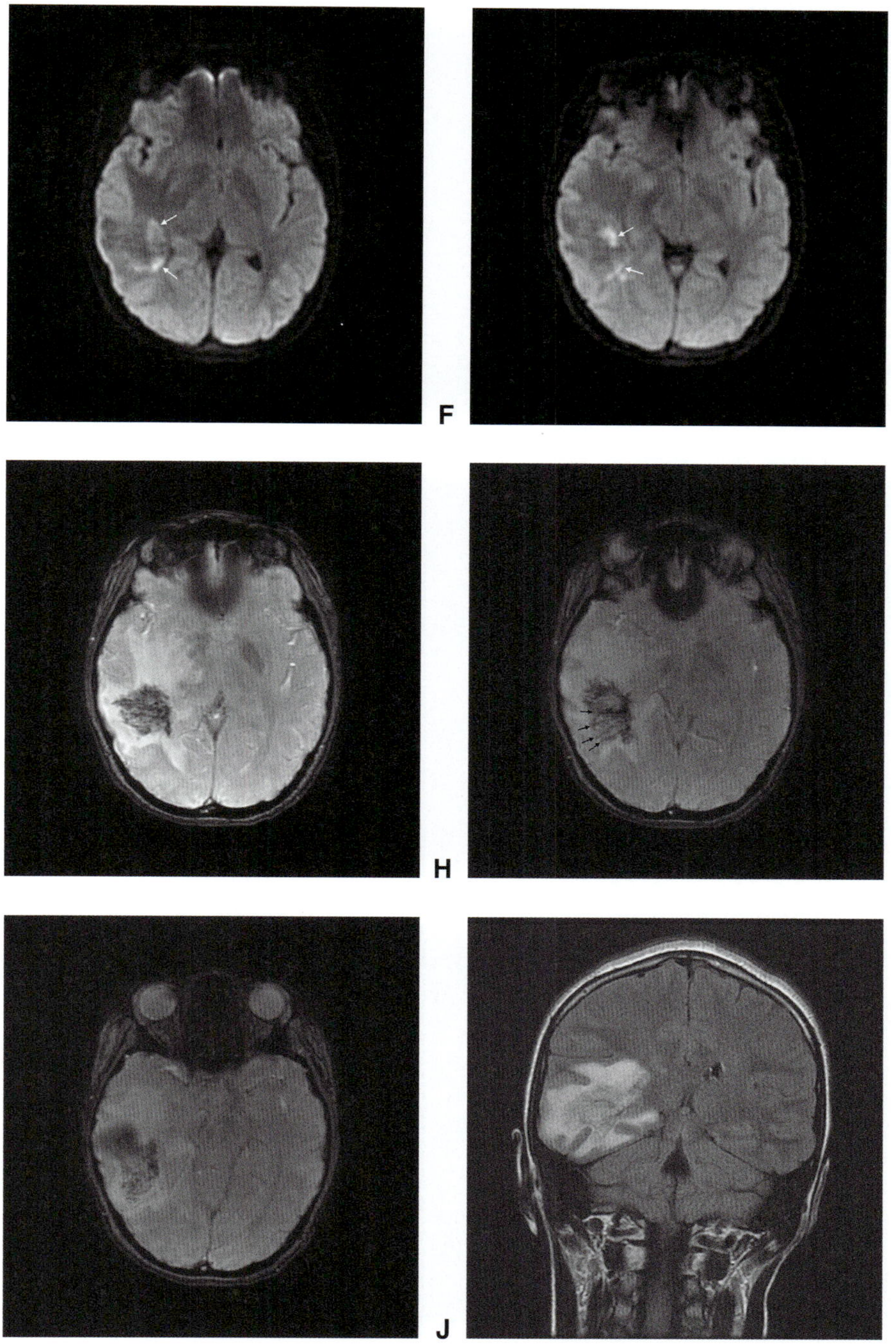

E F G H I J

Figure 20.11. ***(continued)*** **G–I.** Axial SWI: Stacked appearance (black arrows) of susceptibility within the lesion. **J–L.** Coronal FLAIR: Ill-defined lesion in the right posterior temporal lobe with surrounding edema.

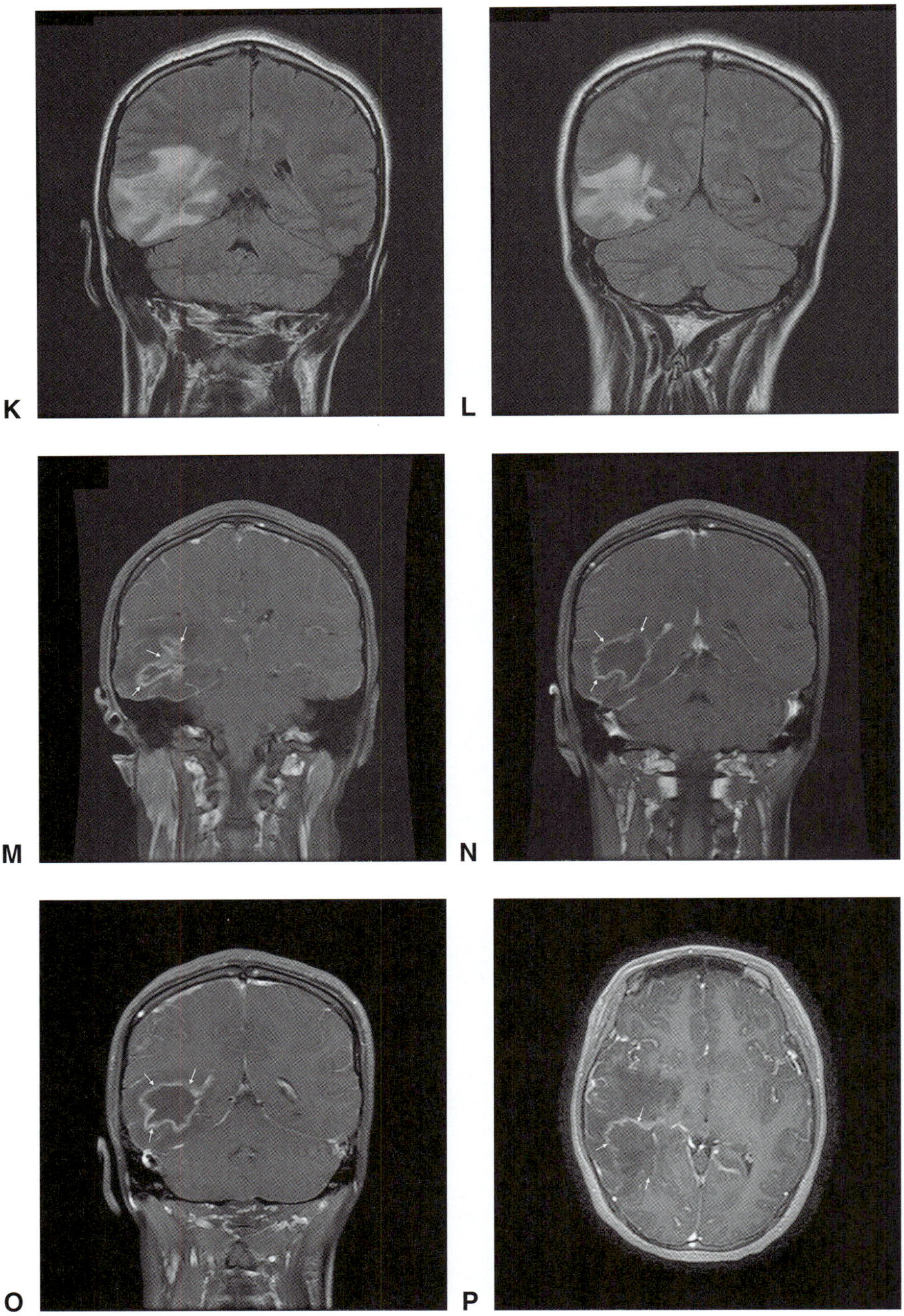

Figure 20.11. ***(continued)*** **M–O.** Coronal T1-postcontrast: Irregular and incomplete rim enhancement (white arrows) and centrally necrotic mass. **P–R.** Axial T1-post-contrast: Irregular and incomplete rim enhancement (white arrows) and centrally necrotic mass.

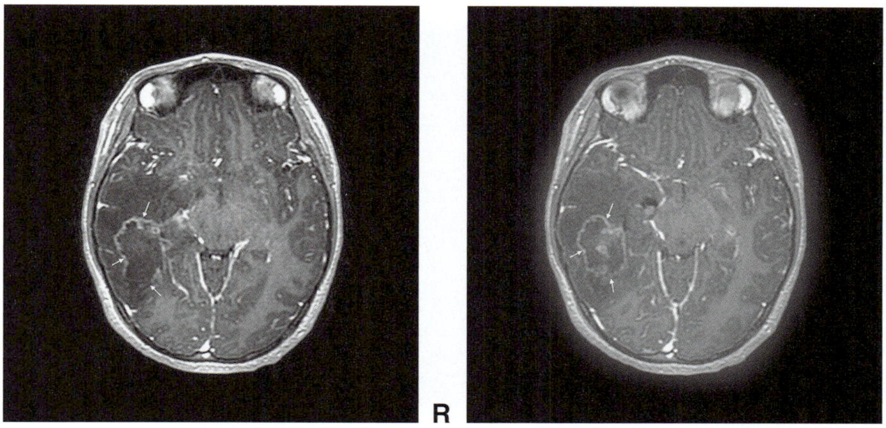
Q R

Figure 20.11. ***(continued)***

Bibliography

Abdel Razek AA, Alvarez H, Bagg S, Refaat S, Castillo M. Imaging spectrum of CNS vasculitis. *Radiographics*. 2014;34:873–894.

Carmo RL, Simao AKA, Amaral LLF, et al. Neuroimaging of emergent and reemergent infections. *Radiographics*. 2019;39:1649–1671.

Cartes-zumelzu FW, Stavrou I, Castillo M, et al. Diffusion-weighted imaging in the assessment of brain abscesses therapy. *AJNR Am J Neuroradiol*. 2004;25(8):1310–1317.

Orr SL, Dos Santos MP, Jurencak R et al. Central nervous system venulitis presenting as migraine. *Headache*. 2014;54:541–544.

Starkey J, Li Y, Tihan T, Cha S. Clinical series: five simple MR imaging features to identify tumor mimics. *Neurographics*. 2016;6:229–236.

Index

Note: Page numbers followed by *f* and *t* indicate figures and tables respectively.